WOMANCARE

WOMANCARE

A GYNECOLOGICAL GUIDE
TO YOUR BODY

BY LYNDA MADARAS AND
JANE PATTERSON, M.D.,F.A.C.O.G.
WITH PETER SCHICK, M.D.,F.A.C.S.

AVON
PUBLISHERS OF BARD, CAMELOT, DISCUS AND FLARE BOOKS

WOMANCARE: A GYNECOLOGICAL GUIDE TO YOUR BODY is an
original publication of Avon Books. This work has never before appeared in
book form.

This book was current to the best of the authors' knowledge at publication, but before
acting on information herein the consumer should, of course, verify information with
the appropriate physician or agency.

AVON BOOKS
A division of
The Hearst Corporation
959 Eighth Avenue
New York, New York 10019

Copyright © 1981 by Lynda Madaras
Illustrations Copyright © 1981 by Avon Books
Text illustrations by Christine Bondante
Cover design Copyright © 1981 by Roger Whitehouse
Published by arrangement with the author
Library of Congress Catalog Card Number: 80-69608
ISBN: 0-380-77123-3

First Avon Printing, April, 1981

AVON TRADEMARK REG. U.S. PAT. OFF. AND IN
OTHER COUNTRIES, MARCA REGISTRADA, HECHO EN
U.S.A.

Printed in the U.S.A.

DON   10 9 8 7 6 5 4 3 2

DEDICATION

For my mother, Margaret Reilly Vogel, my sister, Carol Vogel Martin, my daughter, Area Madaras, and Pam Rousseau, who is not a member of the family but might as well be.

Table of Contents

Gender: The He, She, It Problem

In the first draft of this book, we used the masculine pronouns *he* and *him* whenever we wanted to refer to the doctor. In the next draft we decided to strike a blow for feminism by using the female pronouns *she* and *her* to refer to the doctor, but since 97 percent of the doctors in this country are males, this seemed a bit of wishful thinking. Next we tried *he* or *she* and *him* or *her* and then, putting the female first, *she* and *he* and *her* and *him*, but this got a bit too cumbersome. Then we invented some new, neuter pronouns, but how many readers would know what a *shim*, *herhim*, *sherm* or any of the other combinations of *her* and *him* meant? In the end we struck a compromise: We simply eliminated most of the *hers* and *hims* and used *s/he* instead of writing *she* or *he*. Not a perfect solution, perhaps, but at least it's better than assuming that all doctors are men, or pretending that most are women.

Acknowledgments

This book would not have been possible without the generous support of many people, too numerous to mention here. We would, however, like to acknowledge the contributions of certain individuals. Before doing so, we should make it clear that inclusion in these acknowledgments does not necessarily mean that those individuals mentioned agree with the opinions expressed in the book.

Dr. Peter Schick of Brotman Memorial Hospital in Culver City, California, provided invaluable assistance in preparing the information on cancer. We are particularly grateful for his contributions to the section on breast cancer. Diane Levy, a nurse-practitioner from Los Angeles, made substantial contributions to the section on pregnancy and fertility. Carla Hines of the American Social Health Association assisted in our efforts to gather information on sexually transmitted diseases. Sam Knox, also of the American Social Health Association, was kind enough to review the section on sexually transmitted diseases and offer his comments. Nancy Adess of DES Action shared her expertise, reviewed the sections on DES, vaginal adenosis and clear cell adenocarcinoma and offered many comments. Nancy Kaswell from the Emma Goldman Clinic reviewed a draft of the material on cervical caps and offered valuable criticisms. Dr. Richard Small, a radiologist from Daniel Freedman Hospital in Inglewood, California, was kind enough to answer questions and provide background information on radiation therapy of cancer.

A number of people were helpful in our efforts to gather information on the cervical cap, including: Dr. James Koch, a physician from Brookline, Massachusetts; Renee Potik, a nurse-practitioner from Los Angeles; Jan

Scolastico and Lynn Dockworth from the Emma Goldman Clinic; Sarah Brendt, Sandra Malaski and Peg McElroy from the New Hampshire Feminist Women's Health Center; and Dr. Robert Goeppe of the University of Chicago, who, along with Dr. Uwe Freeze, has developed a new type of cervical cap.

Dr. James Heine of Lubbock, Texas, and Dr. Milos Chapvil of the University of Arizona were helpful in our efforts to learn about the cervical sponge. In addition, a number of other members of the medical profession assisted our research efforts, including: Dr. James Bouquet, Dr. Anthony Koerner, Dr. Val Davajan, Dr. Gerald Bernstein, Dr. Raymond Kaufman, Dr. John Frey and Dr. Walter Henderson.

Although they were not directly involved in the production of this book, there are some individuals and groups whose work in the field of women's health care provided inspiration, information and direction, including: Carol Downer, who introduced us to the concept of speculum self-exam; Rose Kushner, health-care activist and author of *Why Me?*, an outstanding book about breast cancer; Barbara Seaman, health-care activist and co-author of *Women and the Crisis in Sex Hormones*; the women of the National Women's Health Network, an organization dedicated to improving health care for women; and the women of the Boston Women's Health Collective, authors of *Our Bodies, Ourselves.*

A number of friends provided encouragement and support, assisted our research efforts and read and reviewed sections of the book, including: Pam Rousseau, Richard Johnson, Bill Happecook, Patti Pinto, Suzanne Thiele, Peter Tarbox, Pam Rodgers, Annie Sobieski, Jean Madsen, Ann Mulkey, Romaine Alhstrom, Susan Day, Lisa DePalma, Cynthia Pearson, Chris Smith, Sandy Kimball, Clark Bridges, Phil Capobianco, Deborah Capobianco, George Anderson, Carol Depew, David Wright and Leigh Adams.

Without the work of Anita Horvath, Alma Collins, Carol Eden and Gloria Shallcroft, who typed the manuscript, this book, quite literally, could not have been written. The copy editor, Christine Samuels, also made valuable contributions to the manuscript. We would also like to thank our agent, Harold Moscowitz, and our editors at Avon, Beth Rashbaum and Susan Moldow, for their support and unending patience. Last, but not least, we would like to thank the many women who shared their medical histories and problems with us.

WOMANCARE

How This Book Came to be Written

Way back, and it seems like eons ago, when we first conceived the idea behind this book, we wrote what is known in the publishing business as a book proposal. A proposal tells your editor what you're planning to write and is designed to convince the editor that your book fulfills a crying and desperate need and will therefore sell millions of copies.

The primary intent of this book, as we thought of it then, was to teach women how to use a speculum (the medical instrument used by doctors) to examine their own bodies. On the surface, the idea of women practicing gynecological self-exam, although it may sound a bit bizarre, is hardly earth-shattering. In reality, looking at your own vagina and cervix is about as exciting as looking down your throat. Indeed, in the not-too-distant future, gynecological self-exam will probably be a rather ho-hum topic, a routine matter of personal hygiene, about as controversial as brushing after meals or flossing your teeth. But for the time being, gynecological self-exam remains a rather revolutionary practice, for it brings us up against some very basic cultural taboos and makes us confront the negative attitudes about our bodies that have been socialized into us since infancy.

Most women think of their genital organs as unclean, smelly and ugly, which is hardly surprising, since we have been taught to think just that from earliest childhood. The negative images that most women have about this part of their bodies were formed early on, way back when they were toilet-trained, if not before.

Consider the differences between the experience of little boys and that of little girls. Small boys who manage to make it to the bathroom in time,

1

wrestle their pants down and, after taking careful aim, hit the pot are immediately rewarded with lavish praise. In contrast, little girls are told to wipe themselves clean. Equally lavish praise may follow, but for little girls the reflex parental response is "wipe yourself." The implication is clear—that area down there is dirty. Brother, on the other hand, doesn't have to wipe himself after he urinates. He just gives his penis a nonchalant shake, with his bare hands, no less, and puts it back in his pants. Little girls must use a wad of protective tissue lest their fingers touch that caustic mess. For women, it is clear right from the beginning that we've got something really unclean between our legs—such a mess, in fact, that we shouldn't even touch it with our bare hands.

As we grow older, the message remains unchanged. Boys may gather in groups and stage contests to see who can pee the farthest or write their names in the snow and dot the "i." Size and development of genital organs are gleefully compared. To be sure, many a late bloomer becomes the butt of cruel taunts in the gym locker room, but at least the matter is openly discussed. For adolescent girls there are no such public locker-room comparisons of who has the most protruding clitoris, the greatest number of pubic hairs, or whatever (and, as we all know, if it's too terrible to talk about, then it's *really* terrible). Girls have long since learned that there is something unclean and hence unmentionable about their genital organs.

The situation continues unchanged into adulthood. Nancy Friday points this out in her book *My Mother, My Self* when she says: "We all have something to hide. Why else would society build us stalls and cubicles with locks to undress and urinate in, when men are left to get on with it in large, communal, open locker rooms?"[1] The fashion and cosmetic industries make fortunes exploiting women's insecurity about and dissatisfaction with their bodies. But, Friday argues, it is not really our breasts, thighs or waistlines we are concerned about when we complain that we are ugly (and even the most beautiful woman finds something to complain about). These nagging worries are just displacements; our fears are actually about something more central—our genitals. Complaining about our breasts, calves, thighs and so forth only serves to distract our attention from "that other area that mother would never mention, that had no name, that made her face *distort* with disgust if we got it dirty."[2]

Changing our negative attitudes about our bodies, developing what one psychiatrist has called "genital self-respect," is central to coming to view ourselves as fully acceptable and equal human beings. Or, as Nancy Friday puts it, "Convince woman that her vagina is beautiful and you have the makings of an equal person. I believe this with all my heart."[3]

Practicing self-exam is one way of changing all this, of reversing these negative attitudes. As strange as it may sound to the uninitiated, many women discover that this part of their bodies holds a certain beauty, a beauty, for instance, as delicate as an orchid's, which, unlike other forms of beauty in our culture, can be appreciated for itself, for it does not have to measure up to some highly stylized, Madison Avenue standard of attractiveness.

Practicing gynecological self-exam also has other far-reaching consequences. For one thing, it challenges the traditional relationship between women and their doctors. Once a woman learns to use a speculum, she begins to view doctors differently. She has, literally and figuratively, a whole new perspective on the ritualized practice of the gynecological exam. And gynecological exam is a highly ritualized phenomena. It has been compared to the rites performed by medicine men, shamans and priests of supposedly more primitive societies: The supplicant/woman/patient is brought in to be examined by the priest/shaman/holy man/gynecologist. She is depersonalized by the removal of her clothes and/or other marks of personal or tribal identity. The priestly attendant/assistant medicine man/nurse then places her in a vulnerable position, on her knees, flat on the floor or, in our cultural ritual, in the examining table stirrups. The head honcho, in his characteristic garb, then makes an appearance on the scene; the supplicant/patient is draped in the ritual robes—in our culture, the white examining sheet—and the magic rite is performed. But for women who practice self-exam, this whole ritual is demystified. Gynecological self-exam is a sure cure for what we have come to call the M.D.eity syndrome.

The M.D.eity syndrome is a condition that affects vast numbers of doctors in this country and is generally transmitted to their all-too-susceptible patients. Perhaps the most characteristic symptom of the M.D.eity syndrome is the use of esoteric and incomprehensible language. A woman appearing before the M.D.eity with an irritating red rash on her inner thighs might, for instance, be told that she has erythema intertrigo, for which the doctor might prescribe an ointment with a multisyllabic Latin name. This too has its purposes. Such a woman might gratefully pay $50 or $75 to learn she had such an impressive sounding condition that could be so easily cured. But were she to visit a shirt-sleeved doctor who told her that her problem was chafing (a less impressive term for erythema intertrigo) and that she should rub a soothing ointment on her thighs, the woman might, understandably, balk at paying $50, much less $75, for "professional services rendered."

As long as you're not on the short end of the stick, the M.D.eity syndrome, with its overblown language and affected postures of authority, has a certain pompous humor. But the M.D.eity syndrome also has its more serious side.

In 1976 there were 794,000 hysterectomies (an operation in which a woman's uterus is removed) performed in this country.[4] Approximately

3

1,600 women died that year as a result of this operation.[5] But the really upsetting statistic is that, by conservative estimates, some 30 percent to 40 percent, or as many as 300,000, of these operations were unnecessary.[6] Why did 300,000 women risk their lives to have an unnecessary operation? Because the M.D.eity syndrome affects patients as well as doctors. Women too are convinced by the priestly rituals, the medical jargon, the white uniforms, and they fall prey to the delusion that the doctor is an elevated, superior, almost godlike being. The doctor has access to secret knowledge, for s/he can see what we cannot. We have to depend on the doctor for knowledge about this essential part of our bodies. This special knowledge imparts power and gives the doctor control over us, so that when s/he tells us to have our uteri (plural of uterus) removed, far too many of us do not question that judgment. One does not, after all, question the judgment of those in charge. No one wants to find out that the judgments of those one relies on are faulty; the implications of such a finding are far too threatening to our sense of well-being and security.

Self-exam is the first step in changing all this. The knowledge is no longer secret. Practicing self-exam will not magically enable a woman to make sense of all that medical jargon, nor does it take the place of a doctor's examination, but it does begin to demystify the M.D.eity and allow women to deal with their gynecologists in a new way. It is probably a safe bet to say that a woman who practices self-exam will not find herself among the estimated 300,000 women who will have unnecessary hysterectomies this year. She knows too much and is too much in control to allow herself to be manipulated in this way.

This alone was enough to convince us that self-exam was an important topic, vital to every woman. But we had to convince a publishing company of this. Book companies, like most companies, are generally run by men. We were concerned that male readers of our book proposal wouldn't have a gut reaction to it, that it would be difficult for them to understand the impact our book might have on women. So we asked the male readers of our proposal to imagine for a moment that their genital organs were located on their bodies in such a way that they could not see them without making a conscious effort with the aid of a mirror to do so.

"Even then," we continued, "you could only partially see them. In order to see all of them, you would need a special instrument available only to doctors, almost all of whom, not incidentally, are members of the opposite sex. Also imagine that you have grown up in a culture that teaches you that it is nasty and not 'manly' to mention, much less look at or touch, these genital organs. Moreover, these organs have a thin membrane at the orifice which 'nice boys' are cautioned to keep intact for their future wives and to guard from lascivious females who 'only have one thing on their minds.'

"At the age of about 13, you are taken to a female doctor who drapes you in a white sheet and pokes about in this mysterious area, much to your embarrassment and, possibly, pain. Later on, your lovers or wives may familiarize themselves with this part of your body. You may even bear children through it, but you will still never have seen it. From time to time, you are troubled with infections and other ailments in this area, but unless you are especially bold, you are too embarrassed to ask your female doctor any questions. Even if you are so bold, you are too ignorant to ask intelligent questions about this unseen and mysterious part of your body. If, in spite of all this, you do manage to ask questions, she only pats you on the head and tells you 'not to worry your sweet little head about it, dearie, just do as I say.' "

To add to their imaginary problems, we asked our male readers to further pretend that they lived in a society in which one of the burning questions of the day is whether or not people equipped with genital organs such as theirs are competent to deal with positions of leadership and power due to the raging hormonal imbalances produced by those never-seen genital organs: "In this society, you and all other men are conditioned from birth to think of yourself as passive, dependent and weaker than women. As you grow older, though, times change. A Men's Liberation Movement started by some courageous men who feel that biology should not control your destiny gains momentum. At first it seems a bit of a joke, but as the years pass, it begins to exert a pervasive influence on your society. Men, even the most conservative, begin to conceive of themselves and their roles in society differently. Health care, because men by their genital makeup are so dependent on it, becomes a major issue in the liberation movement. Groups of men band together to demand that more men be admitted to medical school and that men be given the legal right to control their reproductive organs. Other groups come together to study and research the working of your still mysterious body. Numerous books denouncing the women-dominated medical profession are written. Others that teach you how your own body works are published and read by millions of men. Even the effectiveness with which your lovers and wives manipulate these still unseen genitals is scrutinized in print. Then one day, you, with the aid of a mirror, an inexpensive plastic speculum and the latest of these 'male-lib' health care books, take a look at these genital organs that have caused such a hullabaloo all of your life. Imagine how you would feel."

As it turned out, the editors who read our proposal were, by and large, women, who had no problem whatsoever in imagining all of this and recognizing the impact the book might have. So the contracts were signed and work began immediately.

But that was only the beginning, and like all beginnings, was only a glimpse of what lay ahead. Buried in the back of our book proposal was a brief book outline. Not only would this book teach women how to practice self-exam, but since women who practiced self-exam would be in a position (no pun intended) to detect abnormalities and diseases in the earliest stages, when they are more curable, we would include information on common gynecological problems, the symptoms a woman might notice and the ways in which these conditions might be treated. Since women who practiced self-exam would also have a greater understanding of their bodies and, consequently, new feelings of control and mastery, we thought it would be worthwhile to include information on the barrier methods of birth control—the diaphragm, spermicidal foams and rubbers—which, unlike the Pill and the IUD, are not beset by a host of risks and complications. Women who were familiar with their bodies would, we felt, have more confidence in using these safer, woman-controlled, methods of birth control, which are highly reliable when used properly.

All this sounded quite sensible and not too terribly difficult, but as we began to talk with women and to review the available materials about gynecological problems and birth control, it became apparent that the emphasis of our book would have to shift and that the scope would have to enlarge. It became obvious that although gynecological self-exam was important, it was just the first step for women who wanted to gain control over their own bodies.

There were whole shelves of gynecologist-talks-to-the-laywoman books, but the majority of these books provided only the most superficial, Mickey-Mouse sorts of explanations of gynecological problems. None was of much use in helping a woman navigate her way through the medical marketplace, for even the best of them had a basic fault: They failed to inform women about their options and alternatives. As we talked to more and more women, we came to realize that what was really needed was a sort of consumer's guide to gynecology, a book that would let women know what choices existed so that they could make informed decisions about health care and birth control.

Consider, for example, what happened to Susan, who is just one of the many women we came across in the course of writing this book. Susan is 36, divorced and the mother of two children, 12 and 9. It hasn't always been easy for Susan, raising two kids and trying to establish herself in a paying career after years as a homemaker. But when we met Susan, things were looking pretty good. Although her job as assistant director at a daycare center wasn't by any stretch of the imagination lucrative, she was making ends meet. And, finally, after hectic years of shuffling schedules and juggling the responsibilities of breadwinner, solo parent and homemaker, she was about to complete her thesis and receive her master's degree in early-childhood education.

To add to all this satisfaction was her relationship with a man. The relationship, which was of some years standing, had, after some fits and starts, progressed from friend to lover to live-in roommate. Now, after some serious thought, she and her lover were considering marriage and, more to the point, a baby—which suited Susan, who found mothering a rewarding experience, just fine.

At this time Susan, who neither smokes nor drinks and is very conscientious about health matters, went to the doctor for her annual physical, which included a Pap smear, a test which involves collecting cells shed from the cervix and which is used to screen for cervical cancer. Susan's Pap smear showed some irregularities, so she had to return to the doctor for further tests called biopsies, in which a number of tissue specimens are taken from various parts of the cervix. Susan's biopsy specimens were sent to a laboratory where they were examined by a pathologist, a doctor who specializes in this field of medicine. The biopsy, which gives the pathologist an actual piece of tissue rather than just a few isolated cells to study, confirmed the diagnosis suggested by the Pap smear.

Susan had cervical cancer. Luckily, the doctor told her, she had caught the disease in its earliest stages, for her biopsy indicated that she had carcinoma in situ, a condition in which cells with all the abnormalities of cancer cells are present, but in which there is no sign that the cancer has invaded the surrounding tissue. The doctor told her that her condition was virtually 100 percent curable, but that she would have to have her cervix, uterus and ovaries removed, an operation known as a hysterectomy.

Susan was, understandably, quite shaken. Although it was a relief to know that her condition was curable, the prospect of losing her uterus and her ability to bear children, especially now when she wanted so much to have another child, was extremely upsetting. Losing her ovaries was especially scary. She knew that having her ovaries removed meant menopause, and even though menopause itself didn't upset her (after all, her mother had never had any problems), she'd heard that having a premature menopause could pose serious health risks.

When she called her mom to tell her the bad news, Susan's mother insisted that she get a second opinion from another doctor. Susan promptly made an appointment with a second doctor and arranged to have her biopsy reports and medical records transferred. After reviewing her records and examining her, the second doctor confirmed the diagnosis and again recommended a hysterectomy, although this time the doctor recommended that her ovaries be spared. Reluctantly, Susan allowed herself to be scheduled for surgery.

It just so happened that one of Susan's coworkers, who knew about her situation, also knew about the book we were writing. We had been spreading the word around, hoping to find women who had personally experienced the various conditions we were writing about and who would be willing to read and review what we had written. We had found that

7

women who had gone through the experience of having an illness often had questions or comments that never really occur to you until you are actually faced with the problem. Susan's friend suggested that she contact us.

Anxious to learn all she could about what was happening to her, Susan called the writer half of the gynecologist/writer team that put this book together. By reading the part of the book that deals with carcinoma in situ of the cervix, Susan not only gained a clearer understanding of what was wrong with her but also discovered something that was to prove very important to her.

What both of her doctors had failed to tell Susan was that there were alternative forms of therapy for her condition. One of these therapies was a relatively new technique known as cryosurgery, which involves destroying the affected cervical tissue by freezing and which doesn't require the removal of any organs. Nor does it affect a woman's ability to conceive or bear children. The other alternative was a procedure known as conization, in which a core of tissue is removed from the center of the cervix, a surgical process somewhat akin to removing a core from the center of an apple. Conization would significantly reduce Susan's chances of being able to have children, but a fair number of women are still able to conceive following the procedure.

There was, however, a catch: Not all women with carcinoma in situ are suitable candidates for these less destructive forms of therapy. We cautioned Susan not to get her hopes up, but we could see she was excited. She was definitely ready for a third opinion. This time Susan saw a gynecologist who was also an experienced cryosurgeon. As it turned out, Susan was an ideal candidate for cryosurgery, although it was necessary to repeat all the diagnostic tests before this was determined. The doctor who originally performed Susan's biopsy had put all of the biopsied tissue specimens into the same container when he sent them to the laboratory for analysis, so there was no way of knowing exactly where on the cervix any given tissue sample had originated. Knowing precisely where the tissue samples have come from is a critical factor in determining whether or not a woman is a suitable candidate for cryosurgery. So, Susan had to suffer the mental anguish of waiting extra days for the repeat lab tests (not to mention the additional expense involved in repeating the tests).

The lab tests looked good and Susan decided to go ahead with the cryosurgery. Instead of spending a couple of thousand dollars or more and losing her reproductive organs, her ability to have children and a significant amount of time from work, Susan spent less than a hundred dollars, didn't lose any time at all from work and was eventually able to go ahead with her plans to add to her family.

Why didn't the other doctors tell Susan about cryosurgery? We can't tell you for certain, although the writer half of this book team did try, with Susan's written permission, to find out. Not surprisingly, both doctors refused to discuss the matter. There are a number of possibilities.

Perhaps it was the old M.D.eity syndrome. Doctors do get to thinking of themselves as rather godlike, and gods, having a wider view of things, are, of course, wiser than we mere mortals. Susan was 36 and already had two children. Some population-conscious doctors feel that no one should have more than two children. (Some doctors feel that minority women on welfare, in particular, should not have more than two children, but Susan was white and didn't collect welfare, so this was probably not a factor in her case.)

Susan was a divorcee and not married, and even in this day and age there are doctors who don't approve of pregnancy in unmarried women and who feel they have the right to inflict their unannounced moral judgments on their patients.

Or, their failure to inform Susan of her options and alternatives may have been motivated by some combination of ignorance and greed. The doctors may have known about cryosurgery, but may not have had the training, experience and equipment necessary to perform this procedure. Instruction in cryosurgery has only recently been added to the medical school curriculum for gynecologists. Unless a gynecologist were a fairly recent graduate of medical school, s/he would have had to go back to school, that is, take a special training seminar in the technique. This training takes time and money, and there is also the added financial outlay for the equipment. If the doctor were not skilled in cryosurgery, this might mean referring the women to another doctor and thereby losing a fee. Doctor's fees for hysterectomies range from about $1,000-$3,000.

Thanks to the Pap smear, cervical cancer is being discovered in its earliest stages. A doctor with a busy practice might see five to ten patients a year with carcinoma in situ. A doctor who saw ten such patients a year and who charged an average fee of $1,500 for a hysterectomy could be faced with referring away $15,000 worth of business annually. If the doctor's fee were $3,000, referring ten patients might mean a loss of $30,000, a rather hefty chunk of money to forego.

Maybe it was simple ignorance. The first two doctors Susan saw may not have been up-to-date on the latest techniques. Even though most states have some sort of continuing education requirement designed to keep doctors abreast of the latest developments, these requirements are generally pretty laughable. Attending a few luncheons presided over by a speaker from the medical society can pretty much fulfill these requirements. Or, better yet, a doctor can take one of the numerous cruises to exotic locations that are designed specifically for doctors and offer continuing-education credits sandwiched in between shuffleboard and other shipboard attractions. At any rate, state requirements by no means guarantee that a doctor is up-to-date, and Susan's doctors might just have been a bit behind the times.

Even if a doctor is a skilled cryosurgeon, s/he still has a financial interest in performing hysterectomies rather than cryosurgery. The cost of cryosurgery runs from about $60-$150. At $60 per patient, ten patients per year with carcinoma in situ treated by cryosurgery would net the doctor $600, while ten hysterectomies at $1,000 per operation would pull in $10,000, a more than ten-fold increase in annual income.

This is not to suggest that all doctors are greedy monsters who are eyeing your uterus with dreams of yachts or Aspen condominiums in their heads; however, the estimated 300,000 unnecessary hysterectomies* performed in this country each year do give one pause. Still, it is probably a rare doctor who actually sits around and says, "Ah, ha! I think I'll give this woman a hysterectomy and make some extra bucks." The process is somewhat more subtle than that. Doctors, like the rest of us, tend to develop rationalizations for what they do. For instance, a doctor who recommends hysterectomies for carcinoma in situ may argue that cryosurgery is not an adequate form of therapy, that it is too new for its effectiveness to have been conclusively proven.** But how much of this is sincere and how much is rationalizing and self-justifying?

If a doctor were to explain to a woman with carcinoma in situ that there are alternatives but that, personally, s/he did not recommend these forms of treatment, we would not doubt his or her sincerity. But this is often not the case. Neither of the first two doctors that Susan contacated even so much as mentioned the fact that these other forms of therapy existed. In situations like Susan's, the financial motivations of a doctor who fails to fully inform a woman of the options available to her are suspect.

Women must realize that this is a "for-profit" medical care system, which is very different from a socialized medical care system, where doctors are paid a flat salary by the government. In our system there is a financial incentive for doctors to recommend more drastic and hence more profitable treatments. This is not to suggest that medical care under a socialized medical system would be any better or worse; both have their problems, and this is a complex issue beyond the scope of this book. Let it suffice to say that for right now, and for the foreseeable future, medical

---

*Unnecessary hysterectomies are those operations in which a healthy uterus is removed. A hysterectomy done for carcinoma in situ would not be considered an unnecessary hysterectomy in the medical sense of the term, even if there were alternative forms of treatment available.

**The risk involved in cryosurgery treatment for carcinoma in situ is discussed in greater detail elsewhere in this book. See the index for page numbers.

care in this country will operate on a "for-profit" basis and this undeniably influences the type of health care women receive.

Susan's case is not unusual. In fact, doctors who fully inform their patients of the options available to them and then allow the patient to make her own decisions are the exception rather than the rule. Many gynecologists feel that informing women about their options and letting them make a decision is a waste of time. Their patients, they tell us, don't want to assume responsibility for such decisions. They want the doctor to do it for them. As one doctor put it, "I used to spend time carefully explaining things to my patients. They didn't want to hear it. They wanted me to tell them what to do. So, I don't bother with all that anymore. I just tell them what to do. That's what they want, that's what they expect from you."

We don't doubt that there are women who don't want to be informed, who want to leave it all in their doctors' hands. Given the cultural barriers that keep women from knowledge about their bodies, the M.D.eity syndrome and the general sexism in our society, it is not surprising that some women feel that they are too incompetent and too ignorant to make decisions about their own bodies. We are so alienated from our bodies that some of us feel we cannot even venture opinions—much less make judgments—about what is in our best interests; however, our work with women has convinced us that, given the choice, most women opt for an active role in making decisions about their own bodies. The growing women's health movement is evidence of the fact that women not only want, but are actively demanding, a role in health care decision-making. We suspect that, in reality, doctors who feel that women want decisions made for them enjoy the paternalistic relationship they establish with their patients. There is after all a certain ego satisfaction to be derived from playing the M.D.eity. It's also less trouble. No need to waste time bothering with explanations. It's much easier to pat a patient on the head and tell her not to worry about it.

Moreover, many doctors think of women as rather hysterical, not-terribly-bright creatures who really aren't capable of understanding the alternatives, let alone making responsible decisions. It is a popular myth in our society that sexist attitudes are held by truck drivers, construction workers and rednecks. The well-educated doctor is, supposedly, beyond all that. But one has only to take a look at medical textbooks to discover that sexism is rampant in the medical profession. The failure of many doctors to inform women of their options and to include them in decision-making stems from their sexist views of women.

Another explanation for why women are not informed of alternative forms of therapy is that many doctors simply don't see this as their responsibility. They see their job in quite another light. Their function, as

11

they perceive it, is to provide their expert opinion and recommendations for therapy. Medicine, they argue, is a complex, highly technical field. Women simply don't have the background and knowledge to intelligently evaluate the alternatives available to them. According to this school of thought, that's the doctor's job.

At first glance this point of view seems fairly sound, but these doctors forget one very important thing. Experts disagree, and they disagree much more often than most of us outside the field of medicine realize. Susan's case is just one example. There are myriad others. Consider, for example, breast cancer. The same women could consult three different doctors and get three different opinions. Doctor A might recommend a lumpectomy, a simple removal of the lump. Doctor B might recommend a modified radical mastectomy, which involves removal of the woman's breast and the lymph nodes in her armpit. Doctor C might recommend the significantly more disfiguring radical mastectomy, which entails removal of the breast, the lymph nodes in the armpit and the muscles of the upper chest wall. None of these doctors could be called a quack. Indeed, each of these procedures is endorsed by top-flight doctors at the nation's most renowned medical schools, and the debate about which treatment is best is argued passionately in medical circles—and probably will be for some time to come.

Those doctors who argue that women cannot make their own decisions about which form of therapy they should have ignore the fact that there is not uniform agreement among experts. When the experts disagree, the decision comes down, as it always must, to one person, the patient herself. In order to make these decisions women need to understand the issues and the options. Then, and only then, are they in a position to do what they must: Weigh the facts and, depending on their own personal values, make a decision.

Are the issues so complex that women cannot understand them? We think not. In our opinion many doctors have an inflated view of the complexity of what they do. This is not to say that the issues in medical debates are not at times rather convoluted, but the complexities can be simplified so that they can be understood by laywomen without undue distortion.

As we worked with more and more women, it became obvious to us that women were not getting the information they needed from their doctors. What was necessary, it seemed to us, was a book that provided this sort of information. Second opinions are fine, and we heartily support them, but, as we saw in Susan's case, second opinions are too often just rubber stamps of approvals. Second opinions do not always assure that women will hear the whole story or be informed of all the available options. Thus we began to shift the emphasis and redefine the scope of this book.

We still felt that women needed basic information about their bodies.

12

The first section of this book is designed to provide that information. The following chapter explains the external anatomy of the genital organs and teaches women how to practice gynecological self-exam. Chapter Three discusses the anatomy and function of the breast and teaches women how to breast self-exam. Chapter Four explains the changes that take place in a woman's body over the course of a menstrual cycle and over the course of her lifetime.

The second part of this book discusses birth control, for this is another medical area in which women are frequently misinformed. There is clearly a great deal of bias in the medical profession in regard to birth control. Doctors often push the more dangerous, physician-controlled methods, such as the Pill and the IUD, and downgrade the safer, user-controlled barrier methods, such as the diaphragm, foam and condoms (rubbers). As we explain in Chapter Five, statistics have been used—or rather misused— to create the impression that the Pill and the IUD are vastly more effective than the barrier methods, but this is simply not true. There have been studies of the condom in which the actual-use—effectiveness rate was better than the commonly quoted theoretical rate* for the Pill and the IUD.

This part of the book also includes a reference section that provides detailed information about the various methods of birth control, so that women can be well informed when making decisions about this matter.

The third section of this book deals with doctors and disease. Chapter Six discusses the doctor-patient relationship, how to find a good doctor and how to get a second opinion. This section also includes a reference section, which contains information about virtually all the ills that female flesh is heir to, with descriptions of causes, symptoms, diagnostic steps and the various treatment options. The conditions described in this reference section are categorized according to the organs they affect. Thus, diseases of the breast are found under the heading The Breast, problems relating to the ovary are discussed under the heading The Ovary and so forth. There are separate headings for sexually transmitted diseases, for problems relating to pregnancy and fertility and for problems related to the menstrual cycle. There is also a separate subdivision that deals with general information about cancer, but specific information about cancer of a particular organ is discussed along with the other diseases of that organ.

Each of the various subdivisions in the reference section on diseases is prefaced with a short introduction, which contains valuable general information about diseases of the particular organ or the set of problems discussed in that subheading. For instance, the introduction to the section

---

*The theoretical rate is the effectiveness rate one could expect if that method were used perfectly, with none of the forgotten pills, broken condoms or other problems that occur in actual use.

on vaginal diseases includes information on the prevention and diagnosis of vaginal infections that applies to *all* of the vaginal infections in that section. Rather than repeat that information in the discussion of each and every vaginal infection, we have included it in the general introduction to vaginal diseases. So, be sure to review the material in the introductions before reading about the specific problem that interests you.

An index of symptoms of the diseases described in this section of the book is included in the appendix. Instructions for using this index are also included in the appendix.

This reference section is not designed to take the place of your doctor or of second opinions. Rather, it is designed to provide you with basic information, so that you will be aware of your options and will have sufficient knowledge to be able to ask the right questions.

The last section of the book deals with gynecological operations, tests, procedures and drugs. Chapter Seven talks about unnecessary surgery and tests and explains how to avoid them. Detailed information about the various operations, tests and procedures mentioned in other parts of the book is included in the accompanying reference section, along with information about some of the more controversial drugs used in gynecological medicine.

A standard format is used for the descriptions of birth control methods, diseases and operations, tests and procedures, and may include any of the following:

Name: The most widely used name of the birth control method, disease, drug, operation, test or procedure is given at the beginning.

AKA: "AKA" stands for "also known as." There is generally more than one name or term used to refer to any given disease, birth control method, drug, operation, etc. For example, yeast infections of the vagina may also be referred to as fungus infections, moniliasis and candidiasis, to mention just a few alternate names. We have included all such alternatives in the index so that women will be able to locate the desired information regardless of the name they look under.

Types: This entry, which is found most often in the discussions of gynecological disease, includes a breakdown of the various categories or types of diseases.

Associated terms: This also appears most often in the discussions of gynecological disease and is a sort of catch-all category used for terms that are not actually synonyms for a disease or types of the disease but are closely associated with that particular gynecological problem. These too are listed in the index in the back of the book.

This index can also be an important tool in helping you become more fully informed. As mentioned above, you can use it to locate information on a birth control method, or a disease, regardless of which of their various names you may know. It may also serve you as a sort of dictionary or glossary of terms. Although we have tried to avoid medical jargon, you may at times come across terms that are not familiar to you. If you will then turn to the index, it will direct you to an explanation of the term elsewhere in the book. In addition, you may also use the index as a sort of guidepost to help you find your way to important, related information. If, for instance, you are reading about a condition that is treated with a hysterectomy, you might want to consult the index and find a page number reference for the discussion of the pros and cons of various types of hysterectomies. By turning to those pages, you would discover that a hysterectomy can involve just the removal of the uterus or removal of the uterus and the ovaries as well. If you require a hysterectomy, will you want your ovaries removed too or will you ask your doctor to spare them? Since some doctors routinely remove the ovaries when doing hysterectomies on women over a certain age, this sort of additional information can be very important. We've made the index quite extensive, to enable you to find all relevant information quickly and easily. We encourage you to use it.

While the index is the main tool we have used to help our readers locate related information, we were concerned that in certain instances it alone might not suffice. There were times, we realized, when no matter how much common sense a reader had, it simply might not occur to her that she should look in the index for related information or that there was in fact additional material of interest to her elsewhere in the book. We were further concerned that in other instances a reader might not be entirely clear on exactly which term in the index would lead her to the related information she needed. Because of these concerns, we devised a cross-reference system to use in these instances. At various points in the text you will see a page number preceded by the word *see* and enclosed in ( ). Related information that may be of interest can be found on the pages given. By using the index *and* the cross-references, you should be able to locate all the information you need to become an informed consumer.

Perhaps we should also mention that metric measurements—centimeters, millimeters, etc.—are generally used in medical literature and that we have often used them in this book. A list of metric abbreviations and a table that will help you convert measurements to more familiar standards is included in the appendix at the back of the book.

We have tried to organize this book so that the information is easily accessible. We hope that it will help to break down the barriers that make medical information accessible only to members of the medical profession, for we believe that every woman should have access to all available knowledge before making any health-care decision.

You may find that your doctor disagrees with some of the things we have written. Such disagreement is unavoidable, for medicine is not an exact science. You, as a consumer of medical services, have a right to a full explanation of medical controversies before giving your consent for any type of treatment. Only in this way can a woman's consent be truly informed; only then can you weigh the alternatives and make the decision you feel to be right for you.

Although the medical information in this book represents the most up-to-date findings at the time of writing, some information will need revising before the ink has a chance to dry, for things change quickly in the field of medicine. We have tried to indicate areas where ongoing research may provide answers or new insights. We hope that there will be revised editions of this book in the future. Nothing would be more helpful in preparing future editions than comments, questions and criticisms from readers. If you have thoughts to share, please contact us by writing to Lynda Madaras, c/o Avon Books, 959 Eighth Avenue, New York, New York 10019.

2

Gynecological Self-Exam

"A book about what?" squawks our friend and neighbor, whom we'll call Doctor Tom (although he is a doctor, his name is not actually Tom).

"Gynecological self-exam, you know, teaching women how to use a speculum," we repeat, making a mental note to call somebody else next time we want to borrow a medical dictionary. From Tom's reaction, you'd have thought somebody had just called him to say she was writing a book on how to perform brain surgery at home in your spare time and wanted to know if she could borrow his scalpel.

In a few moments, Tom, now a man with a mission, is at the front door, medical dictionary in hand. "But, it's dangerous," he sputters.

"Dangerous, how?" This stops him cold. "Come on, it's not dangerous; it's not any more dangerous than cleaning your ear with a Q-tip."

"You could puncture your eardrum with a Q-tip," counters Tom, who works in an emergency room and has a flair for medical oddities.

"What could you puncture with a speculum?"

After some hemming and hawing, Tom is forced to concede that self-exam isn't dangerous, but now he argues that it's much too difficult. Actually, a speculum is about as difficult to use as a shoe horn or a can opener. An adroit five-year-old could probably handle the mechanics of it. The thousands of women in this country who practice self-exam are living proof that it's not too difficult. After a while, Tom, who by now has had to concede that self-exam is neither dangerous nor too difficult, comes up with another objection.

"Yes, but what about cancer?"

Cancer? Tom was obviously clutching at straws. He couldn't possibly think that someone could develop cancer as a result of practicing self-exam. As it turned out, Tom's concern was that women who practiced self-exam might come to feel that it was no longer necessary to have an annual Pap smear, a test that can detect the presence of cervical cancer before there are any visible signs or obvious symptoms.

We don't believe that women who practice self-exam will come to neglect basic health care; quite the contrary. It seems to us that fear and ignorance, not knowledge, are what keep women from having annual Pap smears, breast exams and general physicals. But, just to keep Tom happy, we'll say it: Gynecological self-exam is not meant to be a substitute for going to the doctor. The doctor can perform tests like the Pap smear and other types of examinations that you cannot. Rather, gynecological self-exam is an addition to your regular medical check-ups. By practicing self-exam, women can learn to detect abnormalities and seek treatment when diseases are most curable, in their earliest stages, before they become full blown illnesses. For example, a woman who practices self-exam, is familiar with her own vaginal discharge and knows what is normal for her and can detect a vaginal infection (the most common gynecological problem, the chief symptom of which is an increase in vaginal discharge) right away, before the discharge is so copious that it leaks out onto her underclothes. Vaginal infections, although they are generally not serious, can be difficult to get rid of. Not infrequently, they require more than one course of treatment, which means more doctor's visits, lab tests and medications, which can be quite costly. Women who practice gynecological self-exam can nip these infections in the bud and avoid the necessity for extra courses of treatment, saving themselves both time and money.

Not only can gynecological self-exam save you money, but as discussed in the first chapter, it can also change your whole attitude about your body and yourself and about doctors, medical care and your role in making health-care decisions.

Consider one friend's description:

One evening several years ago, a woman I know invited me to attend what I thought was going to be a meeting of a consciousness-raising group. It was, but not in the way I had expected. Instead of the usual rap session, I found a group of women teaching each other to give themselves gynecological self-examinations. My initial reaction was one of acute embarrassment. It was, after all, a fairly bizarre scene. One by one, the women climbed up on the table, inserted plastic speculums and, with the aid of a flashlight and a mirror, took a look at their own cervixes. My curiosity proved stronger than my lingering Victorianism and, when it came my turn, I hopped up on the table too.

As it turns out, looking at your cervix is no big deal. But the first time I did it, my emotional reaction was overwhelming. Here was a part of my own body intimately connected with my sexual identity, my psychological being, my very self, and I had never seen it. Moreover, the men in my life and my all-male string of gynecologists had more experience with this part of my body than I did. My body, and *they* knew more about it than *me*.

The effect of looking at my cervix was mindblowing. I had an incredible feeling of personal power and competence. I left that evening, speculum tucked under my arm, walking tall, literally strutting down the street. I knew what was happening. I could take care of business. I was in charge, on top, heavy-duty...yes, ma'am!

This chapter describes the anatomy of your genital organs and explains how to go about giving yourself a gynecological exam. We hope that taking this guided tour of your own body leaves you feeling equally in charge, on top and heavy-duty, yes, ma'am!

Equipment

You will need three simple pieces of equipment: a mirror, a light source and a speculum. A mirror with a stand is good because you won't have to hold the mirror and thus both of your hands will be free. A "make-up" mirror with two sides, one of which enlarges your reflection, is also more convenient, but a regular hand mirror will work fine. A gooseneck lamp with a 100-watt light bulb provides a good strong light and is also convenient, since it is easily adjusted to the proper angle and also frees your hands; however, a flashlight will do if you don't happen to have a gooseneck lamp.

The speculum is a little harder to come by. Most doctors use a metal speculum, but this is a fairly expensive piece of equipment. Because these speculums are metal, they can be sterilized after each use and can be used over and over again on the doctor's patients. There are also inexpensive plastic speculums that cost about 50 cents apiece wholesale. These speculums are often used by hospitals and clinics. Since they are plastic and cannot be sterilized by heat, they are intended for one-time use only. It would be unthinkable for a doctor to use these disposable speculums on different patients. You certainly wouldn't want to be examined with a plastic speculum that had been used on another patient, especially someone who had a vaginal disease. However, because your speculum will be used by you and only you, it needn't be heat sterilized after each use. Your plastic speculum can be used without fear of infection as long as simple sanitary precautions are observed. After each use, wash your speculum thoroughly with an antiseptic soap (a number of good ones are available without prescription from the pharmacy) or with isopropyl alcohol. Wrap it in plastic and store it in a clean, dry place after each use.

If you are feeling less than certain about sanitary conditions, please remember that millions of women insert diaphragms into their vaginas regularly as a method of birth control, and there is nothing unsanitary about this. As long as simple sanitary rules are observed, there is no danger of infection. If at some point you should develop a vaginal infection, you might feel more comfortable switching to a new speculum, but as long as you wash the speculum thoroughly, there is really no need to discard your old speculum.

Although there are inexpensive plastic speculums available, it is not always easy to get ahold of one. According to a federal law that regulates any instrument inserted into a bodily orifice, a speculum cannot be sold without a doctor's prescription. It is, to say the least, a curious law. You are much more likely to do yourself bodily harm with a Q-tip (perforated eardrums and so forth) than you are with a speculum. It seems clear that this law is a legacy of bygone days and old attitudes about women and sexuality.

It is sometimes possible to buy speculums direct from medical supplies distributors, who are listed in the yellow pages of your telephone book. The largest manufacturer of plastic disposable speculums is Barnett Instruments, a division of C. R. Bard, and their speculum is registered under the trade name Sani-Spec. The Sani-Spec is sold in packages of ten and comes in three sizes—small, medium and large. The sizes vary both in the width and length of the speculum blades. The small and medium Sani-Specs are about the same length, but the small is only half the width of the medium. If you are a virgin, you would probably use a small size. If, however, you are a virgin and are also not used to inserting tampons in your vaginal opening, it may be difficult to comfortably insert even the small speculum. Using tampons for a few months prior to trying self-exam will widen the vaginal opening and make a speculum exam easier.

Most women can use a medium speculum, especially if they have borne children. If you feel any discomfort upon inserting the speculum, you are probably using too large a size. Your doctor can help you if you are uncertain as to size. There are also special classes available in self-help given by women's clinics across the country where you can obtain a speculum and learn how to give yourself an exam. The appendix at the back of the book lists some of these clinics. Some women prefer to learn about self-exam in the group setting provided by these clinics, where there are other women with experience in self-exam to help. Other women prefer doing this with a friend, by themselves or with their doctor.

Of course, if your doctor is willing to help, this is the most logical place to obtain your speculum. Not only can s/he write you a prescription or provide you with a plastic speculum, but your doctor can also help you find and identify your cervix, which can be a bit tricky the first time. Unfortunately, not all doctors are receptive to the idea of their patients examining themselves. One woman who got interested in self-exam tells of asking her family doctor, a kindly old gent who had brought her into the world and who had delivered one of her own children, for a speculum. "He was," she reports, "vaguely horrified. You'd have thought I'd asked him for a scalpel so that I could perform a hysterectomy on myself. Luckily, I had a good relationship with him and was able to talk to him and explain my reasons. He finally came around to my point of view and got me a plastic speculum from the hospital. In fact, he now uses a speculum and mirror with his patients whom he is teaching to use a diaphragm and claims it is ten times easier to teach them now."

In the course of writing this book, we've talked to many doctors, most of whom have been very enthusiastic about the idea of self-exam. There were, however, some doctors who had an initial resistance to the idea. It's a new idea, and like all new ideas it takes some getting used to for some people. One way to find a gynecologist who will be sympathetic to self-exam is to call a women's clinic, a women's center at a local college or university or a free clinic. Such places will normally have referral lists of gynecologists who are apt to be more sympathetic to the concept of self-examination. (For more information on finding a doctor, see Chapter Six.)

In any case, once you've managegd to get hold of your speculum, spend a few minutes practicing opening and closing it so you are familiar with how it works and are able to operate it smoothly (Illustration 1). You will insert the speculum into your body with the duckbill closed, as shown here. Once it is inside, you will clasp the handles together, which opens the duckbill and allows you a view of the walls of your vagina and cervix. To open it wider and lock it in the open position, simply press down with your thumbs. As you push down, you will hear three clicking noises. This clicking is the ratchet mechanism that opens the duckbill wider with each progressive click. The plastic disposable speculum is not a precision instrument. Since it is designed for one-time use, you may find that it tends to stick a bit with repeated use. Don't give up, it's the instrument, not you, that's at fault; with a bit of perseverance and practice, you can learn to make it work fairly smoothly.

Exploring Your External Anatomy

Before you insert your speculum and take a look at your internal anatomy, take some time to familiarize yourself with your external genitals, also known as your vulva or, as granny used to call them, your "private parts."

Illustration 1   *Working the Speculum*

Illustration 2 will help you recognize and identify the various parts of your external genitals. Some women have told us that these kinds of gynecological drawings are often confusing or misleading. One reason for this is that such drawings typically show only those parts of the female anatomy that doctors are concerned with—the parts that are subject to infection or other ailments. If a feature of the anatomy isn't a typical site of infection or abnormality, then it usually is not named and, for a doctor's purposes, doesn't exist. This can be confusing, especially in regard to the vestibule (see below), where there are several folds and layers of skin that are often not shown in gynecological illustrations. Many women, looking at the typical medical illustration, become worried that they have a growth or some spare parts because they are unable to distinguish the medically

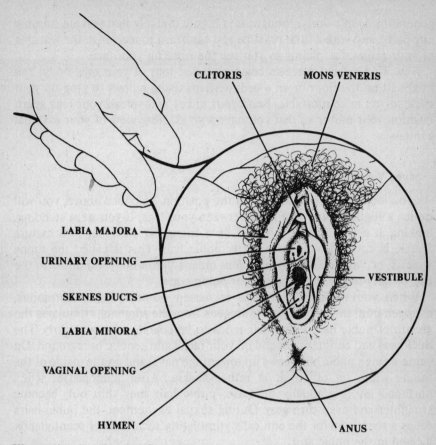

CLITORIS   MONS VENERIS

LABIA MAJORA

URINARY OPENING

SKENES DUCTS

LABIA MINORA

VAGINAL OPENING

VESTIBULE

HYMEN   ANUS

Illustration 2   *External Genitals*

named features from the unnamed but nonetheless present anatomical features. We have provided more detailed drawings of this area in an attempt to avoid this confusion.

Another reason that it is sometimes difficult to identify parts of your genitals from drawings is that each individual is different. Also, the appearance of your genitals changes in the course of your lifetime. A young girl's genitals do not look the same as a mature woman's. So, don't expect to look exactly like the illustration in this book.

However, just as your face has recognizable features (nose, mouth, eyes), so your vulva has identifiable parts that you can learn to recognize. Of course, we are quite used to looking at faces, so it is easy for us to generalize from a stylized drawing of a human face and recognize the salient features on a particular individual. Most of us, however, are not quite so used to looking at female genitals; therefore, it is not as easy to generalize. Don't worry, though; it is highly unlikely that you are missing any parts, and with a little practice you can learn to recognize the features of your genitals as plainly as you see the nose on your face.

Now, find a quiet place to begin a guided tour of your own body. You might sit on the floor or on a bed, perhaps using pillows to prop up your back so you're comfortable. Bend your knees and spread your legs apart. Position your mirror so that you have a good, clear view of your external genitals.

Mons Veneris

As you look down your body from the position described above, you will notice a slight mound that rises between your legs. If you were standing, looking at a wall mirror, it would be a triangular area that in a mature female is covered with short, curly pubic hair. This is called the mons veneris, or "mound of Venus." *Mons* means "little hill" and refers to the pad of fatty tissue that covers your pubic bone.

When you reach puberty, the increased output of two hormones, estrogen from the ovaries and androgens from the adrenals, stimulates the growth of pubic hair. Pubic hair tends to be coarse, crisp and curly. The thickness and curliness depend on your racial and genetic background. On some women pubic hair grows up toward the navel and on the inside of the thighs while on others it is rather sparse. After menopause, when hormone levels gradually decrease, pubic hair may thin out, become straighter and even turn gray. During sexual excitement, the pubic hairs act as a scent trap for the erotically stimulating secretions of scent glands located in the pubic area.

Labia Majora

As you move downward from the mons, you will notice that the area covered with pubic hair divides and continues down toward the anus, the rectal opening. The hairy areas on either side of this division are the labia majora or outer lips. These two folds of fatty tissue protect the urinary and reproductive tract openings that lie between them. These outer lips change in size during the course of your life and also vary in size from individual to individual. If you have never had children, these outer lips may actually touch each other. After childbirth, many women find that these lips are slightly separated, so that the area between is exposed. If you separate these outer lips with your fingers, you will notice that the insides of them are hairless and are dotted with small, slightly raised bumps, which are oil glands that help keep the area moist. The color of the skin in this area may vary from a light pink to a brownish black hue.

24

Labia Minora

If you separate the outer lips, you will see two long ridges or folds of skin. These are the labia minora, or inner lips. They are hairless, quite sensitive to touch and vary greatly in color and texture from light pink to brownish black and from very smooth to very wrinkled. They usually protrude less than the outer lips, although in some women they may actually protrude beyond the outer lips. During sexual excitement, they swell and darken in color.

If you follow the inner lips up towards the mons, you will notice that they come together or fuse. The upper fold of this fused portion forms a sort of hood that covers the bud-shaped clitoris and is called the prepuce, clitoral hood or clitoral foreskin. In some women this hood will completely cover the clitoris; in others the clitoris will protrude slightly. The fold of skin that passes beneath the clitoris or may seem to extend from the lower sides of the clitoris is called the frenulum.

The labia minora, or inner lips, serve to protect the reproductive and urinary tract openings that lay between them, to lubricate the area with their oil-producing glands and to stimulate the highly sensitive clitoris. Any contact or movement of the inner lips moves the clitoral hood, which in turn stimulates the clitoris as it moves across it.

Clitoris

Now you come to the sexiest part of your anatomy, your clitoris. If you pull back the clitoral hood, you will see a small bud-shaped piece of tissue, the glans clitoris, or the tip of the clitoris, which is usually about the size of an eraser on the end of a pencil. The clitoris is made of erectile tissue, which fills with blood and swells during sexual arousal. As you touch yourself in this area, you may well have very pleasurable feelings of sexual excitement.

The rest of the clitoris is hidden from view underneath the surface of the skin. If you press gently just above the clitoral hood in an upward direction toward your mons, you will feel a firm, rubbery, movable cord under the skin. This is the shaft of the clitoris. For some women, this is a very sexually sensitive area. The rest of the clitoris, including the crura, two wing-shaped extensions of the shaft that spread in wishbonelike fashion and are attached to the pubic bone, and two bundles of erectile tissue called the bulbs of the vestibule, lie too far under the skin and muscle of this area for you to feel. These, along with the rest of the clitoris and a system of connecting veins throughout the pelvis, become firm and filled with blood during sexual arousal and account for the warm, tingling feelings we often experience. Some women experience a similar type of

25

pelvic congestion just before their period, and for some women, this creates a heightened sexual desire at that time.

The clitoris is involved directly or indirectly in all female orgasms. Before the pioneering work of Masters and Johnson, two doctors who have done groundbreaking research into female sexual response, it was thought that there were two types of orgasms, vaginal and clitoral. A vaginal orgasm was supposed to be a more mature type of response, while a clitoral orgasm was judged to be an "infantile" response to sexual stimulation. Women who experienced orgasms only in response to clitoral stimulation were said to be "frigid," "sexually immature," "less feminine" and "neurotic."

The so-called vaginal orgasm has been shown by the clinical work of Masters and Johnson to be a myth. All female orgasms are related to the clitoris. Even when an orgasm results from penile penetration, the clitoris is involved, for movement of the inner lips serves to stimulate the clitoris. Also, the vaginal opening lies near the shaft of the clitoris, and the shaft may thus be stimulated orgasmically. For most women, though, penile penetration alone doesn't stimulate the clitoris enough to produce orgasm.

Vestibule

If you separate your inner lips with your fingers, you will be able to see a smooth boat-shaped area that is called the vestibule. The opening of your urinary tract—the urethral meatus, through which you eliminate liquid wastes, or urine, from your body—is located here. The opening to your reproductive tract, through which you insert a tampon, through which a baby is born and into which the penis is inserted in sexual intercourse, is also located in the vestibule. Two small glands known as the Bartholin's glands, are located just inside. The ducts of these glands will probably be too small for you to see. They are generally not noticeable except when the duct of the glands becomes blocked and swells as the result of infection. It was once thought that these glands were responsible for lubrication of the vagina during sexual arousal. It is now known that they secrete only a few drops of fluid at this time and that their function is to keep the opening of the vagina moist.

Urethral Meatus

The urethral meatus may be difficult for you to find unless you have the obvious, protruding kind. To find the urethral meatus, start from the clitoris and move down. If you stay in a straight line, the first dimpled area you find will be the urethral meatus. It usually resembles an inverted v.

You have to stay dead-center while you are moving down from your clitoris or you might mistake the ducts of the Skene's glands, two little niches on each side of the urethral meatus, for the urethral opening.

To make certain you have found the urethral meatus, stand in your bathtub or shower, spread your inner and outer lips and position a mirror so you have a clear view of the vestibule; then urinate. This will teach you beyond any shadow of a doubt where your urethral meatus is located. Furthermore, you will learn how the inner lips help to direct your urine flow and that urine does not hurt mirrors. Wash up and get back in position for the rest of your self-exam.

Hymen

As you continue in a downward direction from the urethral meatus, you will come to the opening of the vagina. At the entrance, you will find the hymen, or maidenhead, as it is sometimes called. It is here that you may have some difficulty making a correspondence between your anatomy and the drawings. This is true for two reasons. First of all, as indicated by Illustration 3, the appearance of the hymen varies considerably from individual to individual. Moreover, most of us have been taught to think of the hymen as some sort of disposable plastic seal that is broken the first time we have intercourse (or by some accident) and somehow disappears or dissolves afterward. This is a complete misconception.

In some women the hymen is a semicircular strip of mucus membrane that fringes the lower edge of the vaginal opening. In some women it encircles the entire rim of the vaginal opening. In still others it may be a semicircular membrane covering the lower half or three-fourths of the vaginal opening. It may have one large or several small openings. The variations are endless. In some rare cases it may entirely block the vaginal opening and it may then become necessary for a doctor to open it to allow for the passage of menstrual flow.

At any rate, the hymen does not break the first time we have intercourse. Rather, it stretches and may tear as it does so, causing some bleeding. And it does not disappear. Irregular fringes or folds of mucous membrane remain and can be seen surrounding the vaginal opening. Some women mistake these irregular bits of membrane for growths of some sort, but they are merely hymenal tissue and are known in medical circles as hymenal caruncles.

Many myths or wives' tales surround these small bits of tissue. One widespread myth is that a broken or stretched hymen indicates that a woman is no longer a virgin, that is, that she has had sexual intercourse. It is just that—a myth. The hymen may be broken or stretched by exercise, masturbation, a tampon or any number of accidents that can occur in a

Illustration 3 *Hymen Variations*

Cervix

The cervix is shaped like a rounded cabinet knob and is one to two inches in diameter. It feels fairly firm, like the tip of your nose, or, if you have had children, it may feel as firm as your chin. The firmness/softness of the cervix varies according to what phase of the menstrual cycle you are in. If you have difficulty locating the cervix, bear down as if you were making a bowel movement or bring your knees closer to your chest. Push the cervix around a bit with your fingers and you will see that it is not a rigid, immovable organ but one with quite a bit of give. In fact, your cervix changes position frequently during different stages of your menstrual cycle and also moves farther back during sexual excitement. So your cervix may not be in the same position each time you examine yourself; however, it is undoubtedly there (unless, of course, it has been surgically removed).

You may be able to feel a small depression or hole or an indented ridge in the center of your cervix. This is the opening to the cervical canal, which leads into the uterus, and is known in medical jargon as the cervical os. In women who have not had children it may be rounded or oval in shape and about the size of the head of a kitchen match. If you have had children, it may be slightly larger. As we said before, tampons and other objects cannot pass through this opening into the uterus. Sperm, however, can pass through the cervical os, and it is through this opening also that the menstrual blood passes.

Speculum Exam

Now you are ready to take a look at the inside of your vaginal cavity with the aid of your speculum. You may find the examination much more comfortable if you urinate first and, of course, wash your hands afterward. Assume the same position, with your back propped up by pillows and your knees drawn up and separated.

Next, position your mirror so that you have a clear view of your vaginal opening. Direct your light toward the mirror, not toward your vaginal opening. The light will reflect off the mirror into your vagina so you will have a clear, well-lighted view of the inside of your vagina.

Now you can insert your speculum. The speculum should be inserted with the duckbill sideways, that is, with the blades of the duckbill perpendicular to the floor, as shown in Illustration 5. Then, once the blades are inserted to the hilt, turn the blades up so that they are parallel to the floor and open the speculum. Some women find it easier to insert the speculum in the upright position with the blades parallel to the floor. Do whichever is most comfortable for you.

If it feels more comfortable to you, lubricate the blades of your

Illustration 5 *Speculum Self-Exam*

speculum with a lubricator like K-Y jelly or Lubrifax, both of which are available at a pharmacy without a doctor's prescription. Do not use too much lubricating jelly or you may not be able to distinguish between it and your vaginal secretions. You can also lubricate your speculum with water. Many women do not need any lubrication at all. Some prefer to soak the speculum in tepid water for a few minutes before insertion to bring it to body temperature, which makes it feel more comfortable for them.

Once you have inserted the speculum all the way, so that the blades are up against the pubic bone, and, if you have inserted the speculum sideways, have turned the blades upright, you will open the speculum by clasping the handles together. Then, with your thumb pushing down on the speculum, lock your speculum in the open position. The speculum locks open in three progressively wider positions. You will hear three clicking noises to correspond to these three positions. Your view will be much better if you open the speculum to its widest position.

Inserting the speculum is apt to be a rather awkward process the first time, indeed the first several times you do it. (Remember the first time you used a tampon!)

Simple mechanics has a lot to do with this awkwardness. Unfortunately, no one has yet devised a speculum to be used by a woman to inspect her own body. The speculum you are using was designed for one person to insert into another's body. Thus. from a mechanical-design point of view, you'll be doing things a bit backward when you use a speculum on yourself. If you find yourself having difficulties, take a closer look at how the speculum works, then practice opening and closing it some more. Remember, it's the speculum that's at fault, not you.

In addition to the mechanical problems encountered because you are using the speculum a bit differently from the way it was designed to be used, you may feel a bit nervous about exploring your own anatomy, which can make speculum exam more difficult. For most of us, this area of our bodies is unfamiliar, even forbidden, territory. We have been conditioned since early childhood to feel uncomfortable about touching our genitals. Although it is socially acceptable for doctors (generally males) or our husbands/lovers to insert something into our vaginas, we ourselves are not given that kind of societal permission. Thus, most of us have only a vague, black-hole sort of image of this area of our bodies.

If you are having difficulties, try to relax, which, of course, is much easier said than done. Remember, however, that if you are not successful the first time, you can always try again. If you are tense, you may feel pain. Pain could also be caused by using too large a speculum, and you might want to try a smaller one. If you are feeling tense and uncomfortable and therefore experiencing pain or discomfort, you need not continue. Put your speculum away and spend some time learning about and exploring your external anatomy. Once you feel comfortable with this, you can try speculum exam again.

If you experience difficulties with speculum exam, finding a sympathetic doctor or a women's self-help group is a good idea. If you aren't successful at first, don't despair. In our experience, we have never found a woman who was unable to learn how to do speculum exam. Even if you don't have difficulties, finding a self-help group or sharing the experience with a group of friends can be a valuable experience.

Finding Your Cervix

Once your speculum is inserted and opened all the way, you can look for your cervix, which appears as a raised, knoblike projection at the end of your vagina. The cervical os is a good landmark to look for. It may appear as a round dent or hole or it may look more like a slit, a smaller version of the slit your lips make if you press them together. It is especially apt to look this way in women who have had children. Illustration 6 shows some of the different ways the cervical os may look. If you use an IUD as your method of birth control, you should be able to see the string of the IUD coming out of the cervical os or opening.

Some women may have difficulty finding and recognizing the cervix. Medical textbooks invariably illustrate the cervix seen through a speculum as if it were on a straight bull's-eye visual path. However, many times this is not the case. The cervix, as we have seen, is a movable organ that is not always in the same place. At various points in your menstrual cycle, it may be higher or lower in the vaginal cavity. Moreover, in some women the cervix may characteristically lie a bit to the left or right. If you do not immediately see your cervix, try moving the speculum to the left or right or position it at a higher or lower angle. Changing the position of your body by bringing your knees closer to your chest or bearing down as if you were making a bowel movement may help to bring the cervix into view. Massaging your lower abdomen may also help. If none of this helps, remove the speculum and use your fingers to locate the cervix. Then reinsert the speculum, angling it in that direction.

If you still haven't found your cervix, using a larger speculum may help. Also check to make sure you actually have the speculum open to its widest position. Women who have particularly long vaginas may want to try examining themselves just before or just after their menstrual period, for the cervix is generally at the lowest position in the vaginal cavity at this time. Examining yourself during your period on the lightest day of flow, which for some women may be the first day and for others the last day, can also help because it will be easy to see the blood coming out of the cervical

A   B

C   D

Illustration 6   *The Cervix: In a woman who has never borne children (A); in a woman who has borne children (B); in women whose cervixes were torn during childbirth (C and D).*

os. On heavier days, there may be too much blood to see clearly, but on the lighter days it is quite easy to see the cervical os.

Women who are heavy may also have fleshy vaginas. Even some women who are quite thin may have fleshy vaginal cavities. Although the speculum will separate the vaginal walls, pads of fat may still bulge around the blades of the speculum, making it hard to see the cervix. Inserting the speculum sideways and using the large-size speculum, which has wider blades, may help. Here again, finding a doctor or a women's self-help group can be helpful.

Once you have located your cervix, make note of the appearance of your cervix and vaginal walls. What color are the tissues of your vaginal walls? In most women the tissue will be a pink color. If you are pregnant, the cervix might have a faint bluish tinge or might even be a bright blue color. In older women, the tissue is apt to be a paler shade of pink. Also take note of the position of your cervix. Is it to the left or to the right? Is it higher or lower in your vagina? The os itself may be more or less open at different points in your menstrual cycle. You may notice that when you are sexually excited, the cervix may be higher in the cervical canal than when you are not aroused.

You will also see some discharge coming from the cervical os. This is quite natural. The os is the opening to the cervical canal. This canal, which is called the endocervical canal, is about one inch long and leads into the uterus. It is lined with tiny mucus-secreting glands whose secretions change character over the course of your menstrual cycle.

The Uterus, Ovaries and Fallopian Tubes

The uterus (Illustration 7), which is about the size and shape of an inverted pear, is a hollow organ lined with a special type of tissue called endometrial tissue that thickens and is shed each month during your menstrual period.

Extending from the upper portion of the uterus on either side are two four- to five-inch-long tubes with tiny fingerlike projections on the end. These are the Fallopian tubes. Near the ends of each of these tubes on either side of the uterus lie two small organs about the size and shape of a Brazil nut. These are the ovaries. They produce substances called hormones that stimulate the uterine lining to grow thicker. They also produce a ripe egg approximately once a month during a woman's reproductive years. Contrary to what many people believe, the ovary is not actually attached to the Fallopian tube, but is suspended by its own bands of supporting tissues called ligaments. The ovary releases a ripe egg every 28 to 32 days. The projections at the end of the Fallopian tubes reach out like fingers to grasp the egg and pull it into the tube. If a man's sperm meets and fertilizes the egg in the Fallopian tube, the egg may then travel to the uterus and implant itself in the rich endometrial lining there. If this happens, you are pregnant, and the uterine lining will not shed since it is needed to nourish the developing egg, which is called the embryo. If, however, pregnancy does not occur, the lining breaks down and is shed. (These processes are discussed in greater detail in Chapter Four).

Even when you are not menstruating, the uterus is constantly sloughing off cells. These, along with the secretions from the mucus-producing glands of the endocervical canal, make up the cervical discharge you see. In addition, the walls of your vagina are constantly secreting fluids. These

OVARY

FALLOPIAN
TUBE

UTERUS

VAGINA

Illustration 7   *The Uterus, Fallopian Tubes and Ovaries* vaginal secretions and the cervical discharges make up the discharge you may see during your speculum exam and which you may notice on the blade of your speculum after you remove it.

The character of these vaginal and cervical discharges will vary from woman to woman and in each individual woman over the course of her menstrual cycle as well as over the course of her lifetime. The discharge also changes as you become sexually excited. Examining yourself at different points in your menstrual cycle, at different times of the day and at different stages of sexual arousal will help you learn how your particular body works.

The discharge may be clear to milky white in color and thin and watery to thick and creamy in consistency. It will taste, smell and feel different at various points in your menstrual cycle. As you examine yourself, note the details of the appearance of your secretions. Are the vaginal walls wet or dry? How much discharge do you have? What color is it? What consistency? How does it smell, taste, feel? Is it slippery or sticky?

In Chapter Four, we will show you how to chart your menstrual cycle and keep a record of the various changes that occur in your body each month or so. By doing this, you will learn to recognize what is normal for you. You will be able to spot abnormalities or disease, perhaps before they become full-blown illnesses requiring expensive medical treatment. You can also learn how to identify those days of your menstrual cycle on which you are most likely to get pregnant, which may be an important factor in helping you choose a method of birth control.

Other Things You May Notice

Some women may notice small fluid-filled cysts on their cervix. These are called Nabothian cysts and are nothing to worry about. Some women may see a reddish circle around the os or red patches on their cervix. In all probability, these are simple cervical erosions or eversions. These are discussed in greater detail elsewhere in this book. They are usually nothing to be concerned about. Indeed, about 20 percent of all women are born with cervical eversions. Occasionally, however, red spots on the cervix will be the result of something more serious. Don't hesitate to discuss these or any other things you notice with your doctor.

Chapter Six provides information on gynecological conditions, and the appendix contains a list of various signs and symptoms that a woman practicing self-exam may notice. If, after you have consulted these sections and read Chapter Four, which details the type of changes you can normally expect to see over the course of the menstrual cycle, you are still concerned about something you have noticed during your speculum exam, feel free to discuss it with your doctor.

You should also feel your vaginal walls and cervix for any lumps, bumps or rough, sandy areas. If, after you have learned what is normal for your body, you are concerned about a possible abnormality, again, don't hesitate to consult your doctor. In all probability, s/he will tell you that everything is OK, but this is part of the process of learning about your own body.

Sometimes we feel hesitant about discussing a "nonsymptom" or something that is only a vague feeling or apprehension with our doctors. We may fear that the doctor will think we are silly, overly worried or perhaps a bit crazy. But there is absolutely nothing wrong with saying to your doctor, "I've learned how to use a speculum and I've noticed (this, that or another thing) and I'm wondering why, or what, or if. . ." If your doctor isn't willing to discuss this with you and fully answer your questions or dismisses you with a pat on the head, assuming a "Don't worry your pretty little head about it, dearie" attitude, find yourself another doctor.

Removing the Speculum

After you've completed your speculum exam, remove the speculum from your vagina. Some women prefer to close the duckbill before removing the speculum by pulling up on the outer rim of the speculum handle. Other women find that it is easier to simply remove the speculum with the duckbill in the open position. After removal, clean the speculum with your antiseptic soap or alcohol, let it dry and store it in a plastic bag in a safe place. Before calling it a day, however, you should also examine your breasts. Breast anatomy and breast self-examination are discussed in the next chapter.

3

Breast Self-Exam, or
How to Save Your Own Life

Breast self-exam (BSE) can save your life and maybe your breast as well. Women who discover breast cancer through BSE have higher survival rates than those whose tumors are detected by the doctor or found only by chance. This is a reflection of the fact that BSE-detected tumors are more likely to be found when the disease is in its earlier, more curable stages. Studies have indicated that deaths from breast cancer might be reduced by as much as 18 percent if women practice BSE regularly.[1] Self-exam is, quite literally, a way to save your own life; yet despite the undisputed value of early detection, relatively few of us routinely practice BSE.

Why don't we? The answer to that question, like the answer to so many questions in the field of women's health care, is complicated. First of all, there's the old It-can't-happen-to-me syndrome. We all prefer to think of breast cancer or, for that matter, any serious problem as something that only happens to other people. But the fact is that one out of every 14 women in this country will develop breast cancer at some time in their lives, and three-fourths of these women will die from the disease.[2] The fantasy that breast cancer is something that only happens to other people is just that—a fantasy—at least for the 7 percent of us who actually develop the disease.

To put the whole thing in a less abstract, more personal and concrete way, make a list of women that includes you and the thirteen women with whom you have the closest personal contact. Your list might include female relatives, Mom, sisters, daughters, close friends, neighbors, business associates, whoever.... OK, now think about the fact that,

40

statistically speaking, one of the women on your list is going to get breast cancer and odds are three to one that she'll die from it. You may have to mourn the loss of a dearly beloved friend or relative or at least regret the passing of a close acquaintance. Actually, you may not have to worry about the funeral arrangements at all; those you leave behind may have to take care of all that. Also consider that your friend/relative/acquaintance/self could significantly reduce the chances of having to attend the funeral if she simply got into the habit of spending a few minutes a month checking her breasts.

If it sounds like we're trying to push your panic buttons, that's because we are. But we can't step out of the pages of this book and do a personal presentation of our Breast-Self-Exam-Can-Save-Your-Life routine. And besides, scare tactics, more than just being a cheap shot, are notoriously ineffective. Perhaps we should try a different approach. How about considering the fact that breast self-exam, in contrast to gynecological self-exam, is a socially acceptable habit. Indeed, it is actively encouraged. Planned Parenthood, the American Cancer Society and other such organizations distribute vast quantities of pamphlets urging women to practice monthly breast exam and explaining how to do so. Part of the reason for this active support of BSE lies in the fact that it has proven to be effective in the early detection of breast cancer.

But, more than that, breasts themselves and the idea of touching them are infinitely more acceptable than vulvas, vaginas and cervixes and the idea of touching them, especially when it's the woman herself who's doing the touching. Unlike our vaginas, vulvas and cervixes, or, to borrow granny's phrase, our private parts, breasts are, to put it mildly, quite public. Close-ups of bulging breasts are plastered across billboards, movie marquees and magazine layouts. We are a breast-obsessed culture. From the time we are prepubescent we are inundated with the message that our breasts are an incredibly important part of our anatomy. Most of us got the message, early on, standing in junior high gym class, elbows bent and arms winging out at shoulder level, pumping furiously as we chanted:

We must! We must!
We must increase our bust!
We may! We may!
We may get big some day!
It's better! It's better!
It's better for the sweater!

Despite—or perhaps because of—the fact that the breast is such a public part of our anatomy, many women fail to practice BSE. Oftentimes we're afraid of what we'll find. If we find a lump, it could be cancerous and if it's cancerous, that could mean losing a breast. In our culture the breast is so tied up with our notions of sexuality, of femininity and of our very worth as female people that the thought of losing one immobilizes many of us. Of course, the thought of losing any part of our bodies is a scary notion, especially if we lose it to the big C, cancer. But, if one out of every 14 of the women in this country contracted cancer of the thumb and if three-fourths of those who did died from the disease, you can bet that a lot more women would practice monthly thumb self-exam than currently practice BSE.

It is important, then, for women to realize that 80 percent of the breast lumps that are biopsied are not cancerous. Moreover, having breast cancer does not necessarily mean that a woman will lose her breast. Today there are less disfiguring forms of therapy that leave the breast largely intact. Although these methods have not yet been proven to be as effective as the older methods, which involve removing the entire breast, there has been enough convincing preliminary data to suggest this possibility, and large-scale studies to determine the effectiveness of these less disfiguring treatments are now underway. Then, too, great strides have been made in breast reconstruction, so that it is now possible in many cases to create a new breast using plastic surgery techniques. Having breast cancer no longer means that a woman's anatomy will be forever disfigured.

However, in order to be a candidate for these less radical therapies, a woman's cancer must be discovered in the early stages of the disease. Common sense will tell you that a woman who practices monthly BSE is 11 times more familiar with her breasts than a doctor who examines them only once a year. More than 90 percent of breast lumps are first discovered by the woman herself, either in the course of routine BSE or by chance, which is why self-exam is so important. The woman who examines her breasts each month has a better chance of discovering the tumor in its early stages. This means that not only is she more likely to save her life but that she may also be able to save her breasts.

Some of us are reluctant to examine our breasts because we are not happy with the way they look. If our breasts do not conform to the bulging, air-brushed, blemishless breasts that adorn the pages of *Playboy*, we may feel that they are inadequate. Careful examination of our breasts may only serve to remind us of our feelings of inadequacy; hence, we may simply choose to ignore them. But it's important to overcome these feelings. Try to let go of the cultural images of what your breasts should or should not look like and enjoy the uniqueness of your own anatomy. Doing this can be a valuable exercise for your mental and emotional—as well as your medical—health.

Breast self-exam is, then, incredibly important. None of us can afford to let fantasies of invulnerability, fears of losing a breast or feelings of inadequacy deter us from developing this life-saving habit.

Breast Anatomy and Function

Knowing a bit about the anatomy and function of the breast will help you in learning to do breast self-exam. In the center of each breast is the nipple, which is surrounded by a pigmented circular area that is known as the areola (see Illustration 8). The color of the nipple and areola varies from individual to individual, ranging from a light pink to a deep brown or almost black color. Generally the color deepens after a woman has had a child. The base of the nipple is ringed with tiny oil-producing glands that help keep the nipple supple. Some women have hairs around the areola.

The nipple is made up of erectile tissue. In some women the nipple is constantly erect; in others the nipple only becomes erect when stimulated by cold, physical contact or sexual activity. The nipple is almost always erect during a woman's orgasm. Most women's nipples protrude beyond the areola, but some women have inverted nipples. This, in and of itself, is not a problem, but if a formerly protruding nipple becomes inverted, this may indicate some underlying disease and should be brought to a doctor's attention.

The interior of the breast is divided into several sections called lobes. These lobes are further subdivided into lobules, each of which contains milk-secreting glands cushioned by fat and fibrous connective tissue. An intricate pipeline system of numerous tiny ducts arranged like the branches of a tree carry the milk produced by the glands to the ampulla, a collecting chamber immediately below the nipple. The entire breast is richly supplied with blood vessels.

The connective fibrous tissue attaches the breast to the muscles of the chest wall, which are known as the pectoral muscles. The breast itself contains no muscle tissue. Those breast exercises you learned in junior high gym class were designed to develop the pectoral muscles so they would become thick and bulging, creating the impression that the breast was larger. But no amount of exercise will make the breast itself larger.

The pectorals extend up into the armpit area, which in medical circles is referred to as the axillary area. The axillary area also contains lymph nodes. Lymph is a transparent bodily fluid that is found in tissue spaces throughout the body. Like blood, lymph is circulated through the body in tiny vessels. These lymph passageways are punctuated by accumulations of lymphatic tissue called lymph nodes. Lymph nodes relating to the breast are found in the axilla (the armpit), in the hollow above the collarbone, along the blood vessels beneath the breast bone and at the neck of the ribs. Lymph is part of our body's immunological, disease-fighting system. The lymph nodes act as sieves filtering bacteria, cast-off cells and other substances from the lymph fluid.

The breast also contains sensory nerves that are exceptionally sensitive.

FAT AND CONNECTIVE TISSUE

LOBULE { MILK GLAND
DUCT

AREOLA

NIPPLE

PECTORAL MUSCLE

RIBS

Illustration 8   *The Anatomy of the Breast*

They account for the sexual sensitivity of some women's breasts. An infant's sucking also stimulates the nerves and triggers the production of breast milk. In fact, the sensory nerves in the breast are so sensitive that the sound of an infant crying in the next room is sometimes enough to trigger a woman's "let-down" reflex and cause a flow of milk.

The production of breast milk is actually quite a complicated process. Tens of thousands of tiny cells inside the milk glands absorb basic substances—like water, salts, sugar, fats and small nitrogen-containing molecules—from the blood stream and use them to synthesize milk. Although actual breast milk is not produced until the infant begins sucking, preparation for the possibility of pregnancy occurs each month. In response to the monthly ebb and flow of hormones, the breast begins to gear up for milk production.

During the first half of the menstrual cycle the hormone estrogen is produced by the ovaries in increasing quantities. The estrogen stimulates the growth of new cells in the glands, ducts and fibrous tissues of the breast. This increase in cell activity is accompanied by an increase in blood flow to the breast, which may be experienced as a fullness, warmth and, sometimes, tenderness. At about the middle of the monthly cycle, a ripe egg is released from the ovary, and as a result the second ovarian hormone, progesterone, is released into the blood stream. The progesterone starts the secreting process in the gland cells. Even this small amount of stimulation can be felt by some women. Part of the swelling and feeling of fullness is due to an increase in the blood supply, but part of it is due to a greater amount of fluid seeping into the tissues from the ducts.

If pregnancy does not occur, the hormone levels shift again. The changes which the hormones stimulated in the breast are reversed. New cell growth is slowed, and the blood supply to the area is diminished. Secretions and cells are reabsorbed by the body to make room for the new cells and secretions that will be produced during the next menstrual cycle. The swelling of the breast tissues diminishes and the breast softens. If pregnancy does occur, the build-up of the duct, gland and fibrous tissue continues. After delivery another hormone, prolactin, which is produced by the pituitary gland at the base of the brain, is released and this triggers the actual production of breast milk. As a baby sucks, more prolactin and, hence, more milk is released. As the baby is weaned, the prolactin levels fall and the production of breast milk tapers off.

Breast Self-Exam

Most doctors recommend that women start to practice BSE after they have had their first menstrual period and continue the habit throughout their lives. Because breast cancer is extremely rare in women under the age of 25, some doctors recommend that women not start BSE until the age of 25. These doctors feel that if a girl starts BSE at the age of 13 and practices for so many years without ever finding abnormalities, she will develop a false sense of security and will drop the habit in later years, when it is most important. Personally, we feel that BSE should be started at the time of the first menstrual cycle. While it is true that breast cancer is rare in women under the age of 25, it does happen. Moreover, there are benign breast conditions that occur in younger women which, although generally not serious in and of themselves, may increase the chances of developing breast cancer later in life. Knowing that she may be at increased risk for breast cancer could influence a woman's decisions about methods of birth control. For example, a woman at increased risk might opt to select a method of birth control other than the Pill.* In addition, a young girl having her first period is often living with, or in close contact with, her mother; if their menstrual cycles are close together, they can practice BSE together, which can be a valuable and special experience for a mother and daughter to share. But regardless of the age at which BSE is begun, it should be continued on a monthly basis for the rest of the woman's life.

Many women become discouraged about their ability to practice self-exam. As we have seen, the breast is an extremely glandular organ. The glands may feel like lumps. At first, it is difficult to know what is normal lumpiness and what is abnormal. This is especially difficult for women whose breast tissues are particularly responsive to hormone stimulation since they are apt to have a periodic increase in the lumpiness and swelling of the breast. Many women have a condition known as fibrocystic disease, which is an exaggeration of the normal, hormone-induced changes in the breast. In its milder forms fibrocystic disease may only produce periodic lumpiness, swelling and breast tenderness. In some cases, one or more distinct lumps, sometimes fairly large ones, may be felt as soft, tender, movable lumps in the breast tissue. These lumps may wax and wane with the cyclical ebb and flow of hormones. At other times, these lumps may last throughout the menstrual cycle. These persistent lumps require a doctor's attention. Generally they are simple fibrocystic cysts, collections of secretions and old cells that were not successfully reabsorbed by the body. The doctor may apply a local anesthetic to the breast, attempt to aspirate the contents of the cyst with a needle and examine the aspirated fluid microscopically to rule out the possibility of cancer. The aspiration usually will cause the cyst to collapse; however, these cysts sometimes reoccur. Women with fibrocystic disease or periodic lumpiness in their breasts should make a chart like the one pictured in Illustration 9 to help familiarize themselves with the lumpy areas of their breast. Any large, definite lumps in the breasts of a woman with a history of fibrocystic disease should be examined by a doctor.

Women with periodic lumpiness in their breasts, in fact all women in their menstruating years, should do BSE at the beginning of their menstrual cycles, that is, right after the menstrual flow stops, for that is when the levels of hormones are lowest and the lumpiness is least noticeable. Younger women who have only recently begun to menstruate often have very irregular menstrual cycles. They may go for months at a time without having a period. If this is the case, it's a good idea to pick a certain day, perhaps the first of the month, and do BSE on that day. Women who are no longer menstruating should also set aside a certain day. The first of the month, payday or any significant day will do.

___

*The debate over the relationship between the birth control pill and breast cancer is discussed in more detail in the section on the Pill.

Illustration 9   *Women with fibrocystic disease may want to make a chart like this, with X's marking the areas where there is periodic lumpiness.*

All women, especially those with periodic lumpiness or fibrocystic disease, should enlist their doctors' help in learning to do BSE. This may require more than one doctor's visit. After the doctor examines your breasts, repeat the exam yourself. If you find an area that you're not sure about, have the doctor feel it. Explain that you're not sure whether what you feel is normal or abnormal and ask the doctor to feel the questionable area. It's not always easy to feel comfortable about doing this. We are apt to feel that we are taking up the doctor's valuable time with silly, vague, half-formed questions, but BSE is an important, even life-saving process, a preventive measure well worth the time and effort of any conscientious doctor. Besides, the doctor is being paid—and being paid quite handsomely—for his or her time. If your doctor is impatient with your questioning or is otherwise not supportive of your attempts to learn BSE, consider findng yourself another doctor. In fact, if your doctor is a really good one, you won't have to ask for help with BSE. Either the doctor or one of the doctor's staff, perhaps a nurse, should ask you if you practice self-exam and should encourage you to do so, offering help and advice. Studies have shown that one of the most effective means of getting women to practice BSE is to have their doctors actively encourage them to do so.

Part One: Inspection

BSE should be done at a time when you are relaxed and not rushed or distracted. The examination consists of two parts: inspection and palpation, or feeling. To begin the inspection portion, stand in front of a well-lighted mirror and let your arms hang at your sides, as shown in Illustration 10. Note the size and shape of your breasts. No one's breasts are identical to each other, but being familiar with the appearance of each of your breasts will help you spot any changes in subsequent months. Pay attention to the contour of the breast, looking for depressions or bulges. Moles or any dimpled, dark or reddened areas, swellings, sores or areas of the skin with a rough or orange-peellike texture should be noted. Some women have prominent blue veins in their breasts. Changes in the appearance of the veins are important. The nipples and areola should also be observed for color changes, scaling, dimpling or retraction. Also note the direction in which the nipples point.

Next, place your hands on your hips and press inward and down so that the pectorals, the muscles of the upper chest, are contracted. Check to see if the chest muscles contract about the same amount or if any bulging or dimpling appears in this position. While your hands are still on your hips, turn to each side and check again for any dimpling or bulges.

Now put your hands in front of your chest at about heart level, press your palms together and check for muscle contraction, bulges, dimpling or unevenness. Rotate to each side, checking for the same signs. If your breasts are large or hang down, you may have to cup each one to check the undersides of the breast.

Next, raise your arms, flex your elbows and place your hands behind your head. Once again check for dimplings and bulges, rotating to each side and making the same type of check.

This all sounds like a rather elaborate set of gymnastics, but once you have the routine down it's really quite simple. To complete the first part of your exam gently squeeze each nipple, looking for signs of discharge. It is not uncommon to have some discharge after childbirth, abortion or miscarriage. A few women have a small amount of discharge at certain points in their menstrual cycle. Many of us may notice dry, crusted secretions in the cracks of the nipple. This is normal. Some women on birth control pills have a bit of nipple discharge. Discharge is not always a sign of disease, *but any nipple discharge should be brought to a doctor's attention*. In fact, all of the signs and symptoms mentioned here deserve a doctor's attention, because any change in the appearance or functioning of the breast is significant.

Part Two: Palpation

This part of the exam is done while you are lying down, as shown in Illustration 11. In this position the breast tissue will spread out against the rib cage and it will be easier to feel the deeper tissue. Women with large breasts may find that placing a folded towel under the shoulder of the side being examined helps distribute the breast tissue and makes palpation

Illustration 10   *Part One—Inspection: Stand in front of a mirror and inspect your breasts in each of the four positions shown here. Finally squeeze each nipple, looking for signs of discharge.*

Illustration 11 *Part Two—Palpation: Lie down with one hand behind your head. With your other hand, start on the outside of the breast and, using a circular motion, palpate the entire breast. Repeat on the opposite breast.*

easier and more comfortable. Lotion or oil applied to the fingertips cuts down on skin friction and heightens the sense of touch. Some women do this part of the exam floating on their backs in the bathtub. The soap and water acts as a lubricating oil.

To begin, bend one arm and place your hand behind your head. This will stretch the chest muscles so that you have a firmer surface to press down on. Use the fatty pads of your fingers rather than the fingertips and, starting on the outside of the breast, using a circular motion, carefully feel the entire breast with the opposite hand. Press down to the chest wall. Women with large breasts may have to hold the breast in place with their other hand, especially when examining the lower part of the breast, which typically has more fat tissue. Also feel the upper part of the chest wall and the armpit area. Repeat the process on the other side. Women who have had a breast removed should palpate the chest, paying particular attention to the scar area. What you are looking for is any lump or thickening in the breast or enlarged lymph nodes, which may feel like hard, rounded, firm bumps. This sounds quite simple, but it's not always easy to learn to recognize lumps. First of all, the whole process is somewhat akin to feeling for a marble in a plastic bag full of Jell-O. This is why you may have to use two hands, especially on the fatty part of the breast, or else that elusive marble will constantly slide away from the pressure of your fingertips. Secondly, most women's breasts are not smooth but instead are rather bumpy. This is especially true of small breasts, which tend to be more glandular than larger ones. The upper outer portion of the breast is usually the most lumpy area. In addition to the glands, ribs, breastbone and underlying muscles can also be mistaken for lumps. Don't hesitate to report any lump, thickening or grainy areas to a doctor. You may think that you feel something, but the sensation is sometimes rather vague. Nonetheless, don't ignore it—see a doctor. It's probably nothing, but investigating your sensations is part of the process of learning self-exam. If it's of any comfort, one of the women who wrote this book (the writer, not the doctor) discovered a suspicious lump and trotted off to the doctor, only to find out that she had discovered her rib. Ah, well, better silly than sorry.

There is nothing to be gained, and everything to be lost, by waiting to see if the lump will go away. Any symptom, sign, change in the appearance or feel of the breasts or persistent ache or pain deserves attention.

If, after your first few exams, you feel uncertain about your ability to distinguish what's normal from what's abnormal, don't give up. You'll feel more confident when you've done fifty exams than when you've done only five. Reading the information on breast diseases in the reference section of this book may be helpful. Find a good doctor and get him or her to assist you. Forge ahead—you *will* get good at BSE, and it just may save your life.

The Monthly Miracle: Menstruation

Each month, deep inside our bodies, the ovary begins, ever so slowly, to turn. A tiny bubble on its surface contains the one egg that has, for some mysterious reason, been chosen out of a field of some 250,000 to ripen that month. The funnellike opening at the end of the Fallopian tube, lined with thousands of undulating cilia, moves toward the ovary, which turns to meet it.

Suddenly, the bubble bursts. Triggered by a spurt of lutenizing hormone, an eloquent chemical messenger from the brain, the ovary contracts sharply and the ripe egg bursts forth. The fringed projections at the end of the Fallopian tube reach out like fingers to grasp the ripe ovum and draw it into the narrow tunnel of the tube. In a dreamlike, slow motion ballet, the tiny cilia caress the ripened egg and gently move it along on its four-inch, four-day journey to the womb.

Through a precise two-way communication system, so complex that it makes the technology of beaming planet-wide transmissions off orbiting satellites look like child's play, the uterus is notified of the impending arrival of the egg and is prepared. The blood vessels in the area swell, flooding the uterus with a rich supply of blood to nourish the soft, spongy tissue of the uterine lining, which will cushion the egg when it arrives. The uterine glands pour forth a banquet of nutriments that will nourish the developing egg. The entire lining of the uterus has thickened to twice its normal depth—a luxuriously rich topsoil in which the egg, if fertilized during its journey through the tube, will implant.

For the first three days after its arrival, the tiny egg floats freely within the plush uterus. If fertilized, it will embed itself in the uterine lining by the seventh day. Meanwhile, on the surface of the ovary, the remnant of the burst bubble, the corpus luteum, which has turned a bright yellow in the wake of its explosive spasm, awaits a message from the uterus. While it waits, it transmits a continuous stream of chemical messages that direct and sustain the elaborate preparations of the uterus.

If, in the upper reaches of the dark, narrow Fallopian tube, no sperm cell meets and joins the egg, the egg will not implant in the uterine wall. The corpus luteum does not receive the message it awaits and ceases transmitting its chemical messages. Without the continued instruction of the corpus luteum, the swollen network of blood vessels shrinks, restricting the flow of blood. This deprives the newly grown tissues in the surrounding area of their support and nourishment. Over a period of days the whole structure is dismantled as small pieces of the lining fall away. Within hours of this dismantling, the now weakened blood vessels open, a few at a time. Each tiny vessel empties its droplets. More and more droplets are released and the flow of menstrual blood empties the uterus.

It takes approximately seven days to complete this journey—from the moment the egg bursts out of the ovary and begins to move through the darkness of the tube toward the possibility of the creation of life and the implantation of the fertilized egg in the lush garden of the uterus. It is a journey we all know. It is engraved upon our genetic memories and etched inside each tiny molecule of DNA in every cell in our bodies. It is a tale that our species tells over and over again in the ancient archetypal legends of heroic gods and goddesses who traveled from darkness into light and renewed life and in the primal myths of creation that form the basis of all our religions. It is the story of our personal and racial creation. It is, indeed, a holy story.

We are clearly creatures of incredible lushness, the very source of life. Yet we do not honor our lushness. There are no puberty rites for women. Hardly anywhere in anthropology or in the histories of the kaleidoscope of cultures this planet has spawned are there societies where mothers take their daughters out on moon-full nights to celebrate the ripening of the seeds we carry in our blood-lined wombs.

Instead, both individually and as a culture, we are rather embarrassed about menstruation. Even today, in an era when the most bizarre of sadomasochistic sexual practices are the subject of newspaper headlines, cocktail chitchat and television specials, the natural bodily process of menstruation remains an unmentionable subject. Indeed, when the topic finally did come up on a segment of the well-known TV show *All in the Family,* the network received more letters protesting public mention of "such a thing" than had been received as a result of the airing of any other segment of the controversial show. And this from a show that had broached such topics as premarital sex, racial prejudice, impotence and homosexuality!

This is nothing new. Throughout recorded history, in culture after culture, menstruation has been taboo. The menstruating woman has been regarded as something unholy and unclean. The taboo has taken myriad forms: One must not eat food cooked by a menstruating woman, touch objects she has touched, pronounce her name, look her in the eye, touch her, share sex with her.

Today we no longer believe that a menstruating woman's glance will wither a field of crops. We know her touch won't poison the water in the well and that having sex with her won't really make a man's penis fall off. We are no longer banished to menstrual huts as were our ancestral mothers in more primitive societies. But our release from monthly exile does not necessarily represent a more enlightened attitude toward menstruation.

As Nancy Friday suggests in her book *My Mother, My Self,* it is more likely that our release is due to the fact that as a result of centuries of conditioning we have so completely internalized the menstrual taboo that it is simply no longer necessary to bother with menstrual huts. Our modern tribe needn't go to such lengths to remove all disturbing reminders of menstruation from its collective consciousness. We do it ourselves with our meticulous, toilet-paper mummification of our bloodied rags as we carefully wrap up and dispose of our used sanitary napkins or tampons. We might drop a used Kleenex in the ashtray without a second thought, but a used Tampax? None of us would think of hiding our toothbrushes under the sink or in the back corners of our bathroom cupboards, yet it is rare to find a box of sanitary napkins prominently displayed next to the deodorants, toothpaste, hairsprays and such that line the bathroom shelves of most homes.

No, the menstrual taboo is not dead. Judging from the resounding silence that surrounds the topic, it is obvious that the menstrual taboo is alive and well. And because of this taboo, we are remarkably ignorant about even the most basic facts of menstruation. Most of us couldn't give a coherent explanation of the menstrual cycle to a fifth grader. Our embarrassment and the cultural taboo conspire to keep us ignorant and to make us think of menstruation in largely negative terms. Indeed, we are so embarrassed about menstruation that we can't even call it by its rightful name, relying instead on negative terms like "the curse" and "falling off the roof." One male writer of a review of a book about menstruation put the situation in a particularly telling perspective when he wrote:

If men menstruated, they would probably find a way to brag about it. Most likely, they would record it as a spontaneous ejaculation, an excess of vital spirits. Their cup runneth over. Their sexuality superogates. They would see themselves as "spending" blood in a plenitude of conspicuous waste. Blood, after all, is generally considered a good. "Blood" sports used to be a true test of manhood. And at the conclusion of a boy's first hunt, he used to be "blooded." All that is turned around when it is the woman who bleeds. Bleeding is interpreted as a sign of infirmity, inferiority, uncleanliness and irrationality.[1]

It is certainly true that we don't often hear women boasting about their periods. If our tissues swell up with retained water as our periods approach, we don't call it "ripening." Instead, we use a negative term like "bloating." While it is true that some women experience pain and discomfort at certain periods in their menstrual cycles, it is also true that many women experience extra energy, heightened sexual desire and a general feeling of well-being.

If women are to become informed consumers of medical practice, we must overcome these negative attitudes and cultural taboos about menstruation. No woman can hope to understand what is wrong with her and to evaluate the medical alternatives unless she understands how her body works. The information in the following pages is designed to provide a basic understanding of the workings of the female reproductive system.

Fetal Development

The logical place to begin is, of course, at the beginning—conception. The female egg, the ovum, and the male egg, the sperm, meet and join together, a process known as fertilization. Then, the fertilized egg, which is called an embryo at first and later a fetus, implants in the uterine wall and continues to grow and develop throughout pregnancy, nourished by the rich blood supply to the uterus.

All ova carry what are called X chromosomes. Sperms may have either an X or a Y chromosome. If a sperm carrying an X chromosome joins with the ovum, the outcome will be a baby girl. If the sperm carries a Y chromosome, the baby will be a boy.

The mass of fetal tissue grows larger and divides itself into sections from which specific organs will develop. As early as the fourth week after fertilization, there is evidence of a gonad, a specific sex organ, but it is not easy to tell at this point whether the fetus is male or female. By about the sixth or seventh week of fetal life, differentiation of the sex organs becomes apparent. By the fetal age of three months the differentiation of the external genital organs is complete.

By five months the ovary is recognizable in the female fetus, and by the fifth or sixth month the internal changes that produce the uterus, Fallopian tubes and vagina are completely effected. In males the gonad, called the testis, produces a hormone that further influences the development of the fetal tissue. The presence of this hormone stimulates the development of the male reproductive organs. The clitoris, under the influence of this hormone, grows larger and becomes a penis. In a sense, a male is a female that has been transformed by hormone stimulation into a male. Contrary to the biblical concept that women derived from Adam's rib, the female seems to be the basic type and the male a variation on that basic theme.

At birth, the female ovaries contain about two million primitive eggs. By the age of seven, about 300,000 remain. Unlike the testicle, which continually manufactures new sperm, the ovary contains at birth all the eggs it will ever have and does not manufacture new ones. However, these eggs lie dormant in a sort of state of hibernation throughout childhood until the time of puberty.

Puberty

Puberty is the phase of the life cycle during which a young woman's reproductive organs mature in size and function. Menarche is the name given to the time when a girl has her first menstrual period, which usually occurs between the ages of 10 and 16, with the average age being about 13. Actually, body weight is a much more accurate predictor of menarche than age. Most girls menstruate when they reach a body weight of from 92 to 101 pounds.

Menarche is just one of a series of changes that occur during puberty, changes that first began to take place a few years earlier. The first changes are invisible ones. No one knows exactly why or how they occur. Somehow the hypothalamus, the master switch in the brain that controls the body's production of hormones, gets switched on. It then sends substances called gonadotropin-releasing factors (GRF) to the pituitary gland, which is located at the base of the brain. In response to this hypothalamic stimulation, the pituitary begins to produce hormones called gonadotropins. The word *gonadotropin* means "acting on the gonads, or sex organs." There are two principal gonadotropins. One of them, called the follicle-stimulating hormone, or FSH, travels via the bloodstream to the ovary, where, as its name implies, it stimulates the follicles of the ovary, the sacs inside which the ova, or eggs, have been resting. Specialized cells in these follicular sacs begin to secrete the ovarian hormone estrogen, which helps the eggs to mature. As more and more follicles are stimulated, more estrogen is released into the bloodstream.

By the age of eight most girls are producing small amounts of estrogen in their bodies. Over the course of the next few years increasing levels of estrogen and other hormones will cause certain noticeable changes in the girl's body. The first of these is a growth spurt just prior to puberty. The average girl grows about two inches per year after the age of two. However, just before puberty this rate doubles. The proportions of the body also change. The head gets larger and the length of the trunk relative to the legs increases. The pelvic bone structure also changes during these years, and fat pads develop over the hips, giving the body a fuller, more mature shape.

The breast also goes through dramatic changes. First the nipple begins to stand out more. Then a small mound develops beneath the nipple and the areola, the ring of tissue around the nipple. The areola gets darker and continues to enlarge. The breast itself also continues to increase in size until finally, in the mature breast, the areola recedes into the general contour, leaving only the nipple protruding.

The entire vulva also enlarges and changes shape. The outer lips enlarge and tend to cover over the inner lips. The hymen, formerly a thin rim of tissue around the vaginal opening, gets thicker, and the entire vaginal opening looks larger. A fat pad develops under the mons veneris, or "little hill," of the vulva. The skin on the inside of the lips gets darker. The clitoris enlarges. Soft, long strands of hair, at first rather sparse and straight but later denser and curlier as well as darker in color, begin to grow on the lips and mons. Approximately two years after the first appearance of the pubic hair, hair also begins to grow in the underarm area.

The internal female organs also undergo changes. The vaginal cavity becomes deeper. The outer layer of tissue on the vaginal walls, formerly only a few cell layers deep, becomes thicker. Vaginal secretions may be noticed for the first time. The entire uterus, both the cervix, or neck, and the fundus, or body, grows larger. The major change is in the fundus. In the years prior to puberty, the cervix is rather elongated in comparison to the fundus, but during puberty the fundus enlarges until it accounts for three-fourths of the total size of the uterus. The lining of the uterus, called the endometrium, also begins to thicken.

The ovary enlarges in size, and the blood vessels in the area develop. As these vascular channels develop, the hormones from the pituitary begin to have more and more of an impact on the ovary. As more follicle-stimulating hormone from the pituitary reaches the ovary, increasing numbers of follicles produce more and more estrogen. At first, this stimulation is sporadic. The follicles start to grow, but then regress. Finally, though, the amounts of estrogen become more constant. The rising levels of estrogen in the bloodstream affect both the hypothalamus, the control center in the brain, and the pituitary. In the hypothalamus, the rising levels of estrogen trigger the release of another of the hypothalamic gonadotropin-releasing factors (GRF) called the luteinizing-hormone releasing factor (LHRF).* The LHRF travels to the pituitary, where it, along with the direct stimulation of estrogen on the pituitary, causes the pituitary to release a surge of another of its gonadotropins, this one known as lutenizing hormone, or LH.

The LH travels via the bloodstream to the ovary, where it causes one of the follicles to burst open and release its egg. The remnants of the burst follicle, which are referred to as the corpus luteum, then begin to secrete the hormone progesterone. The progesterone causes the lining of the uterus, which has already grown thicker as a result of the rising levels of estrogen, to grow even thicker and richer. If pregnancy does not occur, the corpus luteum dies and ceases producing progesterone. Without the continued support of the progesterone the uterine lining breaks down and is shed, and the girl has her first menstrual period.

If all this sounds a bit complex, that's because it is. And we've only covered the highlights. The interactions of hormones in the body are not fully understood. Even many practicing doctors don't have a good grasp of what is presently known. However, the system is a very logical one and once you get past the terminology and become familiar with the names of the various hormones and the organs they affect, the whole thing becomes a lot clearer.

Before we consider the workings of the menstrual cycle in the mature female, a word or two about menstrual periods in the early years following menarche and about menopause, the cessation of menstrual periods.

Menstrual periods tend to be rather irregular in the first few years. The interval between periods varies. For instance, the second menstrual period may not occur for six months or it might occur in three weeks. The amount of bleeding and the duration of bleeding vary too. It usually takes about 40 cycles, or three or four years, before the pattern is set. Some researchers believe that in the early years of menstruation the girl does not actually release an egg from the ovary, that is, that she doesn't ovulate. Others feel that she releases an egg but that no corpus luteum forms from the remnants of the follicular sac. In either case, the bleeding that occurs is not the result of diminishing levels of progesterone; rather, the lining of the uterus simply grows so thick from the constant estrogen stimulation that parts of it break off and are shed. However, in some cases the girl may actually be ovulating and may actually have a functioning corpus luteum, which means that she can get pregnant.

---

*Most current research indicates that there is one gonadotropin-releasing factor that releases both LH and FSH, but many scientists think there are actually two, one for each pituitary hormone, although only one has been isolated.

Menopause

"Menopause" is the term used to refer to the time in a woman's life when the monthly cycle gears down and she stops having menstrual periods. Actually, menopause is just one of the events of what is called the "climacteric," a broader term that encompasses menopause and all the other changes taking place at this time in a woman's life.

An incredible amount of nonsense, full of medical inaccuracies, has been written by both doctors and laypeople on the subject of menopause, so perhaps an explanation of the physiological events of this time of life is in order. During menopause the ovaries cease producing eggs (that is, they become anovulatory), so the levels of progesterone and estrogen drop. The pituitary, no longer held in check by the ovarian hormones, produces increasing amounts of FSH and LH in an effort to stimulate the ovary and trigger ovulation.

Typically, the ovary gears down slowly. Women may ovulate one month and have anovulatory cycles the next. Periods may be skipped for a month or two and then start up again. These irregular bleeding patterns are normal and are nothing to be concerned about. If, however, a woman's periods stop for more than a year and then start again or become heavier than normal, this may be an indication that something is wrong and she should consult a doctor.*

Eventually, the periods stop altogether. In the past, the average age for menopause in American women was 48, but nowadays it is not unusual to find women who are still menstruating in their mid-50's. Some doctors speculate that this may be due to improved nutrition. There is also some indication that women whose mothers have a late menopause also tend to have late menopauses. Whether this is a hereditary phenomenon or a reflection of the fact that mothers and daughters may tend to have similar patterns of nutrition or other environmental factors is not known.

In addition to the cessation of their menstrual periods, climacteric women may experience other changes, including hot flashes (short episodes of profuse sweating characterized by a feeling of intense heat), a thinning of the vaginal and urinary tissues, which makes them more susceptible to infections and other problems, and osteoporosis, a condition which involves a loss of bone density and may make a person more susceptible to bone fractures. These changes seem to be related to the changing hormone levels.

Although many women experience hot flashes, for most women the

---

*For a more detailed description of normal and abnormal menopausal bleeding patterns, see the section on menopause.

problems mentioned above do not present serious difficulties. In the past, women who did experience severe menopausal symptoms were labeled "neurotic" by the medical profession. Medical textbooks often described the typical menopausal patient with severe hot flashes as being a thin, high-strung, emotional and nervous personality type. Actually, it's not too surprising that women with severe hot flashes should appear to be psychologically distraught, for hot flashes often occur at night, causing insomnia. Any woman whose sleep is interrupted five or ten times a night might well appear to be high-strung, nervous or emotional. However, her psychological tensions are more likely the result, rather than the cause, of her hot flashes.

It is interesting to reflect on why the thumbnail sketches of the typical woman with menopausal symptoms invariably describe her as being thin. It may turn out that body weight has more to do with the severity of menopausal symptoms than any psychological factor.

Although we are not aware of any research either confirming or denying this theory, it may not be as farfetched as it sounds. Until recently, the fact that some women seem to pass through menopause with virtually unaltered levels of estrogen and continue to produce fairly high levels of it well into old age was a puzzle to medical researchers. Now, however, we know that certain substances can be converted into estrogen in the fatty tissues of the body, which may explain, at least in part, why some of these women—presumably the heavier ones—were able to maintain such high postmenopausal estrogen levels. Conversely, perhaps women who are thin and therefore have less of this fatty tissue in which to convert estrogen are more apt to suffer estrogen-related menopausal symptoms such as hot flashes than other, heavier women. Thus, rather than being psychiatric in nature, their problems may be related to the amount of fatty tissue in their bodies.

It may also be that, regardless of their body size, women who suffer severe menopausal problems simply don't produce as much of these other substances that are converted into estrogen in the fatty tissue. But at this point it is impossible to confirm or deny these possibilities, for there has been very little in the way of scientific studies of hot flashes. As Barbara Seaman points out in her excellent book *Women and the Crisis in Sex Hormones*, only five studies of hot flashes were recorded in the medical literature in the 70-year period from 1903 to 1973![2]

Despite the fact that so little research has been done on the postmenopausal woman, a wide variety of symptoms has been attributed to the declining levels of estrogen. Indeed, menopause was—and by some doctors still is—considered a deficiency disease. To "cure" this deficiency disease, many doctors prescribe estrogen replacement therapy, which is supposed to keep women from growing old, prevent wrinkling, boost the spirits, ward off depression and keep women slim and sexy, to mention just a few of the benefits claimed for it. Estrogen replacement therapy does none of these things, however. As it turns out, what it does do is increase a woman's chances of developing uterine cancer.[3] The pharmaceutical industry has played on women's fears about aging in our youth-worshipping culture and promoted the widespread use of a dangerous drug. Menopausal women who are considering the use of estrogens should read the sections on menopause and estrogen replacement therapy and consider alternative therapies before making a decision about using these drugs.

The Menstrual Cycle in the Mature Woman

Once a woman matures, the cycle becomes more regular but never totally regular. All women have some irregularity in their cycles. One month the cycle may be 28 days long, another month it may be 26 or 32 days long. Cycles as short as 20 or 21 days and as long as 35 or 36 are considered within the normal range. Some women even have cycles longer or shorter than these, and as long as the amount of bleeding is not excessive and the cycles are fairly regular, this is not usually cause for alarm, though any persistent irregularities should be discussed with your doctor.

The classical medical-textbook menstrual cycle is 28 days long. This does not mean that most women have 28-day cycles; indeed, probably fewer than 10 percent of the women in their peak reproductive years actually have regular 28-day cycles. This 28-day figure was arrived at by measuring the length of the menstrual cycle in a group of women and then dividing the total number of days by the number of women in the group. Thus, the majority of women may actually have 31-day or 27-day cycles; the group average can be thrown off by a relatively small number of women with exceptionally long or short cycles. So don't fret if you don't have the classic 28-day cycle; you're not alone.

There are many things that can cause a woman's cycle to become irregular. The hypothalamus, the brain center that acts as the master switch for the hormone system, is also part of the nervous system and is probably responsible for coordinating the two. Your nervous system collects information from the outside world through your five senses and from the rest of your body as well. The hypothalamus is sensitive to the stimuli collected by the nervous system. Physical and emotional stress can cause menstrual irregularities, probably though the mediation of the hypothalamus. This is undoubtedly a mechanism designed by Mother Nature to prevent us from becoming pregnant when there is already too much stress on our systems.

The intricate relationship between external stimuli picked up by our senses and the menstrual cycle is still largely a mystery. Interestingly enough, there is now some evidence that our sense of smell may play a role in the timing of our menstrual cycles. It has long been a common piece of womenlore that women who are close friends or who live together tend to menstruate at the same time. This was confirmed in a study done at Harvard University in which the menstrual patterns of women living in a college dormitory were carefully studied.[4] After ruling out other factors, such as common light/dark cycles (light also has an effect on menstrual cycles, at least in some animals) and stress patterns, the researchers speculated that the sense of smell might be a factor in the observed coincidence of menstrual cycles among close friends.

This is not as implausible as it sounds. Scientists have long known that odor particles control the mating and reproductive behaviors of insects. (A squirt of a fertile female moth's odor particles is enough to set all the male moths within a five-mile radius on the wing.)

The notion that smell stimuli play a role in regulating human menstrual cycles received further support from another study, done in California, in which a female volunteer was asked to wear a tampon on each day of her menstrual cycle.[5] Odor particles were then isolated from each of her tampons by an elaborate process known as gas chromotography. Next, the women involved in the study were divided into two groups, a control group and a test group. Each day all of the women were asked to rub a cotton pad under their nose. The women in the control group were given odorless pads, but those in the test group were given pads impregnated with the smell particles that had been obtained from the female volunteer. On Day 1 of the study the women in the control group were smelling the odors isolated from the first tampon the volunteer had worn. On the second day they smelled the odors isolated from the volunteer's second tampon, and so on. At the end of five months, a significant portion of the women in the test group, unlike those in the control group, were menstruating in synch with the female volunteer.

The timing of the menstrual cycle, then, is influenced by a number of factors, many of which we are hardly aware of or only dimly understand. We do know, however, that when variations in the menstrual cycle do occur, they are most apt to occur in the first part of the cycle. The menstrual cycle can be divided into four phases. The first phase is the bleeding phase, the time of the actual menstrual flow. The second phase is called the proliferative phase and is dominated by the hormone estrogen. This is followed by the ovulation phase, when the ripe egg is released from the ovary. It is in the first two stages, prior to ovulation, that variations in cycle length occur. Once ovulation has taken place, the fourth stage of the cycle, called the secretory phase, begins and usually lasts for 14 days, after which the menstrual flow starts and the cycle begins again.

The hormones that govern the menstrual cycle are in a constant state of fluctuation. Low levels of all these hormones are produced throughout the menstrual cycle, but these levels are constantly rising and falling, triggering or suppressing levels of the other hormones as they do so. As you can see from the chart shown in Illustration 12, the relationships between these hormones are rather complex. The exact ways in which these hormones interact is not yet fully understood, but let's take a broad look at how these hormones behave during the various phases of the cycle. For convenience, we'll use the classic 28-day cycle, although your cycle will probably vary somewhat.

Phase I: The Bleeding Phase (Days 1–5)

The first day of menstrual flow marks Day 1 of your period and the beginning of the bleeding phase. The bleeding may last from two to eight days, usually between four and six, or an average of five days. The total

Illustration 12 *Hormone Activity in a Typical 28-Day Cycle*
Illustration from *Clinical Gynecological Endrocrinology and Infertility,* edition 2, L. Speroff, R. H. Glass, N. Kase, Williams and Wilkins (publishers), Copyright © 1978. Used with permission.

volume of the flow is usually about four to six tablespoons, or two to three ounces of blood. Women who have light flows may use as few as one or two menstrual tampons or sanitary pads a day, while women with heavy flows might require eight to ten pads a day. (In addition to pads and tampons many women are now using natural sponges, which can be purchased at cosmetic counters. These sponges can be rinsed, wrung out and reused.)* The volume of a woman's flow, incidentally, has nothing to do with her fertility.

The menstrual flow is made up of vaginal and cervical secretions, endometrial tissue and blood. Some women pass clumps of menstrual tissue that look like blood clots, and, unless these are excessive, this is normal. You may be more apt to notice these clots after you have been lying down for a while, for the blood has been pooling in the upper vagina and has had a chance to form these clotlike clumps of tissue. Menstrual blood has no odor until it comes in contact with air and vaginal bacteria.

During this phase of the cycle, the endometrial lining of the uterus sheds most of its thickness until, on the last day of the flow, only the thin innermost level remains. The ovary is producing only small amounts of its hormones, and both progesterone and estrogen are at their lowest levels during this phase.

Phase II: The Proliferative Phase (Days 6–13)

During the second phase of the menstrual cycle, which is called the proliferative, or follicular, phase, the hormone estrogen predominates. The low levels of hormones during the first phase cause the hypothalamus to produce its releasing factors, which then stimulate the pituitary to produce its hormones, particularly the follicle-stimulating hormone, FSH. The FSH, along with a little LH, travels via the bloodstream to the ovary, where it causes a number of follicles to start to develop and produce estrogen. (If all this is confusing you, try humming it to the tune of "the hip bone's connected to the leg bone" while studying the chart shown in Illustration 13.)

Throughout this phase the levels of estrogen increase. By Days 7 and 8 the levels are noticeably rising, and they reach their peak by about Day 13. These rising levels of estrogen act on the uterus, causing the lining to proliferate, that is, to grow thicker—hence the term "proliferative phase." The cells of the gland and duct tissue of the breast also proliferate. The cells of the tissue that lines the vagina likewise multiply, and the cell layers thicken. The vaginal discharge increases.

---

*Natural sponges may, however, be associated with certain problems. See the section on toxic shock syndrome for details.

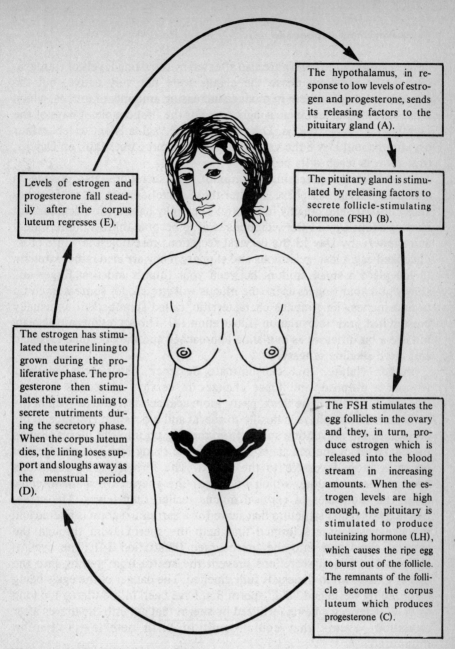

The hypothalamus, in response to low levels of estrogen and progesterone, sends its releasing factors to the pituitary gland (A).

The pituitary gland is stimulated by releasing factors to secrete follicle-stimulating hormone (FSH) (B).

Levels of estrogen and progesterone fall steadily after the corpus luteum regresses (E).

The estrogen has stimulated the uterine lining to grown during the proliferative phase. The progesterone then stimulates the uterine lining to secrete nutriments during the secretory phase. When the corpus luteum dies, the lining loses support and sloughs away as the menstrual period (D).

The FSH stimulates the egg follicles in the ovary and they, in turn, produce estrogen which is released into the blood stream in increasing amounts. When the estrogen levels are high enough, the pituitary is stimulated to produce luteinizing hormone (LH), which causes the ripe egg to burst out of the follicle. The remnants of the follicle become the corpus luteum which produces progesterone (C).

Illustration 13   *The Menstrual Cycle*

The glands in the cervix are also affected by the rising levels of estrogen. During the previous phase the glands were not very active, but the estrogen stimulates them to produce increasing amounts of mucus, which makes the vagina feel increasingly wet. For the first couple of days of the proliferative phase, that is, Days 6 and 7, the vagina is apt to feel rather dry; from about Day 8 the vagina starts to feel more wet, until, on Day 13, this wetness reaches its peak.

In addition to increasing in amount, the secretions also change in character during this phase. At first these secretions are apt to be rather sticky or pasty and creamy in texture. They may have a whitish color. But starting about Day 11 the secretions tend to become thinner, more watery and slippery. By Day 13 the cervical secretions resemble the white of an uncooked egg: clear, gelatinous and slippery. They are also rather stretchy. If you place a small amount between your thumb and first finger and slowly pull your fingers apart, the mucus will stretch, for some women up to four inches. This mucus characteristic, called spinnbarkeit, is usually present just prior to ovulation (Illustration 14). The secretions are also apt to taste a bit different as ovulation approaches and they become less acid and more alkaline (sugary).

Mother Nature, that consummate designer, never does anything without a purpose, and these changes in cervical secretions have an important function. The thick, pasty, more acid cervical mucus seen in the early days of this phase is hostile to sperm and blocks the entrance to the cervical canal, preventing sperm from moving up into the uterus. But as the character of the mucus is altered by the rising levels of estrogen, it becomes more favorable to the sperm. The formerly acid secretions become more alkaline, which nourishes the sperm. On a microscopic level, the molecules of cervical mucus realign themselves. The cross-hatched molecular structure that served as a barrier to sperm is altered and tubelike passages are formed that help the sperm swim through the cervical canal and into the uterus (see Illustration 14). The cyclical changes in cervical secretions prevent the sperm from getting into the uterus except when the egg is fully ripened. The danger of the egg's being fertilized by weakened "old" sperm that have been in the uterus too long or of an older egg's being fertilized by sperm that get into the uterus after ovulation—events that could result in birth defects—is thereby minimized.

The cervix also changes position within the vaginal cavity and becomes softer and the opening to the cervical canal dilates, all of which make it easier for the sperm to penetrate. Not coincidently, many women experience an increase in sexual drive during this phase of the menstrual cycle that peaks right before ovulation.

Meanwhile, back in the ovary, certain changes are also taking place. As the egg follicles are stimulated by the FSH from the pituitary, they move

FERTILE MUCUS   **INFERTILE MUCUS**

Illustration 14   *As ovulation approaches, your cervical mucus becomes slippery and can be stretched into a clear, delicate strand before breaking. Prior to ovulation the molecules of your mucus have a cross-hatched pattern. During the most fertile part of your cycle, the molecules realign themselves, forming passageways to aid the sperm on their journey to the uterus.*

toward the surface of the ovary. For some unknown reason, only one of these follicles normally continues to develop. The other follicles fail to mature fully and regress. The chosen follicle pushes against the outer capsule of the ovary, stretching the capsule and forming a bubblelike protrusion on the surface of the ovary.

Phase III: Ovulation (Day 14)

During Phase I, the rising levels of estrogen reach a certain point and then cause the suppression of the pituitary hormones FSH and LH. When rising levels of one hormone cause a suppression of the production of another hormone, the term "feedback mechanism" is used. The feedback mechanism is extremely complicated. In the case of estrogen, for instance, we know that it can suppress the production of LH, but we also know that once the estrogen reaches its peak level, it can trigger the release of a spurt of LH. This occurs just before ovulation, and this burst of LH causes the bulging egg follicle on the surface of the ovary to rupture and release its egg (see Illustration 15).

In the mythical 28-day cycle, ovulation is supposed to occur at the midpoint, on Day 14 of the cycle. But even in women with regular cycles there is often a variation of one or two days either way. Thus, a woman with a regular 28-day cycle might ovulate anywhere from Day 12 to Day 16.

The standard textbook 28-day cycle has served to confuse a lot of women about when ovulation occurs. We are often told that ovulation occurs at the midpoint of the cycle, which is fairly accurate for the woman who has a 28-day cycle; however, if a woman has a 36-day cycle, this midpoint would be Day 18. But that probably is not when she ovulates, for the midpoint is not really a guide to calculating the date of ovulation. A more reliable way of figuring your ovulation date would be to count backward 14 days from the first day of your cycle. In other words, the woman with a 36-day cycle probably ovulated on Day 22 (36 − 14 = 22). Since there is often a two-day variation in ovulation dates, even in women with regularly occurring cycles, a woman with a constant 36-day cycle may have ovulated anywhere from Day 20 to Day 24. Similarly, a woman with a 22-day cycle would have a midpoint of Day 11, but she probably ovulated on Day 8 (22 − 14 = 8) of her cycle or, allowing for the standard two-day variation, anywhere from Day 6 to Day 10.

Some women are able to pinpoint the time of ovulation because they experience a sharp, cramplike pain at the time of ovulation. This is called mittelschmerz, or middle pain. Some women also experience midcycle

Illustration 15 *The follicles within the ovary are stimulated and begin to develop (A). They migrate toward the surface of the ovary (B). The chosen follicle bursts open and releases its egg at ovulation (C).*

bleeding at the time of ovulation, either with or without mittelschmerz. The bleeding is the result of a rapid drop in estrogen levels. The follicle may literally be so shaken up by the act of ovulation that it stops producing hormones for a while. Without the continued support of the hormones, the thickened endometrial lining starts to break down and shed. Such bleeding is usually only a slight spotting that lasts for a few hours, but it may be heavier and persist for a few days. This type of midcycle bleeding is, however, extremely rare and may be the symptom of a more serious problem, so you should report it to your doctor.

In order for pregnancy to occur, a fresh, live sperm must meet and fertilize a live ovum. Actually, a woman can get pregnant only for a period of, at the most, 36 hours a month, for the egg lives for only 12 to 36 hours. But, you can get pregnant by having sex up to 72 hours prior to ovulation and for 36 hours following ovulation. This is because sperm can live for up to three days (there is now some evidence that they can survive for as long as five days, but it is highly unlikely that a sperm would be vital enough after three days to fertilize an egg). If you were to have intercourse three

69

days prior to ovulation, that sperm could still be in your reproductive tract and could fertilize the egg. Likewise, if you had intercourse within 36 hours after ovulation, the sperm could meet and fertilize the egg.

For many of us, this business about when ovulation occurs isn't terribly important, but if you're pregnant, have more than one lover and are trying to figure all that out, it could be very important. Similarly, if you're trying to get pregnant or are using a birth control method that requires you to figure out when you ovulated, then calculating your ovulation date is of prime importance, for the time preceding and following ovulation is the only time when you can become pregnant.

Just prior to ovulation the levels of estrogen have reached such a high level that they are no longer suppressing the production of LH by the pituitary. Instead, there is a surge of LH, which triggers the release of the egg from the follicle and initiates the next phase of the cycle.

Phase IV: The Secretory Phase (Days 15−28)

The final phase of the menstrual cycle is the secretory, or luteal, phase. During this phase the remnant of the burst follicle, which is called the corpus luteum, begins to produce the hormone progesterone. The corpus luteum is also producing estrogen, but progesterone production predominates. The preovulation surge of luteinizing hormone from the pituitary is responsible for transforming the burst follicle into the progesterone-producing corpus luteum. Although the egg follicle always contains cells capable of producing progesterone as well as estrogen, it is not until the levels of LH rise to a sufficient degree that these progesterone-producing cells receive the stimulation they need to begin to make significant amounts of this hormone. By Day 16, however, these cells are producing a quantity of progesterone, and they continue to do so throughout the first half of the secretory phase.

One of the major effects of the progesterone is to stimulate the cells in the estrogen-primed endometrial lining of the uterus to secrete nutriments that will nourish the egg if pregnancy should occur—hence, the term "secretory phase." The progesterone also initiates the first steps in the secretory process in the milk-producing tissues of the breast, although actual milk production doesn't normally occur until after delivery. This may cause the vels breast to swell and become tender as progesterone levels reach their peak on about Day 22. From that point on, progesterone levels drop and if the breast tissues have trouble reabsorbing these secretions, you may notice increased tenderness and lumpiness in your breasts in the days preceding your menstrual flow.

As the progesterone levels continue to rise, the endometrial lining thickens, reaching its maximum thickness on about Day 21 or 22. After about Day 21, the corpus luteum begins to decline because the increasing amounts of hormones it produces have forced a decline in luteinizing hormone from the pituitary. Without the pituitary LH, the hormone-producing cells in the burst follicle, the corpus luteum, are no longer stimulated. If, however, pregnancy occurs and a fertilized egg implants in the rich endometrial lining, the corpus luteum does not regress. The fertilized egg begins to produce a hormone similar to LH called human chorionic gonadotropin, or HCG. Throughout the first few months of pregnancy the corpus luteum, stimulated by HCG, continues to produce estrogen and progesterone until the fetus and its hormone-producing organ, the placenta, are mature enough to produce these hormones on their own.

In nonpregnant cycles, however, no HCG is produced and the corpus luteum regresses. Without the support of the progesterone, the rich secretory endometrium breaks down. The blood vessels shrink, depriving the endometrial tissue of its nourishment, and pieces of tissue begin to fall away. By the end of Day 28 these pieces of tissue are being shed through the cervix, and the menstrual flow (Phase I) of a new cycle has begun (see Illustration 16).

In addition to its effects on the breast and endometrial tissue, progesterone has a number of other effects. Throughout the proliferative and ovulatory phase of the cycle, the uterus undergoes mild rhythmic contractions, but within a day or two of ovulation the rising levels of progesterone inhibit these muscle contractions. On about Day 27 or 28, this inhibiting effect is lost and the contractions, which aid the expulsion of menstrual blood, begin again. For some women this resumption of contractions causes cramps just prior to menstruation, one of the main symptoms of the premenstrual syndrome experienced by many women.

The hormone progesterone is thermogenic, which means that it causes your temperature to rise. Once you have ovulated, your body temperature rises about six-tenths of a degree and generally remains elevated for a number of days. The cervical mucus is also affected by progesterone. In this phase it tends to be rather scant, thick and pasty. On a microscopic level, the molecules realign themselves once again. The molecular tubes or tunnels that aided the sperm on their journey into the uterus are again replaced by the cross-hatched type of structure that blocks the sperm and prevents them from moving into the uterus.

A wide variety of changes is noticed by women in the later half of the secretory phase. These changes, which are discussed in more detail elsewhere in this book, are given the name premenstrual syndrome because they occur in the "premenstruum," which is the medical term for the days preceding the menstrual flow. These changes may include acne, cramps, skin problems, eye problems, asthma, allergies, urinary tract problems, heightened sexual desire and breast tenderness, to mention just a few. Some researchers feel that these changes are directly related to

PHASE I

PHASE II

PHASE III

PHASE IV

Illustration 16   *Phase I: The lining of the uterus is shed. Phase II: The lining grows thicker. Phase III: The lining is about 2 mm thick at the time of ovulation. Phase IV: The lining begins to secrete nutriments.*

progesterone, but others question whether it is the progesterone itself or an imbalance between the levels of the various hormones. This question is also discussed more fully in the section on premenstrual syndrome.

Charting Your Menstrual Cycle

As you can tell from the preceding discussion, your body undergoes a complex set of changes over the course of a menstrual cycle. At first it may be a little difficult to get this all straight in your mind and remember which hormones are doing what during the various phase of your cycle. That's why we prefer a "hands-on" approach to learning about these changes. By using your speculum and making other simple observations of your body, you can learn to recognize cyclical changes. Keeping track of these changes on a chart like the one shown in Illustration 17 will help to make the somewhat abstract concepts of fluctuating hormone levels and feedback mechanisms more concrete and comprehensible.

How to Use the Chart

The first horizontal line on the chart is used to record the date. The second line indicates the days of your menstrual cycle. The first day on which you notice menstrual bleeding is Day 1 of your menstrual cycle. Write that day's date above the Day 1 column on your chart and continue dating the days of your cycle until your next period begins. The days on which you are actually bleeding can be recorded by marking those days with an X as the woman who kept the sample chart shown here has done.

On the first day of bleeding, this woman had mild cramps, which she noted by drawing a line from the Day 1 column and making a numbered comment to that effect. On Day 2 her flow was the heaviest, and by Day 4 it was tapering off. Some women bleed quite heavily throughout their periods; others start with a heavy flow and taper off; still others start out light and build up to a heavy flow. There are numerous individual patterns of menstrual bleeding. You may find that yours is fairly constant or that it changes from month to month.

Vaginal Secretions

The third section of your chart, which is headed Secretions, is used to record information about your vaginal secretions. As explained earlier, your vaginal secretions, which are composed of cells shed from your vaginal walls and cervix, secretions from your cervical glands and a small

73

MENSTRUAL CYCLE CHART

MONTH August 12 thru September 8

Day of cycle	Date	Secretions	Ovulation / Pain / Pressure	Cervical changes
1	Aug 12	✗		
2	13	✗		
3	14	✗		
4	15	✗		
5	16	✗		
6	17	dry		
7	18	dry		
8	19	dry		
9	20	wet, thin, white, milky		
10	21	lots, milky, sweet		
11	22	wet, translucent		cervix low, soft
12	23	clear, wet, salty		cervix slippery, os open
13	24	Spinnbarkeit		
14	25	wet, clear, abundant	X	
15	26	less wet, but clear, very salty		
16	27	less wet, cloudy		
17	28	creamy, wet		
18	29	creamy, wet		
19	30	tacky, wet		
20	31	tacky, wet		
21	Sep 1	tacky, wet		
22	2	less wet, sticky		
23	3	less wet, cloudy, sticky		
24	4	white, pasty, scant		cervix high, hard
25	5	scant, sweet		os, closed, cervix dry
26	6	dry		
27	7	wet, very		
28	8	cloudy, sticky		
29		✗		
30				
31				
32				
33				
34				
35				
36				
37				
38				
39				
40				

Comments

(1) mild cramps for a few hours.

(2) scanty flow

(4) tapering off

(7) heavy flow

(13) sexual desire ↑ must be about to ovulate

(14) mild pressure on right side over ovary

(21) ough! two pimples on my face, breast tender.

(22) breast sore

(23) larger cramp, breasts more sore, fluid retention, weight gain

(27) ovulation done, just before menstruation, probably sexual lubrication not just vaginal secretions, breast increasing tender; sexual desire ↑ about to menstruate; must be

Illustration 17 *Menstrual Chart*

amount of secretion from the vaginal walls, change character over the course of your menstrual cycle. In the days immediately following your period, when estrogen levels are low, your vagina is apt to feel rather dry. The woman who was keeping the chart shown here noted three dry days, Days 6, 7 and 8.

These dry days are followed by the expulsion of a mucus plug from the opening of the cervix. It is unlikely that you would notice this small, sticky plug, but following its expulsion the vagina begins to feel wet. For some women the first secretions following the dry days are whitish in color and sticky or tacky. Women use words such as *creamy, wet, milky, cloudy, abundant, scant, pasty* to describe these secretions.

As ovulation approaches and estrogen levels continue to rise, these secretions become more slippery and clear until, just prior to ovulation, they resemble the white of an uncooked egg and have the stretchy, spinnbarkeit quality. Note how the changes in vaginal secretions during the proliferative and ovulatory phases (Days 6-14) are noted on this wo-woman's chart.

The woman who kept the chart also experienced a sharp pain, the mittelschmerz discussed earlier, at the time of ovulation that she noted by placing an X on the chart under the appropriate day in the row labeled Ovulation. Some women experience a mild pain or a feeling of tenderness or pressure; others do not have any ovulation symptoms.

Following ovulation, during the secretory phase, the vaginal secretions continue to undergo changes, which you may be able to notice. The secretions become less slippery and more creamy. Some women experience a few dry days following ovulation, when estrogen levels are dropping. Progesterone, the hormone that predominates during this phase, is apt to produce thicker, pastier secretions that are hostile to sperm. Many women notice, as the woman who made this chart did, that they have whitish, sticky or tacky and creamy or pasty secretions that become less abundant after ovulation. The first few days following ovulation are usually dry, and this may be followed by a random pattern of dry days interspersed with sticky days.

In addition to noticing changes in the amount and character of your vaginal secretions, you may also notice changes in the taste of these secretions. Most of the time your vagina is apt to taste somewhat salty, but at times it may taste rather sweet. This is because the acid/alkaline (that is, acid/sugar) balance, or the pH balance, as scientists call it, of your vagina changes over the course of your menstrual cycle. During the secretory phase of your cycle, as estrogen levels are rising, the vagina gradually becomes more alkaline. This happens for two reasons. First of all, the estrogen not only stimulates greater quantities of cervical secretions, but the secretions it stimulates have greater amounts of sugar in them.

Secondly, the estrogen also causes changes in the composition of the cells that make up the vaginal wall, causing the sugar content of these cells to increase. As we noted earlier in the discussion of the secretory phase, the rising levels of estrogen also cause the cells that make up tissues of the vaginal walls to multiply and grow thicker. As they do so, greater numbers of cells are shed from the vaginal walls. As these vaginal cells are shed and break down, they release their sugar and this also makes the secretions more alkaline. For some women this gives a sweet taste to their secretions that is especially noticeable just prior to ovulation. Conversely, some women notice a more acid or salty taste at this time. This quality depends on the woman's personal body chemistry.

Each of us have bacteria that normally live in our vaginas. These bacteria, which are called lactobacilli, or Doderlain's bacteria, are essential to maintaining vaginal health. As the vaginal secretions become more alkaline, these bacteria, which thrive on sugar, multiply. They eat the sugar and secrete a mild acid. This restores the acid balance to the vagina and keeps disease-causing organisms, which prefer sugary environments, from thriving. Women whose lactobacilli are very active and get to work right away will notice an acid taste in their vaginas when the sugar content of the secretions increases. Others will note a sugary taste for a while. The mechanism of the acid/alkaline balance of the vagina is not well-understood, but we do know that some women experience a distinctly acid, salty taste or a particularly sweet taste at certain points in their cycles. Note how our chart woman recorded these taste changes on Days 10, 12 and 25.

For those of you who are having qualms about the sanitary aspects of tasting your vaginal secretions, remember that your vagina is probably a less infectious environment than your mouth. Of course, if you had an infection in your mouth or a cold sore on your lips, you would want to take precautions. The same is true of your vagina. If you have an abnormal discharge (abnormal in terms of unusual color, texture, odor or amount), you may have an infection and so should not taste your secretions. For instance, it is theoretically possible for a couple engaging in oral-genital sex to transmit a yeast infection from the woman's vagina to the mouth of her partner. In order for this to happen, the woman would have to have a roaring yeast infection and we have never seen this. Still, it is possible to orally pass some of the sexually transmitted diseases, such as herpes, gonorrhea or syphilis, from one person to another, so if you have an infection of any type or think you may have been exposed to one of these diseases, let common sense prevail and don't do any tasting.

There is a great deal of variation in the pattern of vaginal secretions that different women notice. Your individual pattern may change from month to month. Women who use birth control pills will probably not notice cyclical changes in their vaginal secretions, for the synthetic hormones in the pill alter the body's normal fluctuations in hormone levels. Similarly, women who have anovulatory cycles, that is, cycles in which they don't actually ovulate, also will not have the usual sort of hormone fluctuations and may not notice changes in their secretions. Anovulatory cycles often occur in women who have just begun to menstruate and in women approaching menopause. They also occur in women with certain gynecological conditions and, on occasion, in all women. Some women, even though they have normal ovulatory cycles, do not notice these changes in secretions.

Women who use spermicidal foams, creams or jellies for birth control may have difficulty in distinguishing between their secretions and the spermicide. Sexual activity can also make it difficult to observe the quality and quantity of your secretions. When you become sexually excited your vagina produces lubrication that has a stretchy quality similar to the spinnbarkeit type of secretion seen just prior to ovulation. Moreover, ejaculate, or "come," deposited in the vagina when a man has an orgasm can also obscure the true nature of your secretions. One way to avoid these confusions is to examine yourself when you are not feeling sexually aroused. If you have had sex the previous night, especially if you use spermicidal creams, foams or jellies, wait until late the next afternoon or evening to allow time for the ejaculate or spermicides to leak out of the vagina before making your observations.

Having a vaginal or cervical infection can also alter the character and amount of your cervical secretions. Infections can cause a change in the color, the texture, the amount and the odor of your secretions. By becoming familiar with your normal secretions you will be able to recognize abnormalities and seek treatment for infections early, when they are easiest to treat.

It is not necessary to perform speculum exam each day in order to keep a chart like this. Some women can tell the wet/dry condition of their vagina merely by observing; others feel the vaginal lips; still others insert a finger into the vaginal cavity to get a sample of secretions.

Recording Cervical Changes

The fluctuating hormone levels throughout your cycle also have an effect on the position of your cervix. Around the time of ovulation, when you are most fertile, the cervix is high in the vaginal cavity; when you are not fertile, it tends to occupy a position lower in the vaginal canal. You may notice that speculum exam is easier during these infertile days, when the cervix is lower and therefore easier to find.

If you practice speculum self-exam at these times, you may also notice other changes in your cervix. For instance, during the fertile times, when the cervix is higher in the canal, it is apt to feel softer (like your fingertip) and the cervical os, the opening to your cervical canal, is apt to be more widely dilated. The whole surface of the cervix may be shiny and may feel rather slippery. When the cervix is lower in the canal, it tends to feel firmer (like the tip of your nose or chin), the os will be closed and the shiny appearance and slippery feeling of the cervix won't be as noticeable. Your os is likely to be dilated again just before your period begins, and the cervix may be lower in the canal at that time. You can record these changes in the section of the chart marked Cervical Changes.

Comments

The last section of the chart, the one labeled Comments, can be used to record other changes that you may notice over the course of your menstrual cycle. Individual patterns vary considerably, and many women are not able to find consistent patterns. But if you record the physical and emotional changes that you experience over the course of your cycle, you may begin to note certain characteristic patterns.

Perhaps a few words about emotional changes and phases of the menstrual cycle are in order. Many women experience emotional changes that seem to be related to the phases of the menstrual cycle. The feminist movement has shied away from this topic, perhaps because feminists fear that this will feed into the cultural stereotype of women as creatures subject to raging hormonal imbalances who are unfit to hold positions of leadership in society because they suffer from periodic bouts of emotional instability. The truth of the matter is that beyond the folklore about "women on the rag," we really know very little about emotions, moods and phases of the menstrual cycle.

The small body of supposedly scientific research that has been done consists of studies analyzing groups of women who have attempted suicide and committed murder or other crimes to see if there was a correlation with a specific phase of their menstrual cycle. The assumption behind these studies is that women become emotionally unhinged at certain points in their cycle. Some of these studies "prove" that these things happen more often during the bleeding phase; others "prove" that they happen more often in the days preceding menstruation; still others find no correlation.6 So much for raging hormonal imbalances. . . .

However, the fact remains that many women do notice changes of mood that seem to be related to their cycles. Given the negative attitude about menstruation in our culture, it is not surprising that we generally hear about these negative emotional changes. This is not to suggest, however, that women who experience depression, irritability or other negative emotions are merely responding to the general cultural attitude about menstruation. There may be a very real physiologic basis for their feelings.

But what we do want to point out is that many women also experience positive emotional changes during this time—increase in sexual desire, extra energy, a generally elevated mood, for example—and yet we hear very little about these things. So, if you are noting emotional responses on your menstrual chart, be aware of this bias and record the positive changes as well as any negative ones.

In addition to emotional changes you may note a number of other variations in yourself, including increased sexual drive, different levels of energy, a craving for sweets, changed sleep patterns, weight gain and acne or clearing of the skin, to mention just a few. Any of the changes listed in the discussion of the secretory phase may be noted. Recording such observations in the comment section of your chart will help you to learn more about your particular body cycles and rhythms.

The Value of Keeping a Chart

In addition to helping you learn to understand the workings of the menstrual cycle, these charts can be useful in other ways. An expanded version of the chart that includes a daily body temperature record can be used as a method of birth control or to determine the optimum time for intercourse if you are trying to become pregnant. This is discussed in detail in the section on birth control methods under the heading Natural Family Planning.

An accurate history of your menstrual cycles can be especially important if you develop certain gynecological problems and may aid your doctor in diagnosis. Knowledge of the length of your cycle and whether or not they are regular may be an important factor in your choice of a method of birth control. Familiarity with your vaginal discharges and the appearance of your cervix can help you spot abnormalities and diseases in their earliest stages, when they are most curable.

Perhaps even more important is the fact that the chart can help you learn more about your body's rhythms and cycles. Once you have this sort of knowledge, you are in a much better position to wend your way through the medical marketplace, to make informed decisions about birth control and health care. Armed with knowledge about your body, you are not likely to fall prey to an unnecessary hysterectomy or other form of medical mistreatment.

Birth Control: The Statistical Lie

There are three kinds of lies, white lies, black lies and statistics. . . .

Mark Twain

Mark Twain probably wasn't thinking about birth control when he made the above observation, but it certainly applies. Statistics have been used, or rather misused, to create false impressions about birth control, in particular about the relative effectiveness of the various methods. Somewhere, somehow, somebody has managed to pull the wool over everybody's eyes.

In order to understand the statistical lies told about birth control effectiveness, a few definitions are in order. Basically there are two types of effectiveness rates: theoretical rates and actual-use—effectiveness rates. The theoretical effectiveness rate is just that—a theory. It tells us how many women would probably get pregnant if that method of birth control were used correctly and consistently, without mistakes: if, for instance, the Pill were taken at the same time every day and no pills were ever missed or if the diaphragm were inserted correctly each and every time a woman had intercourse. The use-effectiveness rate, on the other hand, includes all the mistakes. It is based on studies of groups of women who actually used that particular method over a period of time. The actual-use—effectiveness rate is less impressive than the theoretical rate, for it reflects all the method-failures—condoms that break, diaphragms that slip out of place, IUDs that are unknowingly expelled—and all the user-failures—the women who forget to take their pills or who don't use the foam or diaphragm each time they have sex.

Both actual-use and theoretical rates are given in terms of a group of 100 women using that method for a year. If a method is said to be 98 percent effective, this means that 98 out of 100 women using that method for a year would not get pregnant, but two would. If a method is said to have a failure rate of two per 100 woman-years of use, this means that we could expect that two women out of a group of 100 using this method for a year would get pregnant.

Most American women are laboring under the misconception that, in terms of effectiveness, the Pill and the IUD are vastly superior to the older barrier methods, such as the diaphragm, the condom, spermicides or foam. But, as we shall see, t'aint necessarily so.

This whole issue of effectiveness deserves careful consideration, for as everybody knows, or should know by now, deciding which method of birth control to use is a game of trade-offs. There is no perfect method, so we have to deal with what's available. Basically there are three cards in the deck: safety, convenience and effectiveness. Each of us must shuffle the cards, arrange our hands according to our priorities and pick a method from the pile. It often seems like a no-win game, for no matter what method we choose, we win some but we also lose some.

The Safety vs. Convenience Trade-Off

Methods like the Pill and the IUD, which have the worst safety records, are more convenient. All we have to do is swallow a little tablet once a day or, in the case of the IUD, have the doctor insert a small plastic device into the uterus. What could be easier? On the other hand, the older barrier methods of birth control—diaphragms, spermicides or condoms—are undeniably safer; one doesn't hear about women who die from heart attacks (pill complication) or massive uterine infections (IUD complication) because they used one of the barrier methods. But the barrier methods are messy and, as anyone who's ever chased a springing diaphragm around the bathroom or tried to unroll a condom the wrong way at the critical moment knows, they are definitely less convenient to use. With them there's clearly a trade-off between convenience and safety.

In the past, many women felt comfortable about choosing convenience over safety. The Pill and the IUD were the most widely used forms of birth control. But, over the years, this has begun to change. The ever-growing list of known and suspected side effects and complications from the IUD and the Pill (a list that now contains some 50-odd items) have made many women reconsider the safety vs. convenience trade-off. The fact that the list of complications and side effects keeps growing and that neither the Pill nor the IUD has been around long enough for anyone to judge its long-term effects has contributed to our uneasiness about the safety of these methods.

81

The Long-Term Effects

The biggest concern about the long-term effects of the Pill and the IUD is the possibility of cancer. The Pill in particular is suspect. Indeed, one type of Pill, the sequential pill, was withdrawn from the market because of its possible association with uterine cancer.[1] In recent years, studies have shown that women who take estrogen (one of the components of the Pill) for menopausal symptoms have a risk of developing uterine cancer that is 4.5 to 13.9 times greater than women who do not.[2] There is no evidence to indicate that the lower doses of estrogen used in the birth control pills now on the market will have the same effect, but women on the Pill are younger than the women who took estrogen for menopausal symptoms. Most women who develop uterine cancer are postmenopausal. What will happen to Pill users once they reach that age? Will women who used the Pill during their reproductive years be more likely to develop uterine cancer than their sisters who did not? We don't yet know the answer to these questions; only time will tell.

The relationship between estrogen and uterine cancer is not the only disturbing information to come to light in recent years. In the early 70s it was discovered that the daughters born to women who had taken a synthetic estrogen called diethylstilbestrol (DES) during their pregnancies in order to prevent miscarriage were at increased risk for the development of a rare form of vaginal cancer.[3] The risk was small, but it was undeniably related to the use of estrogen. This discovery has lead to intensive study of women who took DES and their offspring. Abnormalities in the reproductive tract have been found in both DES daughters and sons.[4] There is also some preliminary evidence to suggest that DES mothers may be at increased risk for the development of breast and other cancers.[5] Some authorities believe we may see an increased risk for cervical cancer in DES daughters as they grow older.[6] Except for the association with a rare form of vaginal cancer, the relationship between the use of the synthetic estrogen DES and increased rates of cancer has neither been confirmed nor denied. Will these women be at increased risk for cancer? If so, what implications does this hold for the women who take the lower doses of estrogen contained in the Pill—but for longer periods of time? We don't know the answer to these questions; again, only time will tell.

There have been conflicting reports about the relationship between cervical cancer and the Pill. Most of the studies have failed to indicate a relationship; however, the follow-up time in these studies was often limited.[7] One longer-term study has indicated that women who have a cervical condition known as dysplasia, which is possibly a precursor to cancer, are more likely to have their dysplasia progress to cancer if they use the Pill.[8] The conflicting data about cervical cancer and the Pill makes it impossible to evaluate the relationship between the two at this time; again, only time will tell.

The possibility of a relationship between the Pill and breast cancer has engendered a great deal of heated controversy. On one side are those who point out that all of the studies that have evaluated the Pill and breast cancer have failed to establish a relationship between the two.[9] In fact, several studies have shown that Pill users are less likely to develop noncancerous breast diseases.[10] Since having a noncancerous breast disease increases a woman's chance of developing breast cancer, some doctors theorize that use of the Pill could decrease breast cancer risk.

On the other side of the debate are those who point out that cancers take many years to develop. The Pill has not been used for a long enough period of time by a large enough group of women for anyone to determine whether or not there is a relationship. Some of these experts worry that the slight increase we seem to be seeing in the incidence rates for breast cancer in younger women may be the early warning signs of a problem whose dimensions will become more apparent in future years. But many doctors deny that there is an increase in incidence rates for breast cancer and attribute any apparent increase to earlier detection or changes in methods of collecting statistics. Others concede that there is an increase in incidence but feel that factors other than the Pill are to blame. Let's hope they are right.

There are other reasons for concern about the Pill and breast cancer. Even though there is no proof that the estrogen in the Pill can act as a "seed" for breast cancer, there is ample reason to believe that estrogen may act as a fertilizer, accelerating the growth of certain preexisting breast cancers. Some breast cancers have "estrogen receptors" that make them responsive to stimulation by estrogen produced in the body. What is the effect of the synthetic estrogen in the Pill on estrogen-sensitive cancers in the breast? If a woman with an undetected estrogen-sensitive cancer of the breast takes the Pill, will her cancer be more likely to spread to other parts of her body faster? Since one out of 14 women in this country will develop breast cancer and some 40 to 60 percent of them will have estrogen receptors, this is an important question, but, unfortunately, one that also cannot be answered at this time.

Although studies have shown that Pill users are less likely to get benign breast disease, other studies have shown that those women who already have benign breast disease before starting on the Pill or who develop benign breast disease while on the Pill may be more likely to develop breast cancer.[11] There has also been some disturbing evidence indicating that women who used estrogen to treat menopausal symptoms may, after a time lapse of some 15 years, and regardless of how long they took the estrogen, be at an increased risk for breast cancer.[12] This association was discovered in one study that involved only small numbers of women. What are the implications of this study for women who use birth control pills? Again, the answers to these questions are not yet known.

There has been less concern about the IUD and cancer, but even here questions are raised. The upper two-thirds of the uterine lining are shed each month, but the bottom one-third, the basal layer, remains. Could the presence of the IUD cause cancerous or precancerous cell changes in the basal layer of the uterine lining? Again, nobody knows; only time will tell.

The Pill has other effects on the system whose long-term impact is not known. Indeed, the Pill may modify biochemical processes in all body tissues. More than 50 metabolic changes have beeen recorded.[13] The levels of fats in the blood, including cholesterol, are elevated.[14] Sugar metabolism is altered, causing some Pill users to test out like diabetics.[15] The metabolism of essential vitamins and minerals is altered, and the blood plasma often has a greenish tinge due to increased copper.[16] The ultimate effect of these changes on the user's health is still a question.

Safety

So far, we have been talking about *possible* problems. There are, in addition, definite, clearly documented complications and side effects associated with use of the Pill and the IUD. Fatal and nonfatal heart attacks, strokes, liver tumors, gall bladder disease, high blood pressure and diabetes are just a few of the health problems in which the Pill has been said to be a factor.[17] The IUD has also caused the death of a number of women. One IUD in particular, the Dalkon Shield, the tail (the strings that protrude through the cervix into the vaginal cavity) of which was twined like a candle wick, apparently served as a ladder that allowed disease-causing organisms to ascend into the uterus. It was later banned after being implicated in the deaths of some young women.[18] Other IUDs have also been associated with death, sterility and serious illnesses.[19]

When reports of Pill and IUD deaths and complications first began to appear in the medical literature and the popular press, advocates of these methods were quick to point out that, despite the risks, these methods were still safer than pregnancy. The chances of dying from use of an IUD or the Pill were considerably lower than the chances of dying from a complication related to pregnancy.

Many women have objected to looking at things from this point of view, however. If the Pill and the IUD were the only methods of birth control available, comparisons of pregnancy versus Pill or IUD risks might be relevant. But the IUD and the Pill are not the only available methods; there are other, safer methods, which should be considered in estimates of comparative risks.

Moreover, we now know that the Pill and the IUD are not safer than pregnancy for certain groups of women. Table 1 shows the leading causes of death for American women aged 15-44 years. Table 2 shows the deaths associated with birth control and pregnancy complications in these age groups. In the 40-44-year-old age group, women who use the Pill *and* who smoke are more likely to die from Pill complications than from pregnancy complications.

These tables tell us that for younger women the risks of birth-control—related deaths are relatively small. (Of course, this is all relative; the risks don't seem so small if you're the one who dies.) For all age groups the safest method of birth control is a barrier method, with a back-up abortion should the method fail. Women under the age of 30 are more likely to die as a result of a traffic accident (the second most common cause of death in women of all ages) than as a result of birth control complications. After the age of 30, the likelihood of dying from a Pill complication for users who smoke approaches the risk of dying in a traffic accident, and by the age of 40, Pill users who smoke are more likely to die from a Pill complication than in a traffic accident. Because of the risks reflected in these charts, many doctors no longer prescribe the Pill for women over 30 who smoke; others won't prescribe it for women over 40, regardless of whether or not they smoke; and no one should prescribe the Pill for smokers over the age of 40.

These safety features include only the risks of death from complications that have been clearly documented. They do not reflect possible complications. Five or ten years ago safety figures for the IUD and especially for the Pill looked a lot better than they do today. Back then we didn't realize the risks involved for women, or how dramatically they increased for Pill users over 40. What will these safety figures look like in another five or ten years? Once again, only time will tell.

Table 1
Leading Causes of Death: American Women Aged 15 to 44 Years

Cause	Deaths per 100,000 Women per Year
All causes	91.20
Cancer	18.80
Motor vehicle accidents	14.50
Heart disease	7.25
Suicide	6.95
All other accidents	6.50
Homicide	5.70
Stroke	3.95
All other causes	Less than 3 per 100,000 each

SOURCE: Mortality Statistics Branch, Division of Vital Statistics, National Center for Health Statistics, US Department of Health, Education and Welfare.

Table 2
Birth Control and Risk of Death

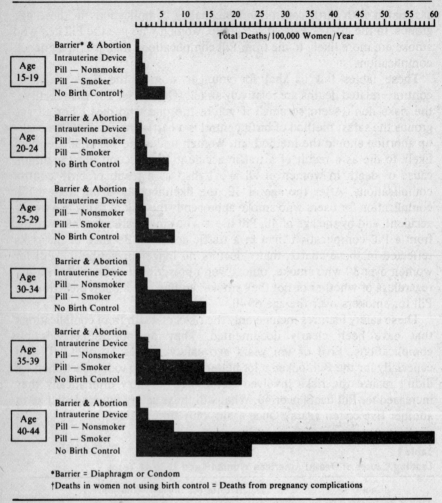

*Barrier = Diaphragm or Condom
†Deaths in women not using birth control = Deaths from pregnancy complications

SOURCE: FDA-approved package insert

Moreover, these figures reflect only death rates. Although the IUD is safer than the Pill in terms of risk of death, each year as many as one in every 300 IUD users will have IUD-related complications serious enough to require hospitalization.[20] These complications generally involve perforation of the uterus by an IUD or an IUD-related infection, both of which often can be successfully treated without further difficulty. At other times, however, these complications may cause infertility, constant pelvic pain and recurring episodes of pelvic inflammatory disease.

Reexamining the Safety vs. Convenience Trade-Off

In light of the new information about relative risks and possible long-term effects, informed women began to reconsider the safety vs. convenience trade-off. Many women thought that it was high time to overhaul old images and attitudes about lovemaking anyhow. The fuzzily romantic fantasies of swooning passion and orgasmic ecstasy on which most of us were weaned and which, of course, couldn't be interrupted by anything so prosaic as inserting a diaphragm, were due for replacement, especially in light of Masters and Johnson's research findings about female sexuality.

Women began to develop, or admit to having, a "hands-on" (pun intended) approach to sexuality. These and other changes began to pave the way for a resurgence of interest in the older, safer methods of birth control. Many couples began to incorporate the placing of the condom, foam or diaphragm into their lovemaking ritual and found a deep sense of satisfaction in sharing birth control responsibilities. Although we Americans haven't become as adventuresome as our European neighbors, who use condoms that come in a bright rainbow of colors (there are even ones that glow in the dark!), a few shy, pastel-colored condoms have made their way to the market, and one American company has recently begun to produce a raspberry-flavored spermicide.

By 1978 trends in birth control usage were beginning to change. Use of the Pill was declining and the number of women using barrier methods has increased.[21] Still, in terms of absolute numbers, the Pill and the IUD remain the most popular of the reversible forms of birth control, for safety and convenience are not the only factors on which a birth control decision is based. Effectiveness is also considered, and most women believe that the Pill and the IUD are vastly superior in terms of effectiveness. Although some women are willing to trade convenience for safety, many women are not willing to trade effectiveness for anything. Thus, many women, although aware of the risks, nonetheless opt for the Pill and the IUD, because they believe these methods to be far superior in terms of effectiveness.

Effectiveness

But are the Pill and the IUD really more effective? The medical profession has certainly tried to create this impression, but a close look at the situation reveals that this impression is actually based on some subtle—and not so subtle—statistical lies.

One way in which women are hoodwinked into thinking that the Pill and IUD are more effective than the barrier methods involves the misuse of theoretical-effectiveness and actual-use—effectiveness rates. Studies have shown that medical professionals tend to quote theoretical-effectiveness rates for the Pill and the IUD and actual-use—effectiveness rates for the barrier methods when informing women about birth control.[22] Not only that, but they often quote figures better than the theoretical rates for the Pill and IUD and worse than the actual-use—effectiveness rates for the barrier methods. Hardly a fair comparison!

Theoretical rates are themselves an example of the bias against barrier methods, for the way in which they are determined begins, upon examination, to seem like a bit of a mystery. It is easy to see how one could come up with a theoretical rate for a device like the IUD or for the Pill. One could insert the IUD and check the woman regularly to make sure that it had not been expelled or hadn't perforated the uterus and then get a pretty good idea of its theoretical-effectiveness rate. With the Pill, one could run a study in which it were administered to women each day at the same time and again come up with a good idea of its theoretical-effectiveness rate. But how does one establish a theoretical rate for the condom, the diaphragm or foam? One could, we suppose, assign a researcher to every woman in the study who would check the placement of the diaphragm prior to each act of intercourse. While this has certain comic possibilities, it is hardly a practical experiment. So the solution seems to involve pulling a figure out of a hat and calling it the theoretical rate. The theoretical-failure rate commonly quoted for foam is three pregnancies per 100 woman-years of use.[23] Yet there are foam studies with actual-use—failure rates of 1.55 per 100 woman-years of use,[24] so it simply does not make sense to say that the theoretical-failure rate is 3. Many birth control experts feel that theoretical rates are totally meaningless and should be disregarded. We agree.

When comparing the effectiveness of various birth control methods, the important figures to look at are the actual-use—effectiveness rates. But here again we run into statistical shenanigans. The Food and Drug Administration (FDA) publishes a pamphlet entitled *Contraception: Comparing the Options* that is the official word on birth control.[25] It too is heavily biased against the barrier methods, telling us that we can expect anywhere from 3 to 36 pregnancies in a group of 100 condom users in a year. The idea of 36 pregnancies is hardly reassuring. Given a figure like this, no one who seriously wanted to prevent conception would use a condom.

Yet the facts behind these statistics tell a very different story. As it turns out, the figure of 36 pregnancies is taken from a study done in West Virginia in 1942[26]—and how applicable is a study done almost 40 years ago to today's situation? For one thing, the quality of condoms has improved dramatically since the time of this study. Traditionally the objection to condoms was that they decreased sexual pleasure for men. Using a condom was likened to taking a shower with with a raincoat on. In the past this reputation was probably a well-deserved one, but with the advent of latex rubber, condoms became much thinner and far more pleasant to use. As a result, they are used much more now than previously.

Moreover, condom manufacturers today must meet strict quality-control standards. Each batch must be tested for pinholes and other defects. Some manufacturers even test each condom individually, although this is a fairly recent innovation. Condoms manufactured in the 40s did not have to meet such rigorous quality-control standards. The fact that condoms in the 40s were not tested for manufacturing defects and were unpleasingly thick undoubtedly accounts for the high pregnancy rates.

The time during which the study was done may also have been a factor in the high pregnancy rates. Published in 1942, the actual study probably took place a year or two before. The country was about to enter a war, men were being drafted left and right and a lot of young men were undoubtedly in a hurry to become family men before they were grabbed up. Of course it's impossible to say whether any of the men in that West Virginia study had draft evasion on their minds, but given this possibility and the fact that the condoms used were not quality-controlled and were rather primitive forerunners of the modern condom, the study hardly seems applicable to today's situation. More to the point would be studies done using the newer, quality-tested, latex-rubber condoms or, better yet, the natural-skin condoms, which allow for better heat transfer and superior sensitivity. One of the most recent studies of condom effectiveness, cited in the prestigious work *Contraceptive Technology* (Emory University), was a study done in 1975 with an actual-use—failure rate of only 0.83, which is better than the *theoretical*-effectiveness rate of the Mini-pill and within a few tenths of a percentage point of the *theoretical* rate for the regular Pill.[27] But these sorts of effectiveness rates are not reflected in the FDA's official 3 to 36 pregnancy failure rate for the condom.

The FDA figures are supposedly an objective and fair representation of the data available in the medical literature. Yet the FDA's effectiveness rates for the rhythm method are derived, in part, from studies done years ago on a group of Tongan women.[28] Again, how applicable are the results of a study done in a South Sea island community whose cultural attitudes about pregnancy and sense of urgency about birth control may be very different from ours? If the FDA's figures are a fair presentation of the available data, then why is a rate of only one pregnancy per 100 woman-years of use cited for the Pill when, in fact, there are reports in the medical literature in which actual-use—failure rates for the Pill are as high as 25 percent?[29] If studies of South Sea Islanders and of men using condoms that bear about as much similarity to today's condoms as a Model T to a Mustang are going to be included, then in all fairness the FDA pamphlet should tell us to expect anywhere from 1 to 25 pregnancies among women using the Pill for a year. But it doesn't.

Why does the medical profession downgrade the barrier methods? Why does the FDA present such biased effectiveness statistics? There are a number of plausible explanations.

First of all, back in the 50s and early 60s, when the Pill and the IUD first made their debut, Americans were having a love affair with technology. Science had ushered in the era of gadgets galore. With just the flick of the switch and a push of the button, we could automatically wash the dishes, dispose of the garbage, brush our teeth, Osterize the morning juice, remotely tune our TVs and open the garage door. If that wasn't sufficient testimony to the incredible efficiency of modern technology, one had only to consider the seemingly endless array of consumable, disposable, throw-away convenience products that were rolling off production lines across the nation. To top it all off, we counted backwards from ten, pushed a button, launched a rocket and landed a man on the moon. If science and technology could perform such miracles, certainly they could produce wonderfully effective methods of birth control.

Of course, less than a decade later, knee deep in nonbiodegradable garbage and choking on industrial pollution, many of us were wondering whether the new era of technology was such a dandy thing after all. But that was later on; at the time when the IUD and the Pill first appeared on the scene, Americans still possessed an incredibly naive faith. Science and technology were in effect the new gods, and one does not question the efficacy of the gods—or look a gift horse in the mouth.

In the era of gadgetry and man-on-the-moon technology, it simply was not believable that age-old methods like the diaphragm or the condom could be as effective as the wondrous new manmade chemicals that could stop a woman's body from ovulating or the clever plastic doodad that could prevent a fertile egg from implanting in her womb. We were so busy admiring our technological accomplishments that we never stopped to take an objective look at the realities of the situation.

Besides, the birth rate was declining, a phenomenon attributed to the widespread use of the Pill and IUD. But here again the facts were ignored by technology-bedazzled family planners. In actual fact, the lowest birth rate this country ever experienced was in 1930, long before either the Pill or the IUD was available.[30] This fact *could* be interpreted as a sign of the efficiency of the barrier methods—the only birth control options available at that time.

On the other hand, the low birth rate might not have been a reflection of their efficiency at all. Perhaps the Depression depressed people's sex drives as well as the economy. Maybe people simply didn't have sex very often; this certainly could account for the low birth rate. In the same vein, perhaps the lower birth rate that occurred during the time of widespread use of the Pill and the IUD was also just a coincidence. Were the Pill and the IUD really responsible for the lower birth rate or were factors like the legalization of abortion, the opening up of jobs for women, improvements in infant and child survival (because most children now live to maturity, women no longer have "replacement" children for those they once expected would die) more directly responsible? Without a clear answer to this question, we can hardly consider lower birth rates a testimony to the effectiveness of the Pill or the IUD.

Yet the myth that the Pill and the IUD are vastly superior methods of birth control persists and is actively supported by doctors. Doctors consider themselves scientists and are perhaps especially apt to place faith in the wonders wrought by science. Then, too, the Pill and the IUD appeared on the scene at a time when abortion was still illegal. Doctors were all too often forced to deal with the aftermath of illegal abortions. Then along came two methods that were so easy and carefree to use that consistent and proper usage seemed assured. It is understandable that doctors who had watched women die from back-alley abortions didn't cast too critical an eye on the statistical data concerning the effectiveness of these new birth control methods.

Abortions are now legal, but despite this fact doctors still tend to downgrade barrier methods. A less benevolent explanation for their continued put-down of these methods has been suggested. After all, it is easier to simply push a prescription for the Pill across the desk than to take the time to carefully fit a diaphragm and teach a woman how to use it. It's also more profitable. The diaphragm takes more of the doctor's time and does not involve the annual or semiannual checkup that women on the Pill must have. In addition, during the heyday of the Pill and the IUD in the 1960s, many medical schools dropped diaphragm-fitting from their curricula, so that many doctors today simply do not know how to fit one properly.

Moreover, the other major barrier methods are not physician-controlled. Condoms and foam can be purchased at pharmacies without a doctor's prescription. Perhaps both ego (the doctor's assumption that anything that only s/he can provide is better than anything a woman can do for herself) and financial considerations have contributed to doctors' tendencies to downgrade barrier methods.

Sexism is also a factor. The simple truth of the matter is that many doctors think women are too dumb to learn how to use the barrier methods. So they downgrade the effectiveness of these methods, hoping to convince women to use the Pill and the IUD instead.

It is true that there is an overwhelming cultural ignorance imposed on women about their bodies. We are taught from early childhood to believe that someone other than ourselves has the knowledge, the expertise and the right to control our reproductive organs. But the barrier methods are childishly simple to use, and anyone with a modicum of knowledge about how her body works can be taught to use these methods if the person doing the teaching speaks the same language.

We are not being facetious when we add the qualification that the teacher must speak the woman's language. A number of studies of barrier methods involved women who did not speak the same language as those people running the study. Follow-ups of some studies of foam effectiveness in which there were unacceptably high failure rates have shown that some women used the foam after making love or applied it to the outer genitals instead of to the inner, vaginal cavity.[31] Not surprisingly, the studies showing the best rates for the barrier methods are those in which the women in the study were taught to use the method by someone of the same racial or ethnic background who spoke the same language.

The pharmaceutical companies have also played a role in creating the impression that the IUD and Pill are vastly superior methods of birth control. Birth control is, after all, a big business. About 325 million monthly cycles of oral contraceptives were sold in 1977.[32] Retail prices for a single monthly cycle may run from five to ten dollars. Not all of that money goes back to the manufacturer, but a hefty chunk of it does. The IUD is also a profitable little item, retailing to doctors for $15 to $25. Of course, the IUD is not as profitable as the Pill, but when you consider that the device contains only a few cents worth of materials, the profit margin isn't bad.

A diaphragm, on the other hand, sells for five to ten dollars and, with proper care, may last for years. Although foam and condoms are consumable items, supplies of which must constantly be replenished, they are used only when they are actually needed, unlike the Pill, which must be taken every day regardless of whether or not a woman is having intercourse.

About half of the dozen or so major world-wide manufacturers of the Pill are American companies. A couple of large U.S. pharmaceutical companies make IUDs. These companies have spent considerable sums of money advertising their products in medical journals, promoting the notion that these methods of birth control are superior to other methods. Doctors, primed by their faith in technology, by their financial and ego interests and by biased statistics from the FDA, have been all too willing to accept these advertising claims and pass erroneous information about relative effectiveness rates on to their women patients.

The fact that the FDA's official statistics on birth control are biased against the barrier methods and favor the methods heavily promoted by the pharmaceutical industry will not come as a shock to women active in the health-care movement. The FDA is the government agency responsible for regulating the drug industry, and their performance of their regulatory duties has come under sharp criticism. Although the agency does a stunning job of stamping out snake-oil salesmen and other smalltime quacks, their track record as far as regulation of the major drug companies is somewhat less admirable. To cite just one example, it took at least seven months for the FDA to act on the unquestionable proof it had about the relationshp between the synthetic estrogen DES and cancer.[33] Having the FDA regulate the drug industry has been compared to having the fox guard the chicken coop. As Barbara Seaman points out in her fine book *Women and the Crisis in Sex Hormones*, it is not unusual for officials in the FDA to wind up as executives in the drug industry after leaving their government posts.[34]

At any rate, regardless of the reasons, one thing is clear: Women in this country have clearly been receiving biased information about birth control effectiveness from both their doctors and the FDA, the very sources women should be able to rely on for objective facts.

What is the truth of the matter? How do the various methods of birth control actually compare in terms of effectiveness? No one knows. Unfortunately, there has never been a well-designed, sound, scientific study comparing the different methods, nor is it likely that one will be done, for such a study would be impractical, if not downright impossible. First of all, such a study would require a number of different groups of women, each of which would use one of the methods for a period of time. The women in the different groups would have to be carefully matched. They would all have to have had at least one child, thus indicating that they were indeed fertile, and they would have to be matched according to age, since 25-year-old women are much more fertile than 35-year-old women. All of the women's sexual partners would have to have fathered at least one child, indicating that they too were fertile. The women would have to have intercourse about the same number of times per week. They would also have to be matched in regard to their intentions, for studies have shown that couples who are using birth control with the intention of merely postponing pregnancy are much less successful at birth control, regardless of the method used, than couples who have completed their families and don't intend to have any children in the future. The study would also have to involve large numbers of women in order to be statistically significant. The differences in actual-use—effectiveness rates, if indeed there are any, are going to be small ones, and the laws of statistics tell us that when we are looking for large differences between groups, only relatively small numbers of people have to be studied, but when we are looking for more refined data and smaller differences, large numbers of participants are necessary in order for the statistics to be valid.

In addition, the study would have to be randomized, which means that the participants could not choose which method of birth control they were to use but would be assigned to a method at random. Randomization would be necessary in order to prevent bias; otherwise, the fact that more

93

motivated users might tend to pick a certain method could bias the results of the study. Finding large groups of well-matched subjects who would be willing to use a birth control method assigned to them at random would be—to say the least—rather difficult.

Lacking such a study, the best that can be done is to hunt through the medical literature and catalog the highest and lowest use-effectiveness rates that have been reported. Table 3 lists the highest and lowest rates we have been able to find. We feel that some of the low figures are probably not too meaningful. For instance, the lowest condom rate of 64 percent comes from the 1942 study discussed earlier. The high rates may be a bit more meaningful, for they represent results that can be expected from highly motivated users who are conscientious about using that method. Depending on your own motivations, you can expect to fall somewhere between these two extremes.

As you can see from looking at Table 3, there is less than a 1 percent difference in actual-use—effectiveness rates when these methods are used in the best of circumstances, that is, when used by women who have been well-educated about the method and who are highly motivated. These facts will probably come as a surprise to most women, for, as we have seen, women are rarely informed about the high effectiveness rates of the barrier methods. Instead, we are fed a collection of statistical lies, with two very serious consequences.

First, the widely held but erroneous belief that methods like the Pill are vastly superior has slowed research into the development of barrier methods that could be even more effective and more convenient to use. Research funds have been funneled into the development of hormonal, Pill-type methods and improvements on the IUD that, it is hoped, will result in their having fewer side effects, thus lowering their high discontinuation rates (large numbers of IUD and Pill users stop using these methods within the first year because of their side effects). Only a minuscule amount has been allocated to the development of barrier methods. Yet it is not beyond the scope of technology to develop a longer-lasting spermicide that could be inserted several hours prior to intercourse so that the spontaneity of the sex act would not be interrupted (one of the major drawbacks to the use of spermicides and diaphragms).

Table 3
High and Low Effectiveness Rates Reported in the Medical Literature

Method	Highest (%)	Lowest (%)
Pill	99+	75
IUD	99+	91.7
Condom	99+	64
Foam	99+	60
Diaphragm	98.6	80.3

The Cervical Cap

The cervical cap is an excellent case in point. It is a diaphragmlike device that is loaded with spermicide and then placed right over the cervix. It is smaller than the diaphragm and, in contrast to it, is held in place by an airtight suction seal. Because of this seal, the spermicide remains active for a longer period of time, for at least three days and possibly even as long as seven days, according to some authorities. This means that the cap, unlike the diaphragm and other barrier methods, can be inserted well in advance of intercourse, so that there is no need for a couple to interrupt their lovemaking. The spermicide is contained within the cap, so the vaginal cavity is not full of spermicide, which also makes the cap less messy to use than the diaphragm. Because the spermicide stays in the cap and therefore it is not necessary to insert more spermicide before each act of intercourse, there is none of the excess lubrication from spermicide that decreases friction and sexual pleasure for some diaphragm and foam users. Nor is there excess spermicide to interfere with oral lovemaking.

The cap has been used in Europe for years and was introduced in this country in the late 50s and early 60s, but it was eclipsed by the Pill and IUD, so the manufacturer discontinued making them here. Because research funds have been funneled into Pill and IUD research, no government money has been available for cap research, so little is known about its effectiveness, use and safety, although Planned Parenthood considers its efficacy to be probably on a par with that of the diaphragm.[35]

Current Status

At the present time, cervical caps are manufactured only in England, so they are not widely used in this country. However, with the growing evidence of side effects and consequences from use of the Pill and the IUD, there has been a renewed interest in the cervical cap, which, unlike the other barrier methods of birth control, doesn't require insertion immediately prior to intercourse.

Recently, an oral surgeon, Dr. Robert Goeppe, and a gynecologist, Dr. Uwe Freese, of the University of Chicago, developed a custom-fitted cap with a one-way valve to permit the flow of cervical and menstrual secretions.[36] A wax impression of the woman's cervix is made, and a special machine is being developed that will laminate the cap in a matter of a few minutes. Since it has the one-way valve, this cap can be left in place throughout the menstrual cycle. Initial testing indicates that this cap, which may not require spermicide, is highly effective; however, large-scale testing is needed to determine use-effectiveness rates. Long-term studies are also needed to determine whether or not use of this cap, which is made of a special material that is sometimes used by orthopedic

95

surgeons to promote healing after bone surgery (the material is sewn into the wound and then removed at a later date), might have detrimental effects (although there are some preliminary indications suggesting that the cap might in fact improve vaginal health).

Women's groups across the country have been experimenting with caps imported from England. As of now, the FDA has not approved the cap as a method of birth control because of large-scale effectiveness and safety studies have not yet been done. If more government funds in the past had been devoted to barrier methods, we might have a perfected cap of proven effectiveness today. Thanks to the efforts of author Barbara Seaman, a nurse-practitioner named Irene Snair and groups like the New Hampshire Feminist Women's Health, the Emma Goldman Clinic in Detroit and others, the FDA is now considering funding these large-scale studies.

The Cervical Sponge

Another exciting and long overdue development in barrier methods is the cervical sponge. The sponge is another diaphragmlike device and is made from highly absorbent natural collagen sponge. Like the cap, the cervical sponge can be inserted well before intercourse and left in place for considerable periods of time. The sponge has been safety tested on female volunteers who had previously been sterilized. These women were able to wear the sponge for up to six weeks without experiencing any irritation. The sponge, with and without spermicides, is now being tested on female volunteers under the direction of Dr. James Heine, of the Texas Institute of Technology in Lubbock, Texas.[37] In the next couple of years, another highly convenient, safe barrier method may be available.

The Effectiveness vs. Safety Trade-Off

While these new advances in barrier methods are exciting, it is unfortunate that bias against these methods has delayed their development. Misinformation about barrier-method effectiveness has also had the unfortunate effect, as we pointed out earlier, of causing many women, who are led astray by the statistical lies about birth control effectiveness, to opt for the more dangerous Pill and IUD. Current trends in birth control usage are changing, however, and the Pill and the IUD are today declining in popularity.

Many couples, concerned about safety yet wanting maximum effectiveness, have chosen sterilization—either tubal ligation for females or vasectomy for males. In fact, sterilization is now the most widely used method of birth control for married couples in their 30s.[38] Although vasectomy appears to be a simple operation with very few serious side effects, there has been some concern about the fact that a number of vasectomized men develop antibodies to their own sperm.[39] Antibodies are substances produced by the body to attack germs and other foreign bodies. The long-term effects of this irregularity in the body's immune response is not known.

Female sterilization, despite the nickname of "Band-Aid surgery" given to certain sterilization procedures, is major surgery that has serious potential complications, including death. The risks are small, but they do exist. Moreover, there have been some recent studies indicating that women who have been sterilized have subsequent menstrual pain and excessive menstrual bleeding, as well as higher rates of hysterectomies and premature menopause than do nonsterilized women.[40]

Thus, although sterilization is undeniably the most effective method of birth control, it carries some risks and may have long-term effects whose ultimate impact on a person's health is unknown. In light of this, many men and women are rethinking sterilization decisions. We cannot help but feel that objective information about the effectiveness of barrier methods might be an influential factor for those considering sterilization.

As you may have gathered by now, we are fans of the barrier methods and encourage their use. On the other hand, we are not what we call "no freaks"—medical professionals who refuse to prescribe the Pill or the IUD. Our basic belief is that every women should be informed of the facts and then allowed to make her own decisions. If a woman is aware of the facts and chooses the Pill or the IUD, we support her right to make that decision and would not deny her access to the option she chooses. But we feel it is vital that she be well informed before making that decision. In the following reference section, we provide detailed information about each of the major methods: the Pill, the Mini-pill, the IUD, the diaphragm, the condom, foam, the cervical cap, abortion and postcoital contraception. We also include a section on natural family planning, a method of birth control that depends on a woman's learning to recognize when she is fertile and abstaining from intercourse during that time. This method may be particularly suitable for women who practice speculum self-exam. We do not include information on withdrawal, or coitus interruptus, in which the man withdraws before ejaculation, or on breastfeeding as methods of birth control because both of these methods are notoriously ineffective.

Reference Section:
Birth Control Methods

BIRTH CONTROL PILLS

AKA: the Pill, oral contraceptives, OCs

Types: combined pills or estrogen/progestin pills
Mini-pills or progestin-only pills

Birth control pills are tablets containing synthetic (manmade) hormones similar to the ones made by a woman's ovaries. Presently, there are two types of birth control pills marketed in this country: the combination pills, which contain both synthetic progesterone (progestin) and synthetic estrogen; and the Mini-pills, or progestin-only pills, which do not contain estrogen.

The Pill works by preventing the ovary from maturing an egg and releasing it at ovulation. By taking a daily dose of hormones, a woman's normal cyclical fluctuations in hormone levels are stopped and the complicated feedback mechanism that controls ovulation is interrupted. As you may recall from Chapter Four, the low levels of the ovarian hormones in the early part of the cycle stimulate the hypothalamus to produce its releasing factors, which in turn causes the pituitary to release two essential hormones, FSH, the follicle-stimulating hormone, and LH, the luteinizing hormone. The FSH acts on the egg-containing follicular sacs in the ovary, causing the eggs to mature. As they do so, the cells lining the inside of the sacs produce estrogen. Once the levels of estrogen are high enough, they trigger a spurt of LH, which causes the ripe egg to burst out of the ovary at ovulation.

The combined pill prevents this from happening by providing a daily dose of estrogen high enough to prevent the triggering of the hypothalamus and, indirectly, of the pituitary, which therefore doesn't produce FSH. Without FSH, there are no mature eggs, so fertilization cannot occur.

The Mini-pills don't contain estrogen, and they don't completely suppress the pituitary hormones, but the constant daily dose of progestin blocks or at least blunts the surge of LH. The majority of Mini-pill users, then, don't ovulate. A significant proportion do, but pregnancy is nonetheless prevented, for the pills also work in the following ways.

The progestin in both the Mini-pills and the combination pills alters the character of the mucus secreted by the glands in the cervix. Normally, the cervical mucus becomes more alkaline (sugary) at the time of ovulation, which nourishes the sperm. On a microscopic level, the molecules of the mucus realign themselves, forming tunnels to aid the sperm on their journey into the uterus. After ovulation, when the hormone progesterone is produced by the remnant of the burst follicular sac (the corpus luteum), the cervical mucus becomes hostile to sperm—more acid and thicker, with a cross-hatched molecular structure that blocks the sperm (see Illustration 14). The progestin—synthetic progesterone—in birth control pills has this same effect on the cervical mucus.

The uterine lining is also altered by the hormone stimulation of the Pill. Normally, the estrogen in the first part of the cycle stimulates the development of the uterine lining. The process is then completed by the progesterone in the second half of the cycle. With the combined pill and its continual stimulation of both estrogen and progesterone, there is not the normal alternation between the two hormones that is necessary in order for a uterine lining that is capable of nourishing a fertilized egg to develop. Similarly, the continual progestin stimulation of the Mini-pill alters the endometrial lining, making it impossible for a fertilized egg to implant in the uterus.

The hormones in both the combined and the Mini-pills may also change the normal contractions of the Fallopian tubes, which help the fertilized egg move through the tube into the uterus. In order to develop properly, the egg must spend a certain amount of time in the tubes, nourished by special tubal secretions. The Pill speeds up the tubal contractions, so that the egg reaches the uterus before it has matured properly. Therefore, it cannot successfully implant in the uterine wall.

Effectiveness

We are often told that the pills are 99 percent or "practically 100 percent" effective. This is a theoretical-effectiveness rate for combined pills containing at least 50 micrograms (mcg) of estrogen. Pills containing 35 mcg or less have a slightly lower theoretical rate of about 98 to 99 percent. Mini-pills have a theoretical rate of about 97 percent.

Actual-use—effectiveness rates may be considerably lower, for these rates reflect all the user-failures, that is, forgotten pills. Actual-use—effectiveness rates for the Mini-pill range from 87 to 97 percent.[1] Actual-use—effectiveness rates of 90 to 96 percent are generally quoted for the combined pill[2] although there have been studies with rates as low as 75 percent.[3]

How to Use the Pill

Combination pills are packaged in three different ways, 20-day, 21-day, and 28-day packs. The most common is the 21-day pack, which contains 21 hormone pills. With it, your schedule would be 21 days on, 7 days off, 21 days on, 7 days off and so forth. The 28-day pack contains 21 hormone pills and 7 blanks, which are tablets containing sugar and iron. With this pack you take the 21 hormone tablets first and then the 7 blanks. Once you have finished the pack, you begin a new pack immediately, with no days off. In the 28-day pack the 7 blanks are your seven days without hormones. You may start the 21- or 28-day packs any time during the first seven days of your normal menstrual cycle (Day 1 of your cycle is the first day of menstrual flow). If you start before Day 8, chances are you won't ovulate during that cycle, but most doctors recommend that you use a back-up method of birth control, such as foam, diaphragm or condom, for the first 14 days that you are on the Pill.

If you are using a 20-day pack, begin each new pack on the fifth day after your period starts or on the eighth day after you took your last pill, whichever comes first.

If you are using Mini-pills, you take a pill every day for as long as you want to prevent conception. There are no off days; you must take the Mini-pill during the time of your menstrual flow as well. To start on Mini-pills, take the first one on Day 1 of your menstrual period.

☐ Do not start on pills if there is any chance that you might be pregnant. If your last menstrual period seemed too light, too early or too late, tell your doctor.

☐ Try to take the pill at about the same time each day. This is especially important if you are taking Mini-pills.

☐ If you miss one combination pill, take two the next day. Take the missed pill as soon as you remember it and take your regular pill for that day at the usual time. If you are on Mini-pills, use another method of birth control in addition to the Mini-pill until your next period starts. (This is not necessary if you are using the combination pill.)

☐ If you miss two pills, take two each day for two days until you are caught up. Take the first missed pill as soon as you remember it and your regular pill for that day at the usual time. Take the second forgotten pill along with your regular pill at the normal time on the following day. Use a back-up method of birth control until your next period starts.

☐ If you miss three or more pills, stop using your pills until you have your period. If you are using combination pills, start a new pack as you normally would after your period starts. If you are using Mini-pills, begin a new pack on the first day of your period. Use a back-up method as soon as you discontinue the pills and continue to use the back-up method for two weeks after you have started your new pack.

☐ If you lose, damage or run out of pills, call your doctor. You can usually arrange for a refill with a telephone call so you won't have to interrupt your pill schedule. Many family-planning clinics, such as Planned Parenthood, will provide emergency refills if you are traveling or are unable to reach your doctor.

☐ If you have nausea, try taking your pill with dinner or in the evening. If you vomit within one hour of taking a pill, take another from a separate pack.

☐ If you are on combination pills and want to alter your menstrual cycle to avoid having your period at a certain time (during vacation, for example), you can change your cycle length by taking as many as seven additional pills (one pill per day) or by discarding one or two from your regular pack. Your period should start about 48 hours after you take your last pill. Regardless of whether you've brought your period on two days early or have delayed it for seven days, you must allow for your usual seven no-hormone days before starting your new pack.

☐ If you are using combination pills and do not have a period during your seven no-hormone pill days and are *absolutely sure* you have taken all your pills correctly, there is very little likelihood that you could be pregnant, so most doctors recommend that you go ahead and start your new pack as scheduled. We feel that this advice is acceptable for women who do not have religious or moral objections to abortion. But if you would not have an abortion under any circumstances, then, because there *is* a slight chance of being pregnant, you should use another method of birth control and have a pregnancy test before starting a new pack, since there is evidence that use of hormones during pregnancy can cause birth defects. If you have missed a period and are *not* sure that you have taken your pills correctly, there is a greater chance that you are pregnant. Stop taking the pills and see your doctor for testing. Similarly, if you miss two periods, regardless of whether or not you have taken your pills correctly, also stop the pills and see your doctor.

☐ If you are taking Mini-pills and do not have a period within 45 days of your last period, stop taking the pills and see your doctor for pregnancy testing.

☐ If you have spotting or bleeding while you are taking combination pills, continue on your pill schedule. This bleeding will usually stop after a few days and is not uncommon during the first couple of months of Pill usage. But if the bleeding is heavier than the bleeding you have on the heaviest days of your period, if you soak more than three sanitary napkins in an hour or if the spotting continues for more than one cycle, call your doctor so that s/he can examine you to rule out the possibility that the spotting is being caused by something other than the Pill. If you are using Mini-pills and have persistent spotting, you will also need to discuss this with your doctor. If you have a fever or abdominal pain along with the spotting, call your doctor at once, as you may have an infection or other serious problem.

☐ If you develop any of the following danger signs, see your doctor right away:

* Chest pain	* Dizziness or faintness
* Shortness of breath	* Muscle weakness or numbness
* Unusual coughing	* Speech disturbance
* Pain in the legs	* Vision changes or loss of vision
* Severe headache	* Severe depression
* Breast lump	* Yellowing of the skin

☐ Since certain drugs, including ampicillin, sulfa drugs, antihistamines (both prescription and over-the-counter varieties), tranquilizers like Librium, some antidepressants, sedatives like phenobarbital and some drugs taken for epilepsy, tuberculosis and arthritis, can decrease the effectiveness of birth control pills, you should switch to another method or use a back-up method while you are taking these drugs.

☐ Pills can also interact with insulin, anticoagulants, certain tranquilizers, Demerol (a pain medication) and tuberculin skin tests. Pills can alter the results of laboratory tests, so be sure to tell the doctor that you are a Pill user, even if you are being tested for a totally unrelated problem.

Advantages

The chief advantage to combination birth control pills is that, with the exception of sterilization, they offer the most effective method of birth control if they are used properly. The Mini-pills, while less effective, are still a highly reliable form of birth control. Another advantage is that they do not interfere with the spontaneity of lovemaking.

Pills offer other benefits in addition to contraception. For many women the greatest advantage of the Pill is that it offers them freedom from heavy bleeding and painful menstrual cramps. With the Pill, periods are regular, light and predictable. The Pill also allows women to manipulate their periods to allow for vacations or other such events in their schedules.

Because there is a reduction in menstrual blood loss, deficiency anemia is less common among Pill users. Since the Pill suppresses ovulation, Pill users have a lower incidence of ovarian cysts. Ovulation pain (mittelschmerz) doesn't usually affect Pill users. Many women find that acne improves.

Problems and Disadvantages

As more time has passed and greater numbers of women have used the Pill, our knowledge about side effects and complications has grown considerably. There are now more than fifty side effects and complications that may be associated with Pill usage. In some cases, the association between Pill usage and a side effect or complication has been clearly established. In other cases, the evidence for a cause-effect relationship is strong but not conclusive. In still others, the relationship is only speculative. There may also be other as yet undiscovered side effects and complications. Research is still being done. Something that is thought to be a possible complication today may be either confirmed or refuted in the future. For example blood-clotting disorders, which are responsible for most Pill-related deaths, were at one time only a suspected complication. There was no proof that Pill usage actually increased a woman's risk for such disorders. But today that relationship has been well documented. Women who choose to use oral contraceptives should keep up to date on the latest findings.

Some Pill-related problems are thought to be associated specifically with the estrogen in the Pill, and some with the progestin, but often it is not possible to say which hormone is responsible. The Mini-pill is generally considered safer than the combination pill, but most of the side effects and complications listed below may be caused by either type of Pill.

Changes in the Menstrual Cycle

The menstrual period usually becomes shorter, and the blood flow is usually lighter. Normally, the uterine lining is built up by the rising levels of ovarian hormones at different points in the cycle. Since women on the Pill do not experience these same peaks of hormone production, they don't build up as much of a lining; hence, there is less menstrual flow. Pill users may experience spotting or bleeding between periods, which is called breakthrough bleeding. This happens because there is not enough hormone present to maintain the endometrial lining, so some of it sloughs off. This may also happen if you miss a pill. Such bleeding does not mean that the contraceptive effect is not working, however. It is most common in the first few months of Pill use, as the uterus is adjusting to altered hormone levels. If, however, it persists, you should see a doctor.

Some women on the Pill cease to have menstrual periods and do not resume menstruation after discontinuing its use, a condition known as ammenorrhea. This is most likely to happen to women who had menstrual irregularities before going on the Pill.

Many women experience relief from menstrual cramps on the Pill since ovulation no longer occurs. Many also experience relief of premenstrual syndrome symptoms; for other women, however, menstrual cramps and other menstrual symptoms may be intensified by the Pill.

Breast Tenderness and Swelling

Breast tenderness and swelling are not uncommon side effects. Sometimes this problem passes after one or two months, but it may persist.

Skin Changes

A Pill high in estrogen often improves acne; the Mini-pill or a Pill high in progestins may increase skin oiliness. Some women have an allergic reaction to the Pill and break out in skin rashes; others become more sensitive to sunlight (become sunburned more easily, for example). The Pill may affect the pigment (color) cells of the skin and a few women develop a condition called chloasma, in which areas of the skin become darker.

Vaginal Discharge

The estrogen in the Pill may cause an increase in vaginal discharge. The Pill also alters the acid/alkaline balance of the vagina, making the vaginal environment more conducive to disease-causing organisms. Women on the Pill seem to be particularly susceptible to yeast infections. They may be more susceptible to other forms of vaginitis and certain sexually transmitted diseases as well.

Weight Gain, Bloating, Fluid Retention, Headaches, Nausea and Vomiting

These symptoms are common side effects in Pill users. For some women they are not serious problems; for others they are and cause these women to discontinue using the Pill.

Cervical Problems

Cervical erosions and eversions are all more common in Pill users. In one large-scale study Pill users had a rate of cervical erosion and ulcerations of 9.4 per 1,000, whereas diaphragm users had a rate of 4.82 and IUD users 3.03 per 1,000.[4]

Bronchitis and Viral Infections

Women who use the Pill have higher rates of bronchitis and of virus infections like flu, chicken pox and colds.[5] The reason for these increased rates is not known. Some theorize that since the Pill decreases the level of infection-fighting gamma globulin protein in the blood, users are more susceptible to illness. On the other hand, some argue that perhaps Pill users are simply more likely to have intercourse with greater frequency and are therefore exposed to more disease-causing organisms.

Urinary Tract Infections

Some reports indicate that women on the Pill are more susceptible to urinary tract infections, that is, bladder and kidney infections. Some women report relief of chronic urinary tract infections after discontinuing the Pill.

Fibroid Tumors

Fibroid tumors, benign tumors of the uterus affecting perhaps as many as one in every five women, are estrogen-sensitive and their growth may be stimulated by the estrogen in the Pill. Although these tumors are benign, they can cause problems if they grow large and may necessitate a hysterectomy.

Sex Drive

Reports of the Pill's effect on sex drive are contradictory. Some women report an increase, some a decrease; others don't notice any change. Some researchers point to studies showing that many women experience an increase in sex drive at the time of ovulation and theorize that the Pill's suppression of ovulation might account for a lessened sex drive.

Circulatory Disorders

Women who use birth control pills are at greater risk for the development of circulatory disorders such as abnormal blood clotting, heart attack and stroke. Whether it is the estrogen or the progestin in the Pill that is responsible is not entirely clear. Most Pill-related deaths are due to circulatory disorders.

Several different types of clotting disorders have been associated with Pill usage, including:

Thrombophlebitis: This is a condition in which plugs, clots or pieces of blood are attached to the wall of a vein or artery. These clots may become detached and travel to other parts of the body, in which case they are called emboli, and can cause crippling or even fatal complications, depending on where they lodge. Symptoms include a knot or swelling and heat or redness in the calf or thigh.

Pulmonary embolism: If a clot travels to the lung, it may cause a heart attack. Symptoms include chest pain, cough and shortness of breath.

Myocardial infarction: This blood-clot—related heart attack can produce such symptoms as chest pain, pain in the left arm and shoulder, difficulty in breathing and weakness.

Cerebral infarction: Also called a stroke, this blood clot in the brain can cause headaches, numbness, weakness, visual problems and intellectual impairment.

Retinal vein thrombosis: This is a blood clot in the eye, which can cause symptoms such as loss of vision and headaches.

Pelvic vein thrombosis: This is a blood clot in the pelvic veins that may produce lower-abdominal pain and cramps.

Any of these conditions may have serious or fatal consequences. The Pill definitely increases the risk of developing these conditions. For instance, for Pill users ages 15 to 34 the risk of death due to a circulatory disorder is about one in 12,000 per year, while for nonusers it is only about one in 50,000. The risk of hospitalization for a clotting disorder is also increased. Nonusers ages 20 to 44 have about a one in 20,000 risk, while Pill users have a one in 2,000 risk, a ten-fold increase.

The use of oral contraceptives may double the risk of heart attack. That's bad enough, but if a woman is both a Pill user and a smoker, her chances of having a heart attack are even greater. Such women are five times more likely to have a heart attack than users who do not smoke and ten times more likely to have a heart attack than women who neither smoke nor use the Pill. Age is also a factor in this risk equation. If you are a Pill user between the ages of 30 and 39, you have a one in 10,000 chance each year of having a fatal heart attack if you smoke and a one in 50,000 chance if you are a user but don't smoke, as compared to a one in 100,000 chance for women who do not smoke or use the Pill. For older women the odds are more frightening. In the 40 to 44 year-old age group, a woman who neither uses the Pill nor smokes has a one in 14,000 chance of having a fatal heart attack, but if a woman both uses the Pill and smokes, her chances are one in 1,700. For this reason women who are smokers or are over 35 (some say 40) should not use this method of birth control. Risk also seems to increase for women who have used the Pill for five years or more, so some doctors limit the years of Pill usage. The risks continue as long as you use the Pill and may continue for some time afterward as well.

In addition to blood-clotting disorders, women who take the Pill are twice as likely as nonusers to have a stroke due to rupture of a blood vessel in the brain.

Gallbladder Disease

A number of studies have documented the fact that Pill users are at increased risk for developing gallbladder disease. In one study an increased risk was evident after two years of use and doubled after four or five years of use. In another study increased risk was apparent between six and twelve months of use.

Liver Problems

Women who use birth control pills have an increased risk of developing benign liver tumors. It is not entirely clear whether this is solely an estrogen effect or whether both estrogen and progestin are to blame. Although these tumors are noncancerous, they have been known to rupture and cause death. Cancerous liver tumors have also been reported in women taking the Pill, but whether these rare cancerous tumors actually occur more frequently in Pill users is not yet known.

Women who have a history of jaundice, a liver problem that leads to an accumulation of yellow pigment in the eyes and skin and thus gives the skin a yellow tinge, may get jaundice again if they take the Pill. Since the liver is responsible for breaking down estrogen and eliminating it from the body, women with impaired liver function should not use the Pill.

High Blood Pressure

Large studies involving thousands of women have indicated that 5 to 7 percent of all women on the Pill will develop abnormally high blood pressure, a condition known as hypertension, which puts a woman at higher risk for heart attacks and a type of stroke caused by burst blood vessels in the brain. Though only 5 to 7 percent develop hypertension, many women on the Pill experience some elevation of blood pressure. The long-term effects of having elevated blood pressure that is still within the normal range are not known. The blood pressure usually reverts to normal within six months following discontinuation of the Pill, but there is some evidence that some of the changes associated with Pill-related high blood pressure may persist, at least in some women.

Certain women are more prone to Pill-related hypertension: those with a family history of hypertension, women over 40 and overweight women. Black women in general are more prone to hypertension; whether they are more prone to develop hypertension when on the Pill than white women are is not known. There are contradictory reports as to whether women with a history of toxemia, a type of hypertension found during pregnancy, are more prone to develop a rise in blood pressure if they use the Pill.

All women on the Pill should have their blood pressure checked once every six to twelve months.

Birth Defects

Estrogen can cause birth defects. Some of these defects have been caused by the use of synthetic estrogens during pregnancy. Others have been associated specifically with birth control pills, and it is not entirely clear whether these are due to the estrogen or the progestin in the Pill. In any case, neither of the female hormones should be used if pregnancy is a possibility.

Women whose mothers took certain estrogens during pregnancy have an increased risk of developing some forms of cancer later in life. They also face an increased risk of certain benign diseases of the vagina and cervix, some of which may be precancerous. Fertility may be affected as well. The sons of such women may also develop certain abnormalities. This topic is discussed more fully under the heading DES.

Not only are risks of birth defects increased if hormones are taken during pregnancy, but there is also evidence that taking birth control pills *prior* to pregnancy can also cause problems in the embryo. One study showed a dramatic increase in a rare type of chromosomal aberration in the aborted embryoes of women who conceived within three months of discontinuing the Pill.

Recent studies have refuted the claim that hormones taken *prior* to conception can cause birth defects or higher rates of miscarriages.[6,7,8] Despite these new, more favorable reports, most doctors still suggest that women who stop the Pill in order to become pregnant use another form of contraception for three months before they attempt to conceive.

Since pills have been implicated in birth defects, these hormones should never be taken during pregnancy. Women who miss one or more pills during a cycle and then don't have a period after the last pill, should get a pregnancy test prior to starting a new box of pills. If a woman accidentally takes a pill after becoming pregnant, she should consider the possibility of abortion.

Ectopic Pregnancy

The likelihood of ectopic pregnancy, in which the fertilized egg implants in the Fallopian tube or some other inappropriate location, is higher if you become pregnant while using the Mini-pill. Ectopic pregnancies can have serious complications, including death. Any Mini-pill user who suspects pregnancy should insist on the most sensitive type of pregnancy test (p. 756) since routine pregnancy tests may fail to detect an ectopic pregnancy.

Infertility

As noted earlier, some women do not resume normal ovulation and menstruation after discontinuing the Pill. One recent study suggested that temporary infertility may be a problem for some Pill users who have never had previous pregnancies.[9] After 30 months the former Pill users had 5 percent fewer pregnancies than former users of other methods of contraception; however, after 40 months there was no difference between the groups. A delay of 40 months, or about three-and-one-third years, might not be a significant problem for a woman in her 20s, but since the chances of conception decrease and the chances of birth defects increase as a woman gets older, this might be a problem for a woman in her 30s.

Breast Milk

The use of birth control pills may reduce the quantity and quality of breast milk. Small amounts of Pill hormones have been found in the breast milk of nursing mothers using oral contraceptives. The effect of these hormones on the infant is unknown, so it is suggested that nursing mothers not take the Pill.

Depression

Some Pill users experience depression. Studies designed to investigate the relationship between the Pill and depression have produced contradictory results. Some studies, including one of the largest and most thorough studies ever done, reported a 30 percent increase in depression in oral contraceptive users. Other studies have reported a decrease in depression, and still others have failed to find any difference in the incidence of depression between users and nonusers.

The depression experienced by some Pill users may be related to the fact that some Pill users are deficient in vitamin B_6. Depression may subside when such women take supplementary vitamin B_6.

Thyroid Gland

The Pill can cause changes in the results of some of the tests used to measure thyroid function. Although these test results are altered, the thyroid gland itself is apparently not affected, for other, more sensitive thyroid tests do not indicate changes in its function.

Pituitary Tumors

Recently there has been some evidence that estrogen in the Pill can, if not cause them, at least stimulate the growth of preexisting benign tumors in the pituitary gland.[10] As many as 5 to 10 percent of the population probably have microscopic pituitary tumors that never become large enough to cause problems. If a woman with a microscopic pituitary tumor takes the Pill, however, tumor growth may be stimulated and the tumor may eventually require treatment.

Eye Problems

The Pill, on rare occasions, has caused inflammation of the optic nerve, loss of vision, double vision, pain and swelling. Because the Pill causes fluid retention, the shape of the eyeball may be altered, with the result that some women who use the Pill may have to have their contact lens prescriptions changed; other women find that they can't use contacts at all.

Lipid Content

The Pill alters many metabolic and chemical processes in the blood. Lipid content, for instance, is increased. Lipids are potentially harmful chemical substances found in the blood. Fatty acids, cholesterol, phospholipids and triglycerides are all lipids that may be affected by the Pill. It has been theorized that these substances contribute to arteriosclerosis, or hardening of the arteries, which makes the arteries more prone to blockage by a blood clot and may account, in part, for the blood-clotting problems experienced by Pill users.

Vitamin and Mineral Metabolism

The Pill may affect the way in which the body uses vitamins and minerals. Studies of Pill users have indicated deficiencies in folic acid, trace minerals, riboflavin, thiamine and vitamins B_6, B_{12}, C and E.[11,12,13] As noted earlier, depression has been relieved in some Pill users by the use of a vitamin-B supplement. Some doctors prescribe vitamin supplements for Pill users.

On the other hand, the Pill increases the levels of certain other nutriments. Vitamin K levels, for instance, are higher in some Pill users. Since vitamin K influences blood-clotting factors, some researchers have linked these higher levels of K to the blood-clotting disorders that are the source of most Pill-related deaths.

Sugar Metabolism and Diabetes

The Pill alters the way in which the body metabolizes sugar. Women on the Pill with previously normal test results may develop abnormal glucose tolerance, or sugar tolerance, tests like those of women who have diabetes, a disease in which the body is unable to metabolize sugar properly. These women do not, however, have the symptoms of diabetes, but no one knows what the long-term effects of this stress on the body will be. Test results usually return to normal after the Pill is discontinued; however, in a few cases, abnormal test results have persisted.

Because of the Pill's effect on blood-sugar levels, most doctors will not prescribe the Pill for women who have borderline test results prior to going on the Pill.

Skin Cancer

A recent study showed that Pill users were more likely than nonusers to develop a form of skin cancer that involves skin pigment cells.[14] The difference between the groups were small, and the finding may have been coincidental. Further studies must be done in order to confirm or deny this relationship. The fact that the overall rates for this type of skin cancer are increasing and that the Pill is known to affect the skin pigment cells (see Skin Changes, above) suggests that there may be a relationship between the Pill and skin cancer. Any suspicious sores, moles or other growths should be brought to a doctor's attention.

Cervical Cancer

Most studies have failed to demonstrate a relationship between cervical cancer and Pill usage; however, a recent long-term study indicated that women with precancerous conditions, such as dysplasia, are more likely than non-Pill users to have their dysplasia progress to the more serious carcinoma in situ.[15] Many doctors feel that women with a history of dysplasia should not use birth control pills.

Uterine Cancer

The sequential birth control pills were withdrawn from the market because they were linked with the development of cancer of the endometrial lining of the uterus. The combination pills now on the market have not been associated with endometrial cancer. However, estrogen used by postmenopausal women has been strongly linked to the development of uterine cancer. Some researchers feel that this should not alarm women who take birth control pills since the Pill also contains synthetic progesterone and progesterone has a counterbalancing effect that is sometimes used to reverse precancerous changes in the uterus. Other researchers, however, point out that women who are on the Pill do not ovulate and women who do not ovulate have a higher incidence of endometrial cancer. The evidence regarding the Pill and endometrial cancer is somewhat contradictory, and firm conclusions cannot be drawn at this time.

Breast Cancer

Thus far, most studies have not indicated a relationship between Pill usage and breast cancer. Critics of these studies argue that not enough time has yet elapsed for any cancerous effects on the breast to have become obvious.

Some disturbing facts have come to light in recent years. A preliminary study has indicated that women who took estrogen for menopausal symptoms may be at increased risk for the development of breast cancer.[16] Women who took synthetic estrogens during their pregnancies may also be at increased risk.[17] The implications that these studies may have for Pill users are not yet known.

Many studies have shown a decreased risk for the development of benign breast diseases in Pill users. Since having benign breast disease decreases the risk of developing breast cancer, some authorities have felt that Pill usage would decrease breast cancer risk; however, this has not been demonstrated. Moreover, one study suggests that women who already had benign disease and then took the Pill had a greater chance of developing breast cancer than non-Pill users with benign disease.[18] It may be that the Pill can act as a fertilizer—if not a seed—for breast cancer, perhaps stimulating the growth of preexisting cancers.

Contraindications

A contraindication is a medical condition that makes the use of a certain type of drug or form of treatment inadvisable. Because of the controversy that has surrounded the Pill, there is a good deal of disagreement as to exactly who should and shouldn't use birth control pills. The following list of contraindications is divided into three parts: 1. absolute contraindications, with which all doctors would agree; 2. strong contraindications, with which most doctors would agree; and 3. relative contraindications, with which many, but not all doctors, would agree. Since the combination pills contain estrogen, they are sometimes contraindicated where the Mini-pill would not be.

Absolute Contraindications (Women with these conditions should definitely not take the Pill):

☐ Blood-clotting disorders, such as thrombophlebitis and pulmonary embolism
☐ Heart attack, stroke or angina (heart pain)
☐ Impaired liver function
☐ Coronary artery disease
☐ Known or suspected cancer of the breast, uterus, cervix, ovaries, vagina or elsewhere in the female reproductive tract
☐ Pregnancy or suspected pregnancy

Strong Contraindications (Women with these conditions who take the Pill may be vulnerable to serious health problems):

☐ Pregnancy within the last 10 to 14 days, including childbirth, abortion or miscarriage
☐ History of severe headaches
☐ High blood pressure now or during pregnancy in the past
☐ Diabetes or a strong family history of diabetes
☐ Gallbladder disease or gallbladder surgery now or in the past
☐ Jaundice during pregnancy in the past, a condition known as cholestasis

☐ Mononucleosis now or in the recent past
☐ Sickle-cell disease
☐ Undiagnosed abnormal uterine bleeding
☐ Major surgery planned in the next month
☐ Leg casts or major injury to the lower leg
☐ Fibrocystic breast disease or fibroadenoma of the breast, abnormal breast X-rays in the past, or close family history of breast cancer.
☐ Age 35 to 40 or older
☐ Heavy smoker (15+ cigarettes a day)
☐ Cervical dysplasia

Relative Contraindications (Women with these conditions may want to avoid the Pill):

☐ History of serious heart or kidney disease
☐ History of heavy smoking
☐ Failure to have established regular menstrual cycles or history of irregular menstrual patterns
☐ Breastfeeding
☐ Five or more years of Pill use
☐ Previous exposure to DES-type drugs
☐ Fibroids (tumors of the uterus)
☐ Severe asthma
☐ Severe varicose veins
☐ Epilepsy
☐ Serious depression or suicidal feelings
☐ History of hepatitis
☐ History of hair loss or chloasma (darkening of the facial skin during previous pregnancy or Pill use)
☐ Sickle-cell trait
☐ High cholesterol levels
☐ Recurrent urinary tract infections

INTRAUTERINE DEVICE

AKA: IUD, loop, coil

Types: Lippes Loop
Saf-T-Coil
Copper-7
Copper-T
Progestasert, or progestin-releasing device

Intrauterine devices, or IUDs (Illustration 18) are small plastic devices that are inserted by a doctor or a trained medical person into the uterus. They prevent pregnancy as long as they remain in place. Most IUDs may be left in the uterus for considerable periods of time and should be removed only by a doctor.

How the IUD Works

Despite the fact that they've been around for some time, no one is quite sure how IUDs work. One theory is that the IUD irritates the uterus so much that it triggers the body's defense mechanisms, which literally "eat up" either the sperm or the fertilized egg. Another theory is that the fertilized egg may not be able to attach itself to the irritated uterine lining. Still another theory holds that the IUD works by mechanically dislodging the implanted egg, a sort of miniabortion. There is also the theory that the IUD somehow speeds up the movement of the egg through the Fallopian tube. Since the time the egg spends moving through the tube is critical to its proper development, too short a time in the tube will result in an egg too immature to successfully implant in the uterine wall.

Types

There are several types of IUDs currently available. The most widely used are the Lippes Loop, which comes in sizes A, B, C and D; the Saf-T-Coil, available in the nulliparous size for women who have never had children and the standard size for women who have given birth; the Copper-7, which is also called the Copper-7-200, 7Cu200 or CU7 Gravigard, available in one size; the Copper-T, also known as the Copper-T-200 and Tu200; and the Progestasert, or Progesterone-T, which contains a synthetic progesterone.

The original IUDs were made of plastic. Later models also included copper or a synthetic form of the hormone progesterone (progestin) embedded in the plastic. The copper was added to the Copper-7 and Copper-T and some Lippes Loops to enhance the contraceptive abilities since copper has sperm-killing effects. Also, it was thought that the copper would relax uterine contractions and would therefore relieve cramping problems. The progestin was added because it changed the character of the cervical secretions (*see* page 70), making it difficult for the sperm to pass through the cervix and into the uterus, and because it was thought that the progestin would reduce the bleeding problems associated with IUDs.

Three other types of IUDs—the Majzlin Spring, the Birnberg Bow and

Illustration 18   *Types of IUDs*

the Dalkon Shield—were formerly available in the United States but have now been withdrawn from the market because they were associated with some of the serious problems discussed below.

The Dalkon Shield

The Dalkon Shield has received the most publicity. The device was withdrawn after a somewhat lengthy battle between the manufacturer, the Food and Drug Administration and women's health-care activists.[19] It was thought that the strings of this particular IUD, which were twined together like a candle wick, served as a ladder to permit infection to travel up the strings into the uterus, causing serious pelvic infection that necessitated hysterectomy in some women and resulted in infertility and even death in others (see below).

When the bad news about the Dalkon Shield first became public, Planned Parenthood encouraged all women under their care to have the device removed. Many gynecologists throughout the country have not followed this policy, so there are still many American women who still have Dalkon Shields. Any woman who has a Dalkon Shield should contact her doctor or a Planned Parenthood clinic. It is our policy to explain the situation to women who have Dalkon Shields or other banned devices and to encourage removal. Most women, apprised of the facts, decide to have their Shields removed.

Recently, the Dalkon Shield has become the subject of even more controversy.[20] The device, though no longer available in the United States, has been exported to other countries with the aid of American-based population control groups. These devices were sold at reduced rates in unsterilized bulk packaging for use in Third World countries. Normally the devices are sterilized and packaged individually with inserters. Women in other parts of the world who have IUDs inserted are still receiving Dalkon Shields.

The Dalkon Shield is not the only IUD that has raised doubts in the medical community. Recently, the use of the progesterone devices, which seem to be associated with higher rates of ectopic pregnancies, that is, pregnancies that implant in the Fallopian tube or other abnormal location, has been questioned.[21] The Lippes Loop also came under scrutiny at the time of the Dalkon Shield investigations; however, the Food and Drug Administration did not consider the data sufficient to ban it as well.[22]

The National Women's Health Network has established a registry for IUD-related problems. Women who have suffered such problems can contact them by writing to NWHN, 2025 I Street NW, Suite 105, Washington, DC 20006.

Effectiveness

The effectiveness rates quoted by the FDA tell us that somewhere between one and six pregnancies will occur in a group of 100 women using the IUD for a year.[23]* For some types of IUD, this figure may be as low as two to three pregnancies per 100 women-years of use.[24] Though the rates of effectiveness seem to vary depending upon which particular device is used, it is hard to evaluate relative effectiveness since the women in these various studies are not well-matched in terms of age, background, proven fertility and other important factors.

This is the one method of birth control in which the theoretical rate most closely matches the actual-use rate, for there is no pill to take each day, no diaphragm and foam or condom to put into place. The failures occur because the woman has an ectopic pregnancy, the IUD has been expelled without the woman's knowing it or the device has perforated the uterus or has simply not done its job. The failures are method- not user-failures.

Insertion

The IUD must be inserted by a doctor or other medical person specifically trained to do so. It is important to have an experienced person insert the IUD, for improper insertion can cause the IUD to perforate, that is, to make a hole in the uterus. Unfortunately, it is difficult for a woman to be sure the person inserting her IUD is experienced. Even if she goes to a family-planning clinic or a Planned Parenthood clinic where IUD insertion is done frequently, it might be her lot to get an intern who has relatively little experience. One rule of thumb is to not accept an IUD from someone who tries to talk you out of that method of birth control, for their negative attitude, although perhaps justifiable, will probably mean that they don't routinely insert IUDs.

Insertion of the IUD should require two office visits. A woman should never accept an IUD from a doctor who offers to fit her on the first visit, for a thorough medical history, physical exam, blood test for anemia, Pap smear, wet smear and gonorrhea culture must be done first. These tests will rule out the possibility of undiagnosed pregnancy or disease or abnormality of the uterus, all of which could cause serious complications if an IUD were inserted.

Once the results of these tests are in, assuming everything is OK, the doctor can determine the position, shape and depth of the uterus with an instrument called a uterine sound. This step should not be ignored, for it is important in preventing perforations of the uterus (see below).

*For an explanation of birth control effectiveness terminology, see Chapter Five.

Once all of this has been done and the cervix has been washed with an antiseptic solution the IUD is retracted back into an inserter tube, which is a hollow tube about the diameter of a straw. The tube is then gently pushed through the cervical os, the opening into the uterus. The IUD is then released from the inserter tube (Illustration 19). If the cervical opening is quite narrow, it may be necessary to dilate it with a special instrument before insertion.

Insertion may be painful. The degree of pain varies from woman to woman. There is usually less pain for women who have had children or when the device is inserted immediately after delivery. For some women, especially for women who have never given birth, the pain may be quite intense. Some doctors inject a painkiller into the cervix, which blocks most, if not all, of the pain. Some women need to take a painkiller for the first few days following insertion.

There is usually some bleeding after insertion, lasting anywhere from a few hours to several days. About one-half of all new IUD users have bleeding between their periods for the first couple of months.

There is some controversy about when an IUD should be inserted. Many doctors favor inserting the IUD during a woman's period since the cervical os is more open at this time and insertion is therefore less painful. Moreover, there is less chance of a woman's having an undiagnosed pregnancy. Other doctors feel that there may be a greater chance of infection at this time. Some doctors will insert an IUD immediately after an abortion or after childbirth, when the cervix is softened and more open, which makes insertion easier and less painful; but others point out that there is a higher rate of expulsion when IUDs are inserted at this time and that the risk of perforation is greater since the uterus is softened. Some feel that the risk of infection is higher as well. Moreover, the bleeding that occurs after delivery or abortion may mask the more serious bleeding that may accompany perforation.

After the IUD is inserted, the doctor clips the strings, leaving a few inches of string protruding from the os so that the woman can feel strings with her fingers and thus check that the IUD is still in place.

Some women's sexual partners complain that the strings of the IUD can be felt or, in some cases, that they actually cause them pain. This problem may be alleviated over time as the strings are softened by vaginal and cervical secretions. If the problem persists and is a serious concern, some doctors will snip the strings off. We do not recommend such a procedure. It is better to switch methods of birth control, for without the strings a woman has no way of knowing whether or not the IUD is still in place.

It is important to check the IUD strings regularly—at least once a month, right after the menstrual cycle (when some authorities feel expulsion is more likely), and preferably more often, especially during the first few months, when expulsion rates are highest. Checking is

Illustration 19 *Insertion of the IUD: The IUD is placed inside the inserter tube (A). The tube is inserted through the cervix into the uterus (B). The IUD is released into the uterus and the inserter tube withdrawn (C).*

important, for if the strings cannot be felt, this may mean that the IUD has been expelled, that it has become embedded in the uterine wall or that it has actually perforated (made a hole in) the uterus, which can lead to an unwanted pregnancy or other serious problems (see below).

A change of string length is also important. If the strings suddenly seem longer, this indicates that the IUD is too low in the uterine cavity—possibly embedded in the cervix—and if so, is less effective in preventing pregnancy. Shortened strings may mean that the IUD is embedded in the uterus or is in the process of perforating the uterus.

The cost of IUD insertion may run anywhere from a low of around $10 at a family planning clinic to a high of $100 at a Park Avenue gynecologist's office.

How Long Should an IUD Be Left in Place?

Another area of controversy surrounding the IUD concerns the question of how long the device should be left in place. It is generally agreed that the progestin-releasing devices (Progestasert) should be removed every year. The manufacturers recommend that the copper devices be removed every three years because the IUD tends to become covered with calcium deposits that prevent the release of the copper upon which the device partially depends for its effectiveness. Because of the dangers of perforation and infection involved in IUD insertion (see below), we recommend that other types of IUDs not be removed unless there are problems or the woman wishes to become pregnant or to use another method of birth control.

Advantages and Benefits

The chief advantage of the IUD is its convenience. There is no pill to remember to take. It is put in once and can remain in place for a considerable amount of time. It does not require any interruption of lovemaking, as do the condom, diaphragm and foam. In addition to the fact that it is convenient, the IUD is also highly effective.

Problems and Disadvantages

There are a number of problems involved in using IUDs.

Contraindications

Not all women can tolerate an IUD, and certain women should not use one. There is some difference of opinion among doctors as to what exactly these contraindications are; however, it is universally agreed that IUDs should not be used by women with the following conditions:

☐ Gonorrhea or any other acute infection of the organs of the pelvic cavity
☐ A known or suspected pregnancy
☐ Abnormal uterine bleeding
☐ Cancer of the pelvic organs
☐ Severe obstruction of the cervical canal
☐ Certain congenital deformities of the uterus
☐ Certain heart diseases involving the valves
☐ Fibroid tumors of the uterus
☐ Use of anticoagulants
☐ Sickle-cell disease
☐ Anemia
☐ A small uterus (less than 6.5 cm)

Some doctors would add to this list of contraindications a history of repeated pelvic infections, recent childbirth or abortion and abnormally heavy or prolonged menstrual periods. The reasons for their feeling this way are discussed below.

Safety

One of the biggest concerns with the IUD is safety. The FDA's official estimate is that the mortality (death) rate from the intrauterine device is between one and ten deaths per million women-years of use.[25] While the odds of even ten per million do not seem too risky, the odds on complications serious enough to require hospitalization are less reassuring, ranging from one in 300 to one in 100 per year.[26] Moreover, this figure includes only complications serious enough to require hospitalization. If complications not requiring hospitalization were added, the figures would be much higher.

Bleeding and Pain

The most common problem for IUD users is increased bleeding, often accompanied by cramplike discomfort or lower back pain. This increased bleeding may take the form of a greater volume of flow, longer duration of menstrual periods and/or spotting between periods. It is estimated that between 5 and 15 percent of all IUD users will have their IUDs removed within 12 months because of these types of problems.[27]

The amount of blood lost may increase as much as two- or threefold for some women. The blood loss is related to the type of IUD. The copper devices increase the bleeding, but not as much as the Loop, Saf-T-Coil and other nonmedicated IUDs. The progestin-releasing IUDs do not increase the overall volume of flow and in some cases may even decrease it, at least temporarily, but they may prolong the length of the menstrual period.[28]

Some evidence suggests that women with heavier than normal periods before IUD insertion experience a smaller increase in bleeding than do other women after IUD insertion.[29] In some cases, there may even be a decrease in bleeding. So, while some doctors think women with heavy periods should not use IUDs, others, with this evidence in mind, feel that IUDs are an acceptable form of contraception for such women.

The length of the menstrual period is also prolonged, anywhere from one-half day to four days, depending on which study you read and which IUD is used. Some researchers now feel that the progestin devices are more likely to cause longer periods.

Bleeding between periods may occur with any type of IUD, but again seems to be somewhat more frequent with the progestin devices. This bleeding is usually of the spotting type.

IUDs have also been associated with increased menstrual pain. This usually takes the form of increased cramplike pain in the lower abdomen and back and is thought to be associated with the contractions caused by the uterus as it attempts to expel the foreign body.

Besides the inconvenience associated with prolonged and heavier periods and the discomfort of increased cramps, anemia may be a problem if too much blood is lost. If a woman becomes anemic as a result of blood loss from her IUD, she should have the IUD removed and use another form of birth control.

Vaginal Discharge and Infection

IUD users tend to have a characteristic discharge that is watery, mucuslike and odorless. It causes no itching or burning and is believed to be due to the IUD strings stimulating the mucus glands in the cervix.

Women who wear IUDs may be more susceptible to the common vaginal infections, which, though not serious, can be extremely bothersome.

Pelvic inflammatory Disease

Many authorities feel that women using an IUD run a greater risk of pelvic inflammatory disease than do non-IUD users. Their estimates of increased risk run from 1.7 to 9.3 times higher for users than nonusers.[30]

Those who believe that there is an increase in pelvic inflammatory disease in IUD users theorize that either the chronic state of inflammation associated with IUD usage makes the uterus less able to defend itself against infection or that the strings of the IUD serve as a ladder for infections to ascend into the uterus. It is also thought that a woman who has an IUD and contracts gonorrhea may be more likely to have the disease progress to its more serious stage, in which it moves beyond the cervix into the uterus, the tubes and the pelvic cavity.

Pelvic inflammatory disease, whether gonorrheal or nongonorrheal, can be a serious disease requiring hospitalization. If the bacteria spread beyond the uterus and infect the tubes and other pelvic structures, the tubes and ovaries may become matted together in a ball of pus (tubo-ovarian abscess), which, if it ruptures, may produce an overwhelming reaction and a dramatic drop in blood pressure. This condition, known as septic shock, may be fatal. Fertility may also be impaired. Pelvic inflammatory disease doesn't always produce such dramatic symptoms, but even if the symptoms are so mild as to go unrecognized, the disease can still cause infertility. The question of IUDs and pelvic inflammatory disease is an important one. Some doctors feel that women who have a history of recurring pelvic infections should not use an IUD. In any case, it is important to have a test to rule out gonorrhea and other infections before an IUD is inserted, for insertion could cause an infection to spread up into the uterus.

Expulsion and Perforation

Another problem with the IUD is that some women's bodies don't tolerate the IUD very well and the device is expelled. Sometimes, a woman is aware that the device has been expelled, but in about 20 percent of the cases she is not.[31]

Studies have shown that between 5 and 20 percent of IUD users will have expelled it by the end of one year.[32] The expulsion rates are influenced by the age of the user, whether or not she has had children, when the device was inserted, the amount of time that has elapsed after insertion, the skill of the person inserting the device and the size and type of the device.

Since a woman may become pregnant after expulsion of her IUD, any woman considering an IUD should be aware of the possibility that she may expel the device and should check the IUD strings regularly. Women who have never had children and women with small uteri do not tolerate the IUDs as well as other women. Older women are among those who tolerate them better. Even among women who have had children, the expulsion rate is higher for women under 30 than for those over 30.[33]

The skill of the person inserting the IUD also affects expulsion rates, as demonstrated by the fact that certain centers report expulsion rates of only one or two per 100.[34] The longer a woman successfully retains her IUD, the greater the chances that she will continue to do so. Because the highest incidence of expulsion is within the first three months of use, many doctors feel that women should use another method of birth control for the first few months. After three years, the expulsion rates drop to practically zero.[35]

Expulsions occur more frequently when the IUD is inserted four to six weeks after childbirth or in the first 17 days after the menstrual period.[36] Generally, the larger the device, the greater a woman's chance of retaining it; unfortunately, the larger devices are also associated with increased bleeding and pain and more difficulty in insertion of the device.

Another problem with the IUD is that it may perforate the uterus either partially or completely and can move out into the pelvic cavity, where it may cause problems. Some authorities say that perforation occurs only at the time of insertion, even though it may not be evident for quite some time, and is due to faulty technique on the part of the inserter. Others feel that perforation can occur even with the most conscientious of inserters. It is hard to say exactly how often perforations occur since many times there aren't any obvious symptoms. Some studies estimate a rate of two perforations per 1,000 insertions, while others report a rate as high as 8.7 per 1,000.[37] Always insist that the uterus is sounded (measured) before insertion to help avoid perforations.

If the IUD is expelled or perforates the uterine wall, the woman is, of course, susceptible to pregnancy. The first step in dealing with a missing IUD is to do a pregnancy test. The problems of the IUD in pregnancy are discussed below. If the pregnancy test is negative and the woman knows for certain that the device has been expelled, she may choose to have the IUD replaced or select another method of birth control. The problem arises when the strings are no longer visible and it is not clear whether the IUD has been expelled, whether the strings have merely been drawn up into the uterus or whether the device has actually perforated the uterus.

There are a number of ways in which a doctor can check to see if the IUD is still in the uterus. After injecting anesthetic into the cervix, the doctor can insert a special instrument into the uterus to feel for the IUD. Most of the time, if the IUD is still in the uterus, it can be located and the string pulled back down, but if the IUD is not in the uterus the doctor doesn't know whether it has perforated or has been expelled.

Another alternative is to do an ultrasound examination, which like an X-ray, is a method of taking pictures of the interior of the body, although it does not involve any exposure to radiation. Ultrasound is painless and can tell the doctor whether or not the IUD is still in the body, but the procedure is expensive (about $75) and doesn't retrieve the strings, should the IUD still be in the uterus.

Still another alternative is to do a hysteroscopic examination, which requires using a local anesthetic and inserting a specialized viewing instrument into the uterine cavity to look for the IUD or signs of perforation. If the IUD is in the uterus, the string can usually be retrieved at the time of the hysteroscopic exam. This procedure has the advantage of direct visualization and string retrieval, but is new and is not yet widely available.

Yet another alternative is to locate the IUD by X-ray, with a probe or a second IUD inserted into the cervix. The X-ray will confirm the presence of the IUD and its relationship to the probe or second IUD will help the doctor decide whether or not the IUD is still within the uterus. (Remember, the uterus itself is soft tissue and will not show up on an X-ray.) This alternative might be suggested if the doctor suspects perforation or has been unable to find the IUD by probing.

If these methods fail to locate the IUD, the woman can safely assume the device was expelled without her knowing it. If the device is still within the uterus, the woman has the choice of having the device removed or leaving it within the uterus. There is some controversy about what to do if the device has perforated the uterus. Devices with copper or progestin *must* be removed because these substances can irritate the pelvic cavity. Similarly, it is universally agreed that certain closed devices (no longer marketed) that have perforated the uterine wall must be removed because they can obstruct the bowel. We feel that any perforated device should be removed because the IUD could cause an infection to flare up any time the woman's general resistance to infection was lowered. Moreover, there has been evidence that all devices, closed or open, can cause obstruction and perforation of other organs. Although most doctors favor removal, there are, nonetheless, still some doctors who feel it's all right to leave an IUD that has perforated the uterus in the pelvic cavity unless it starts to cause problems. A woman whose doctor doesn't counsel removal would be wise to seek a second opinion (*see* page 226).

Most of the time, an IUD that has perforated the uterus can be recovered by laparoscopy, a procedure in which a small incision is made in the abdomen and a tube-like viewing instrument, a laparoscope, is used to locate the IUD. A tool for removing the IUD can likewise be inserted through this tube. However, if the IUD is not located in a place accessible via laparascopy, a larger incision is made and a more major form of surgery must be done.

The IUD and Ectopic Pregnancy

Another controversy centers around the IUD and ectopic pregnancies, that is, a pregnancy in which the fertilized egg implants outside the uterus, usually within the Fallopian tube. An ectopic pregnancy is a potentially life-threatening situation that, when diagnosed, calls for immediate surgery.

When pregnancy occurs in an IUD user, she has roughly a seven to ten times greater chance of having an ectopic pregnancy; that is, approximately one in 30 pregnancies of IUD users will be ectopic as compared to one in 250 of non-IUD users.[38]

All women wearing an IUD should be alert to the possibility of an ectopic pregnancy (*see* page 647), the symptoms of which include abdominal pain and bleeding. Unfortunately, these symptoms may be caused by the IUD itself or by a number of other gynecological problems as well. In fact, IUD users with ectopic pregnancies are frequently misdiagnosed on the first doctor's visit. This delay is important, because the larger the fetus grows, the greater the chance that the Fallopian tube will rupture, causing a medical emergency that could result in sterility or even death.

The higher ratio of ectopic to uterine pregnancies in IUD users could be explained in two ways, and this is where the controversy arises. Some authorities have argued that this higher ratio is simply a reflection of the fact that the IUD, while it does a fairly good job of preventing uterine pregnancies, doesn't do very well at preventing ectopic pregnancies. Others feel that the IUD actually causes ectopic pregnancies, by so inflaming the uterine lining that the fertilized egg is forced to find another place to implant.[39]

Strong and convincing arguments are made on both sides, and at this point, there is not enough good, clear-cut data to settle this debate. Should it be decided that the IUD actually causes ectopic pregnancies, it would be unwise for any woman to use the IUD as a method of birth control. Some doctors feel that until the final verdict is in, women with a history of ectopic pregnancies should not use an IUD. Other doctors are particularly reluctant to use the Progestasert IUD, which some studies have implicated as being associated with particularly high rates of ectopic pregnancies.[40]

Still other doctors feel that because of the increased risk of ectopic pregnancy and of pelvic inflammatory disease, both of which can result in sterility, women who have never had children and who, according to some studies, are therefore more at risk for these sorts of problems than users who have had children, should not use the IUD if they hope some day to conceive. (See IUD and Subsequent Fertility below.) Still other doctors feel that the chances of ectopic pregnancy, especially of ectopic pregnancies that result in death or permanent effects on fertility, are so low that the IUD, which is so convenient to use, is worth the risk. This risk/convenience trade-off is one each woman must weigh for herself.

IUDS and Pregnancy

If the IUD does fail while remaining in place and the woman becomes pregnant, there are other reasons for concern beside the possibility of an ectopic pregnancy. About 50 percent of the women who continue their pregnancies with IUDs in place will have a miscarriage.[41] This is about three times the normal rate. However, if the IUD is removed, this will cut the risk of miscarriage to 25 percent.

Moreover, the question of septic spontaneous abortion (that is, infected miscarriages) and the IUD must be considered. In the early 70s, attention was focused on a small number of deaths from septic abortion in IUD users. A survey conducted by an FDA committee uncovered 289 cases of septic midtrimester abortion in IUD users, including 21 deaths.[42] A later analysis of data collected between 1972 and 1974 showed that of the 50 women in this country who died of spontaneous abortions, 23 were IUD users.[43] The news of these septic-abortion deaths led to the withdrawal of the Dalkon Shield, a device that, at the time, was thought to be particularly associated with such deaths. However, some researchers have questioned whether the attention focused on the Dalkon Shield might not have obscured the fact that septic abortion, with the risk of death, can apparently occur with any IUD.[44]

There is also some evidence that the continued presence of an IUD increases the risk of premature delivery[45] and stillbirth[46]. There has been some concern expressed about the copper and progestin IUDs being close to the developing fetus. There has been some evidence that *progestin* may also cause birth defects; however, no deformities have been reported in the small number of infants born following exposure to a Progestasert IUD.[47] There has been a report of two copper-IUD users, both of whom gave birth to infants with limb deficiencies, but it is not clear that these birth defects were related to the IUD.[48] Another study showed no limb deformities and only one minor vocal chord abnormality.[49] The final verdict is not yet in, for the number of infants thus far born under such conditions is too small to make any definite judgments.

Until fairly recently, most doctors recommended leaving the IUD in place if the woman wished to continue the pregnancy; however, with the information now available about increased rates of miscarriage and septic abortions and the possibility of premature labor, birth defects and stillbirths, most doctors now advise removing the IUD if the strings are still visible or having an abortion if the strings are not visible.

If the strings are still visible, there generally isn't a problem, for the IUD can usually be removed without disturbing the pregnancy. Although on occasion removal will cause a miscarriage, the increased risk of miscarriage due to this procedure is more than offset by the increased risk for miscarriage and other problems if pregnancy is continued with the IUD in place. Sometimes the strings will be visible, but the IUD won't come out or the strings will break off, making removal impossible. In these cases abortion is usually recommended.

If a pregnant woman whose IUD strings are missing or whose IUD strings break off during removal does have an abortion, the contents of the uterus will be examined. If the IUD is found, no further treatment is necessary. If the IUD is not found, the question of whether it was expelled or has perforated the uterus remains and the doctor may do one of the procedures described previously.

Although we advise abortion if the strings are not visible (especially if the woman has a Dalkon Shield), a woman who would like to avoid abortion on the chance that the IUD was expelled without her knowing it might choose to have an ultrasound exam to see if the device is still in the body. If no IUD is visible, she can assume the device was expelled and continue her pregnancy without worrying. Since ultrasound does not involve radiation, there is no problem about radiation exposure to the fetus, although there have been some questions about the possible effects of ultrasound on a fetus. In this instance, when a decision about abortion is being made, the benefits probably outweigh the theoretical risks of ultrasound.

Women who are absolutely opposed to abortion and choose to continue the pregnancy with the IUD in place should be followed carefully and should be alert to the signs of impending miscarriage (*see* p. 637).

IUD and Subsequent Fertility

Still another area of controversy is the question of the effect of an IUD on a woman's ability to become pregnant after the IUD has been removed. We have already discussed the relationship of pelvic inflammatory disease and ectopic pregnancies to the IUD. Both of these conditions can cause infertility. For this reason, some doctors have been reluctant to prescribe IUDs for women who have never had children.

Even beyond the question of pelvic inflammatory disease and ectopic pregnancy, there has been some debate about IUDs and fertility. There are basically three points of view in this controversy. The first holds that there is no effect on subsequent fertility. This has been the generally accepted viewpoint, based on a number of studies, including large-scale studies done in 1970 and 1971.[50]

The second viewpoint holds that although women who use IUDs may be slower to achieve pregnancy after removal, the overwhelming majority eventually do recover their fertility. This point of view is supported by a study done in England in 1978 with smaller groups of women.[51] The study showed that 48.7 percent of 258 women who had had their IUDs removed in order to get pregnant had not given birth after 12 months, compared to 29.4 percent of 1,085 women who had abandoned diaphragms or other traditional methods. After three-and-one-half years, however, only one former IUD user (0.4 percent) compared to 13 women from the other group (0.8 percent) had not given birth.

The third viewpoint holds that the longer a woman wears her IUD, the less chance she has of getting pregnant after removal of the IUD compared to a group of nonusers of the same age. This viewpoint is supported by a large study of former IUD users done in Taiwan in 1977, which followed women for a period of six to nine years and showed a significant decrease in fertility among former IUD users even in the absence of obvious pelvic inflammatory disease when compared to nonusers of the same age.[52] This was particularly true of women over the age of 30 at the time of removal who had been using the IUD for more than three years.

Obviously, this question needs more study before it can be resolved. In the meantime, women who are using the IUD to delay pregnancy rather than to prevent it altogether, especially long-term users over the age of 30, should consider the possibility of reduced fertility after IUD use when weighing the various birth control possibilities.

IUD and Cancer

None of the studies done on IUD users has demonstrated any link-up between IUDs and cancer. However, some critics of the IUD argue that cancer is a slowly developing disease and that sufficient time has not yet elapsed for cancerous effects to be obvious.

DIAPHRAGM

Types: coil spring
flat spring
arcing
bowbent

A diaphragm is a shallow cup of thin latex rubber with a rim of flexible metal under the rubber. It looks like a rounded lid or dome and is about three inches in diameter. Sperm-killing cream or jelly is placed inside the dome. The diaphragm is then inserted into the vagina prior to intercourse.

The diaphragm works in two ways. First, when properly inserted, it fits up around the cervix, covering it so that it forms a mechanical barrier to block the sperm. Second, it holds the spermicidal cream or jelly up against the cervix, so that any sperm that do manage to swim up around the rim and into the diaphragm are killed before they can reach the cervical opening.

Types

Diaphragms are available in varying diameters, or sizes, and in a number of different varieties. Ideally, a woman should have a chance to try the different kinds or at least should have a choice between several types, since some women will find one type more comfortable or easier to use. Women with certain physical irregularities or medical problems, such as a tipped uterus, cystocele, rectocele or poor vaginal muscle tone, may require a diaphragm specially fitted to their anatomy.

Spermicides

The diaphragm should be used with a spermicidal cream or jelly. Some spermicidal creams and jellies are specifically made to be used with a diaphragm; others are made to be used alone. Research has shown that creams and jellies do not disperse as well as foams, so we therefore do not recommend using these alone. However, the ones manufactured to be used alone may be stronger than those made to be used with a diaphragm, so some authorities feel it makes sense to also use these stronger ones with a diaphragm.

If the choice is between jellies and creams, it may be a matter of individual taste. Masters and Johnson have shown that creams disperse better than jellies when used alone.[53] Whether this makes any difference when the creams or jellies are used with a diaphragm is still a question. Some women, on the basis of what is known, prefer to use the creams. You needn't use a spermicide manufactured by the same company that manufactures your diaphragm. A new, flavored spermicide (raspberry, for some reason) has recently come on the market, and couples who enjoy oral lovemaking can order this product from Nova Corporation of America, 475 Park Avenue South, 12th Floor, New York, New York 10016. Try various products until you discover which is most pleasing to you.

Some women find that they can use the diaphragm successfully without a spermicide, but this is not recommended at present since too little is known. We do know that the upper two-thirds of the vagina balloons during intercourse. This ballooning can cause the diaphragm to slip. This is especially likely to happen when the woman is in the superior position (on top) and when couples experience simultaneous orgasm. By using a cream or jelly with the diaphragm, there is still some protection should one of these situations occur. If a diaphragm with spermicide is too objectionable, a woman would do better to try a cervical cap, or perhaps her partner should wear a condom.

Effectiveness

The official Food and Drug Administration figures on diaphragm effectiveness rates tell us to expect anywhere from 2 to 20 pregnancies per 100 women using the diaphragm for a year.[54] Unfortunately, these odds are rather wide-ranging, with a spread of from about one in five chances to one in 50. A woman concerned about the possible side effects of the pill and the IUD, a woman willing to trade off an increased risk of pregnancy or abortion for greater long-term safety or one whose sexual contacts are rather infrequent might be willing to accept a one out of 50 set of odds, but one out of 5 would probably be unacceptable to anyone who seriously wanted to prevent conception. It is necessary to take a closer look at the effectiveness rates and the studies from which they are derived in order to figure out whether you as a particular individual are more likely to have the one in 50 chance of getting pregnant—or the one in 5 chance.

It must be remembered when considering these studies that even when there were 20 women who got pregnant, there were 80 who did not. What makes the difference? Why does the method work for some and not for others?

First of all, there are problems with the method itself. That is, even if you used your diaphragm each and every time you had intercourse, you still might get pregnant. This is due to a number of factors:

☐ Your diaphragm may not have been properly fitted, you may have lost or gained more than ten pounds or you may have had a child, miscarriage or abortion that has affected your fit.

☐ Your diaphragm may have a manufacturing defect (unlikely). Or you may have made a hole in it when removing it or cared for it improperly, resulting in leaks or in deterioration of the rubber.

☐ Your diaphragm may have become dislodged during intercourse, because the vagina expands during orgasm. As noted earlier, this is most likely to happen when the women is on top during intercourse or when couples experience orgasm at the same time. It also may occur when there are multiple mountings, that is, when the penis slips out and is reinserted, either accidentally or deliberately, during lovemaking.

But when one looks closely at the studies, it becomes apparent that despite these possible drawbacks, the diaphragm can be highly effective.

As it turns out, the critical factors seem to be the age of the woman, how long she has used the diaphragm, proper instruction in its use, proper fit and whether or not she has completed her family or is merely using the diaphragm to delay pregnancy (that is, her motivation). In a large study done in England in 1974, over 4,000 diaphragm users were tested, for a combined number of months of use that totaled over 70,000 months. Not surprisingly, this recent, large-scale, long-term study came up with the 2.4 failure rate per 100 woman-years of use.[55] However, this study was limited to women over the age of 25 who had been carefully instructed in diaphragm use, carefully fitted and who had used the method for at least five months prior to being included in the study. When the data from this study was further analyzed, it showed failure rates as low as 1.1 per 100 for women ages 35-39, 4.1 for women ages 25-29 and 1.4 for women who'd been using the diaphragm for five years. In 1976, the largest study ever done in this country showed rates as low as 1.9 per 100 women under 18[*] to a high of 3 per 100 women ages 30-34.[56] When fitted and used properly the diaphragm can have an effectiveness rate on a par with the Pill and the IUD.

Fitting a Diaphragm

A diaphragm requires a doctor's prescription. The initial kit, which comes with a diaphragm case and a small tube of spermicide, costs about $5 to $10. The doctor's visit can run anywhere from $10 to $75, depending on whether you get your diaphragm at a clinic or from a private doctor.

A diaphragm should be fitted by someone who is well trained and experienced. This person need not be a doctor. A paramedic, nurse, nurse-practitioner or other medical personnel can fit a diaphragm and often have more time to help you learn to use it properly.

Proper fitting is important since too small a diaphragm will tend to slip out of place when the upper part of the vagina swells during sexual excitation. Most diaphragms vary only about one inch in size, but these small variations are critical. Too large a diaphragm may buckle or lie vertically in the vaginal canal, leaving the cervix uncovered and causing discomfort.

The fitter will estimate the proper diaphragm size by inserting two fingers into the vagina and determining the distance between the pubic bone and the cervix. Then a sample diaphragm is inserted. The fitter should insert the next larger and next smaller size to make sure there is a proper fit. Ideally, there should be two or three types of diaphragms available so that a woman can select the one that is easiest and most comfortable for her to use.

Once the fitter has selected the proper size, the woman should practice

---

[*]This low rate for women under 18 may be a reflection of the fact that although women in this age group menstruate, some are not actually producing eggs and cannot therefore get pregnant.

inserting it herself and the fitter should then check to see that she has inserted it properly. Women with tipped uteri should be particularly fussy about their fitting and the qualifications of the fitter, since they, along with women who are virgins, are the most likely to be fitted badly. A second or even a third visit to check the fit is a good idea for such women.

If you are a virgin, it might be wise to use another method of birth control, like foam or condoms, for a while before having a diaphragm fitted since sexual intercourse tends to enlarge the vaginal cavity.

If you were particularly tense or uptight during your first fitting, as many women are, it is especially important to arrange a second visit after you have practiced at home with your diaphragm, for nervousness may have made you tighten your vaginal muscles, thus altering the normal contours of your vagina.

If you have decided that the diaphragm is the method, or one of the methods, you would like to use for birth control, scout around for a doctor who is a diaphragm enthusiast and who has had a good deal of experience in fitting them. Since the Pill and the IUD came into vogue, instruction in the techniques of fitting a diaphragm was dropped from many medical school curriculums. Since proper fitting is so important to successful diaphragm use and since many doctors tend to downgrade the effectiveness of the diaphragm, it is important to find a diaphragm "fan," who is much more likely to be experienced with them, when making your choice. Never have a diaphragm fitted by a doctor who has tried to talk you out of using this method of birth control.

How to Use the Diaphragm (Illustration 20)

☐ Put about a tablespoon of spermicidal cream into the cup of your diaphragm. Apply a thin film on the inside of the rim. Do not put the spermicide on the top of the rim as this may make the diaphragm more prone to slipping out of place. Some women coat the outside of the diaphragm as well, for extra safety.

☐ Pinch the opposite sides of the rim together so that the diaphragm folds in the middle.

☐ The diaphragm can be inserted while you are in a number of different positions: sitting on the edge of a chair, lying flat on your back with knees bent, squatting or propping one leg up on a toilet or chair. If you are standing, the diaphragm is inserted almost horizontally; if you are lying down, it is inserted almost vertically.

☐ The diaphragm is then pushed up along the back wall of the vagina as far as possible. This insures that it is actually covering the cervix. It

Illustration 20 *Using a Diaphragm: Place spermicide in the dome of the diaphragm and rub it on the dome and the rim (A). Fold the diaphragm so the rims are touching (B). Insert the diaphragm into the vagina (C). Guide it along the back wall of the vagina until it covers the cervix (D). Use your finger to check that the cervix is under the dome of the diaphragm (E).*

should then lock into place, fitting snugly against the pubic bone in the front. Check to make sure the cervix is actually covered by feeling for it beneath the rubber dome of the diaphragm. (Your cervix feels like a knoblike projection and is firm, like the tip of your nose.)

☐ Traditionally, diaphragm users are told that the diaphragm may be inserted up to two hours prior to intercourse. There is some debate on this subject. In the most recent and largest diaphragm study done in this country, the participants were told that they could put the diaphragm in as much as six hours ahead of time and they still achieved results of only three pregnancies per 100.[57] It may be that the increased convenience of the six-hour method results in fewer diaphragms being forgotten at the last minute and is, therefore, worth the risk that the spermicide will be more diluted and thus less effective after this longer period of time.

☐ The diaphragm should be left in place for eight hours after intercourse.

Advantages and Benefits

The diaphragm has many advantages. When fitted and used properly, it has a high rate of reliability. Not a single hospitalization or death has ever been related to a diaphragm (and that's saying something). For women who have sex only infrequently it is particularly well suited, especially as compared to the IUD and the Pill, which must be worn or taken even if a woman is not having sex very often.

There are no long-term effects on fertility, and a woman may use a diaphragm during breastfeeding without worrying about its effect on her milk.

There seems to be a lower incidence of cervical and vaginal infections and of sexually transmitted diseases among women who use diaphragms as opposed to IUDs or the Pill.[58] Although it is not certain, it is thought that the antibacterial effect of the spermicide and/or the fact that the cervix is protected by the diaphragm may help in preventing these infections. Some studies have shown that cervical cancer, which may be associated with herpes type II (*see* p. 350) or some other sexually transmitted virus, occurs less often in women who use diaphragms than in women using nonbarrier methods such as the Pill and the IUD.[59]

Women who experience an upsurge in their sexual desire at the time of menstruation like the diaphragm because it catches the menstrual blood and makes sex at that time less messy. Others like the diaphragm because they involve their mates in the insertion of the diaphragm, and they find that sharing the responsibility for the birth control is very satisfying.

Disadvantages and Problems

Certain women cannot wear a diaphragm because of their particular anatomy or poor muscle tone in the vagina. The following conditions may also make it impossible for a woman to use a diaphragm:

- ☐ Prolapse of the uterus
- ☐ Fistulas
- ☐ Severe cystocele or rectocele
- ☐ Severe retroversion or anteflexion of the uterus
- ☐ Septate vagina

Some women experience cramps and pressure on the bladder or rectum when the diaphragm is left in place for eight hours following intercourse as recommended. A smaller size or a different type of diaphragm may correct this problem, but if it persists, the woman should use another method of birth control.

There is some evidence that women who use diaphragms are more apt to develop urinary tract infections.[60] It is theorized that the pressure of the diaphragm on the bladder or on the urethra causes this increased susceptibility to infection. A smaller-size diaphragm may eliminate the problem, but women who have repeated infections should use another method of birth control.

In addition, in certain rather rare cases a woman or her partner may be allergic to the latex rubber or to the spermicides. Some men complain that they dislike the sensation of hitting up against the diaphragm during intercourse, but this should not be a problem if the diaphragm is properly fitted.

Others find the diaphragm too messy or too inconvenient. Still others say it interferes with the spontaneity of their sex lives. There are plastic inserters available. Women who don't like to touch their genitals may find that the use of the plastic inserter makes this method of birth control more acceptable. Some couples incorporate the placement of the diaphragm into the lovemaking ritual so that spontaneity is not compromised.

If a couple tends to reach orgasm simultaneously, if they prefer the woman-superior position or if the male tends to slip out during intercourse or prefers to withdraw and reenter (multiple mounting), then the diaphragm is more likely to get dislodged and is likely to be less effective as a means of contraception.

Couples who enjoy oral-genital sex often find the taste of spermicides quite unpleasant. They may engage in oral-genital lovemaking and then insert the diaphragm, but if the partners become intensely excited by this form of foreplay, the diaphragm may be forgotten. Once it is inserted, some couples find it impossible to resume oral-genital contact due to the unpleasant taste of the spermicide. Using the raspberry-flavored spermicide mentioned earlier may help alleviate this problem.

Some women have questions about the safety of spermicides. Other than an occasional allergic reaction, there have been no adverse effects reported, and there have even been some studies indicating that spermicides may be antibacterial and may actually promote vaginal health.[61] In the past there has been some question about certain spermicides that included a compound containing mercury, but these compounds are no longer used.

Even though the spermicide may be anti-infective, a diaphragm left in too long may cause irritation to the vagina. To prevent this, be sure to remove the diaphragm at least every 24 to 36 hours and wash and dry it thoroughly before reinserting it.

VAGINAL SPERMICIDES

AKA: spermicides or topical contraceptives

Types: contraceptive foam
  contraceptive tablets
  contraceptive cream
  contraceptive jelly

Vaginal spermicides are chemical mixtures containing a base material and a sperm-killing agent. They are inserted into the vagina just prior to intercourse. They work in two ways: by coating the cervix and forming a mechanical barrier, so that the sperm cannot pass into the uterus; and by killing the sperm within the vagina. There are basically three kinds of spermicide available—foams, creams, and jellies. The creams and jellies are used in conjunction with a diaphragm or a cervical cap. Although some manufacturers advertise their creams and jellies to be used alone, we do not recommend this procedure. While they are excellent when used with a diaphragm or cup, the creams and jellies simply don't disperse and cover the cervix as well as the foam does.[62]

Types

Foam is available in two forms: in an aerosol spray can and in tablets (suppositories) that are inserted into the vagina prior to intercourse. The vaginal secretions activate the tablets and the foam is released (a process somewhat akin to dropping an Alka-Seltzer into a glass of water). We do not recommend use of the tablets, as studies have shown that the tablets do not always dissolve completely.[63]

A special note should be added here about the Encare Oval, a new and highly advertised foam tablet that is well packaged and extremely easy to use. The effectiveness rates cited by the Encare Oval manufacturers, which are extremely high—on a par with the Pill—are based on studies derived from what one rather diplomatic source discreetly called a "very unconventional study design."[64] Our personal experience, having performed a number of abortions on women relying on the Encare Oval, make us skeptical about their effectiveness and we don't recommend them.

Effectiveness

Foam, like all the barrier methods of birth control, has a bad reputation as far as effectiveness goes. One study conducted in Puerto Rico with a group of low-income women indicated that 29 out of 100 women using this method for a year would get pregnant.[65] Yet, other studies have reported rates as low as 1.5 pregnancies per 100 woman-years of use.[66] The wide variance in rates may have to do with the fact that the studies with the high failure rates were done with non-English-speaking women, teenagers and others who had not been properly instructed in the use of foam.[67] Some of these women reported jumping up and applying the spermicide immediately after intercourse. Others applied the foam to the outside— not the inside—of their bodies. Moreover, many of these less successful studies were done with women who did not specifically choose to use the foam. With those who actively decide that foam is the method they want to use, the results are, not surprisingly, much superior. One such study, which included more than 3,000 women who were "medically indigent" (that is, low-income) and who were chronically unsuccessful at birth control, showed a pregnancy rate of only four per 100 women.[68] Moreover, these women were told that the foam could be inserted as long as three hours prior to intercourse, which is a couple of hours more than most manufacturers recommend (see below). The results might have been even better had the product been used according to the manufacturer's directions, although perhaps the freedom to insert the foam prior to intercourse contributed to better rates. A critical difference between this and other studies is that the staff administering the study came from the same background as the women in the study, spoke their language and presumably understood their lifestyles and problems.

Also, many of the studies that yielded high pregnancy rates involved women who wanted to delay, rather than prevent, pregnancy. Other studies have shown that there is a great deal of difference in the effectiveness of any birth control method, depending on whether the users' intentions are to merely delay pregnancy until a later date or to prevent pregnancy, either because their families are complete or because they absolutely do not want children.[69] One study conducted among couples who firmly did not want children showed a failure rate of 1 percent for the Pill, 7 percent for foam, and 6 and 7 percent for the diaphragm and condom, respectively.[70] The latest study, published in 1979, involved 326 "affluent, well-educated and highly motivated" women, all of whom were carefully instructed by private physicians and followed-up at regular intervals.[71] The results of this study showed 0.3 pregnancies per 100 women years of use. If the foam is used in conjunction with a condom, the effectiveness rate should be even higher.

The upshot of all of this seems to be that foam is an extremely effective method of birth control. Its effectiveness can be on par with that of the Pill if it is used properly.

How to Use Foam

First things first—read the directions that come with the foam. Unfortunately, these directions often leave much to be desired, so we've devised a set of our own:

- ☐ Most instructions will include a line like "Shake the can." Really shake it—at least 20 times. This will make the foam about the consistency of shaving cream, so that it is more effective. Shaking vigorously will also assure an even distribution of the spermicide, which tends to settle on the bottom of the container.
- ☐ Most foams come with a plastic plunger and tube device that works like a tampon. In most cases, the applicator tube is filled by pressing down or by tilting it over the nozzle on the container of foam. The foam is released into the tube by pulling the plunger back as far as possible, so that it is ready to insert. Foam can get a bit messy at this point since it takes a light touch and good timing to remove the applicator before it fills and the excess foam spurts out every which way.
- ☐ The applicator is then inserted into the vagina right away, preferably while you are lying down. It should be inserted as far as it can go (about three or four inches), then withdrawn about a half-inch or an inch and the plunger pressed down to release the foam. The reason for the partial withdrawal is to assure that the foam is being deposited

on or near the cervix (which protrudes from the top of the vaginal cavity) and not on the back wall of the vagina (see Illustration 21).

☐ Push slowly while pressing the plunger in so that the bubbles have a better chance of spreading evenly over the cervix and vaginal walls.

☐ The applicator should be withdrawn without pulling the plunger out to avoid sucking some of the foam back into the applicator.

☐ Even though the manufacturers don't recommend it (perhaps to keep the cost from being prohibitive), many women who have had children or have had abortions sometimes use two—rather than one—applicators full of foam. This is because the opening of the cervix is larger in these women. Some women who know when they ovulate (*see* p. 68) also use extra foam around this time since the cervix is more dilated then and they are of course more susceptible to pregnancy.

☐ The foam should be inserted as close to the time of actual intercourse as possible. Some authorities say the bubbles go flat within 15 minutes to a half hour. Some researchers have allowed insertion as

CORRECT

INCORRECT

Illustration 21 *Inserting foam: Insert the foam applicator deep into the vagina so that the foam will cover your cervix.*

long as three hours ahead with good results, but the consensus is that insertion no more than one hour prior to intercourse is optimal.

□ An additional applicator of foam should be inserted before each act of intercourse. Each dose has the capacity to kill the amount of sperm deposited each time a man ejaculates, or comes, but it may not be strong enough to be effective a second time. Then, too, if an hour has passed, the bubbles may have fizzled out, making a second application necessary.

□ If the woman gets up or goes to the bathroom after application but prior to intercourse, she should insert another application since some foam may have been lost. After intercourse, getting up poses no problem since the spermicide has done its work.

□ The applicator should be washed with a mild soap and water. It should not be boiled since it is made of soft plastic, and sterilization is not necessary anyway. Some women keep a glass of water handy and drop the applicator into it. In any case, the applicator need not be washed immediately.

□ Do not douche for eight hours afterward. This may dilute the foam and force any sperm that are still alive up into the womb.

□ Although the foam won't stain and dries or dissolves within a few hours, some women use a sanitary napkin to catch the foam that sometimes leaks out after intercourse. A tampon should not be used for this purpose.

Buying Contraceptive Foam

Contraceptive foam is available in drugstores and in some grocery stores. There is no law regulating how old you must be in order to buy foam. Most of the time the foam can be found sitting on the store shelves. If not, ask for it by one of the brand names listed below. Be sure that the product you are buying is actually contraceptive foam and not one of the feminine hygiene products (douches, deodorants and such) that are often on the shelves right next to the contraceptive foams. Foam is also available by mail in an unmarked envelope from Population Services, Inc., 105 North Columbia Street, Chapel Hill, North Carolina 27514 (919-929-7195).

Contraceptive foam deteriorates over time and has a shelf-life of three years. Most brands are now dated for freshness, but for some manufacturers this is a recent innovation, so you may find older, undated boxes. Shop for a dated brand that has an expiration date and check to make sure you have a fresh batch.

The cost of foam ranges from about 20 to 40¢ per application, which can get rather expensive if you have an active sex life. However, it does not require initial or follow-up doctor's visits. Also, it is used only when it is needed, unlike the Pill, for example, which is taken every day. Moreover, the user does not run the risks of costly complications (except, perhaps, the cost of pregnancy or abortion should the method fail).

There are a number of different types of foam available:

☐ Emko Contraceptive Foam: Available in 30- and 60-application containers. The foam can be purchased in a starter kit, which includes an applicator and carrying purse, or in the slightly less expensive refill kits, which come without an applicator. A dosage cup that lets you know how much foam is left in the container comes with all except the 30-application refill kit; however, the cup from the other kit will fit. This is an important feature since it prevents you from getting an incomplete dose or from suddenly discovering that you've run out.

☐ Emko Pre-Fil Contraceptive Foam: Available in a 25-30 application kit, which comes with an applicator and a carrying purse, or a 50-60-application refill kit. The Pre-Fil foam is in liquid form until the plunger is depressed. This means that the applicator can be filled ahead of time so that lovemaking need not be interrupted by the somewhat messy and more time-consuming process of filling the applicator.

☐ Because Contraceptor: This is also an Emko product. It contains six applications in one easy-to-use, tampon-size applicator.

☐ Koromex II Contraceptive Foam: Manufactured by Holland-Rantos, it is available in 30- and 60-application containers, again with applicator and purse or refill kits.

☐ Delfen Contraceptive Foam: Manufactured by Ortho Pharmaceutical, Delfen comes in a starter kit, which includes an applicator, a purse and a container that holds about 20 applications, or in refills in either the 20- or 50-application size.

☐ Dalkon Contraceptive Foam: Made by the A. H. Robins Company. The starter kit contains applicator, carrying purse and 35 applications of foam. Refills, holding 90 applications, are also available. Like the Emko products, Dalkon also has a built-in device that lets you know how much foam is left.

Advantages and Benefits

One of the biggest advantages that foam has in comparison to methods like the Pill and IUD is that it is harmless. No one has ever died as a result of using foam. Occasionally, there may be an allergic reaction, but this can usually be cured by switching to another brand.

Also, foam does not require a doctor's exam, prescription, supervision or follow-up. It is readily available in drugstores and grocery stores. Unlike the Pill or IUD, which are used on a day-to-day basis, foam is used only when intercourse is actually going to take place. Nor does it involve a device like the cervical cap or the diaphragm.

Moreover, foam may be effective against venereal disease and common vaginal infections.[72,73] As a sidelight of contraceptive research, it was noted that women who had minor vaginal infections at the start of the study were free from infection after using foam. In laboratory studies, various foams have been shown to inhibit the growth of syphilis and gonorrhea bacteria, herpes virus and other disease-causing organisms. However, this was only in laboratory situations. Whether the foam in actual use is concentrated enough to have the same effect is a question now being studied.

Contraceptive foam is often used during the first months of birth control pill usage and the first several months of IUD use. It is good to keep some around in case you stop, run out of or forget to take your pills. It is also a good backup in case your IUD is expelled or a condom breaks (insert several applicators of foam immediately). Foam is also used by some women at midcycle to increase the effectiveness of an IUD or condom. Since many doctors recommend that a woman should not try to become pregnant for the first few months after stopping the Pill (*see* p. 108), foam may be useful at these times.

Foam is also relied upon by diaphragm users who have intercourse a second time, but some professionals feel that the contraceptive jellies or creams are better, fearing that the foam will weaken the rubber of the diaphragm.

Disadvantages and Problems

The biggest drawback to foam as a contraceptive is the fact that it must be applied just before intercourse and thus interrupts lovemaking. Some couples overcome this problem by using a prepared type of foam, so that they aren't bothered by having to fill the applicator. Other couples incorporate the insertion of the foam into their lovemaking. Since the foams have an unpleasant taste, couples who enjoy oral-genital contact must apply the foam after oral sex and may not care to resume this form of lovemaking once the foam has been inserted.

Some women find that the foam provides too much lubrication and consequently reduces their sexual pleasure. On the other hand, women who produce only a minimal amount of lubrication may prefer foam for this very reason.

Since many of the spermicidal products have been on the market for years, some of them have not been subject to the safety tests required of new products. There has been some question about the possible association of foam with birth defects. In a user who was unknowingly pregnant, the chemicals could be absorbed through the vaginal tissues, but there is no proof that this occurs, either in experiments with laboratory animals or in humans, and there hasn't been any increase in birth defects since these products came on the market. It is also theoretically possible that the spermicide could cripple, though not kill, a sperm. Such a damaged sperm could conceivably cause a birth defect, but here again there is no evidence that this occurs.

CONDOMS

AKA: rubbers, prophylactics, safes, French letters, sheaths, skins, trojans

A condom is a sheath made from thin rubber or lamb's gut that fits over the erect penis in a glovelike fashion. Placed on the erect penis just prior to intercourse, the condom acts as a barrier that prevents the sperm from entering the vagina. Some condoms have a plain end; others have a special receptacle at the tip to contain the sperm after the man ejaculates, or comes. The rubber at the open end of the condom is thicker, forming an elastic ring that keeps the condom from slipping off the penis. The condoms available in this country are available only in one size, but since they are considerably elastic, one size is supposed to fit all.

Types

There are three types of condoms: those made from a basic grade of latex rubber; those made from a thinner grade of latex; and those made from the intestines of sheep, which are called skin condoms. Skin condoms are more expensive, but many men prefer them since they transmit body heat much as human skin does and therefore permit more sensitivity. Many men object to using a condom, likening it to "taking a shower with a raincoat on"; however, when questioned, many such men will admit that they have never actually used one or have not used one for many, many years. A number of men, once they've tried them, find that the newer condoms, either skins or those made from a thinner grade of latex, provide a very natural feeling.

Latex condoms are available dry or lubricated with either a dry or wet lubricant. Most users prefer the lubricated varieties since they replace the natural secretions from the penis that are blocked by the condom, thereby facilitating entry and cutting down on the penile or vaginal irritation sometimes experienced with the nonlubricated variety. Some users complain about the medicinal odor of some of the wet lubricants and prefer the dry lubricants, which are odorless and slippery rather than wet.

Most condoms are colorless—opaque or transparent—but recently American companies, following the lead of foreign manufacturers, have been marketing colored condoms. In some countries, even "glow-in-the-dark" condoms are available, but the more adventuresome in this country who would like to try them out will have to wait until an American company manufactures them since the thinner foreign condoms do not meet American standards.

Condoms are also available with ribbed and textured surfaces and with "ticklers" on the end. Such extras are advertised as being sensually pleasing to women (if that's what "drive her wild" is supposed to mean); however, we've yet to meet a woman who has noticed the difference.

The lamb's gut, or skin, condoms are lubricated with a special oily substance that makes them cling to the penis for a snug fit. Still, they don't fit as snugly as the latex type, which makes some first-time users worry that these condoms will fall off. But, despite their seeming looseness, they don't. Although many men find that the skin condom actually enhances penile sensation, others find that the oily, lubricating substance makes them messier to put on.

Effectiveness

Condoms, like other barrier methods of birth control, have long been downgraded as being ineffective methods of birth control, but a look at the facts provides a different picture.

The highest rates of condom contraceptive failure are quoted as being 36 pregnancies per 100 woman years of use.[74] This study, however, was done in 1942. We have already discussed the problems with this study in Chapter Five. A study done in 1969 recorded actual-use rates of 3.1 pregnancies per 100 woman years;[75] rates as low as 0.83 have been recorded in one study.[76] The big factor is, of course, motivation. If the condom is used properly, each and every time a couple has intercourse, it is a highly effective method of birth control.

Using Condoms

Condoms, it's true, are simple devices, but they can be a bit tricky the first time since the directions that come with the condoms (if there are any) tend to be rather brief and leave a lot to be desired. We've created our own expanded version:

☐ The condom purchased years ago by a young boy in junior high school (with high hopes) and carried around in his wallet to impress his friends won't be too useful, since body heat tends to deteriorate the rubber, and even the best-sealed condoms, carefully stored away from heat, should be discarded after two years.

☐ Dry condoms, which may irritate the vaginas of women who don't have a lot of lubrication, should never be lubricated with Vaseline or petroleum jelly since this tends to deteriorate the rubber. Lubrication will help prevent tearing, and spermicidal foam, cream or jelly will lubricate with the additional advantage of adding extra contraception. Saliva works well but is said to increase the chances of contracting vaginal yeast infections.

☐ Although this may seem obvious, especially to anyone who's tried it another way, the condom can be placed on the penis only after the male is sexually aroused and his penis erect. If lubrication is desired, it should be applied after the condom is in place.

☐ Most condoms come prerolled. It is usually rolled around the firm rubber-ring end of the condom. Unless the condom is placed over the tip of the penis and unrolled the reverse way, it will not move smoothly down the shaft of the penis and will become bound up after unrolling an inch or so. Unroll the condom about one-half inch and then place it on the penis (see Illustration 22).

Illustration 22   *The Condom: Unroll the condom on the erect penis, leaving space at the end for semen to collect.*

☐ Some condoms come with a tip at the end to collect the semen. If yours doesn't, leave about a half inch of free space between the tip of the penis and the closed end of the condom, making sure that the air is squeezed out of the tip or half inch of space. This is done so that his come will collect in this area and not be forced down the shaft of the penis, around the rolled end of the condom, possibly finding its way into the vagina. Some manufacturers claim that the tip of half inch of extra space will prevent the condom from "bursting" when the man comes, but this somewhat exaggerated suggestion is probably wishful thinking.

☐ The condom should be unrolled all the way, to the base of the penis if possible. That way, even if semen does leak down the shaft, it is unlikely that it could travel all the way back up the condom to the top of the vagina and cause a pregnancy.

☐ Uncircumcised males should pull the foreskin back from the end of the penis before putting on the condom.

☐ The condom should be placed on the penis prior to any contact with the vagina. Some couples begin actual intercourse without the condom, the game plan being to withdraw prior to orgasm. Needless to say, the game doesn't always go according to plan and the condom may be forgotten until it's too late. Besides, many authorities feel that even the small numbers of sperm that leak from the penis before orgasm can cause pregnancy.

☐ The penis should be withdrawn as soon as possible after intercourse since with most men the penis becomes smaller and softer soon after climax, which might allow semen to leak out of the open end or allow the condom to slip off the penis into the vagina. Hold the condom firmly at the base of the penis when withdrawing so that semen won't be spilled in or near the vagina. This is particularly important for women who have little vaginal lubrication. Pulling out too abruptly may cause the condom to slip off or allow the semen to escape.

☐ The vagina should not come in contact with the penis after it has been withdrawn since there still might be live sperm on the penis. If you have multiple intercourse, a fresh condom should be used each time.

☐ If the condom breaks (which may happen if the woman's vagina is not sufficiently lubricated) or slips off in the vagina (which may happen with condoms that are lubricated on both the inside and the outside), remove it immediately (with the open end held tightly closed) and apply contraceptive foam.

□ If you're the thrifty type, good-quality rubber or skin condoms can be washed, dried and reused several times. Keep a jar of water by the bed and later on, wash, dry and reroll the condom. A dilute solution of household boric acid and water will clean skin condoms. However, condoms are available cheaply, and many couples find it easier to discard used ones (not down the toilet—think of the fishies!).* If you are using a condom for protection against venereal disease, use it only once.

□ Keep the condom handy, by the bedside or in your purse, so that it is readily available.

Buying Condoms

Condoms can be purchased at drugstores, vending machines, family-planning and Planned Parenthood clinics or through mail order. The prices run from about 20¢ to 80¢ per condom, depending upon which kind you buy (natural skins are the most expensive), whether you buy them in packages of three, twelve or economy-sized (six dozen, the cheapest way to buy them) and whether you buy them in a discount or regular drugstore.

Since the Supreme Court decision of 1977, there are no laws prohibiting minors from buying condoms or drugstore owners from displaying them prominently.[77] Sales, not surprisingly, have risen accordingly.[78] Women are making up a larger share of the market, 20 percent according to some estimates, which probably reflects dissatisfaction with the riskier forms of birth control and a growing awareness of the protection against venereal disease that the condom provides.

There is some controversy as to the quality of condoms purchased through vending machines. All condoms must pass strict quality-control standards, but over time and under conditions of heat or direct sunlight, the quality of the materials deteriorates. Some authorities feel that vending machines may contain condoms that are over the generally accepted usefulness age of two years. Other authorities point out that nobody would be in the vending machine business if it took that long to turn a profit. The key factor may be whether or not the condoms are stored in hermetically sealed foil packages. But, if you have to dust off the

*Believe it or not, dead fish, apparently strangled by condoms, have been found floating on the surface of the water!

machine in order to insert your coin, you'd probably better do your condom shopping elsewhere.

Condoms may also be purchased by mail in an unmarked envelope from Population Planning, 105 N. Columbia Street, Department GW-1, Chapel Hill, North Carolina 27514.

Varieties and Brands

Most drugstores have open displays of condoms, usually near the cash register, but ask if you can't locate them. Salespeople may ask what size you want. If so, they are inquiring about whether you want a 3-pack, a 12-pack or a 72-pack, since the condoms themselves come in only one size. The list below, which includes some of the popular brands, will help you make your selection and know what to ask for.

Wet Lubrication: Trojan Brand Guardian and Trojan-enz Lubricated

Dry Lubrication: Trojan Plus, Conceptrol Dry-Lubricated, Trojan Ribbed

Nonlubricated: Trojans, Trojan-enz (with reservoir tip), NuForm Nonlubricated, Ramses Nonlubricated (plain end), Sheik Nonlubricated

Fitted Condoms (body hugging) with reservoir tip: Trojans Plus (dry lubrication, golden colored), Conceptrol Shields (nonlubricated or dry lubricated, transparent)

Ribbed and/or Flared: Excita (flared end, ribbed surface), Nuform Lubricated (flared end, allows for freedom of movement within condom), Trojan Ribbed (golden and transparent)

Natural Skin: Fourex Skins Capsule Pack (lubricated inside and out, comes in blue capsule), Trojan Brand Natural Lamb (lubricated, rolled)

Colored Condoms: Trojan Plus (golden, dry lubrication); Fiesta (pink, yellow, green and black, lubricated)

Advantages and Benefits

The condom has many advantages. It is highly reliable when used consistently. It is readily available and doesn't require a medical examination, supervision, prescription or follow-up. This is particularly important to teenagers who are uncertain about approaching their family doctors about birth control, fearing that their confidence will not be kept. The condom is light, compact and disposable, another feature of value to teenagers worried about their parents knowing about their sexual activity.

There are no side effects other than an occasional minor allergic reaction to the latex or lubricant. The condom is easy to use and totally reversible; that is, if pregnancy is desired, one need only to discontinue use without fear of reduced fertility or birth defects.

The condom may be a particularly good idea for those men who are unable to maintain an erection during intercourse. For them, the rim of the condom may have a slight tourniquet effect, helping them to prolong their erection.

In some rare cases, women have an allergic reaction to their partner's sperm that can cause medical problems for them. In such cases, a condom can help the situation. In fact, couples suffering from infertility for this reason are sometimes treated by using a condom for a few months to decrease the woman's allergic response.

Perhaps the most important advantage to the condom is its role in the prevention of sexually transmitted diseases. Unless there is leakage of the semen during withdrawal, the condom is highly effective in preventing gonorrhea. There is also some protection against syphilis, venereal warts, trichomoniasis, and herpes, but less so because these organisms may enter through the unprotected outer lips of the vulva or from the man's scrotum. Some authorities feel there is less protection against these diseases than against gonorrhea because the organisms that cause these diseases are smaller and can penetrate the condom. Studies of the incidence rate of these diseases among men who use condoms versus those who don't support this decrease in risk,[79] and other studies, like those correlating the rise in condom sales in Sweden with the drop in disease rates, help to confirm it.[80] The protective factor in the case of herpes is especially important since there is evidence linking herpes to cervical cancer (*see* p. 350).

For some women, the fact that using condoms means that the man is sharing the responsibility for birth control is very important. The act of placing the condom can become part of lovemaking. It is a way for a sexual partner to demonstrate his care and concern for a woman by protecting her from the risks associated with other forms of birth control, such as the Pill and the IUD. In long-term relationships, this demonstrated element of caring can be particularly important. In shorter-term relationships, in which you may not know if you'll be having intercourse or not, condoms may be very convenient. If you don't know your sex partner well enough to trust that he'll have a condom with him, it makes sense to carry one with you. It may be hard for some of us to pull out a condom and suggest that our partner use it, but given the fact that we are in the midst of an epidemic of gonorrhea and herpes, such a practice makes a good deal of sense.

Disadvantages

One disadvantage to the condom is the fact that it has such a bad (though undeserved) reputation for effectiveness. Many women, planning to use this method, may fail to do so at the last minute figuring, "Oh, well, it doesn't work very well anyhow, so I might as well not bother." This is not true—the condom is highly effective, but its biggest disadvantage is that it must be placed on the erect penis just prior to intercourse. For some of us, remembering to use it and interrupting our lovemaking to place it on the penis is a problem. Keeping them handy, in our wallets, pocketbooks or by the bed, and making the placement of the condom part of our lovemaking can help.

From a man's point of view, the condom's most serious drawback is decreased penile sensitivity. Trying the newer, thinner latex condoms or the more natural, heat-transferring skin condoms may alleviate this problem.

In rare cases, there may be an allergic reaction to the latex rubber. This reaction is usually milder in women so affected than in men and can often be dealt with by switching brands or using dry condoms. In the case of couples with an active sex life, the cost of natural skin condoms may also be a problem.

CERVICAL CAP

AKA: birth control pessary

The cervical cap is a device that looks like a thimble for a giant-sized finger. It fits right over the cervix and is held in place by suction. The cap works by mechanically blocking the sperm and also by acting as a holder for spermicides (the same type used with the diaphragm), which are put into the cervical cap prior to insertion. The cervix swells slightly from the pressure of the cap and forms an airtight seal. This means that the spermicide stays active for a considerable period of time; therefore, the cap can be inserted well in advance of intercourse and may be left in place for a number of days.

The caps come in a number of different sizes and a few different styles. They are made of plastic or firm rubber and are widest at their open end, which has a thick, semirigid rim. Generally, the rubber caps are preferable, although in hot climates where rubber materials deteriorate rapidly, the plastic cap may be preferable.

At the present time the cervical caps used for birth control are manufactured only in England, so they are not widely used in this country.* They were manufactured here during the late 50s and early 60s; however, the popularity of the Pill and the IUD eclipsed the cervical cap. Since there was not sufficient demand, the manufacturer discontinued making the device. With the growing evidence of the side effects and consequences of the Pill and the IUD, there has been a renewed interest in the cervical cap, which unlike the other barrier methods of birth control, doesn't require insertion immediately prior to intercourse.

Unfortunately, little is known about the cervical cap and there are a number of unanswered questions about its effectiveness, use and safety. It is not known, for instance, how long the spermicide inside the cap remains effective. There is also some question as to exactly how much spermicide should be put inside the cap and how long the cap can be worn without changing it.

At the present time, the Food and Drug Administration has not approved the cervical cap as a method of birth control, for there are no long-term effectiveness and safety studies. The companies that manufacture such items may not want to invest in the required testing for the device, which is a "one-time" item as compared to the Pill or spermicide, supplies of which must constantly be replenished. Moreover, less spermicide is needed in the cap than in the diaphragm, so, from the companies' point of view, the cap may not be a potentially profitable item. Indeed, it might even cut into the profit margin on their spermicide products.

Then, too, doctors are not always open to exploring new developments. The cap requires more of the doctor's time for fitting and instructing the woman in how to use it. It is certainly easier to simply write out a prescription for pills. However, the cap appears to be much safer than the Pill and the IUD and much more convenient to use than the diaphragm, condom or spermicidal foam. For these reasons, it has been championed by concerned doctors and women active in the health-care movement, so the government is now considering funding large-scale studies.

Effectiveness

According to Planned Parenthood Federation of America, the cervical cap is about as effective as a diaphragm.[81] Some authorities believe that the

*A device that is also called a cervical cap and that is used to treat infertility problems is manufactured in this country, but it is not designed to be used for birth control.

cervical cap may actually be more effective than the diaphragm. Since it fits right on the cervix, they feel that the cap is less susceptible to being dislodged during intercourse, as sometimes happens with the diaphragm when the upper portion of the vagina expands during sexual excitement. Others feel that the cap may be more easily dislodged.

Unfortunately, valid effectiveness rates are not available because no large-scale, long-term studies have been done. The last major study was done in 1953 on a group of 143 women using the plastic caps.[82] The overall use-effectiveness rate in this study was 7.6 pregnancies per 100 women-years of use, which included the women who used the cap incorrectly, inconsistently or not at all For those women who claimed to have used the cap regularly and correctly, the rate was 3.2 pregnancies per 100 women using the cap for one year. Some of these failures might have been due to the cap's having been dislodged during intercourse, which is less likely to happen with today's rubber caps since their suction grip is tighter than that of the plastic caps used in this study. Moreover, the researchers were not able to follow up on all the women that they fitted with caps. Those who became pregnant might have been more likely to stay in contact with the doctor than those who did not, and this may have biased the effectiveness rates.

An informal, unpublished study of 165 women fitted with caps found that six of the women became pregnant, all during the first two months of use.[83] In other words, about 96 percent of the women fitted did not become pregnant. Currently, some doctors and women's health groups are conducting informal studies and the government may soon fund studies, so more data may be available in the future.

Fitting a Cervical Cap

Proper fit is essential, and although the person doing the fitting does not have to be a doctor, special training is required. Unfortunately, very few people in this country have been trained to fit cervical caps. The list in the appendix includes some of the people now fitting caps in this country. Fees vary, but many doctors charge more for caps than for diaphragms since proper fitting and instruction in use require more of the doctor's time. The person fitting the cap will first look at the cervix with a speculum to determine its size. After selecting the proper cap, the fitter places it on the cervix and checks the suction to make sure that the cap fits properly. Caps a size larger and a size smaller than the one selected should be tried as well in order to insure the best fit.

After the cap has been fitted, the woman should practice inserting and removing it until both she and the person doing the fitting feel confident that she has mastered the process. The woman should not be aware of the cap once it is in place.

Some women, approximately 20 percent, cannot wear caps. Women with deep cervical lacerations and extremely long or extremely short cervixes can't be fitted with cervical caps. Some doctors feel that women with cervical erosions or eversions, especially those that are congenital rather than acquired, should not wear cervical caps. Others feel that the cap may actually aid in healing erosions. Women with erosions who use caps should practice gynecological self-exam so that they can monitor the effect of the cap on their cervix and discontinue usage if their condition worsens. Such women may not want to leave the cap in as long (that is, they may want to use it like a diaphragm) until the erosions heal.

Some women's cervixes change size over the course of the menstrual cycle. This cervical swelling is usually rather slight and most authorities feel that it shouldn't cause any problems. Others feel that perhaps some women should have two caps, one to be worn at the time of ovulation and the other to be worn during the rest of the month.

Women with active cervical or vaginal infections should not be fitted for a cap until the infection is cleared up, since the infection might cause the cervix to swell, resulting in an improper fit.

Childbirth, miscarriage or abortion can alter the cervix; the cap should be refitted after any of these occurrences. Even though it might become slightly discolored, caps properly cared for are good for a number of years.

How to Use the Cervical Cap

Before the cap is inserted (Illustration 23), it must be filled from one-third to two-thirds full with spermicide. The same spermicides used with a diaphragm can be used with the cap, although some doctors argue that creams are preferable to jellies because they last longer in the cap. Some authorities recommend one-third full because they feel that too much spermicide will affect the suction. Others favor two-thirds full, feeling that the moisture from the spermicide actually tightens the seal and makes for better suction. Some authorities recommend that the spermicide be smeared around the inside rim as well, but others have found that this caused the cap to become dislodged.

The cap can be inserted in a number of different positions. Some women like to stand up with one foot raised and resting on a chair, bathtub or bed. Other women like to squat or to recline halfway.

The cap is compressed between the thumb and forefinger of one hand, while the other hand spreads the lips of the vagina apart. The cap, with the open end first, is then inserted into the vagina and slid along the back wall

Illustration 23   *Inserting the Cervical Cap: The spermicide is placed in the cap (A), inserted into the vagina (B), guided along the back wall of the vagina and fitted over the cervix (C). Use your finger to feel for the cervix under the cap (D).*

until it reaches the top of the vaginal cavity. Use one or two fingers, whichever is easiest for you. Care must be taken not to spill the spermicide out of the cap. The cap is then released and pushed onto the cervix.

If you have difficulty reaching your cervix, squat and bear down as if you were having a bowel movement or push down on the abdomen above the pubic hair. These maneuvers will bring the cervix to a lower position.

The cervix will not completely fill the cap. The extra space in the dome of the cap will hold the spermicide and cervical secretions. This extra space may collapse or it may not, but either way, suction is not affected.

After inserting the cap, check to see that the cervix is covered. You can do this by running your finger around the rim of the cap, making sure that no portion of the cervix protrudes from under the cap. Or you can feel for the cervix above the rim, so that you know the cervix is inside the cap.

After checking, push the cap up onto the cervix again, just in case you pulled it down a little when checking.

You should check the position of the cap before and after each act of intercourse. If the cap should become dislodged during intercourse, push it back on the cervix and insert several applicators of spermicidal foam or cream into the vagina immediately.

Some women find it harder to remove the cap than to insert it, for the cervix swells slightly when the cap has been in place for a while. To remove the cap, the index and middle finger are inserted into the vagina. The rim of the cap is tilted away from the cervix and a finger is hooked under the rim between the cap and the cervix. This permits air into the cap, breaks the suction and allows for easier removal. The positions for easier insertion described above will also aid in removal. A string of unwaxed dental floss may be attached to the thick rubber tab on the rim of the cap before insertion for easier removal later. (Illustration 24).

The cap should not be removed for at least eight hours after intercourse to make sure the spermicide has killed all the sperm. The woman should not douche with the cap in place, as this could dilute the spermicide. The cap should be removed during menstruation because it will fill with menstrual blood, which will break the suction and cause the cap to come off the cervix. Women who wish to have contraceptive protection during menstruation can use a diaphragm or have their partners use a condom.

The cap should be inserted at least a half hour prior to intercourse to allow time for cervical swelling and the formation of the suction seal. Exactly how long the cap can be left in place is a matter of debate. It is thought that the airtight seal created by the cap helps the spermicide to remain effective for a longer time than it does with the diaphragm. Some doctors allow as long as seven days, provided that the first time the woman uses the cap she removes it after three days and checks to see that it is still at least one-third full of spermicide. If so, she then refills the cap to two-thirds full and checks it again after five days. If the cap remains at least one-third full, she repeats the process after seven days. (Always use a condom as backup protection during this "checking period.") If the cap is still one-third full at seven days, her maximum time for leaving the cap in place would be seven days; if not, her maximum time would be shorter. The time the cap is left in place should not exceed seven days, for the effectiveness of the spermicide after then is questionable. Many cap fitters feel that the cap should not be left in place for more than three days.

Some women use the cap in the same way a diaphragm is used, except that they insert it several hours prior to intercourse. Other women like to take the cap out every day or every other day. They feel that replacing the spermicide gives them more protection and that washing the cap is more

Illustration 24   *Removing the Cervical Cap: Hook your finger over the edge of the rim to break the suction. Some women attach a piece of dental floss to the rubber ridge to aid in removal.*

hygienic. It also helps to prevent the odor problems some women have if the cap is left in for too long. If odors do develop, the cap can be washed with soap and water or soaked in a solution of dilute lemon juice. Some women add a drop of chlorophyll to the inside of the cap before insertion to prevent odor problems. Removing the cap also allows the cervical secretions to flow freely, which may prevent vaginal infections. Although some doctors feel that the cap can be refilled and reinserted immediately, some women like to leave it out for at least several hours to give the cervical secretions a chance to flow.

Once the cap has been removed, it should be washed in soap and water, patted dry with a towel and, if it isn't going to be replaced immediately, stored in a clean safe place. The cap should never be boiled. It can be soaked for 15 minutes in alcohol or vinegar to prevent odors. Dusting with cornstarch will make the cap last longer. Talc should not be used, for it could be irritating and is not water soluble, so it can't be washed off easily. Vaseline, cold cream or other greasy products should not be used with the cap, as they will deteriorate the rubber. A water-soluble, nongreasy lubricant like K-Y Lubricating Jelly, which can be purchased without a doctor's prescription, can be used if lubrication for intercourse is desired.

Disadvantages and Problems

One big disadvantage is the problem of availability. At the present time, the caps used for birth control are manufactured only in England, although some American companies have recently expressed interest in making caps. Perhaps as more women learn about caps, the demand will prompt companies in this country to manufacture them. Hopefully, the range of styles and sizes will increase so that more of the estimated 20 percent of women whose particular anatomies do not conform to the caps presently available can be fitted.

In some rare cases, there may be an allergic reaction to the material that the cap is made from or to the spermicide. Changing brands can usually solve allergy problems.

Some women's sexual partners complain that they can feel the cap if they thrust deeply, and in some cases this causes some discomfort for the man. This is probably due to the penis's hitting the little tab of thick rubber on the rim of the cap and can sometimes be avoided by making sure the tab is facing backward, so that the penis doesn't hit it.

Some women don't like to touch their genital organs, and some women have difficulty inserting or removing the cap. This, of course, limits the usefulness of the cervical cap for such women.

The effectiveness rates for the cap have not been clearly established. Since the pregnancies that do occur with the cap seem more likely to occur in the first two months, some cervical cap fitters recommend that women use extra spermicide in the vagina or that the man wear a condom at least around the woman's ovulation time (*see* p. 68) for the first two months.

Advantages

The cap can be inserted well in advance of intercourse and left in the vagina for a number of days, so there is no need to interrupt the spontaneity of lovemaking in order to insert the cap. This convenience also means that the cap is less likely to be forgotten, as might be the case with the condom, diaphragm or spermicidal foam.

Since the vagina is not full of spermicide (as it is with the diaphragm), oral-genital lovemaking is more pleasant than with the diaphragm.

The cap is inexpensive, probably quite effective when used properly and safe. Although there have been a few minor side effects, the cap has not caused a single death. It can be used by many women whose anatomy precludes the use of the diaphragm.

Some medical workers fear that the cap may harm the cervix or vagina. Injury could conceivably occur during insertion or removal. It is possible that long-term use of the cap could cause irritation to the cervix or cervical erosions. Some researchers worry that the cervical secretions build up inside the cap instead of bathing the vaginal walls. Some doctors feel that the free flow of secretions may be important in preventing infection or other problems, and are concerned about the cap for this reason. So far, these concerns are only theoretical. The cap, in various forms, has been used for hundreds of years, so serious effects would, presumably, have become evident by this time—and they haven't.

NATURAL FAMILY PLANNING

AKA: NFP, periodic abstinence, fertility awareness, natural or organic birth control, cooperative birth control

Associated Terms: rhythm, or calendar rhythm, method; cervical mucus, or Billing's, method; basal body temperature, BBT, or thermal method

Natural family planning (NFP) can be used either to prevent pregnancy or to maximize the chances of conceiving for those women who want to get pregnant. Women can get pregnant only during a certain period of time in each cycle, and that period generally occurs about two weeks before the onset of the next menstrual flow. Women who use this method of birth control learn to determine when they are fertile and either abstain from intercourse during this time or use another method of contraception.

Natural family planning is based on certain biological facts:

☐ Ovulation occurs quite consistently about 14 days before the next menstrual period begins, regardless of the length of your menstrual cycle.

☐ There is occasionally a two-day variance either way, so ovulation may occur 12 to 16 days prior to the first day of the menstrual flow.

☐ Sperm are capable of surviving for three days or, according to some experts, for five days.

☐ The female ova lives for only 12 to 24 hours or, according to some experts, for 36 hours.

☐ Once ovulation has occurred, the hormone progesterone is produced in increasing amounts, which causes a rise in body temperature.

☐ The character of the cervical mucus undergoes changes both prior to and after ovulation.

Because a woman can get pregnant only for a certain amount of time preceding and following ovulation, natural family planning depends on two factors: **1.** predicting when ovulation will occur, so that a woman can avoid intercourse prior to ovulation for the three (some say five days) of the sperms' lifespan; and **2.** being able to recognize when ovulation has occurred, so that she knows when it is safe to resume intercourse. The days prior to ovulation, when a woman is infertile and it is therefore safe for her to have intercourse, are called the early safe days, and the days following ovulation, when she is again infertile, are called the late safe days.

Natural family planning encompasses three methods for predicting when ovulation will occur and recognizing when it has happened: the rhythm method, the basal body temperature chart and the cervical mucus method.

The Rhythm Method

The rhythm method can be used alone, without the other components of NFP, but unless safe days are calculated by the strictest method (see below), it is not a dependable method of birth control (see Effectiveness below). It can be used to calculate both early and late safe days, but unless a woman is using only this method the late safe days are not as important, for NFP provides other ways of determining these days.

Calculating Early Safe Days

In order to use the rhythm method you must know the length of your menstrual cycles for the previous 9-12 months. To calculate your early safe days, subtract 14 days from the length of your shortest cycle, since ovulation usually occurs 14 days prior to the first day of the following cycle. Now, subtract 2 more days just in case, as sometimes happens, you have ovulated 16 days prior to the first day of your next cycle. Now subtract 3 more days to allow for the lifespan of the sperm since sperm deposited prior to ovulation could still be alive in your reproductive tract 3 days later. There is some evidence that sperm have a lifespan of 5 days, so if you want to be extra careful subtract 5 days. Altogether you will be subtracting 19 days, (or 21 days if you're figuring on a 5 day sperm lifespan) from the length of your shortest cycle. The resultant figure will be the last of the early days of your cycle on which you can safely have intercourse.

This can be expressed in the following formula:

$$(S = \text{the length of your shortest cycle})$$
$$S-19 = \text{last of the early safe days}$$
$$\text{or}$$
$$S-21 = \text{last of the early safe days}$$

Table 4 lists the safe days for various cycle lengths. Example: Jeanenne's shortest menstrual cycle in the past 12 cycles was 25 days long. Subtracting 14 days, puts her at Day 11, the day on which she probably ovulated. Subtracting 2 more days puts her on Day 9, the earliest she is likely to have ovulated. Subtracting 3 more days to allow for the lifespan of the sperm would put her at Day 6. If she allowed for a 5-day sperm lifespan, that would put her at Day 4.

Table 4
Early and Late Safe Days as Calculated by the Rhythm Method

If your shortest cycle has been:	The last of your early safe days would be:	The first of your late safe days would be:
21	Day 2	Day 11
22	Day 3	Day 12
23	Day 4	Day 13
24	Day 5	Day 14
25	Day 6	Day 15
26	Day 7	Day 16
27	Day 8	Day 17
28	Day 9	Day 18
29	Day 10	Day 19
30	Day 11	Day 20
31	Day 12	Day 21
32	Day 13	Day 22
33	Day 14	Day 23
34	Day 15	Day 24
35	Day 16	Day 25
36	Day 17	Day 26

$$S-19 = \text{last of the early safe days}$$
$$25-19 = \text{Day 6}$$

or

$$S-21 = \text{last of the early safe days}$$
$$25-21 = \text{Day 4}$$

Using the rhythm method, Jeanenne could safely have intercourse from Day 1 (the first day of her menstrual flow) to Day 4 or Day 6 without using any protection.

Calculating Late Safe Days

To calculate the late safe days of the cycle, subtract 14 days from the length of your longest cycle. Then add two days to that figure in case you actually ovulated 12 days prior to the first day of the following cycle. Next add one more day to allow for the 24-hour lifespan of the ova. Some authorities feel the ova can survive for 36 hours and suggest adding 2 days. If to be safe you have added 2 days to allow for the lifespan of the sperm, you would then be subtracting a total of 10 days from your longest cycle. If, however, you are using the rhythm method in conjunction with other NFP techniques, this is not necessary since there are other more accurate ways of determining post-ovulatory safe days.

These calculations can be stated in the following formula:

$$(L = \text{the length of the longest cycle})$$
$$L-10 = \text{the first late safe day}$$

Table 4 lists the safe days for various cycle lengths. Example: Jeanenne's longest cycle was 31 days. Subtracting 14 days would put her at Day 17, the day she probably ovulated. Adding two days just in case, as sometimes happens, she ovulated 12 days, instead of 14 days before, would put her at Day 19. Adding one more day to allow for the lifespan of the ova would put her at Day 20, the last day of her cycle during which she would be fertile:

$$L-10 = \text{the first of the late safe days}$$
$$31-10 = \text{Day 21}$$

So Jeanenne could resume unprotected intercourse on Day 21.

The Strictest Method

There is another method of calculating early safe days which is quite simple: no days prior to the ovulation are considered safe. In Jeanenne's case, this would mean that she could only have unprotected intercourse from Day 21 of her cycle on. If she had a 25-day cycle she could have unprotected intercourse for the last 5 days of that cycle. If she had a 31 day cycle, she could have unprotected intercourse for the last 11 days of her cycle. If a woman is using other methods of birth control on her unsafe days, this might be acceptable and has the advantage of greatly increasing the effectiveness of the method (see below), but for women who are abstaining on their unsafe or fertile days, this method of calculating, which would severely restrict sexual activity, might be too limiting.

Basal Body Temperature

The basal body temperature, that is, the temperature of the body when it is at complete rest, drops about 24 hours before ovulation and then rises, usually remaining elevated for at least three days following ovulation. Thus, your basal body temperature indicates when ovulation is about to occur, though it cannot be used to calculate early safe days since it provides only a one-day warning and sperm can survive in the reproductive tract for three or possibly five days. It can, however, indicate

163

that ovulation has occurred and is therefore of use in calculating late safe days.

In order to determine your late safe days by this method, you will need a chart like the one shown in Illustration 25, which is available at pharmacies (or you can make your own with graph paper), and a thermometer. Either an oral or a rectal thermometer may be used, and the temperature may be taken orally, rectally or vaginally. Do not switch back and forth as there may be a variation of a degree or two that could make the chart difficult to interpret.

A standard fever thermometer, which runs from 94°-108°F and has a mark every two-tenths of a degree, can be used, but most women prefer to use a basal body temperature thermometer (BBT), which runs from 95°-100° and is marked off in tenths of a degree, making it easier to read. BBTs can be purchased at a pharmacy without a prescription.

Taking and Recording Your Basal Body Temperature

The temperature reading must be taken first thing in the morning, before you get out of bed, smoke a cigarette, talk or do anything else. Your basal body temperature is the temperature of your body at complete rest. Even slight activity may cause a rise in temperature. Shake your thermometer down the night before (some authorities say the energy required to do this is negligible but suggest that you do it then to guard against breaking the thermometer in the early, groggy hours of the morning).

After leaving the thermometer in your mouth (or rectum or vagina) for about five minutes, take it out, read your temperature and record it on the chart.

It is not necessary to record your temperature on the first few days of your cycle, while you are still bleeding. Mark those days with an X as shown in Illustration 25. Start to record your temperature as soon as the menstrual flow stops.

Once you have read your temperature, record it on the chart by making a dot where the vertical date column joins the horizontal temperature column. Connect the dots with straight lines, as shown. If you miss an occasional day, make a note on the chart. Likewise, if you are forced out of bed before taking your temperature (a ringing phone, a crying child or whatever), are unable to or have forgotten to take your temperature, note this on the chart.

Interpreting the Chart

The chart shown in Illustration 25 is an easy one to interpret. Yours is apt to be more complex, but for now, consider this chart. The Xs indicate the days of the menstrual flow. The first temperature of 97.6°F was recorded on Day 6. After Day 6, the temperature sort of jumps up and down, but

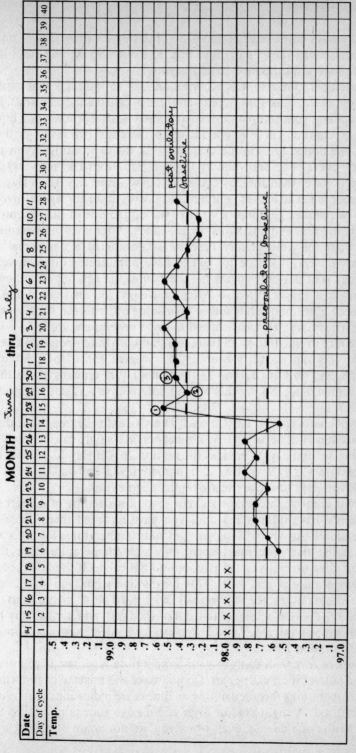

Illustration 25   *Basal Body Temperature Chart*

165

basically stays between 97.6° and 97.9° until Day 15. From Day 15 onward, the temperature shows a definite rise, to around 98.6°, and stays in this higher range until the next period begins.

The temperature rise that occurred on Day 15 indicates that ovulation has taken place. This shift in temperatures is called a thermal shift. If you are ovulating, your temperature should show what is known as a biphasic curve. A biphasic curve is one in which there are two levels or distinct areas. The dotted lines in the chart indicate the two distinct levels of the biphasic curve. The preovulatory temperature, from Day 6 to Day 14, is definitely lower than the postovulatory phase, from Day 16 to Day 29.

In order to get an idea of your biphasic curve, make an "eyeball average" of the two phases and draw a line like the dotted line in Illustration 25 to indicate the pre- and postovulatory baselines. After your temperature has risen from the preovulatory baseline six-tenths of a degree for three successive days, it is safe for you to have unprotected intercourse. The three-day wait not only covers the lifespan of the egg but also allows for certainty of a temperature rise. After three days, you can be sure that it has truly been a hormone shift rather than some other factor, such as a fever or a restless night, that has caused the rise in temperature.

Note that in Illustration 25 there is a slight dip in temperature after Day 15, but this dip is still six-tenths of a degree above the preovulatory baseline, and on Days 17 and 18 the temperature remains above the six-tenth degree range. So, for this woman, intercourse was safe beginning on Day 18.

Not all charts are this easy to read. The six-tenths degree rise indicating that ovulation has occurred may not happen in a single day, but may take a period of several days. Consider Illustration 26. On Day 12, this woman's temperature was 97.7; on Day 13 it jumped to 98.0 and on Day 14 to 98.3°. It took two days to make the six-tenths degree leap.

If your chart doesn't show a single leap of six-tenths of a degree, you should not have intercourse until you have recorded three consecutive temperatures that are .4°F higher than your temperatures for the six days prior to the rise. You may cancel one high temperature from the six temperatures previous to the rise, but do not cancel if there is more than one temperature at that level. This means that when you start counting higher temperatures, the day you call Day 1 must be .4° higher than the six days before the rise began (or five out of six days), and it must stay higher for the days you call Day 2 and 3. You can have intercourse again on Day 3. (see Illustration 27).

Illness or fever can confuse your temperature readings. If you are sick, make a note of it on your chart. Do not make the mistake of thinking that high temperatures recorded during an illness are indications that ovulation has occurred. A slight cold or fever could raise your temperature two or three tenths of a degree, even when you are not aware of having a fever.

BASAL TEMPERATURE CHART

MONTH _April_ thru _May_

Illustration 26 *This woman could not have considered Day 13 to be the first day of temperature rise since her temperature rose only .3 of a degree. Instead she had to use the .4 degree rule and count back six days.*

BASAL TEMPERATURE CHART

MONTH _Oct._ thru _Nov._

Illustration 27   This woman was permitted to cancel Day 12, on which she had a high temperature.

You should not have intercourse for three days after you are *sure* your illness has passed. Remember also that illness during one cycle can cause early or late ovulation during the following cycle, so be especially careful during the subsequent cycle. You might, for instance, want to use the strictest calendar rhythm method and not calculate any early safe days the following month.

The Cervical Mucus Method

The cervical mucus method can be used to predict when ovulation will occur and to confirm BBT evidence that ovulation has taken place. As explained in Chapter Four, mucus secreted by the cervical glands changes over the course of the cycle. In the early days of the cycle, when estrogen levels are low, the secretions are scant and the vagina is dry. As ovulation approaches and estrogen levels rise, the cervical secretions become more abundant and the vagina feels increasingly wet. The character of the secretions also changes from a thick, pasty, tacky texture, gradually becoming creamier, until just before ovulation it changes to a slippery, thinner, more watery type of mucus. The early, pasty, thick secretions are rather acid and hostile to sperm. On a molecular level, the structure of this type of mucus is crosshatched and prevents sperm from passing through the cervix into the uterus. The more abundant, thinner, secretions that occur later, just prior to ovulation, are more alkaline and favorable to sperm. The molecules that make up the mucus have rearranged themselves to form tubes or tunnels to facilitate the sperm's passage through the cervix (see the illustrations on page 67). This type of mucus is the most fertile, and it can be stretched between your thumb and forefinger into a clear, shimmering, delicate strand or thread before breaking. The term "spinnbarkeit," or spinn, is used to refer to this type of mucus.

Illustration 28 shows the four types of mucus conditions you may notice over the course of your menstrual cycle. For purposes of this method of birth control, there are two types of mucus—fertile and infertile. The only time the mucus can be considered infertile is in condition I (Dry), when the vaginal opening is dry. No one is certain whether Condition II (Early Mucus) is fertile or not, so it must be considered as fertile mucus for purposes of birth control.

The Mucus Cycle

The mucus cycle in most women works something like this: Day 1 through 5 there is bleeding from the menstrual period. Right after the period, secretions are almost absent and the vagina feels dry. These two, three or more dry days are followed by the expulsion of a mucus plug from

Illustration 28   *Condition I: dry, infertile mucus; Condition II: pasty, tacky mucus, possibly fertile; Condition III: slippery, wet, fertile mucus; Condition IV: spinnbarkeit, very fertile. Intercourse is safe only during Condition I.*

the opening of the cervix. The small, sticky plug may not be noticed, but following its expulsion, the vaginal lips feel wet. For some women, the first mucus following the dry days is whitish in color, sticky or tacky. Although this creamy mucus is probably not fertile, it can change to slippery fertile mucus quickly. (Besides, "probably not fertile" is not too reassuring when you're talking about birth control, so it should be considered fertile.) By the day of ovulation or the day preceding it, the mucus takes on the classic spinn character. Its appearance has been compared to the white of an uncooked egg—somewhat gelatinous, slippery and translucent.

Following ovulation the secretions become less slippery and more creamy. Some women have dry days following ovulation; others have a more variable pattern that changes from dry to wet to creamy. Illustration 29 indicates a typical mucus cycle.

Observing Your Mucus Cycle

Each woman is different and your pattern may not correspond to the typical pattern described above. Women with very short cycles may not have any dry days following menstruation. Those with long cycles may have five or six dry days. Some women never see spinn mucus. Before relying on this method, you should observe your patterns for a period of at least six months.

You will need to keep a daily record of your secretions. Some women can observe their mucus symptoms by merely noting a feeling of wetness or

MENSTRUAL CHART

Illustration 29 Chart combining BBT, Rhythm and Cervical Mucus Methods dryness. Others touch the inner lips of the vagina or note the discharge on their underclothes. Still others insert a finger into the vagina and take a sample of mucus right from the cervix. If you practice self-exam, you will more easily be able to learn to recognize these changes. Of course, the vagina is never entirely dry, so the term is a relative one, but by observing your symptoms over a period of time and coordinating them with the BBT and rhythm charts, you can learn to tell the difference between fertile and infertile mucus.

The following suggestions should help:

☐ Check your mucus several times a day after you've been awake for a while and before you urinate. If you have short cycles, check on the last couple of days of your period.

☐ Don't check when you are about to make love or are sexually aroused, because this produces vaginal lubrication that could be mistaken for fertile mucus.

☐ Don't check right after lovemaking, because the man's sperm and seminal fluid can obscure the mucus characteristics. Some women learn to distinguish between these two secretions. Unless, or until, you can, you should have intercourse at night on your dry days—and only every other night, since you will probably be a little wet and drippy on the day following lovemaking and will therefore be unable to determine the condition of your mucus. Later on, when you are more experienced, you may be able to stop skipping a day, but only if you always lose all of your partner's sperm and ejaculate before noon and are dry the rest of the day.

☐ If you are anything but dry during a preovulatory time, even if the rhythm method indicates that it should be a safe day, do not have intercourse; your mucus may be warning you of an unexpected, early ovulation.

☐ After ovulation, the mucus will return to the dry or sticky type. The fourth day after it dries up you are no longer fertile. This should correspond to the third day of higher temperatures on your BBT chart. But, if your mucus says you are infertile and your temperature says you are fertile or vice versa, consider that day an unsafe one. The one exception to this is if your mucus gets a little milky later in the month, after it has demonstrated ovulation (spinn, fertile mucus) and your temperature has remained up following this ovulation. You may consider yourself safe at this time. It is not uncommon to experience a few of these wet days and a drop in temperature just before your next period. This is not because you're fertile but because your period is coming.

☐ If you have long cycles and hence a long preovulatory phase, you may show some preovulatory mucus before the true preovulatory mucus build-up. If you do have mucus earlier than you expect it, don't have unprotected intercourse on that day and for three days after you become dry again. Then you can go back to having intercourse every other night, as long as the rhythm method indicates that it is a safe day.

☐ After your temperature and mucus have both demonstrated that ovulation has occurred two days previously, you can resume having intercourse every day, if you choose, until the end of your cycle. Any mucus you might have from then on is not fertile.

Recording and Interpreting Your Mucus Symptoms

You can record your mucus symptoms on a chart like the one shown in Illustration 29. Use descriptive words like creamy, wet, white, clear, sticky, slippery, spinn, milky, scant, cloudy, profuse or translucent.

The cervical mucus method can be used alone. This is particularly valuable for nursing mothers and women approaching menopause whose BBT charts are apt to be rather meaningless, since they may not be ovulating regularly.

Effectiveness

Unfortunately, there are no good studies of how the rhythm, BBT and cervical mucus methods work when used in combination. The calendar rhythm method used alone has produced rates ranging from 14 to 47 pregnancies per 100 women years of use. The BBT method has produced rates ranging from less than 1 to 20 pregnancies per 100 women years of use. The mucus method has produced pregnancy rates ranging from 1 to 25 pregnancies per 100 women years of use. Using the BBT and having intercourse only on the late safe days after ovulation has occurred has produced rates ranging from 1 to 7 pregnancies per 100 women years of use.[84] The combination of all three methods would undoubtedly improve these figures.

How to Use Natural Family Planning

Natural family planning can be used in two ways: by abstaining from sex on the unsafe days or by using one of the barrier methods, such as foam, diaphragms, condoms or cervical caps on the unsafe days. Women who choose to use NFP in combination with a barrier method on unsafe days should be aware that the effectiveness of the barrier methods may be significantly reduced when they are not used consistently during each act of intercourse. Nonetheless, some women who dislike these barrier methods are willing to compromise on effectiveness as long as some days of unprotected intercourse are available to them during each cycle. We would encourage women who decide to use NFP in this manner to calculate their early safe days by the strictest calendar method and not have unprotected intercourse until after ovulation has occurred.

In order to use NFP, you should mark off your early safe days as calculated by the calendar rhythm method on a chart as shown in Illustration 29. This woman's shortest cycle in the previous nine months was 27 days long. She allowed for a sperm lifespan of three days in making her calculations, so her last early safe day would be Day 8. Her longest cycle was 31 days, so the first of her late safe days would be Day 21. The intervening days were marked off with Xs on the line marked Days of the Cycle.

Next, record your mucus and temperature observations each day. This woman had dry days until Day 10. But she could not have intercourse after Day 8, since that was the last of her safe days according to her calendar rhythm calculations. If she had noticed fertile mucus prior to Day 8, she would likewise have had to discontinue having unprotected intercourse. If any of the methods indicate that an early day is an unsafe day, you should discontinue unprotected intercourse.

This woman had a temperature jump on Day 15 and her temperature remained high for three days, so she was able to resume intercourse on Day 17. In calculating late safe days, you may ignore the calendar rhythm days and resume unprotected intercourse after you have recorded three high temperatures. If, however, your cervical mucus shows signs of spinn or maximum wetness on that day, you may not resume intercourse. If, on the temperature rise day that you call Day 1, you still have spinn mucus or a lot of wetness, wait until the spinn has gone or the wetness has dried up before counting Day 1. If your mucus indicates fertility but your temperature chart indicates a safe day, do not have unprotected intercourse. Similarly, if your temperature indicates not safe but your mucus says safe, do not have unprotected intercourse.

Using this method may seem rather difficult, but people who use it claim that it becomes automatic once it is incorporated into the daily routine. We recommend that couples who are interested in this method not rely solely on the instructions given in this or any other book. It is best to have personal instruction from a doctor, medical professional or couples who have successfully practiced the method. We would suggest that people interested in natural family planning contact one of the following sources for information about and training in the use of this method:

Natural Family Planning Federation of America, Inc.
Suite A, 1221 Massachusetts Avenue NW
Washington, DC 20005

Couple to Couple League
P. O. Box 11084
Cincinnati, Ohio 45211

Fertility, Love, Insight Counsel
P. O. Box 464
Piscataway, New Jersey 08854

Natural Family Planning Association of Connecticut
P. O. Box 250
New Haven, Connecticut 06502

Natural Family Living
c/o Mr. James McGill
47 Hill Terrace
Westwood, Massachusetts

Catholic Family Life Program
2021 North 60th Street
Milwaukee, Wisconsin 53208

Family Life Center
Diocese of Pittsburgh
Pittsburgh, Pennsylvania

Planned Parenthood: some chapters offer classes in natural family planning; contact your local chapter for information.

Advantages

Natural family planning is completely safe. It poses no threat to the user's health and has no effect on long-term fertility. NFP is very inexpensive, and it is acceptable to the Catholic Church and religious groups that are opposed to other methods of contraception.

NFP enables women to tune in on their cyclical patterns and to learn more about how their bodies work. It may open couples up to alternative forms of sexual pleasuring on the days when intercourse is not safe. It does not require the use of any apparatus, such as an IUD, or harmful medications, such as the Pill, and is a completely natural, organic method of birth control.

Disadvantages and Problems

Some people find the extra time and attention required to keep these charts too bothersome. Other people have schedules that are too irregular or too hectic to allow them to incorporate this method of birth control into their lifestyles.

Another problem is that you must accumulate many months of records and charts before you begin to use this method of birth control. The Pill, which alters normal BBT curves and cervical mucus patterns, cannot be used during the time you are establishing your charts and records. Using spermicides either with or without a diaphragm may present difficulties in establishing the cervical mucus patterns. IUDs can also distort cervical mucus patterns. This leaves only the condom, the strict calendar method or abstinence as birth control choices during the months while you are learning to establish your cycles.

Douching, infection, semen and lubrications can make it difficult to recognize cervical mucus patterns. Some women do not have recognizable cervical mucus or BBT patterns.

There has been some concern that women using this method might have a higher rate of birth defects.[85] Intercourse is avoided prior to and after ovulation, but should ovulation occur unusually early or late, the egg or sperm involved might not be a fresh one. Studies on laboratory animals have shown that the rate of birth defects is higher in such pregnancies.[86] In addition, the incidence of birth defects is higher among Catholics than among Protestants.[87] Neither of these facts proves that couples using the rhythm method are more likely to give birth to abnormal infants should the method fail. Moreover, chances of such a pregnancy occurring are reduced when the BBT and cervical mucus methods are combined with the rhythm method. Still, the possibility of increased risk of birth defects should be considered by couples using natural family planning.

VASECTOMY

AKA: male sterilization

Vasectomy, or male sterilization, is a surgical procedure in which the vasa deferentia, the internal tubes that carry sperm from the testicles to the penis, are severed. It is considered a permanent, irreversible form of birth control, although in some cases it has been possible to perform corrective surgery to restore a man's fertility. The severed tubes can be rejoined in 40 to 90 percent of cases (this figure varies according to which type of vasectomy was performed and the skill of the surgeon doing the repair), but not all of these men will actually be fertile again. One study involving small numbers of men who were particularly likely candidates found that 69 percent of the men were successfully able to impregnate their partners following corrective surgery. Other studies have reported considerably lower rates. In the largest study the success rate following corrective surgery was only about 19 percent.[88]

There are also sperm banks where sperm can be frozen and stored. More than 500 normal infants have been born as a result of the use of frozen semen, the greatest success being with sperm stored less than six months, although pregnancy has been achieved using sperm stored for as long as ten years.[89] Most investigators, however, question the viability of sperm stored more than three years. Moreover, sperm banks are hard to find and several have gone bankrupt or closed for lack of financial success. Any man considering a vasectomy should not count on the possibility of reversing the operation or of using frozen sperm specimens.

It may be difficult for a young man, especially a single one who has never fathered any children, to find a doctor willing to perform a vasectomy on him. The Association of Voluntary Sterilization (708 Third Avenue, New York, New York 10017) has a referral service.

Finding an experienced doctor to perform the vasectomy is important. Many of the complications, although these are very rare, can be prevented by having the operation done by an experienced doctor.

Effectiveness

Although vasectomy is not completely foolproof (studies in the late 60s reported failure rates as high as four per 100), today, with improved techniques the failure rates are less than one per 100.[90] When failure does occur, it is most often because the cut ends of the tube have rejoined. Occasionally, when done by an inexperienced doctor, the wrong structure is cut or the ends of the tubes are not tied or clipped tightly, permitting sperm to leak through. In some instances, a man will have more than two vasa deferentia (singular form, vas deferens) and thus, one may be missed. Because some sperm remain in the tubes and it takes a number of ejaculations before all the sperm are cleared out, unprotected coitus before two consecutive negative sperm counts could also cause pregnancy.

Procedure

Vasectomy is a minor surgical procedure that takes about 15 minutes and can be done in a doctor's office under local anesthetic. Fees range from about $150 to $300.

The scrotal area is shaved, a local anesthetic is injected and either one or two small incisions are made, as shown in Illustration 30. Next, each of the vasa deferentia is located, pulled out through the incision and cut. The loose ends are then tied, burned or clipped. Most doctors remove a small portion of the vas to assure that the loose ends will be kept apart and won't grow back together. The incision in the scrotum is closed with absorbable sutures that dissolve in seven to ten days.

Following a successful vasectomy, the sperm produced in the testicles are blocked from passing beyond the point of the operation. These sperm

Illustration 30 *Vasectomy: The vas is located and an incision is made directly over it. Ties are placed on the vas and the tube is cut. The incision is sutured, and the process repeated on the other vas.*

are dissolved or in some cases destroyed by antibodies, part of the body's defense system. Antibodies are produced by one-half to one-third of the men who have vasectomies.[91] Hormone levels, sex drive and the ability to achieve and maintain an erection remain the same. (Psychological factors may affect erection in some men; see below). Because sperm accounts for only 10 percent of a man's ejaculate, or come, the volume of ejaculation is not noticeably affected.

There may be some slight problems after the vasectomy. Skin discoloration—a bruise—is common and is caused by blood seepage. This usually occurs in the scrotal area, but may involve the penis or, less frequently, the groin and inner thighs. There may be some associated swelling. Ice packs should be applied to the area for at least four hours following the operation. Neither of these complications requires any special treatment, and both subside within a few days or, at the most, a few weeks.

Although seldom severe, there may be pain or discomfort either when the local anesthetic is injected, when the vas is pulled into view or when the procedure is over. Pain sometimes occurs during the first intercourse following vasectomy, and in some cases it may persist for a few months during both erection and ejaculation. Ice packs will help reduce the initial discomfort, swelling and bruising. Aspirin can be taken for pain. Hot sitz baths taken four times a day will help promote healing and relieve discomfort. One week after the procedure, there should be a postoperative checkup so the doctor can be sure that everything is healing properly.

Most men experience a moderate amount of pain and discomfort on the day of surgery and on the following day. A man should not plan to drive himself home after a vasectomy. Returning to work is not advised for three days following the vasectomy if the man has a sedentary job or for seven days if he performs manual labor. Strenuous activity and intercourse should be avoided for at least a week. It's a good idea to wear an athletic supporter day and night for the first 48 hours and thereafter as long as it is more comfortable to wear it than not to wear it.

After the procedure, there are still some sperm left in the vasa deferentia and seminal vesicles (the sperm "storage tanks") that must be emptied before a man can rely on his vasectomy for contraception. It can take anywhere from six to twenty ejaculations to completely empty all the active sperm. Most doctors will ask a man to bring a sample of sperm after eight to ten ejaculations and then a second one following another series of ejaculations. Not until two negative ejaculation samples can a man consider himself sterile, and other forms of birth control must be used until this is accomplished.

In addition to the minor problems of pain, bruising and swelling mentioned earlier, there are other possible complications from the vasectomy. A hematoma, a mass of clotted blood, may form in the scrotal area. This occurs in less than 4 percent of all vasectomies.[92] This can be prevented by careful surgery and by avoiding heavy straining for the several days after the vasectomy. Most small hematomas reabsorb spontaneously. Ice packs can usually be used to treat those that do not. In less than 1 percent of the cases, it becomes necessary to reopen the scrotum, drain off the blood and tie off the bleeding vessel.

Infections, ranging from superficial skin infections to deeper ones, occur in less than 1 percent of the cases[93] and can usually be prevented by proper surgical sterilization by the doctor and cleanliness on the part of the man; however, a man should not shower or bathe for the first two days following vasectomy. Antibiotics and bed rest can be used to treat these rare cases of infection. Other rare complications include adhesions (scar tissue), hydrocele (a collection of fluid around the testicles due to surgical injury), orchitis (inflammation of the testicles), epididymitis (inflammation and tenderness near the testicles) and sperm granuloma (generally small and harmless accumulations of "leaked" sperm, which in rare instances may become infected). Some of these complications have no symptoms, while others require antibiotics and bed rest or, in some cases, minor surgery. It is interesting but hardly surprising that while these relatively minor complications associated with vasectomy are given a great deal of attention in both medical and lay literature on the subject, complications of similar importance (for example, bruising and subsequent infection of incision scars) are never even mentioned in most discussion of female sterilization procedures.

Advantages and Benefits

Vasectomy is the simplest, cheapest, safest, most effective method* of birth control. There have been no significant long-term side effects, although many millions of operations have been done. The complications rate is very low, only 2-4 percent, and most of these are short-term and minor.[94] The operation takes only about 15 minutes and, in most cases, can be performed in the doctor's office.

Disadvantages and Problems

In addition to the minor problems of swelling, bruises and pain and the rare complications (generally short-term and minor) mentioned earlier, there are several other disadvantages and problems associated with vasectomies.

First of all, not all men can have vasectomies. Men with previous hernia surgery, a thick, tough scrotum, a fixed, undescended testicle, a hydrocele (collection of fluid around the testicle) or a varocele (varicose vein) are not good candidates for vasectomy. Any local infections or problems should, of course, be cleared up before the vasectomy is attempted.

Moreover, about one-half to one-third of all vasectomied men develop antibodies to sperm, that is, their own bodies produce an immunity that inhibits sperm activity.[95] Although similar antibodies have been found in normal fertile men, they are more common in infertile men and in men with vasectomies. There is some controversy as to importance of these sperm antibodies. The immunological response of the human body is not well understood. Although there is no such evidence to date, some authorities theorize that sperm antibodies may attack something other than sperm and note that other irregularities in the immune system have been associated with conditions such as arthritis. Time will tell whether vasectomized males will develop a higher incidence of immunological disorders in old age.

Like the Pill, IUD and sterilization of females, the long-term effects of

---

*Actually, hysterectomy, or removal of a woman's uterus, is slightly more effective, but we do not recommend such a major operation for the sole purpose of birth control.

vasectomy cannot yet be determined. However, given the ever-increasing knowledge of the side effects of the Pill, IUD and female sterilization, it seems unfair to recommend these procedures with their undeniable dangers and then to express hesitancy about the merely speculative dangers of the vasectomy.

Although the vast majority of men who have had vasectomies report an improvement in their sex lives, which is probably due to freedom from the fear of unwanted pregnancies and the bother of other methods of birth control, some men experience a decline in their sex drive or inability to get and/or maintain an erection.[96] This is thought to be psychological, for the procedure, in and of itself, does not have a physiological effect on sexual performance or hormone levels. In some cases, the wife of the sterilized man may experience a decrease in sex drive. For such women, the act of intercourse may be so tied up with conception that once pregnancy is no longer possible, sex becomes less pleasurable.

Most researchers feel that the men who do experience these sorts of problems generally had sexual and psychological problems prior to the operation. The vasectomy merely triggered the problem. Anyone who is having surgery on his sex organs, especially surgery that will impair fertility, is likely to have some normal anxiety; however, anyone who has serious doubts about the procedure should not have the operation.

FEMALE STERILIZATION

AKA: tying the tubes, tubal ligation, tubal sterilization

Types: minilaparotomy, or Pomeroy technique
laparoscopic sterilization, Band-Aid sterilization or
belly-button surgery
colpotomy

Female sterilization is a method of birth control that involves removing or blocking some portion of the female reproductive tract. In the past, hysterectomy, an operation that removes the uterus, tubes and sometimes the ovaries as well, was a standard procedure for the sterilization of a woman. While hysterectomies are, unfortunately, still done by some doctors for the sole purpose of sterilization, we do not recommend them. Federal funds can no longer be used for such hysterectomies. Hysterectomies have considerably higher complication rates, anywhere from 10 to 100 times higher than the less radical procedures now available. While the risks facing a young, healthy woman are not all that great, hysterectomy is more expensive and requires a longer recovery time and may be more difficult to adjust to emotionally than the other types of sterilization. Any woman whose doctor suggests a hysterectomy for sterilization should read the section on hysterectomy carefully and should seek a second medical opinion (*see* p. 226) before consenting to the operation.

In recent years, less drastic procedures, which involve blocking the Fallopian tubes so that the sperm cannot fertilize the egg inside the tube, have been developed and have become increasingly popular. Indeed, for married couples over thirty years of age, sterilization has become the most commonly used method of birth control in this country.

Sterilization Abuse

Women considering sterilization, especially minority and low income women, should be aware of the controversy surrounding sterilization abuse. Since 1970 female sterilization has increased almost threefold, and poor and minority women are heavily overrepresented. Twenty percent of the married black women in this country have been sterilized versus 7 percent of the married white women. Fourteen percent of native American women have been sterilized. In Puerto Rico, one-third of all women of childbearing age have been sterilized. The United States has widely financed and promoted sterilizations in Third World countries as well.[97]

Consent forms have been pushed at women in the throes of labor and women under the influence of anesthesia and drugs. In some cases, written consent was not even obtained or women were mistakenly led to believe that the operation was not permanent and that their tubes could be untied at some time in the future. Other women were told that they would die if the procedure was not done. Still other women have been forced into sterilization by being threatened with having their welfare benefits cut off.[98]

It seems that a number of doctors feel that overpopulation has become such a problem that for them it is acceptable practice to trick or coerce women into being sterilized. Indeed, a survey that polled gynecologists in four major cities indicated that 94 percent of the doctors responding favored compulsory sterilization for welfare mothers with three or more illegitimate children.[99] Women interested in learning more about sterilization abuse and how to prevent it can contact the Committee to End Sterilization Abuse, CESA, Box A244, Cooper Station, New York, New York 10003.

Making the Decision

Meanwhile, every woman considering sterilization should know that it is a permanent method of birth control. It means that such women cannot have children in the future. Although there have been some cases in which the tubes were repaired after sterilization, these reparative operations involve risks and are not successful in most cases. There is at present no dependably reversible form of sterilization, even though some people mistakenly believe that certain types of rings or clip sterilizations are reversible. A woman should never have a sterilization procedure done with the idea that it can be fixed later on. Both she and her partner, if she has one, must be absolutely certain that permanent sterilization is what they want.

A woman should also know that she has the right to change her mind at any point about having the procedure done, even after she has signed the consent form, and that no one can deprive her of any benefits, such as welfare or medical payments, because she has refused the operation.

Through the efforts of female health activists and doctors concerned about sterilization abuse, certain rules for sterilization operations funded by the federal government have now been established. First, you must be at least 21 years of age. You must wait at least 30 days after you have signed the consent form to have the operation, except in some special instances, such as premature delivery or emergency abdominal surgery that takes place at least 72 hours after the consent is obtained. (This is to prevent unnecessary second surgeries in these women.) Also, a woman's consent to sterilization cannot be obtained while she is in the hospital for childbirth or abortion or under the influence of alcohol or any other substance that might affect her state of awareness. A woman may, if she chooses, bring someone with her when she signs the consent form. The consent form is effective for 180 days from the date on which it is signed. If a woman has questions or if something is not clear to her, she has the right to have all of her questions answered and to have a translator available if she speaks a foreign language.

While sterilization has sometimes been forced on minority and poor women, many white middle-class women have had difficulty finding a doctor who will perform the operation on them. It is no longer necessary for a woman to have the legal consent of her husband in order to be sterilized. Still, some doctors are reluctant to perform sterilizations on such women, especially if they have no children and sometimes even if they already have two or three children. Any woman having difficulty finding a doctor to perform a sterilization operation can contact a local Planned Parenthood or Zero Population Growth office or can write or call the Association for Voluntary Sterilization, 14 West 40th Street, New York, New York 10018 (212-524-2344).

Couples considering sterilization should know that despite the publicity surrounding so-called Band-Aid sterilization, female sterilization is a major surgical procedure with significantly higher risks, more potentially serious complications and higher costs than the male sterilization

183

procedure, vasectomy. A couple considering sterilization should seek counseling on both methods before they make their final decision.

Effectiveness

Other than abstinence, that is, not having intercourse at all, sterilization is the most effective method of birth control. Surprising as it may seem, however, it is not 100 percent effective. If failure does occur, it is usually because the tubes have grown back together or because a supporting ligament rather than a tube was cut or tied off. However, these are rather rare occurrences, and the effectiveness rates for all of the various methods of sterilization are said to be about 0.04 percent.[100] Certain techniques will have a slightly higher rate than others, but pregnancy rates for all forms of sterilization are lower than those obtained with any other method of birth control.

Methods of Sterilization

Tubal sterilization procedures, which interrupt the Fallopian tube, are now the preferred methods for female sterilization. Traditionally, this has involved ligation (tying of the tube), which may be accompanied by excision (cutting away) of a piece of the tube. More recently, electric coagulation (burning), elastic bands and rings and/or clips have been used to close the tubes.

Tubal sterilization can be done by either a vaginal or abdominal route, depending on how the doctor decides to get at the tubes to close them off. In the vaginal approach, an incision is made in the vagina and a special viewing instrument, known as a culdoscope, may be used. The two most widely used abdominal approaches are the minilaparotomy, involving an incision in the abdomen, and the laparoscopic tubal ligation, which makes use of another special viewing instrument, the laparoscope.

Prior to Surgery

Before the operation, the doctor will take a detailed medical history, which should include complete information about previous problems with anesthesia, bleeding disorders, allergies and any medications currently being taken. Any history of sexually transmitted diseases, pelvic infections or previous surgery should also be noted, for any of these conditions may result in pelvic scar tissue or adhesions that could complicate certain methods of performing tubal sterilization. Most doctors recommend that IUDs be removed prior to surgery to decrease the chances of infection. Oral contraceptives, which increase the risk of blood clots, should also be discontinued for at least one month prior to surgery. A complete physical examination, including a general evaluation to identify medical conditions that might alter the decision about surgery or anesthesia, is also done prior to surgery. A gynecological exam is given to identify pelvic disease, such as fibroids, that might complicate surgery or indicate the need for alternative surgery. Laboratory tests, including a Pap smear, which should be normal, a blood count and urinalysis are done. Although not all doctors do it, it is a good precaution to have preoperative bleeding and clotting-time tests done and to have a specimen of blood held in the blood bank in case transfusion is needed during surgery. We also recommend chest X-rays, even if a woman is having a local anesthetic, in case some complications during the operation should require a general anesthetic. The chest X-ray will rule out possibly dangerous conditions that could contraindicate general anesthesia.

Prior to the operation, the area where the incision is to be made is scrubbed with an antiseptic solution. If the approach is abdominal, the area is shaved, and if the incision is to be made near the pubic hair, most or all of the pubic hair will be shaved to prevent infection. All food, solids and liquids are prohibited for eight hours prior to surgery so that the stomach will be empty in case an emergency occurs and a general anesthetic is required. Some doctors will also order a preoperative enema. In some cases, the doctor will empty the bladder via a tube known as a catheter prior to surgery. This makes some forms of sterilization operations easier for the doctor. However, the introduction of the tubal catheter also increases the chance of postoperative urinary tract infection, so some doctors will merely have the woman empty the bladder herself immediately before the operation.

Either a local or a general anesthetic can be used for most tubal ligations. If a general anesthetic is used, a tube is inserted down the throat after the woman is put to sleep, which will help the anesthesiologist control her breathing. Local anesthetics may be injected into the incision site. Although there may be a slight prick from the first injection, subsequent injections can't be felt; however, there may be some discomfort when the Fallopian tubes are pulled into view by the doctor. Spinal anesthetic, which temporarily immobilizes the legs, or, preferably, epidural anesthetic, which allows for movement of the legs, may also be used in some tubal sterilization procedures. The anesthetic is injected into the lower back so that there is no pain at the operative site but the woman will still be awake. The epidural doesn't have the disadvantage of the excruciating headache that sometimes follows the spinal, but the epidural is more difficult to administer and not all anesthesiologists are equally skilled at it.

If a general anesthetic is used, a shot is given about a half hour before surgery that contains a tranquilizer and a drug that dries up secretions in the mouth or throat that might cause breathing problems. Even if only a local anesthetic is planned, the drug to dry up secretions may still be given in case serious bleeding complications requiring prolonged surgery occur and a general anesthetic is then needed. Because of the possibility of complications that might require a general anesthetic, some doctors feel that the anesthesiologist should be at hand during the operation. This is particularly important in a laparoscopic tubal ligation, even if it is done under a local anesthetic.

Either a local or general anesthetic can be used for most sterilizations; however, even though a general anesthetic involves more risks, most doctors prefer it, since if emergency surgery is required, there is no time lost giving a woman a general anesthetic and inserting the tube into the windpipe. Moreover, some doctors feel that a woman is apt to move when the tubes are grasped if she has only had a local anesthetic, which could lead to complications in the operation.

Laparoscopic Tubal Ligation

As mentioned earlier, there are a number of different techniques for tubal sterilization. In recent years, the laparoscopic tubal ligation (see Illustration 31), also called Band-Aid sterilization, has become increasingly popular. The laparoscope is a lighted viewing instrument that can be inserted into the abdomen and used to locate the Fallopian tubes. After the anesthetic is given, a tiny incision is made at the bottom of the navel. Next, a long, thin needle is inserted into the abdomen. The needle is then attached to a tube, which in turn is connected to a machine containing either carbon dioxide or nitrous oxide gas. The gas is run through the tubing into the abdominal cavity until the abdomen is so swollen and firm that it sounds like a drum when tapped. The gas moves the intestines out of the way and makes it easier for the doctor to see the pelvic organs and to close off the tubes without injuring any other tissue. If only a local anesthetic is used, the woman may experience a feeling of bloating and a mild to moderate discomfort as the abdomen fills with gas.

An instrument known as a trocar, which is enclosed in a special sleeve, is then inserted through the incision. The trocar is removed, leaving the special tubelike sleeve in place. When the trocar is removed, an audible whoosh of gas may be heard. After the trocar has been removed, the laparoscope is inserted through the sleeve and the light source and gas tubing are attached to it. Most doctors then make a second incision lower in the abdomen and insert a smaller trocar in a sleeve. The electric

Illustration 31   *Laparoscopic Tubal Ligation*

coagulation tool is inserted through this. If a local anesthetic is being used, more anesthetic is first injected, but even with adequate local anesthetic the woman is likely to feel more discomfort from this than from the first incision. Other doctors will use only one incision, and the coagulation equipment is introduced through this incision as well.

The Fallopian tube is then grasped with the forceps of the coagulation tool. Once the doctor is sure that the intestines or other tissues are not near the tube and in danger of being accidentally burned, s/he pushes a button or pedal that activates the electric current from the electric cautery machine. The short burst of electricity causes the Fallopian tube to burn and turn white. The doctor may then pull slightly on the forceps to break the tube in half. Some doctors prefer to burn the Fallopian tube in several locations rather than pulling on it to separate the pieces. A new type of cautery, bipolar cautery, is used by some doctors and has cut down on the dangers of burning other tissue (see below) at the time of the sterilization procedure.

After severing both tubes and checking for bleeding, the doctor releases as much of the gas as s/he can through a valve on the sleeve by pressing on the abdomen. The instruments are removed and the incision or incisions are closed with an absorbable suture and covered by one or two Band-Aids. The procedure takes about half an hour, and regardless of whether a local or a general anesthetic is used, most women can usually leave the hospital within eight hours after their surgery. The Band-Aids are removed the following day. Occasionally, there is a slight tenderness, redness or fluid leaking from the incision. Hot water soaks three times a day will usually clear this up.

Minilaparotomy

Another abdominal procedure, the minilaparotomy (Illustration 32), or minilap, involves inserting an instrument through the cervix and into the uterine cavity in order to push the uterus up against the lower wall of the abdomen. An abdominal incision is then made directly over the top of the elevated uterus. The tubes are then brought into view. Then the doctor cuts, ties, burns or clips the tubes. A special instrument that looks like a small vaginal speculum may be inserted through the incision to help the doctor see the tubes. This operation also takes about 30 minutes, and the stay in the hospital is usually less than 24 hours.

Colpotomy

Vaginal tubal ligation (Illustration 33) can be performed by colpotomy. "Colpotomy" is a term used to refer to any operation in which an incision is made in the vagina just behind the cervix. Once this is done, the tubes may be brought out through the incision and tied. The incision is then stitched up. The procedure takes about half an hour. This operation has the advantage of not leaving any visible abdominal scar. After the operation, the woman can sometimes go home on the same day, but this is not always possible, with an average stay of four days. The postoperative time away from work is anywhere from two to four weeks, although many women will require a longer recovery time. Intercourse is prohibited for three to four weeks after the operation to allow the vagina time to heal.

Women who have enlarged uteri, which includes all women who have just given birth, cannot have this operation, for the tubes would be too far away to be reached through the vaginal incision. If the woman has had previous abdominal surgery or has a history of pelvic inflammatory disease, there may be too much scar tissue for the colpotomy to be done safely. It is also easier to do this operation on women who have had children previously.

Illustration 32 *Mini-Laparotomy: An incision is made just above the pubic-hair line. The tube is pulled through the incision. A loop of the tube is sutured shut with the Pomeroy technique and then the top part of the loop is cut away.*

The problem with this method is that the complication rate is about twice as high as with abdominal tubal ligations. The complications (see below) can include bleeding, acute chronic pelvic infection, chronic pelvic pain and chronic pain on intercourse, even when the operation is done by a well-trained, experienced gynecologist. In the hands of a novice, the complication rates may be extremely high. When complications do develop, they are potentially more serious than those following abdominal tubal ligation, and the postoperative pregnancy rates are slightly higher.

Methods for Closing off the Tubes

With laparoscopic procedures, the tubes are usually coagulated (burned); however, this sometimes involves serious complications, so recently some doctors have been using rings or bands instead of coagulation. Although

189

Illustration 33 *Culpotomy: An incision is made in the vagina, just below the cervix (A). The cervix is lifted up and held steady while a grasping instrument is used to locate the tubes (B).*

this avoids the risks associated with coagulation, such rings and bands are still experimental and may not be as effective in preventing future pregnancies. Coagulation is never used for vaginal approaches. Usually, the Pomeroy technique is used for colpotomy or laparotomy. The Pomeroy technique involves elevating a knuckle of the tube (see Illustration 32) and tying a suture just below the knuckle. By the time the suture is absorbed several weeks later, the two stumps heal, leaving a gap in the tube.

Following Surgery

Most women experience some pain and discomfort. There may be abdominal and shoulder pain as a result of pockets of gas and air pressing on abdominal organs or on the diaphragm, but this shouldn't last more than 24 to 48 hours. There may be soreness around the incision site. With the vaginal procedures, sexual intercourse is prohibited for three to four weeks, to give the incision time to heal. For the abdominal procedures, intercourse can be resumed whenever the woman feels comfortable, usually within a week. Even if a local anesthetic has been used and a less extensive procedure has been done, the woman will need to rest for at least 24 hours and should not expect to resume regular activities for a minimum of two to three days. Women should avoid straining or lifting heavy objects for at least one week. Your doctor will have specific instructions about bathing, showering, intercourse and the use of tampons.

The stitches do not require any removal, for they will dissolve themselves. However, there should be a follow-up appointment within a month so that the doctor can check the incision and healing process. If a woman develops any of the following symptoms, she should contact her doctor immediately, for they may be signs that one of the more serious complications described below has occurred: fever greater than 100.4°F, fainting spells, abdominal pain that is persistent or increasing after 12 hours and bleeding from the incision site.

Advantages and Benefits

Sterilization is the most effective method of birth control. For many women, freedom from the fear of pregnancy and the bother of contraception means increased sexual enjoyment. Although sterilization may cost anywhere from $300 to $700 or even more, assuming there are not major complications, this is a one-time expense. Although there may be some questions about the long-term effects of sterilization on the menstrual cycle, these effects are not thought to be as serious as those that may be encountered with some other methods, such as the birth control pill.

Disadvantages and Problems

The most obvious disadvantage with sterilization is that it must be considered a permanent, irreversible method of birth control. It is important to get good counseling and to consider the question thoroughly before having the sterilization operation. In one study, 30 percent of the sterilized women later regretted their decision.[101] One question that might be helpful for a mother contemplating sterilization is to consider whether she would want more children if something happened to her existing children. Other women might ask themselves if they were to marry or remarry, would they then want to start a family?

191

Aside from the common postoperative problems of pain and discomfort described above, there are sometimes more serious consequences from sterilization. Despite the nickname of Band-Aid sterilization, which implies a minor surgical procedure, sterilization, even laparoscopic sterilization, is a major operation. Although the risks of death are rare, they are not nonexistent. The use of a general anesthetic always carries risks. In addition, arteries may be punctured and blood clots and heart attacks can occur. The overall death rate for women undergoing traditional tubal ligation is estimated at somewhere between 10 to 25 women per 100,000.[102] For laparoscopic tubal ligation, the mortality rate is 2.5 deaths per 100,000 women undergoing the operation.[103]

Aside from death, other serious complications, such as the burning of surrounding tissue, puncture of the bowel or other organs, cardiac arrest, hemorrhage, infection and chronic pelvic pain can also be complications of sterilization. A few women continue to have pelvic pain for months or years after surgery. This is usually localized in the area of the tubes and is described as a tugging, drawing sensation. It is often associated with intercourse or sudden changes in position that stretch the pelvic muscles.

Psychologically, sterilization has its effect as well. Some depression is bound to follow, for childbearing is an integral part of our self image and the loss of this function affects some women in a negative way. Feelings of depression are not uncommon, and most women—the great majority— recover within weeks and months. A few stay depressed and mournful, and a very small number of suicides have been attributed to abnormal psychological adjustment after sterilization.

It has long been assumed that sterilization would not affect the function of the remaining organs—that the egg would pop off the ovary each month and when it reached the obstruction of the tube it would simply be reabsorbed in the surrounding tissue. Recently, information has come to light about the possible long-term effects of laparoscopic sterilization on ovarian function. A study done in 1974 compared the menstrual bleeding patterns of two groups of women, one of which had been sterilized by laparoscopic tubal ligation and the other by laparotomy, with a third group of women whose husbands had been sterilized.[104] Thirty-nine percent of the women sterilized by laparoscopy had increased menstrual blood loss, and another 21 percent had increased menstrual pain. A year after the operation, 7.4 percent of the women who had had laparoscopic steriliza- tions had to have hysterectomies, compared with only 5.4 percent of those who had had the older minilaparotomy, tube-tying method and 1.4 percent of the control group, whose husbands had been sterilized.

There are several problems with this study. First of all, it was a retrospective study. Retrospective means "looking back." Information about menstrual pain and amount of menstrual flow came from what women remembered about their periods before the procedure. It asked subjective questions, like "more or less pain?" or "more or less blood flow?" According to another group of critics, the study fails to take into account the fact that these women may have used different forms of birth control prior to the sterilization. Perhaps it was the long-term effects of the previous birth control method that were responsible for the subsequent differences. Obviously, a better study than this one is needed; still, the fact that there was a striking difference between the laparoscopic group and the other sterilized group, both in terms of bleeding, pain problems and in the higher hysterectomy rates, raises some serious questions about sterilization and its long-term effects. It may be that the blood supply to the ovary is damaged during the operation, especially with the laparoscopic sterilization and cautery. However, this is mere speculation. We are not even sure that a negative effect exists, much less what causes it. We do know that some women who have been sterilized have had premature menopause, which is probably caused by damage to the blood supply at the ovaries at the time of operation, but how frequent this effect is and whether it is actually connected to a sterilization procedure remain to be determined.

Another problem with sterilization is that not all women are candidates for the procedure. A woman with a history of pelvic inflammatory disease, endometriosis or any condition that leaves a good deal of scar tissue in the abdominal cavity may not be suitable for sterilization. Likewise, large fibroids and certain ovarian cysts make some methods of tubal sterilization impossible for some women.

ABORTION

Types: vacuum abortion, early abortion or suction curettage
menstrual extraction, very early abortion, menstrual regulation or menstrual induction
dilation and evacuation, or D&E
amniocentesis abortion or infusion or instillation abortion
prostaglandin suppository abortion
hysterectomy
hysterotomy

Abortion is the deliberate removal of fetal tissue from the uterus. Elsewhere in this book, we have discussed spontaneous abortions or

193

miscarriages. Here we are concerned with therapeutic abortions, that is, the deliberate removal of fetal tissue in order to terminate a pregnancy.

There is a rather widespread misunderstanding about abortion. Many people, women and doctors alike, are apt to feel that a woman who has an abortion has been careless or irresponsible about birth control. Women who have more than one abortion are often viewed as having some deep-seated psychological problem. These attitudes betray an ignorance of the facts. No method of birth control is 100 percent effective, which means that any woman, no matter how conscientious, is liable to face the problem of an unplanned pregnancy at some time in her life.

Consider, for example, what would happen in a group of 1,000 women who were using a 98 percent effective method of birth control like the Pill, IUD or diaphragm. As we explained in Chapter Five, birth control rates are given in terms of 100 women using that method for a year. A 98 percent effectiveness rate means that in the course of a year 98 of those 100 women would not get pregnant, but two would. In a group of 1,000 women using a 98 percent effective method, this would mean 20 unplanned pregnancies a year. Women have an average of 35 years of fertility during their lifetimes. Over a period of 35 years this could mean as many as 700 unplanned pregnancies in a group of 1,000 women! Women faced with an abortion decision should be aware of these facts and should not allow themselves to be made to feel that they have been careless or irresponsible. Although some women who have repeated abortions may not have practiced proper birth control methods or may have psychological problems, repeat abortions, in most cases, reflect nothing more than statistical odds.

Legal Status

In 1973 the Supreme Court handed down a landmark decision that legalized abortion.[105] The Court ruled that, during the first trimester (the first 12 weeks of pregnancy),* decisions regarding abortion are a private matter between a woman and her doctor and that neither the state nor the federal government can place restrictions on how, when or where an abortion procedure can be done. During the second trimester (the second 12 weeks of pregnancy), a state may impose regulations designed to protect a woman's health. For instance, an individual state can require that second trimester abortions be done only in licensed hospitals. According to the same Supreme Court decision, an individual state can also place

*The duration of a pregnancy is measured by counting from the first day of the last menstrual cycle even though conception probably didn't take place for a couple of weeks after that.

restrictions on or even outlaw abortions after the second trimester, when fetal viability begins (the time after which a fetus might possibly survive), except when the mother's life or health is in danger. (Viability occurs at 24 weeks or, according to some, at 26 weeks. In other words, some fetuses aborted as early as 24-26 weeks of pregnancy might be able to live if special care were given.) The Supreme Court decision did not automatically overrule all state laws regarding abortion, at least not those covering late abortions, so in some states late abortions may be difficult to obtain.

There has been considerable opposition to this Supreme Court decision, and the groups opposed to the legalization of abortion, often called Right-to-Life groups, have worked hard to have these laws weakened or reversed, because they feel that abortion is morally wrong.[106] Their efforts have met with considerable success. In 1977 the Supreme Court decided that states had the right to prohibit payment for abortion for poor women receiving state medical assistance. More recently, regulations written for federally funded medical programs have prohibited abortion payments except in cases of rape, incest or risk to the mother's life. Military dependents no longer have insurance coverage for abortion.

The Right-to-Lifers believe that abortion, regardless of the viability of the fetus, is morally wrong, the equivalent of murder. They feel they are protecting the rights of the unborn. The groups who support the legalization of abortion, often referred to as Pro-Choice groups, believe that a woman must have the legal right to control her own reproductive organs and to decide what happens inside her own body. They point to the fact that prior to legalization, millions of women were having illegal abortions, often under dangerous conditions, and that many of these women lost their lives needlessly. Pro-Choicers believe that abortion is a moral decision but one that must be made by the individual woman. They argue that no group of people has the right to inflict their personal moral judgments on others by legally restricting abortion.

We too believe that abortion should remain legalized. Unless the Supreme Court reverses its decisions or a constitutional amendment outlawing abortion is passed, the procedure will remain a legal one. There is, however, a strong movement to pass such a constitutional amendment. Women who want abortion to remain legalized should be aware of this and of the fact that their silence on this issue could allow a vocal minority to change the legal status of abortion. Women interested in working to assure their legal right to abortion can contact Abortion Action Coalition, Box 2727, Boston, Massachusetts 02208.

Legally, a woman need not have the consent of her spouse, her parents or anyone else in order to have an abortion.[107] There are, however, some clinics and hospitals that require the husband's or parent's signature before they will provide treatment. This is more likely to happen with late

195

abortions. In such cases, a woman may either provide the required signatures or seek treatment elsewhere.

Making the Decision

A woman who is pregnant has three basic options:

1. She can have an abortion
2. She can have the baby and keep it
3. She can have the baby and give it up for adoption.*

Many times this is a very difficult decision for a woman to make. In most cases there is not much time in which to decide. By the time most women discover that they are pregnant, they are already four to six weeks pregnant. Although there are now special tests that can detect pregnancy within 22 to 24 days of the last menstrual period, the standard test is not accurate until about six weeks. Since the less risky, simpler abortion procedures must be done before 12 weeks, this usually allows only a month for decision-making.

A woman is likely to have ambivalent feelings when making this very difficult decision about whether or not to have an abortion. The first step for her is to find out for certain whether or not she is pregnant. This can be done through her regular doctor, public-health clinic or Planned Parenthood. Planned Parenthood has chapters throughout the country that provide testing, counseling and abortion referrals.

A good, reputable counselor will not try to influence a woman's decision, but will help her by providing information about her options, by arranging for adoption or medical assistance while she is pregnant and afterward (if she should choose to keep the child) and by giving information about abortion procedures and other important facts.

Somewhere between 5 and 6 percent of the women who at first decide on abortion change their minds before they actually have the abortion. For this reason it is suggested that the counseling and the actual abortion do not take place on the same day.

There may be medical factors that will influence your decision. Now that abortion has been legalized and it is possible to detect certain defects early in pregnancy by analyzing a sample of fluid from the amniotic sac

---

*A cooperative community group known as The Farm (Summertown, Tennessee 38483) has offered to help any woman who is thinking about abortion to deliver her baby by natural childbirth for free. If the woman decides to keep the baby, she may; otherwise they will raise the child for her. If the woman ever decides that she wants the baby back, she can have it. The Farm midwives offer this alternative to the limit of their ability to provide good care.

that surrounds the fetus (a procedure known as amniocentesis), more women are having abortions to terminate defective pregnancies.

Any woman who is 35 years of age or older, has already borne a child with a birth defect, has a personal or family history of birth defects or whose sex partners have such a history should have genetic counseling to determine whether or not she is a candiate for amniocentesis. Your doctor can obtain a free directory of federally supported genetics centers from the National Foundation for the March of Dimes, Box 2000, White Plains, New York 10602.

Many pregnant teenagers wonder whether or not they should involve their parents in the decision-making process. They are reluctant to upset their parents or are afraid that their parents will be angry with them. Despite these fears many teenagers find that their parents are very supportive and helpful in terms of finances and in finding good medical care. However, parental consent is not legally required for pregnancy care or for abortion, and many teenagers handle these problems on their own.

Test and Examinations Prior to Abortion

All women should have a pregnancy test before undergoing an abortion. Although this seems obvious, there have been cases where women were referred to abortion clinics solely on the basis of the fact that they had missed one or more menstrual periods.

It is often a good idea to have the pregnancy test performed at a qualified laboratory and not at the clinic or facility where the abortion will be done. There have been cases where women health activists who were investigating abortion clinics deliberately submitted male urine samples to a number of clinics. Some of these clinics actually told these women that they were pregnant and offered to schedule abortion surgery for them. You can see why it is important for women to have independent pregnancy testing.

Many doctors and clinics do a routine test for gonorrhea on all women undergoing abortions. If you have any reason to think that you might have been exposed to gonorrhea, insist on having this test before the abortion. If you do have gonorrhea and go ahead with an abortion, there is a good chance that the gonorrhea may spread beyond the cervix and into the uterus and tubes. This can cause pelvic inflammatory disease, which can have serious and even fatal consequences.

You also should have your blood pressure taken and blood tests made to check for anemia and to find out whether you have Rh-negative or Rh-positive blood. Most women have Rh-positive blood, which doesn't cause any problems. But if a woman with Rh-negative blood becomes pregnant with an Rh-positive fetus, the Rh-positive cells from the fetus could enter her bloodstream during abortion, delivery or miscarriage. Since the mother's blood is Rh-negative, this may cause an antibody reaction. Antibodies are protein substances that are part of the body's immune system. They attack "foreign invaders" in the body, which, in this case, would be the Rh-positive blood cells from the fetus. If an Rh-negative woman develops these antibodies, they will attack the blood cells of the fetus during each succeeding pregnancy, possibly causing severe jaundice and fetal death.

Luckily, there is now a vaccine that can be given to the mother within 36 to 72 hours after delivery, miscarriage or abortion that will prevent the antibody reaction. After a full-term delivery, the decision as to whether or not to give this vaccine is based on a sampling of the baby's blood. If the baby's blood is negative, there is no need for the drug, but if the baby's blood is positive, then the drug is given. It should be given to all women who have Rh-negative blood following abortion or miscarriage. At one time it wasn't given to Rh-negative women who had early therapeutic abortions, but studies reported in the medical literature indicated that even in early abortions there is a small chance of the mother's developing antibodies, so the vaccine is now given in these cases as well. Women having therapeutic abortions should ask about their blood type, whether the vaccine will be necessary and if so, whether the cost of the vaccine ($35—$55) is included in the price of the abortion.

A chest X-ray and urine tests may also be done, especially if you are having a general, rather than a local, anesthetic. Some doctors and clinics give preoperative enemas or shave the pubic hair, neither of which is necessary. The doctor should do a pelvic exam and take a medical history to find out if you have a history of heart disease, blood-clotting disorders, epilepsy, adverse drug reactions or other medical problems that could influence how the abortion is done. The pelvic exam and the date of your last period will help the doctor decide how advanced the pregnancy is, which will also influence the choice of procedure. Some doctors or clinics do a routine Pap smear on all women undergoing abortion. You should be prepared to make two visits to the doctor or the clinic, one for tests and one for the abortion.

You should not eat or drink anything for eight hours prior to the abortion, regardless of whether you are having a local or general anesthetic. Some doctors allow a woman to eat a light breakfast if a local is planned, but we don't think this is a good idea. If complications requiring a general anesthetic do occur, food or liquids in the stomach could be regurgitated, causing respiratory problems. If a woman is having a general anesthetic, she may be given a preoperative shot of a drug called atrophine to dry up secretions in her mouth and throat, so that she doesn't choke on them. If a local anesthetic is planned, she may be given a shot of tranquilizer before the abortion.

Early Vacuum Abortion (4–12 weeks)

In a vacuum abortion, or suction curettage (Illustration 34), a tube attached to a suction device is inserted through the cervix and into the uterus. Suction is then applied and the contents of the uterus are gently vacuumed out. This procedure is the one most widely used in abortions.

It may be done using either a local or a general anesthetic. Most clinics prefer a local anesthetic, however, and most doctors believe that the local is safer, although there have been deaths associated with locals as well.

The general anesthetic has the advantage of completely blocking any pain. Women may experience some pain with a local, but most feel the pain is tolerable. Not all abortion facilities offer a choice between the two, so if you are adamant about having a general, this may be a factor to consider in deciding where to have the procedure done (see below).

The doctor first performs a bimanual pelvic exam. A speculum is inserted and the cervix is cleaned with swabs that have been dipped in an antiseptic solution. The doctor then steadies the cervix with a special clamplike device called a tenaculum.

If a local anesthetic is used, it is injected into the cervix and ligaments that support the uterus. The anesthetic usually takes effect in a few seconds. Some women experience a numbness in the mouth or fingertips following the injection, but these reactions usually subside in two to three minutes. Some women feel a pinprick sensation when the local anesthetic is injected or a mild cramping; others don't feel anything.

The anesthetic takes effect in five to ten minutes, and the doctor then gently pulls the cervix to straighten it. Next, the opening to the cervix is dilated by the insertion of metal rods of increasing width until the os, the opening to the cervical canal, is open wide enough to accommodate an appropriate-sized vacuum tube (Illustration 35).

For abortions done in the first eight weeks, a tube called a cannula, six mm in diameter, is generally used. After eight weeks, a tube with a diameter equal to or two millimeters less than the number of weeks of pregnancy is used. Most doctors feel that these larger tubes, called curettes, should never be larger than 12 mm in size. Some doctors have used larger ones to abort pregnancies of more than 12 weeks duration. However, most abortions experts believe that the risks of uterine perforation, bleeding complications, cervical injuries or subsequent cervical incompetence, a condition in which the cervix opens up too early in the pregnancy, causing a miscarriage, are increased by use of a curette

Illustration 34   *Dilation: A tenaculum steadies the cervix, and rods of increasing diameter are used to dilate it.*

TENACULUM

DILATING RODS

Illustration 35 *Early Vacuum Abortion: Vaginal retractors are used to keep the vagina open, and the suction tube is inserted through the dilated cervix into the uterus (A). The contents of the uterus are vacuumed out (B). A curette may be used to insure that all of the contents of the uterus have been removed (C).*

larger than 12 mm. This belief is based on studies in which uteri removed surgically for other reasons were dilated with various size curettes and then examined microscopically for signs of damage.[108] The researchers found that there was no evidence of tissue damage with dilators less than eight mm in size. In almost 50 percent of the uteri tested there was some evidence of tissue damage with dilation of 9 to 11 mm. Although there is some question about the applicability of data obtained on surgically removed uteri to processes that occur in live uterine tissue, the point is obvious: the smaller the diameter the better. Women should ask their doctors what size dilators and tubes will be used. If the answer is a nine mm dilator for a pregnancy of seven weeks duration, for example, or a dilator larger than 12 mm at any time, find another doctor or clinic.

Some doctors prefer to use laminaria, rods made of sterilized seaweed, rather than metal dilators to open the cervix. The rods are inserted into the cervix either the night before or several hours prior to the abortion. The rods swell up with fluid, gently dilating the cervix. This gradual dilation over a period of hours seems to be associated with lower risk for uterine perforation, bleeding complications, cervical injury or cervical incompetence. However, some doctors fear that the use of laminaria may cause a higher rate of infection, because the cervix is open for a longer time, allowing more disease-causing organisms to enter the uterus. This is more likely to be a problem with rods left in place for more than 24 hours prior to the abortion. Also, on rare occasions the rods will cause a spontaneous abortion.[109]

The rods, which look like brown tampons, may come out prior to or at the time of the abortion. Be sure to save them to show to the doctor if they come out beforehand, since on occasion they are inserted too far into the cervix and move up into the uterus. X-rays are then necessary to locate them so that they can be removed.

Most women experience a mild cramping sensation when the laminaria rods are inserted. Such cramping may persist for hours, and some women have reported severe cramping. Studies comparing metal dilators and laminaria rods are now underway. Women should discuss these two methods of cervical dilation with their doctors, obtaining up-to-date information before making a decision.

After the cervix has been dilated and the vacuum tube inserted, the tube is attached to a suction machine. The suction machine, the sound of which you will probably hear, is turned on and the tube is moved around in the uterine cavity until its contents have been suctioned out. After the vacuuming begins, women who have had locals may feel a slight tugging sensation. Toward the end of the procedure, the uterus contracts sharply. The procedure takes three to five minutes. Some doctors then insert a curette instrument into the uterus to check it for retained tissue or abnormalities.

Most women experience strong cramping sensations that may last for 2 to 20 minutes. Pain medication may be given. Women who have had locals can usually get up and walk to the recovery room. Some women experience nausea and cramping for a half hour or so, but most can leave in one or two hours. If a general anesthetic has been used, the recovery time may be longer. You should plan to have someone help you home.

Many doctors give six tablets of ergotrate to be taken every four hours for 24 hours. This drug helps to keep the uterus contracted and diminishes the amount of bleeding. There may be some cramping after you take each tablet. Since the drug tends to elevate the blood pressure, it cannot be used by women with high blood pressure.

Most women experience some bleeding following the procedure. The blood may be dark in color and may be accompanied by an occasional clot. The bleeding may stop completely and begin again a few days later. The use of four to five pads a day for ten days following the abortion is not unusual; however soaking two pads with bright red blood in an hour or less or passing several clots over a short period of time may be an indication that something is wrong, and should be reported to the doctor. In addition, severe cramps that begin a day after the abortion, an oral temperature of over 100.4°F, a green or foul-smelling vaginal discharge and burning or frequency of urination should be reported to the doctor. If you do not have a period within 50 days, see your doctor. Always schedule a follow-up exam two to three weeks after the abortion, even if you are feeling fine.

You should rest the day of the abortion, but most women can return to work the following day. Avoid douching or intercourse for two weeks and use napkins, not tampons, for the first week or so.

Fertility returns rapidly. Sixty percent of women ovulate within the first 25 days, so contraception must be used right away.

Deciding Where to Have a Vacuum Abortion

Suction abortions can be performed in a doctor's office, an abortion clinic or a hospital. Several studies have shown that complication rates are lower when early abortions are performed in an abortion clinic rather than a hospital.[110] This may be due to the fact that local rather than general anesthetics are generally used in doctors' offices and clinics.

Abortions done in a doctor's office or clinic are generally less expensive. Having the abortion done in the office of a doctor whom she knows and feels comfortable with is an important factor for some women, but it may be slightly more expensive than an abortion clinic. Moreover, doctors working in clinics perform large numbers of abortions, and they become quite proficient at them.

If the pregnancy is beyond 11 weeks, many doctors prefer a hospital setting because occasionally there will be bleeding complications requiring transfusion when the uterus is this large. Women with fibroid tumors and congenital abnormalities of the uterus may have to have their abortions done in a hospital. Likewise, high-risk women—those with heart disease, blood-clotting disorders, chronic debilitating diseases and anemia—are often treated in a hospital.

Choosing the right doctor or clinic is important. We talk about choosing a doctor in more detail in Chapter Six. Having a board-certified gynecologist is important. Although the family doctor or a general surgeon might be quite competent to perform an abortion, a board-certified gynecologist is apt to do a better job should complications occur.

If you are planning to have your abortion done at an abortion clinic, you will want to make sure that the clinic is a good one. After abortion became legal, a number of clinics were set up for the sole purpose of performing abortions. While the majority of them provide excellent care, there are definitely some substandard ones. One way to locate a good clinic is to contact your local Planned Parenthood chapter. Some Planned Parenthood chapters provide first trimester abortions, and these clinics must meet rigid standards. In addition, those chapters that don't provide abortions can refer you to a doctor or clinic in the area. The doctors and clinics on their referral list have usually been inspected by a representative from Planned Parenthood and they also get follow-up evaluations from women who have been referred to these doctors or clinics. If treatment is below par, the doctor or clinic doesn't stay on the referral list for long. Other family-planning clinics may also have such referral lists. Be sure to ask whether the facilities on their list have been personally inspected and whether follow-up evaluation has been done. Women's health clinics are another excellent source for referrals. These groups often have referral lists that are carefully and scrupulously evaluated.

No matter where you have your abortion done, be sure that there is a 24-hour emergency telephone number so that you can reach a doctor in case complications develop. It is crucial that the clinic or doctor you choose be able to provide immediate access to a hospital should a medical emergency arise. There should be a hospital within a ten-minute drive, and more importantly, the doctor performing your abortion should have staff privileges at that hospital. Be sure to inquire about this when choosing a facility or doctor.

Cost may also be a consideration. Prices range from $125 to about $200, but of course this could change if inflationary trends continue. There may be an extra charge for a general anesthetic, Rh vaccine or IUD insertion.

Complications

The complication rates vary according to the duration of the pregnancy. Problems that may arise include: infection, excessive bleeding, injury to the cervix, perforation of the uterus or other organs, adverse drug reactions and incomplete abortion, in which some of the fetal tissue is left in the uterus.

Mortality figures vary in different studies, but one of the largest and most complete studies reported a death rate of less than one per 100,000 for abortions performed within the first eight weeks, 1.9 per 100,000 in the first nine to ten weeks and 4.1 in the first eleven to twelve weeks.[111] After that point, procedures that carry higher mortality rates (see below) are required.

Other Early Abortion Procedures
(see also Postcoital Contraception below)

Some doctors perform a D&C instead of an early vacuum suction abortion, but this may involve more blood loss and more pain and it has a higher rate of complications. If your doctor does not have access to suction equipment, find one who does.

Menstrual Extraction

Menstrual extraction is a procedure similar to vacuum abortion, only a syringe rather than a vacuum machine is generally used and it is usually not necessary to dilate the cervix. In the past, when pregnancy tests were not accurate until six weeks, this method was used on women whose periods were slightly overdue who thought they might be pregnant. Now that there are special pregnancy tests that can be accurate within one day of a missed period, it is no longer necessary for a woman to undergo this procedure without really knowing whether or not she is pregnant. Many doctors no longer perform menstrual extraction, since there is a chance that the procedure will not succeed in removing all the fetal tissue.

However, menstrual extraction does have advantages. It may not require dilation or an anesthetic, although some women do find the procedure quite painful. It is usually less expensive than an early vacuum abortion and women can usually leave the doctor's office within a half hour. It is important to have a follow-up visit within three weeks to make sure that the pregnancy was indeed terminated and that no complications have developed.

Some women involved in the health-care movement are strong advocates of menstrual extraction. Women in certain self-help groups have developed their own equipment and learned to perform this operation on each other. Since an anesthetic is not required and the cervix is not dilated, this procedure can be done quite simply. A flexible plastic tube is inserted through the os. Gentle suction is applied with a syringe and the menstrual lining is removed, along with the products of conception (if the woman was pregnant). See Illustration 36. Some women extract their menses on a regular basis, regardless of whether they suspect pregnancy, claiming that to do so relieves menstrual cramps. Advocates of menstrual extraction also believe that it is important for women to develop such simple, do-it-yourself methods in case there is an abortion backlash

FLEXIBLE
SUCTION TIP

COLLECTING
JAR

SYRINGE

Illustration 36 *Menstrual Extraction: The flexible suction tube is inserted into the uterus. A vacuum is created by drawing on the syringe, and the contents of the uterus are sucked into the collection jar.*

and abortion again becomes illegal. We do not recommend that women have this procedure done on a regular basis. No one knows what the effect of continually removing the lining of the uterus in this manner will be. Nor do we recommend that women perform this procedure on each other. There is always a risk of uterine perforation, cervical injury and infection with this procedure even when it is performed by experienced personnel in approved medical facilities. Moreover, we feel that political action is a more effective way of safeguarding the legal right to abortion.

Dilation and Evacuation Abortion: (13-18 weeks)

Dilation and evacuation (D&E) is a combination of the suction curettage done in early abortions and a surgical procedure in which a sharp curette is used to remove any remaining fetal tissue. The curette is necessary because of the larger volume of fetal tissue. A general anesthetic is usually required and the cervix must be dilated more widely (12-14 mm or more) than with an early vacuum abortion. The procedure also takes longer (20-30 minutes). Otherwise, from the woman's point of view, the proce-procedure and recovery are similar to the early vacuum abortion.

Some doctors perform this procedure beyond 18 weeks, even up to 24 weeks, but most doctors feel that the amniocentesis abortion described below is preferable after 18 weeks; however, studies are now underway to evaluate the D&E, and recommendations may change in the future.

D&E is a relatively new procedure. Since suction curettage alone will not suffice after 12 weeks because of the greater volume of fetal tissue and since amniocentesis abortion cannot be performed prior to 16 weeks (see below), it used to be that women over 12 weeks would have to wait until 16 weeks to have their abortion, which sometimes was emotionally devastating. Although the D&E involves higher complication rates than an earlier abortion, studies have shown that for a pregnancy of 13 to 16 weeks, it is the safest procedure.[112] Many doctors now recommend that the D&E, which has an overall mortality rate about half that of the amniocentesis procedures, be done on women over 12 weeks, rather than waiting until the 16th week. Women should discuss these alternatives with a doctor who is experienced in performing second trimester abortions before making a decision.

Amniocentesis Abortion (16−24 weeks)

Amniocentesis (Illustration 37) is a procedure whereby a hollow needle is inserted into the fluid-filled amniotic sac that surrounds the developing

207

HYPERTONIC SALINE SOLUTION

AMNIOCENTESIS NEEDLE

Illustration 37   *Saline Abortion: The saline solution is introduced into the amniotic sac through the amniocentesis needle.*

fetus. As mentioned earlier, fluid may be withdrawn from the sac and analyzed in order to detect certain birth defects. In an amniocentesis abortion, a drug that causes fetal death is injected into the sac. Fetal death is followed by a series of uterine contractions, which causes the expulsion of the fetal tissues.

Amniocentesis cannot be done before 16 weeks because prior to that time the amniotic sac does not contain enough fluid for the procedure to be done safely.

This procedure must be done in the hospital. It involves more risk than earlier abortions, and emergency facilities must be on hand in case complications occur. A local anesthetic is used, for the woman must be wide awake and fully alert so that she can report any unusual sensations to the doctor.

Prior to the procedure, the woman is asked to urinate so that her bladder is not distended. This cuts down on the chances of accidentally puncturing the bladder when the needle is inserted. The doctor then examines the abdomen and locates the top of the uterus. A small area of skin may be shaved and the area is then washed with an antiseptic solution. A local anesthetic is injected into the area, which may cause a brief stinging feeling. A long, hollow needle is then inserted through the anesthetized skin and the uterine muscle. Most women experience a feeling of pressure and some discomfort when this is done, but for most of them, this discomfort is alleviated once the needle is in place.

Some doctors insert a narrow, flexible plastic tube called a catheter through the needle and then withdraw the needle, leaving the tube in place. This has both advantages and disadvantages. The advantage is that the tube can be taped to the abdomen and left in place, so that if abortion does not occur within 48 hours, reinjection of the fluid is easier and less painful. On the other hand, leaving the tube in place increases the chance of infection. Since the majority of women will not require a second injection, many doctors don't use the tube.

Regardless of whether the needle or tube is used, some of the amniotic fluid is withdrawn and the drug is introduced into the sac. Many women note a slight sense of fullness or pressure at this time, which is normal; however, any feeling of pain or warmth should be reported to the doctor immediately.

If a needle is used, it is then withdrawn and the puncture is covered with a Band-Aid. If the tube is used, it is closed off and taped to the abdomen. Experiments in which the fluid is introduced through the cervix rather than the abdomen have been tried, but this has proven less satisfactory and is done only in special cases.

Some doctors insert one or two laminaria rods (described above) into the cervical canal after the amniocentesis procedure. Some doctors insert the laminaria 14 to 19 hours before the procedure. The point of inserting the laminaria is to dilate the cervix and thus to avoid tearing the cervix when the fetal tissue is expelled from the uterus. It has also been shown to shorten the time between the injection of the solution and the expulsion of the fetus. While the insertion of laminaria rods 14 to 19 hours before the procedure assures that the cervix will be well dilated by the time the fetal tissue is expelled, the longer they are in place, the greater the chances of disease-causing organism moving past the cervix and into the sterile uterus. If the laminaria rods are inserted right after the amniocentesis procedure, there may not be enough time before the expulsion of the fetal tissue to allow for sufficient dilation of the cervix but there is less chance

209

of infection. Other doctors feel that the cervical dilation that occurs naturally once the fetus dies is sufficient, so they do not use rods at all.[113]

Following the amniocentesis procedure the woman is usually returned to her hospital room. Uterine contractions, similar to labor pains, usually begin with six to eight hours; however, the contractions may begin earlier than this or later.

Some doctors give an injection of Oxytocin, a drug that causes uterine contractions. Again, this has both advantages and disadvantages. It shortens the time between the amniocentesis procedure and the expulsion of the fetus, which reduces the chances of infection and of the placenta being retained (see below). However, it increases bleeding complications, especially in women with certain blood disorders. The drug sometimes causes fluid retention, which if untreated can cause serious complications, including coma and convulsions. (If the drug is used, all fluid intake and output must be monitored carefully.) Some doctors use it routinely, while others prefer to reserve use of it for cases where the contractions are not strong enough and don't seem to be progressing rapidly enough.

The length of time between the amniocentesis procedure and the expulsion of the fetus varies considerably. In most cases, expulsion takes place within 24 to 36 hours, and 93 percent of the women undergoing this procedure will abort within 72 hours.[114]

Most women experience an increasing sense of fullness and pressure as the time for expulsion of the fetus approaches. The degree of pain a woman feels may be slight, moderate or intense. Pain medication can be given. Since the fetus is relatively small, the expulsion itself is usually not painful and doesn't usually require the incision at the vaginal opening (an episiotomy) that is frequently used in the delivery of a full-term pregnancy.

A member of the nursing staff may be with you when the expulsion occurs, or it may happen before the nurse arrives. You should be prepared for the fact that the fetus is recognizable at this stage of development. The nurse will usually handle the situation, so that you will not see the tissue. You may prefer not to look, should expulsion occur before she arrives. On the other hand, some women feel a strong need to see the actual fetus, finding that this makes it easier for them to deal with the emotional aspects of the situation. If you are among the latter, you should make your wishes known beforehand, as most nurses have been trained to conceal the fetus from you.

In three out of four cases, the expulsion of the fetus is followed shortly by the expulsion of the placenta, but sometimes it is necessary for the doctor to remove the placenta. This may be accomplished by pressing on the abdomen or by the use of a blunt grasping instrument. If these techniques don't work, a D&C may be required.

After expulsion, the woman usually remains in the hospital for at least three or four hours. The length of the hospital stay varies, depending on the time between the amniocentesis and the expulsion. Some clinics will send a woman home after the amniocentesis procedure, telling her to return once contractions have begun, but this is a questionable practice, and a woman should seek treatment elsewhere if her doctor or clinic suggests this.

Risks and Complications

The risks and complications involved in amniocentesis abortions depend somewhat on the drug used to cause fetal death. Any of the following substances may be used: urea, a concentrated solution of nitrogen waste products excreted by the kidney; prostaglandins, a class of hormones; and saline, a concentrated salt solution. Saline is the most widely used, but some doctors now prefer prostaglandins. The use of urea is a fairly recent innovation so there have not been as many abortions done using this substance. Each solution has its own particular advantages and disadvantages, and there have not yet been a sufficient number of prostaglandin and urea abortions done for conclusive comparisons to be made.

Infection, excessive bleeding and injury to the cervix can occur with any type of amniocentesis procedure. The complications may be serious enough to be fatal. The mortality rate for saline abortions is about 15.2 per 100,000 cases.[115] Most of these deaths result from infection; however, complications may also occur if the saline is not injected properly. If the saline is injected into the muscle wall of the uterus, this may cause death of the tissue and necessitate a hysterectomy. If the saline is accidentally injected into the abdomen, there is usually instant, severe pain, but this stops when the saline is discontinued. If the saline is injected into a blood vessel, it can cause instant death, though rarely is the reaction that severe. Indications of saline in a blood vessel include headache, restlessness, numbness and a feeling of warmth.

Prostaglandins are associated with a shorter interval between amniocentesis and expulsion of the fetus but with a higher incidence of the fetus being born alive and not expiring until shortly afterward. The mortality rate for the woman appears to be lower—about 10.5 per 100,000—than with saline, but there is a higher proportion of cervical injuries.[116] As many as 50-75 percent of women experience vomiting, nausea or diarrhea.

The complications associated with improper injection are less severe, even if the prostaglandins are injected into a blood vessel. Many doctors now feel that prostaglandins are safer than saline.

Urea is thought to be safer and to have less serious complication rates than either saline or prostaglandins. There is less vomiting, nausea and diarrhea than with prostaglandins and fewer clotting problems than with saline.[117] So far there have been no reports of live births. Bleeding may occur, but so far, these problems have not required transfusions. Infection is infrequent and can usually be treated with antibiotics. The rate of cervical injuries may be lower than with prostaglandins. Unfortunately, urea usually involves a longer time interval before the fetus is expelled and is less potent than saline or prostaglandins. Oxytoxin or the use of a second dose of prostaglandins may be required.[118]

Prostaglandin Vaginal Suppositories

Recently, vaginal suppositories of prostaglandins inserted every 3 to 4 hours have been used to induce abortion. This method is new and has not been widely used. It can cause extreme nausea, intense contractions, diarrhea and fever. It is also associated with relatively high rates of incomplete abortions requiring immediate D&C's. Since prostaglandins are hormones and all of their effects are not yet understood, it is too early to accurately evaluate this method.

Hysterotomy and Hysterectomy

Hysterectomy, an operation whereby the uterus is removed, is rarely used for abortion purposes anymore. It may, however, be used for women who have serious medical problems that prevent them from having an amniocentesis abortion. But since it is a major operation and since we now have alternative procedures, it should be used for abortion only on this and other rare occasions.

Hysterotomy is an operation whereby an incision is made in the uterus through which the fetal contents are removed. It is a sort of mini-Caesarean section. Again, the operation is rarely used today and is reserved for special cases.

Look to the Future

Obviously, there are many questions still be be answered about abortion procedures. The safety of the D&E versus the amniocentesis abortion, the use of contraction-stimulating drugs, the proper method of cervical dilation, the possibility of using prostaglandin suppositories in early abortions, the choice of medications in second trimester abortions—all of these issues are now being studied, so watch for future developments in this area.

Abortion and Subsequent Fertility[119]

Abortion complications such as infection can result in infertility. So far, the research in this country and in Great Britain indicates that other than complication-related infertility, repeated abortions do not have any consequences concerning subsequent fertility, miscarriage, premature births or other pregnancy problems. There are, however, reports from other countries indicating that having repeated abortions may cause decreased fertility and an increased risk for premature birth, infants with low birth weights and other pregnancy problems. It may be that the abortion procedures or the medical care in these other countries is inferior and is responsible for the problems in women who have had abortions. On the other hand, abortion has been legal in this country for only a relatively few years. Perhaps, as more time passes, such problems will become evident in this country as well.

POSTCOITAL CONTRACEPTION

Types: morning-after pill (MAP)
morning-after IUD
menstrual extraction, menstrual regulation or menstrual induction

Coitus means "intercourse," and postcoital contraception is a method of birth control that is used after a woman has had unprotected intercourse, because she has been raped, has forgotten to use birth control, has used it improperly or has used a method that has failed (broken condom, expelled IUD, etc.).

There are basically three methods of postcoital contraception now available: the morning-after pill, the morning-after IUD and menstrual extraction. The first two methods must be used within a few days of the unprotected intercourse. The third may be used around the time of the missed period.

There is some controversy about the use of postcoital contraception. The chance of becoming pregnant from a single act of intercourse may be as little as 2 percent and is probably no higher than 30 percent[120], even if you have intercourse at the most fertile time of the month. (*see* p. 68). The postcoital methods all involve certain risks and in some cases their effectiveness has been questioned or has not been confirmed, so some doctors recommend that women wait until a pregnancy test can confirm the pregnancy before doing anything. The newest pregnancy tests can be accurate in about 22 days after the last menstrual period, so women can find out whether they are pregnant quickly and can then have an abortion if they so desire. However, many women don't want to wait. They may prefer to take the risks without awaiting confirmation of pregnancy. Also, some women who have moral or religious objections to abortion prefer postcoital contraception, which may be viewed as preventing implantation of the egg rather than as actual abortion.

Before making a decision about how to deal with unprotected intercourse, read the following material as well as the above information on abortion and discuss the alternatives with a doctor. In making your decision, you will want to weigh the relative risks and benefits of each course of action against the probability of your actually being pregnant. Remember that your chances of getting pregnant are between 2-30 percent, with the chances being greater if the unprotected intercourse occurred near ovulation. If you are over 30 to 35 years of age, your chances of being pregnant are less than those of a woman who is in her 20s, the peak age for fertility. Similarly, if you are in your early teens, your chances are lower than if you were in your 30s.

We personally do not encourage the use of postcoital contraception and recommend that women wait and have pregnancy tests to make sure they are actually pregnant before taking any action.

The Morning-After Pill (MAP)

A synthetic estrogen, DES, has been approved by the Food and Drug Administration for use as a morning-after pill in emergency cases (rape, incest, etc.). Five pills of five mg. each must be taken twice a day for five days beginning within 72 hours (preferably within 24 hours) of the unprotected intercourse in order for the drug to be effective. Even then there is some question about its effectiveness. Although most studies have indicated that DES is effective as a postcoital contraceptive, a recent study of rape victims who had been given DES has raised serious questions.[121] In this study, the rate of pregnancies was about the same as that in similar groups which had not been given DES.

It is theorized that DES works (if indeed it does work) by altering the endometrial lining of the uterus in such a way that a fertilized egg cannot implant or survive. Some experts theorize that DES interferes with pregnancy by slowing down or speeding up the passage of the fertilized egg through the Fallopian tube.

One problem with the massive doses of estrogen required for postcoital contraception is the fact that these doses (50 times what the body normally produces) cause nausea as well as vomiting in 16-25 percent of the women who take the drug. Many doctors therefore prescribe an antinausea medication to be taken one hour before DES. If vomiting occurs within four hours, another dose of DES must be taken, since there is a chance that not all of the DES in the first pills will have been absorbed.[122]

With DES more than seven out of ten women will experience one of the following problems: nausea and vomiting, headaches, menstrual irregularities and breast tenderness. Some women may also experience vaginal spotting, dizziness, diarrhea, increased vaginal discharge, cramps or bloating. Only about one-third of the women who take DES as a postcoital contraceptive are symptom-free. About 20 percent of the women who take the MAP will have an unusually heavy, unusually light or delayed menstrual period. A late or light menstrual period does not mean that the MAP has failed, but such women should have pregnancy tests to rule out this possibility.[123]

If pregnancy does occur despite MAP treatment, the chances are greater that the pregnancy will be an ectopic pregnancy, a condition in which the egg implants in the tube or some other abnormal location and which can have serious consequences, including infertility and death. It is not clear whether this increased rate of ectopic pregnancies is because the MAP is more effective in preventing uterine pregnancies than ectopic pregnancies or because the MAP actually contributes to ectopic pregnancies by slowing down the Fallopian tube contractions.[124]

DES is an estrogen and may therefore cause any of the side effects and complications associated with the estrogen in birth control pills (*see* p. 98). In addition, DES has been implicated in reproductive tract abnormalities and cancer in the women who used this drug during pregnancy and in their offspring (*see* p. 769). Because DES has caused the development of cancer in some of the daughters of the women who took it during pregnancy, as well as other serious problems in both DES sons and daughters, the drug should not be taken by women who would not consider abortion if the drug were not effective and pregnancy ensued.

Estrogens have been clearly implicated in the development of fatal and nonfatal blood clots. If any of the following signs, which may be symptoms of a blood clot or other serious problems, develop, discontinue the drug and call your doctor IMMEDIATELY:

* severe headaches
* dizziness
* numbness in arms or legs
* shortness of breath
* loss of vision

* severe leg pains
* blurred vision
* chest pain
* abdominal pain
* sensation of flashing lights

Certain women should not take the MAP. Contraindications for it are similar to those for the birth control pill and include:

- ☐ Pregnancy (the MAP will not prevent an already established pregnancy and may harm the fetus)
- ☐ Tumors of the breast or reproductive organs or a family history of these conditions
- ☐ Blood clots or strokes
- ☐ Serious liver conditions
- ☐ Unexplained vaginal bleeding
- ☐ Women who are DES daughters
- ☐ Strong opposition to abortion if the MAP did not work

Some doctors would add:

- ☐ A history of severe migraine headaches
- ☐ Fibroid tumors of the uterus
- ☐ Heart or kidney disease
- ☐ A history of high blood pressure, asthma, diabetes or epilepsy.

Because of these contraindications, women should have certain tests and exams before taking MAP, including:

- ☐ A complete medical history, with special attention to family history and the possibility of DES exposure
- ☐ A breast exam
- ☐ Bimanual pelvic exam
- ☐ A pregnancy test if there is any possibility of a preexisting pregnancy.

There have been some experiments using estrogens other than DES and synthetic progestins as postcoital contraceptives. Some of these have shown promising results, but the risks may be similar to those involved in the use of DES. Only DES has been approved by the Food and Drug Administration (FDA) as a postcoital contraceptive. Despite the fact that the FDA has approved the drug for this use, the major manufacturer of DES publishes a warning in its package insert that says that DES *should not* be used as a postcoital contraceptive. The company apparently feels (as we do) that its use as a postcoital contraceptive is too dangerous and is seeking to avoid future lawsuits with this disclaimer. Nonetheless, private physicians and many college and university health centers continue to prescribe DES as a postcoital contraceptive.

The Postcoital IUD [125]

The intrauterine device (IUD) has also been used as a method of postcoital contraception. So far, only the copper IUD has been tested for this

216

purpose, and only on a relatively small number of women. These tests have indicated that the copper IUDs are highly effective when used in this manner, but larger numbers of women must be studied before firm conclusions can be drawn.[126]

The postcoital insertion of the copper IUD apparently prevents the implantation of the fertilized egg in the uterine wall. Because implantation takes place about six days after ovulation, researchers have inserted the copper IUDs as long as six days after unprotected intercourse, but most experts feel that the sooner the IUD is inserted, the better.

The copper IUDs were chosen for testing because the effect of the metal begins almost immediately after insertion of the device. Other noncopper IUDs may take several days or weeks to reach maximum effectiveness and may therefore be less effective when used postcoitally.

The postcoital IUD has definite advantages in comparison to the morning-after pill. Although IUD insertion may have side effects, such as pain and bleeding, and may cause perforation and other complications (*see* p. 122), the side effects and possible complications are not thought to be as serious or as frequent as those that may be associated with the morning-after pill. Moreover, once the IUD has been inserted, it provides protection against future pregnancies as well. The postcoital IUD is probably a better choice for women who would leave it in place and would continue to rely on the IUD as a method of birth control.

If pregnancy should occur following IUD insertion, removal of the device or abortion is advisable, because pregnancy with an IUD in place involves risk to both the fetus and the mother (p. 127).

Postcoital contraception with an IUD does have definite drawbacks. The usual contraindications to the IUD should be observed. The risks and problems normally associated with IUD use also apply to postcoital IUD use. Many doctors will not insert an IUD except during the menstrual flow (they feel complications like expulsion and perforation are thereby minimized), so they do not use the IUD postcoitally. In addition, the postcoital IUD is not a wise choice for rape victims or women who have multiple sex partners. The chances that such women have been exposed to gonorrhea or other venereal diseases are simply too great. Inserting an IUD in a woman with one of these diseases could cause pelvic inflammatory disease, a condition that can have serious and even fatal consequences.

Menstrual Extraction

Menstrual extraction is an office procedure in which the uterine lining is removed by suction. It is performed at about the time the menstrual period is normally expected. Before the advent of today's pregnancy tests, which are accurate within a day or so of the missed period, this procedure was done on women who had had unprotected intercourse and feared that they might be pregnant. Now that such tests are available, this procedure is not widely used. The advantages and drawbacks of menstrual extraction are discussed in greater detail in the section on abortion.

6

Dealing with Doctors, or How to Survive in the Medical Marketplace

In November 1979 the Commonwealth of Massachusetts signed a bill into law.[1] In some ways it was a pretty silly law, hard to implement, probably impossible to enforce and subject to such a variety of interpretations that it will undoubtedly enrich the lives of dozens of lawyers for years to come if anyone ever tries to file a suit based on it. Still, it was a gesture, and gestures like this one do have a certain significance.

The law says, among other things, that a doctor must inform a woman with breast cancer of "all alternative treatments that are medically viable." Although we're not lawyers, it seems to us that the hook, the catch-22 in this law, lies in the words "medically viable." A doctor who performed a radical mastectomy* on a woman with breast cancer without telling her of the availability of other, less disfiguring treatments, like a simple removal of the lump,** could be sued under this law. However, the doctor could make a defense by arguing that, in his or her opinion, anything less than a radical or at least a modified radical mastectomy† was not a viable medical alternative. At present it's a moot point medically and probably legally as well.

By making this criticism of the Massachusetts law, we aren't trying to rain on anybody's parade, and we certainly aren't intending to belittle the

*Radical mastectomy: removal of the breast, the muscles of the upper chest wall and the lymph nodes.
**Lumpectomy: removal of the cancerous lump; breast left largely intact.
†Modified radical: same as a radical mastectomy, except that chest muscles are not removed.

219

efforts of the dedicated souls who must have worked like maniacs to push the bill into law. They deserve our undying (pun intended) gratitude, for although the law may not offer a completely solid legal recourse to women whose doctors fail to inform them about treatment options, nonetheless, the law is a public and legal statement of the responsibility of the physician. It marks the beginning of the end for the M.D.eity.

The M.D.eity and the Doctor/Patient Relationship

[He] got past the nurses by impersonating a doctor. All he did was clip four ballpoint pens on his vest pocket and march in looking preoccupied.

—Lois Gould, *Such Good Friends,* 1970

In the introduction we talked about the M.D.eity syndrome and poked a bit of fun at the pomposity of doctors, and quite rightly so, for as we also pointed out, the M.D.eity syndrome, which allows to doctors the status of at least a minor god, also has its distinctly unfunny side: the some 300,000 unnecessary hysterectomies performed in this country each year, for instance.[2] And hysterectomies are just one example; gynecological medicine is full of them. What woman doesn't have a gynecological atrocity tale to tell abut a woman misdiagnosed, mistreated, misinformed, maimed or mangled by her doctor?

In all fairness to doctors (and we do want to be fair to them; after all, one of us *is* a doctor), not all of these gynecological horror stories are to be believed, for gynecologists are dealing with sex and reproduction, two extremely sensitive issues. Moreover, most gynecologists are men. In this era of women's liberation, any man trying to deal with a woman on the issues of sex and reproduction in the framework of what had traditionally been an authoritarian, paternalistic relationship between women and doctors—well, it's not surprising that he doesn't always come up smelling like a rose.

Yet even if you discount the horror stories, it's undeniably obvious that there are basic problems with the way in which many doctors relate to patients, which is what the Massachusetts law is an attempt to remedy. The M.D.eity syndrome has reached epidemic proportions. Many, if not most doctors, have convinced themselves that they—and not the patient— should have the final say when it comes to making treatment decisions, so they feel that there is really no point in the patient's bothering her pretty little head about other options. These doctors would oppose the spirit of the Massachusetts law. They don't believe it's their job to inform women of "all the alternative treatments that are medically viable," so that she can make her own decision. They, the experts, the M.D.eities, by virtue of their special knowledge and training, are the only ones qualified to make these decisions. As one noted breast cancer specialist explains:

> Every woman with breast cancer must make the only decision she is capable of making. . . . She must choose which physician will be responsible for her treatment; she cannot choose which treatment to have. She must rely completely on the good judgment of the physician in whom she has confidence.
>
> Philip Strax, M. D., in *Early Detection: Breast Cancer Is Curable*, 1974

According to Dr. Strax's philosophy, a woman who goes to a radical mastectomy proponent must have a radical; if she ends up at the office of a remove-the-lump-and-radiate-the-breast fan, she must be radiated; and if she happens upon a lumpectomy advocate, she must have a lumpectomy. *She* can't choose what treatment to have; she has to trust her doctor.

Peculiar advice. Do you suppose Dr. Strax buys a car this way—if he winds up at a Cadillac dealer, he buys a Cadillac, at a Volkswagen dealer, a Volkswagen?

However strange Dr. Strax's advice may seem, he is by no means an isolated crackpot on the fringes of the medical world. We'd be willing to bet that his views are shared by most card-carrying members of the AMA. In the context of all this, it seems rather petty to criticize the Massachusetts law because it isn't the most airtight legal construct ever devised. Indeed, one is tempted to advocate the passage of similar laws in all states, laws that would require doctors to inform women of all the viable medical alternatives, not just for breast cancer but for all diseases.

But laws alone can't right what's wrong with the doctor/patient relationship. They can't change the hierarchical, authoritarian mode of relating that characterizes most medical training programs, where the medical residents, or "the boys," as they are called by "the king," the chief resident, vie for interesting patients so they can score "brownie points" and maybe, someday, make it to the top of the heap and get to be the chief themselves. (These descriptive phrases are lifted from Dr. William Nolen's bestseller, *The Making of a Surgeon*, a saga of medical training that alternates between sounding like the story of a bunch of adolescent boys working out their personality problems and the melodrama of a Prussian Army training camp.)

221

Nor can the law legislate away sexism in the medical profession. As long as most of the women in a doctor's life are nurses, who are viewed not as partners in the health-care team but as subordinates, it's going to be tough to get doctors to deal with their women patients on an equal footing where the patient is seen as having a right to make her own health-care decisions.

Perhaps we're painting too black a picture. There are plenty of good doctors out there, doctors who are committed to a patient's right to know, who are well informed about the latest developments and who don't dismiss women's complaints as "psychogenic." You just have to know how to go about finding them.

Finding a Doctor

Most of us spend more time choosing a new dress than we do choosing a doctor. While we would never dream of asking a friend to recommend a new dress and then calling the store and ordering it sent out to our house sight unseen, we might very well ask a friend for the name of a doctor and just call to make an appointment without thinking any more about it.

This is another consequence of the M.D.eity syndrome. Just because a person has an M.D. after his or her name, we assume that s/he is competent. Moreover, the idea of shopping around, of comparative buying, is definitely a consumer's notion, and women patients are not encouraged to think of themselves as consumers. We may hire an architect or a lawyer, but one does not "hire" a doctor. Indeed, we are apt to consider ourselves lucky if we manage to get an appointment, particularly if the doctor is highly recommended.

So, begin your search for a doctor at the beginning: by collecting the names of doctors to interview for the job of being your doctor. Remember, just like the butcher, the baker, the candlestick maker or anyone else in the business of selling their services or goods, the doctor is in the business of selling his or her services—in this case, medical care. The doctor is in your employ. You are his or her client, and this holds true whether the doctor is being paid directly by you, by your insurance company or by a state or federal medical care program.

An excellent source of names of prospective doctors is a hospital scrub nurse. These nurses work in the operating room, right alongside of the doctors. They have an inside track, know exactly who's good and who isn't and are generally pretty open about sharing that information. Similarly, an anesthesiologist (a doctor who administers anesthesia) or an anesthetist (a nurse or specially trained person who administers anesthesia) is an excellent source of information. In some areas of the country, women's health groups have files of consumer comments and ratings of doctors in the area. These can be invaluable and can save you a lot of time by steering you away from the less than adequate doctors and towards those that have the qualities and qualifications you are looking for.

Board-Certification

Once you have some possibilities, check these doctors' credentials. Evaluating credentials is only part of the process of choosing a doctor, but such credentials are important factors to consider. One important credential is board-certification. Certification boards are private, nonprofit organizations that offer certification to doctors who meet their standards. There are individual boards for each of the various medical specialties, including general surgery, pediatrics, psychiatry, family practice, obstetrics (childbirth) and gynecology. There are also subspecialties. A surgeon might, for example, specialize in plastic surgery or vascular surgery. Gynecology and obstetrics, or OB/GYN, also has subspecialties, including fertility, gynecologic oncology (cancer of the female reproductive organs) and perinatology (difficult or high-risk pregnancies).

Once a gynecologist has completed residency training, s/he may take written examinations administered by the board. After practicing medicine for at least two years, s/he submits records of all hospital cases to the board for review. Members of the board, which is made up of top-notch gynecologists, then conduct oral examinations. If the written and oral examinations and the review of the hospital cases are satisfactory, the board certifies the doctor.

Not all doctors are board-certified. You may hear the term "board-eligible." This means that the doctor has completed the necessary training but is not yet certified. A young gynecologist who has not yet completed the requisite two years of medical practice would be board-eligible. There has been a movement in recent years to restrict the use of the term, for some doctors who have long since completed their residencies and the required two years of practice continue to call themselves board-eligible even though they either have failed to pass the requirements for certification or don't even intend to try for it. If a doctor claims to be board-eligible, ask how long s/he has been board-eligible and be skeptical if s/he has been eligible for a number of years.

There are many good doctors who are not board-certified, and board-certification does not guarantee competency. But a doctor who is board-certified has subjected him or herself to the rigorous testing required for certification, and his or her technical skill and experience have been evaluated by experts in the field and judged to be outstanding.

You can check your doctor's qualifications in *The Directory of Medical*

Specialists, which gives detailed information including where the doctor trained, membership in professional societies, appointments to medical schools, hospital affiliations and specialties. All doctors listed in this directory are board-certified. *The American Medical Directory* also gives information about doctors' credentials but lists only those doctors who are members of the American Medical Society, regardless of whether they are board-certified. Many public libraries have these books, as do most medical libraries. If you can't get hold of a copy, you can call your local or state health department or medical society and ask whether or not the doctor you are considering is board-certified.

Most people outside the medical profession are not aware of the process of board-certification, but it is widely recognized as a sign of competency within the profession. You can bet that when doctors or their families are operated on, the operations are performed by board-certified surgeons.

In addition to board-certification, there are other factors to consider, including:

Where the doctor served his or her internship and residency: The most coveted intern and residency programs are those associated with university medical schools, for the top-notch doctors work in these hospitals and a wide variety of patients are referred there for care. A doctor who has trained at a university hospital generally has had the opportunity to work under the most skilled doctors in the field and has had more experience with a wider variety of cases than doctors who train at less prestigious hospitals.

Hospital affiliations: Doctors are granted staff privileges at hospitals. The quality of the hospitals with which the doctor is affiliated is important. The most prestigious types of hospital affiliations are with hospitals associated with medical schools. Hospitals are accredited by the Joint Committee on Hospital Accreditation (JCHA). It is preferable that your doctor be affiliated with an accredited hospital. The size of the hospital is also a factor. Generally, hospitals with 200 or more beds are better equipped than smaller hospitals.

Membership in professional societies: Membership in professional societies like the *American College of Gynecologists and Obstetricians* that offer conferences, workshops and other continuing-education programs are an indication of a doctor's interest in keeping up to date and well informed on developments in his or her specialty. If a gynecologist is not only a member, but a fellow of the American College of Gynecologists and Obstetricians, this means that his or her colleagues have accorded the gynecologist special recognition.

Personal style (also known as bedside manner): Your gut reaction to the doctor is of utmost importance. A string of impressive credentials after a doctor's name doesn't mean a thing if you can't communicate.

A doctor you feel comfortable with, even if his or her credentials aren't as impressive, is a better choice. On the other hand, don't let a charming bedside manner obscure a lack of experience, training or skill.

Health Care for Gay Women

Lesbians face special difficulties in finding a doctor with whom they can communicate openly. Many doctors have prejudices about lesbians and consider any sexual preference that is not strictly heterosexual a sign of a deep-seated psychological disturbance. Thus, many lesbians are in a quandary. If they tell their doctors they are gay, they are apt to be put down, lectured, treated with scorn or horror and referred to a psychiatrist. One woman we saw who was having abnormal vaginal bleeding told her doctor that she was a lesbian. He referred her to a psychiatrist, and in his preoccupation with "curing" her of her "problem," neglected the symptom that had brought her to the doctor in the first place. When she finally came to us, it was too late; her undiagnosed vaginal bleeding turned out to be cancer of the endometrial lining.

If, on the other hand, a gay woman doesn't tell her doctor that she is a lesbian, her symptoms are apt to be attributed to conditions related to pregnancy or to diseases like gonorrhea that lesbians rarely develop. Valuable time is lost and needless expense incurred in ruling out diagnostic possibilities that she, because she is a lesbian, is not subject to.

Women's centers and lesbian groups may be able to refer such women to doctors who will treat them in a nonjudgmental way. Recently, a group of doctors sympathetic to the health-care problems of both gay women and gay men has established a referral service in San Francisco and in the Los Angeles area. (In the San Francisco area, contact Bay Area Physicians for Human Rights, P.O. Box 14546, San Francisco, Calif. 94114, 415–673-3189; in the Los Angeles area, contact Southern California Physicians for Human Rights, 7985 Santa Monica Blvd., Suite 109, Los Angeles, Calif. 90046, 213–858-6767.)

The Nurse-Practitioner

All women looking for good health care should be aware of the emerging role of a new health-care professional, the nurse-practitioner. Many gynecologists are taking advantage of the services of nurse-practitioners, who are nurses with special training who can perform many of the routine services usually performed by doctors. In our experience, nurse-practitioners provide excellent care. Their time is less expensive, so they usually have more time to spend explaining things and answering questions. Indeed, they are often better at explaining things to the layperson than doctors are, so don't feel slighted if you spend more time with one of them than with the doctor. In fact, if your doctor incorporates nurse-practitioners into his or her office staff, this is a sign that you've found yourself a forward-thinking gynecologist, one who is probably not so caught up in the M.D.eity syndrome.

Second Opinons

Even if you manage to find an absolute wonder of a gynecologist, one who walks on water, you should still consider getting a second opinion before consenting to any form of treatment for a serious illness. Doctors, even the top-notch ones, disagree, and you owe it to yourself to get all the facts and many points of view before making a decision.

Of course, getting a second opinion falls into the easier-said-than-done category. It is hard for many women to say, "I'd like a second opinion before deciding, so don't write out that prescription or don't schedule me for surgery yet." Let's face it, most of us have difficulty switching hairdressers or garage mechanics, let alone switching M.D.eities. Even though on an objective, rational level, all that a second opinion means is that we want more information before making a decision, the implication is that we are somehow not satisfied with or are distrustful of our doctor.

Undoubtedly, an up-front, honest approach is best. But if you find yourself unable to do this, you've got a couple of other options. You can always shift the responsibility by saying "My mother, my husband (or somebody else in charge of my life) insists that I get a second opinion." Given most gynecologists' view of women, you'll probably find your doctor is remarkably accepting of the notion that someone other than you is doing your thinking for you and is making your decisions. It feeds right into the view of women patients expressed in the quote from Dr. Strax above. Perhaps you're copping out a bit this way, but if you've got a serious medical problem, the paramount thing at this point is to obtain quality medical care. First things first; you can sort out your inabilities to be assertive later on.

Another option is to simply pocket the prescription or hedge about scheduling the surgery date and beat a hasty retreat from the office. Then, schedule a second appointment and simply call your first doctor's office later, speaking to the secretary and getting her to arrange to have the necessary medical records sent to the second doctor. Again, this is not the most up-front way of dealing with the situation, but if that's what you need to do, it's perfectly OK.

226

When making your appointment with the second doctor, just say that you've been diagnosed as having such and such a condition and that you'd like a second opinion or consultation before you make any decisions. You should ask what medical records, test results and so forth the doctor would like to see before consulting with you and arrange to have these available for him or her at the time of your appointment (see Your Medical Records below).

When you see the second doctor, explain your medical history, your problem and symptoms and what diagnostic tests have been done (the results of which he or she should now have). The natural impulse in this situation is for you to say something along the lines of "So my doctor recommended such and such; however, I want a second opinion before going ahead." If that's your impulse, stifle it. We recommend that you not mention the first doctor's opinion, even though it may be stated in the medical records transferred to the second doctor. If it's not stated, your second doctor is likely to ask you what your first doctor said or recommended. If so, simply say, "Before discussing that, I'd rather hear what you have to say."

The reason for this rather secretive approach is that too often the second opinion will simply be a rubber stamp of approval. "Professional ethics" dictate that your second doctor not malign the opinions or professional competency of your original doctor. It is considered extremely tacky in the medical profession for doctors to "steal" each other's patients. (In our opinion extreme tackiness enters the situation when a doctor fails to tell a patient that another doctor has, in his or her opinion, misdiagnosed, misinformed or mistreated a patient, but ethics are always situational, and what any given person sees as ethical depends on his or her particular point of view.) By approaching the matter in this fashion, you are letting the second doctor off the hook and decreasing the chances that the second opinion will merely be a polite affirmation of the first doctor's recommendations.

Many of the medical books written for a lay audience pay lip service to the idea of obtaining second opinions and suggest that you find a doctor for a second consultation by asking the first doctor for a referral. Perhaps it is putting it too strongly to say that this is like asking the fox for advice about guarding the chicken coop. Still, asking the first doctor to recommend a second-opinion doctor and expecting to thereby obtain an unbiased, objective opinion seems a bit foolish.

We suggest that a woman go about getting a second opinion in the same way that we suggested she find a doctor in the first place—by asking for referrals from a number of sources, checking the doctor's credentials and then interviewing him or her. One excellent source for second opinions is a university hospital outpatient clinic. If you live near one of these institutions, call the gynecology department or the women's clinic and ask for a consultation.

If you have been diagnosed as having a specific problem for which there are alternative treatments (see below), you may want to ask if the doctor you are consulting for a second opinion is equipped or trained to perform or provide alternatives to what your first doctor has recommended. If, for example, you have been diagnosed as having carcinoma in situ of the cervix and your first doctor has recommended a hysterectomy, you might ask if the second doctor has cryosurgery equipment. If you are under the age of 35 or 40 and your first doctor has recommended a total hysterectomy (removal of the uterus *and* ovaries) for a benign disease, you might ask the second doctor whether s/he recommends simply removing the uterus or whether s/he routinely removes the ovaries in all women in your age group. But you must be very cagey in wording your questions. The standard response to such questions is, "I'll have to see you to answer that," and it's a fair response. No doctor can be expected to make a diagnosis, recommend treatment or give a second opinion over the phone. If, however, you phrase your question along these lines: "Doctor, I am 36 and have been diagnosed as having (some benign disease) and am considering a hysterectomy. Of course, I want a second opinion before surgery and would like to make an appointment for a consultation. I realize you can't tell me much before you have reviewed my medical records and examined me, but I would like to know, just in general, do you ever consider sparing the ovaries in a woman my age, assuming of course this is possible, or do you feel it's better as a rule to take them out?"

Some doctors will still refuse to answer your question. Most will still hedge a bit, but you can often get at least some indication as to whether they would or would not consider sparing the ovaries. By asking such questions of the doctor when making your consultation appointment, you can make sure that you will be getting a second opinion from someone who will at least consider another point of view on your case.

So far we've been talking about situations in which getting a second opinion is a fairly easy matter. Things get a bit trickier if you're already in the hospital. If you know ahead of time that you're going into the hospital to have a hysterectomy or whatever, the time to get a second opinion is, of course, *before* you are admitted. But you may not always know ahead of time. For example, a woman might be hospitalized in order to receive intravenous (IV) antibiotics to treat pelvic inflammatory disease, an infection that can affect the uterus, Fallopian tubes, ovaries and other pelvic organs. If the antibiotics don't work, the doctor might then suggest a hysterectomy.

In such cases, you can get a second opinion in one of two ways. The first option is to check yourself out of the hospital and seek a second opinion.

This is not always possible. The other alternative, having the second doctor see you in the hospital, may be more feasible. The second doctor must be on staff at the hospital or have consulting privileges there. Most hospitals have some sort of patient advisor or social worker who can help you arrange for a second opinion, or the head nurse may be able to supply you with a list of such doctors.

Getting a second opinion becomes even more complex when the disease involved is a cancerous one. This is discussed in detail under the heading Cancer in the reference section. If you have been diagnosed as having cancer or there is even a possibility that you may have cancer, be sure to read that section.

The cost of a consultation varies but is often surprisingly inexpensive. Many medical and insurance companies and government medical programs will cover the costs of a second opinion, but you may want to check your coverage first, since some companies or government programs still do not do so.

Your Medical Records

In some states the laws have clearly established the fact that a patient has a right to her own medical records. Yet even in these states a woman may have difficulty getting the doctor to release her records to her. They will, however, release your records to another doctor, so you may have to ask the doctor you are consulting to call and request that your records be transferred.

Dealing with Doctors/How to Use This Book

Regardless of whether you are seeking a first or a second opinion or are merely having a routine check-up, there are certain things to keep in mind when you are consulting a doctor. Of primary importance is the fact that *you* are paying the doctor, directly or indirectly, and that by virtue of this simple fact, you have certain rights and a certain amount of consumer power. If you are paying the doctor directly, this fact may be quite obvious.

If, however, like the majority of Americans, you are employed by a company that provides medical benefits or are receiving state or federal medical aid, you may not feel that you are actually paying the doctor. If it's your company that is providing medical coverage, you may feel that you are fortunate to be employed by an organization generous enough to offer its employees such extra benefits. You may believe that your employer provides this as an extra, added attraction, a "freebie." This is not true.

229

When you receive benefits, they are in lieu of extra salary. Instead of paying you a wage that would allow you to seek medical care at your own expense, the company that employs you has made a deal with an insurance company. By insuring all of its employees with the company, the employer is able to get insurance at a group rate that is much cheaper than it would be for an individual. So your medical coverage is not a gift bestowed upon you out of the kindness of the corporate heart; it is part of the wages you earn for the work that you do. If you are paying your doctor indirectly, through a medical insurance plan, it is still you who is paying the doctor and you have the same consumer power as if you were paying directly out of your own pocket.

If you are receiving medical aid from the state or federal government, you are still paying the doctor and you have the same rights as if you were paying out of your pocket. Our national social programs—foodstamps, welfare payments, medical assistance and the like—are an attempt to compensate for the inequities created by racism, sexism and ageism in our society. Contrary to the popular image of the welfare recipient as a shiftless, lazy person unwilling to work, the typical recipient is a single mother with children under school age who is unable to find a job that will pay her enough money to allow her to feed, house and clothe her family as well as pay for childcare. The elderly and the disabled are also typical recipients. Such people have a right to medical care; it should not be considered a gift. Your doctor is paid by the government for the services s/he provides you—and paid well. The doctor does not receive money unless you "pay" him or her with your medical voucher. Again, even though you are paying the doctor indirectly, you have the same rights as people who pay for medical care directly.

Your Medical Rights and Duties

Now that we've got that very important point out of the way, what exactly are those medical rights? First and foremost, you deserve a clear explanation of what is wrong and why, at least to the best of the doctor's ability to give you that information. There are gaps in our medical knowledge, and many times a doctor will not be able to diagnose what is wrong.

The It's-All-in-Your-Head-Dearie Diagnosis

In cases where medical information is less than perfect, you have the right to an honest "I-don't-know" reply from your doctor, although you may not get it. It has long been a medical custom for doctors to attribute diseases for which they are unable to find a cause or cure to "psychogenic factors," the old it's-all-in-your-head-dearie diagnosis. M.D.eities do not like to admit to not knowing, so they fall back on the old I-can't-figure-out-what's-wrong-with-you-so-you-must-be-crazy switcheroo, projecting their problem onto you. Throughout the reference section on diseases, we have tried to alert women to situations in which they may run into these sorts of reactions from doctors.

If your doctor suggests that your symptoms are psychosomatic or refers you to a psychologist or psychiatrist, evaluate this bit of advice carefully. Has the doctor fully evaluated you medically? In the section on menstrual disorders, we talk about a woman who had severe nausea and vomiting during her period each month. Her doctor couldn't figure out what was wrong, decided the woman was neurotic and referred her to a psychiatrist. After months of exploring "her rejection of her female role" with her male therapist, this woman saw a second gynecologist, who didn't dismiss her symptoms. Instead, the doctor took a look at the woman's pelvis with the aid of a special viewing instrument called a laparoscope, which is inserted into the body through an incision in the abdomen. As it turned out, this woman's problem was not in her head but in her pelvis. She had a condition known as endometriosis, and once it was treated, her symptoms disappeared.

So use the symptoms index in the appendix of this book. Read the section on the possible diseases that could be causing your symptoms and check to see that your doctor has done all the diagnostic tests to rule out the various possibilities. Although psychotherapy can be valuable for anyone, you should not let symptoms that may be caused by a medical problem that needs attention be diagnosed as psychosomatic, especially if your medical condition has not been fully evaluated.

Other Medical Rights

Along with the right to a clear explanation of your problems, you also have a right to an explanation of all the treatment options available. Here again, you may not get it. If you have been diagnosed as having a specific problem, look that disease up in the reference section of this book. Find out if there are alternative treatments. Ask your doctor about the possibility of using these other forms of therapy in your case. The questions listed in Chapter Seven may be particularly helpful. And always get a second opinion before submitting to any form of treatment for a serious problem.

Your doctor may disagree with the opinions expressed in this book or may recommend a form of treatment different from the ones outlined here. This is to be expected and certainly doesn't mean that your doctor is wrong. New discoveries are taking place all the time and there may have been advancements in the forms of treatment for your condition since this book was written. In addition, the particulars of your case may rule out a specific mode of therapy for you.

This book cannot be used to diagnose or recommend treatment. Rather, it is intended to make you aware of the existing options and to provide enough information to allow you to ask questions and to evaluate your alternatives. If your doctor disagrees with us, that's fine, but remember, you have the right to a full explanation of his or her point of view. If all you get as a reply to your questions is a because-I'm-the-Doctor-and-I-say-so response, find another doctor.

Similarly, you have the right to a full explanation of any tests the doctor may order. Again, the questions listed in Chapter Seven will be helpful. You may find that your doctor is not terribly pleased with your asking all these questions. If you balk at following orders, you may be made to feel that you are being "difficult," that you are a troublesome sort of person or that you are being silly and overly cautious. Well, so what if you are. If, according to some estimates, 30 percent of the X-rays done in this country each year are unnecessary, then women are quite right to refuse to blindly follow their doctors' orders and submit to all these tests.

Your Responsibility

Along with these rights come certain responsibilities. You must assume responsibility for being informed about the basic workings of the female body. If, for instance, you don't know how the menstrual cycle works, it's unrealistic to expect the doctor to explain why you've stopped having menstrual periods and the various tests s/he wants to do or the various methods of treating your condition. This is where this book comes in; use it to inform yourself. Once you have been diagnosed, read the section on your disease carefully and make notes so that you will remember your questions. Take this book along with you when you see the doctor so you will be able to refer to the appropriate section if the need arises.

If you are confronted with the possibility of a serious disease, you may want to ask a family member or friend to read the section as well and help you frame your questions. Our experience has been that women diagnosed as having something seriously wrong, for example, cancer, are often so shaken and upset that they find it difficult to absorb all the necessary information. A relative or friend may be better able to do this.

When you see the doctor, take notes so that you will be able to refer to them later on. You may also want to bring a friend or relative along with you when you see the doctor. Women's groups often have volunteers who serve as patient advocates and who are usually well informed. They will visit the doctor with you. Having another person along can be particularly valuable. It's more difficult to communicate and receive information when you're upset, and having a friend along assures that you will clearly understand what is being said to you.

A Word About References

As explained in Chapter One, the diseases and conditions described in the following reference section are organized according to the organs that they affect. There are separate subsections for the vulva, the vagina, the cervix, the uterus and Fallopian tubes, the ovaries and the breast. In addition, there are separate subsections that deal with problems related to pregnancy and fertility, the menstrual cycle and sexually transmitted diseases, as well as a section giving general background information on cancer. At the back of the book you will find a list of references.

We have relied on two main sources in preparing this reference section, *Novak's Textbook of Gynecology*, 9th ed., by Edmund R. Novak, M.D., Georgeanna Seegar Jones, M.D. and Howard W. Jones, Jr., M.D. (Baltimore: Williams & Wilkins, 1975), and *Gynecology*, 2nd ed., by Langdon Parsons, M.D., and Sheldon C. Sommers, M.D. (Philadelphia: W. B. Saunders, 1978). These are the two most widely used gynecological texts. Facts and figures given in our text are, unless otherwise noted, derived from these two sources, though to avoid littering the pages with footnotes, we have not cited them explicitly. When other sources were used, appropriate references are given.

Reference Section: Diseases

The Vulva

The Vagina

The Cervix

The Uterus and the Fallopian Tubes

The Ovaries

The Breast

Sexually Transmitted Diseases

Problems Related to the Menstrual Cycle

Problems Related to Pregnancy and Fertility

Cancer

The Vulva

The anatomy of the vulva is illustrated and described in Chapter Two. Reviewing the information in that chapter will help you to understand the vulvar diseases described in the following pages.

Most of the diseases and conditions described in this section are skin diseases, for the skin of the vulva, just like the skin elsewhere on the body, is subject to all sorts of lumps, bumps, pimples and inflammations.

Vulvitis

The vulva is particularly susceptible to inflammations because the area is frequently warm, and moisture there is trapped by clothing. This warm, moist environment is a perfect breeding ground for infection. Moreover, the vulva is subject to a number of irritants, including vaginal and menstrual discharge, sanitary napkins, vaginal deodorants, perfumed soaps, powders, the laundry soap used to wash undergarments and so forth. Additionally, the chemicals used in the manufacture of synthetic undergarments may dissolve due to the heat in the area, also irritating the vulva. "Vulvitis" is the general term used to describe these inflammations, and the various types of vulvitis are described in the first part of this section.

Other Vulvar Problems

In addition to vulvitis, a number of other inflammations of the vulva, including postmenopausal vulvitis; vulvar folliculitis, an infection of the hair follicles; hidradenitis, an infection of the sweat glands; barthlinitis, and skeneitis, infections of the Bartholin's and Skene's glands, respectively; and vulvar dystrophies are included in the following pages. Circulatory diseases of the vulva and congenital and acquired abnormalities are also discussed. Both cystic and solid benign vulvar tumors as well as malignant and premalignant tumors are considered as well.

In addition to the problems discussed in this section, there are other conditions that can cause the same or similar symptoms. These include sexually transmitted diseases, common vaginal infections, genital tuberculosis, endometriosis, lacerations of the vulva and vagina and congenital abnormalities of the ovary.

Vulvar Biopsies

Any itching, sore, lump, swelling, red or white areas, indeed, any abnormality of the vulvar skin that persists after treatment or that does not go away in three or four weeks, needs medical attention. Even as serious a disease as invasive vulvar cancer may produce no more than an itching feeling in its early stages. Too often these symptoms are not given sufficient attention by the woman or her doctor. Yet, any chronic irritation of the vulva needs attention, for untreated it could lead to vulvar cancer. Therefore, any persistent itching, inflamed areas, lumps or sores that do not respond to medical treatment deserve a vulvar biopsy.

In the vast majority of cases, the vulvar biopsy is a simple office procedure that can be done under a local anesthetic. Many doctors will, however, hospitalize a woman and may even use a general anesthetic. This is more dangerous for the woman, since any general anesthetic involves a risk, however slight, of serious complications—and, in some cases, fatal ones. It is also more costly and inconvenient. A few doctors will argue that hospitalization is necessary because of the risk of excessive bleeding, but the most widely respected experts feel that the biopsy should be done in the office. Perhaps the fact that a biopsy done in a hospital and using a general anesthetic is more lucrative for the doctor explains why these procedures are sometimes done there. At any rate, if your doctor proposes to do the procedure in the hospital, and especially if s/he proposes to use a general anesthetic, insist that the reasons be made clear to you. If you are not satisfied with the answers, remember that you have the right to seek a second opinion.

The vulvar biopsy involves cutting samples of tissue that are sent to a lab for microscopic evaluation. Any obvious sores or lumps will be biopsied. The doctor may also paint the vulva with a stain called toluidine blue. This stain is then washed off with a slightly acidic solution. Any areas that retain the blue color should be biopsied. This process helps the doctor locate affected areas that cannot be seen with the naked eye. This is important, for invasive cancer may be lurking at the edges of an area affected by some other, more obvious disease. Without the staining, this more serious condition might go undetected until it was too late.

The biopsy may also include a colposcopic exam. The colposcope is a magnifying instrument that can be used to examine the vulva (and also the vagina and cervix). With the colposcope, the doctor can see abnormal areas that might be missed by the staining method. Although the use of a colposcope is not as critical in vulvar biopsy as it is in cervical biopsy, it is still an important tool; however, many doctors feel that a good magnifying glass is equally effective for vulvar biopsies.

VULVITIS

AKA: vulvar dermatitis

Types: chronic dermatitis, eczema or chronic eczemoid dermatitis
allergic vulvitis, contact dermatitis, drug eruption or dermatitis medicamentosus
seborrhea or seborrheic dermatitis
intertrigo, erythema intertrigo or chafing
vulvovaginitis or secondary vulvitis
tinea cruris
diabetic vulvitis
neurodermatitis

The term "dermatitis" in its broadest sense refers to any inflammation of the skin. When these sorts of irritations occur on the vulva, the term "vulvitis" or "vulvar dermatitis" is used. Vulvitis may be caused by bacteria, fungus, injury, allergic substances or other irritating factors.

Symptoms

Vulvitis is characterized by itching, redness and swelling. The itching is usually followed by scratching; then, if they weren't already there to start with, symptoms like swelling, redness, irritation, oozing, crusting and scaling may appear. In some forms, fluid-filled blisters called vesicles may form. Scratching may cause these to break open. Pus formation, crusting and scaling may then follow. There may be secondary infection. The scratching may also thicken the skin and give it a whitish appearance that could be mistaken for vulvar dystrophy. As bothersome as this all may be, it is generally not serious in terms of general health.

Types

Vulvitis may be acute—sudden in onset and lasting for a relatively short time—or chronic—slow in progressing and lasting for a long time. The terms "eczema" or "chronic eczemoid dermatitis" are sometimes used to refer to chronic dermatitis. Chronic dermatitis frequently affects postmenopausal women in whom a drop in estrogen production causes a thinning and drying out of the vulvar tissues. Minute cracks in the surface of the skin then make the area more susceptible to inflammations, a condition known as atrophic, or senile, vulvitis. There are many different types of vulvitis and a great deal of overlapping in the classifications of these various types by different writers. It would probably take another whole book just to sort through it all; however, the major types are described below.

Allergic Vulvitis

Allergic vulvitis refers to an irritation of the skin of the vulva that results from an allergy to either a natural or synthetic substance. Sometimes the offending substance actually comes in contact with the vulva, in which case the term "contact dermatitis" is used. Vaginal deodorants, sanitary napkins, perfumed soaps, cosmetic powders, laundry detergents and the chemicals in synthetic materials are frequently responsible for allergic reactions. In addition, synthetic undergarments and pantyhose create an environment that will contribute to any existing vulvar irritation. Menstrual blood, feces and other normal bodily secretions may on occasion cause contact dermatitis.

Medications, either those applied directly to the vulvar area or ones taken by mouth or injection may cause allergic vulvitis. Terms such as "drug eruption," or if you prefer medical jargon, "dermatitis medicamentosus," are used to describe this type of allergic vulvitis. These reactions may involve the skin in various other parts of the body or may affect only the vulva and the surrounding area. Interestingly, allergic vulvitis caused by drugs often occurs without fever, joint pains and that generally sick-all-over feeling that usually accompany drug reactions.

The allergic vulvitis reaction may not appear immediately following exposure to the allergen. In some cases, it may be delayed for quite some time; but normally the reaction appears within two to four days. The reaction does not always occur at the first exposure; sometimes the sensitivity develops only after repeated exposure.

240

The symptoms range from a mild redness to severe swelling. Itching is almost always present, which leads to scratching, which in turn may lead to the formation of tiny little blisters and the sequence of events described above.

Seborrhea

Seborrhea, or seborrheic dermatitis, is related to an overproduction of the sebaceous (oil-producing) glands located in the vulva. The reason for this overproduction is not known. Seborrhea can occur in the hairy areas of the vulva as well as on the inside of the vulvar lips. Other areas of the body where there are concentrations of sebaceous glands, such as the scalp, ears and underarms, are apt to be affected at the same time. It is more likely to occur in overweight people. In the typical case, there are greasy, yellow scales covering the glands.

Intertrigo

"Intertrigo" refers to any acute, superficial inflammation of opposing skin surfaces. The condition is also referred to as "erythema intertrigo," which is an even more pompous term for what most of us call chafing. It is caused by moisture, warmth and friction from opposing skin surfaces rubbing together. The labia are subject to this kind of chafing, as are the inner thighs, the anal region, the underarms, the spaces between the fingers and toes and the area under the breasts. Women who are overweight, have diabetes or perspire profusely in hot weather are more likely to be bothered with this condition. Like all forms of vulvitis, this condition, although it is not serious, can become quite uncomfortable, causing redness, itching and burning, especially if the skin is rubbed raw. In more extreme cases, the skin may thicken and turn a white color, in which case the condition may be incorrectly diagnosed as vulvar dystrophy. Monilial and bacterial infections are common complications. If these should occur, treatment of these infections is combined with local treatment to relieve symptoms. Preventive measures include regular use of nonirritating dusting powder and, for overweight women, losing weight. Here again, wearing cotton underwear rather than synthetics and wearing loose clothing rather than tight garments will help prevent the condition.

Secondary Vulvitis

The terms "vulvovaginitis" and "secondary vulvitis" are used to refer to those irritations of the vulvar skin that are secondary to vaginal infections, cervicitis or various sexually transmitted diseases. The symptoms will depend on the nature of the primary infection. Treatment consists of curing the primary infection that is creating the irritating discharge and various creams and lotions to soothe the irritated vulva and relieve the itching.

Tinea Cruris

In some cases, certain fungi may cause vulvar dermatitis. These may be secondary to fungal vaginal infections or may exist solely on the vulva. Tinea cruris is a fungus infection that can affect the upper inner thighs, the vulva, anus and buttocks. It begins as a small red circular patch that has small bumps, pimples or blisters on its outer edges. Sometimes it heals in the center as the edges continue to spread outward. It is contagious and has been known to spread rapidly through schools, prisons and similar institutions. Treatment consists of keeping the area dry and application of antifungal lotions and powders during the day and creams at night. If the condition persists or recurs, oral antifungal medication may be used.

Diabetic Vulvitis

Irritation of the vulva may also occur in women who have diabetes, a disease in which the body is unable to process certain vital nutriments. In this case, the term "diabetic vulvitis" is used. Women with undetected diabetes may complain of itching and burning before there are any observable changes in the skin of the vulva. Eventually, though, the vulvar skin takes on a beefy-red color and looks extremely irritated. Local treatment without diagnosis and treatment of the underlying diabetic condition will not do much to alleviate the irritation.

Neurodermatitis

Just as it is often hard to identify the exact nature and cause of acne on the face, it may be difficult to diagnose irritations of the vulvar skin. Thus, we have the term "neurodermatitis," which is a sort of scapegoat diagnosis. A puzzling case may be diagnosed as neurodermatitis, a condition that is said to have "a large psychogenic component"—it's "nerves," it's psychosomatic or the old it's-all-in-your-head dearie diagnosis.

In some medical textbooks, neurodermatitis of the vulva is said to be common "in women whose life situations create sexual frustrations, such as widows and divorcees."[1] The itching associated with it is said to be worse at night than during the day, when, according to one medical text, "her thoughts are diverted from her genital organs." Such texts often fail to mention the fact that itching from insect bites, drug eruptions and other forms of dermatitis also tend to be worse at night.

Undoubtedly, some women do develop vulvitis as a result of psychological problems, just as some people develop nervous tics or break out in hives as a result of "nerves." Perhaps in the largest sense all disease is basically psychological in origin, for we have yet to figure out why, when two seemingly healthy, robust individuals are exposed to the same bacteria, one gets sick and the other one doesn't. Be that as it may, the diagnosis of neurodermatitis is often not an accurate one. It would be much better for the doctor to simply tell a woman that s/he is unable to find a cause for her condition, rather than falling back on the standard medical ploy, I-can't-figure-out-what's-wrong-with-you-so-you-must-be-crazy. Not only is it unfair to manipulate a woman in this way, but the anxiety created by implying that a woman is psychologically disturbed is counterproductive and contributes nothing to the healing process. In the absence of obvious psychological disturbances, women should be wary of accepting a diagnosis of neurodermatitis and should insist on a thorough investigation of their symptoms.

Treatment

Whatever the cause of vulvitis—insect bites, vaginal infections, drug reactions, vaginal sprays and so forth—the treatment is basically the same. The aim of treatment is to eliminate the causative factor, when possible, and to alleviate the symptoms, particularly the itching, since unchecked it will lead to even more intense itching and bothersome complications. There is a tendency to overtreat, coating the area with creams, lotions and ointments that in turn cause irritations. The simplest treatments, applied locally, are the best.

If the vulvitis is caused by a vaginal infection, any treatment applied to the vaginal canal should also be applied to the irritated vulva. If diabetes is the associated disease, the diabetes and the often accompanying vaginal fungus infection must be treated as well as the vulvitis.

Cleanliness, hot boric acid compresses and hot sitz baths may be helpful. Following compresses or sitz baths, the area should be gently patted dry with soft linen or cotton and allowed to dry in the air. Then, and only then, should drying powders (nonirritating ones) be applied. Simple calamine lotion, available without prescription at pharmacies, will help alleviate the itching. Cortisone creams may be prescribed if the itching is particularly severe.

In cases of chronic vulvitis, that is, vulvitis that recurrs or that is resistant to cure, a vulvar biopsy should be done to rule out the possibility that a more serious type of cancerous or precancerous disease is present. This biopsy can be done in the doctor's office using a local anesthetic. If the doctor proposes hospitalization and a general anesthetic, be sure to read the discussion of vulvar biopsy in the introduction to this section.

POST MENOPAUSAL VULVITIS

AKA: senile atrophy, atrophic vulvitis

To atrophy means "to wither." It is a normal part of the process of aging. Older women past menopause or younger women who for one reason or another no longer have functioning ovaries will notice changes in the appearance of the vulva. Without the stimulation of hormones, the skin becomes less elastic, the layer of fat beneath the skin may be lost, the labia majora and minora (large and small lips) and even the clitoris may shrink in size. The skin may become dry and smooth, and pubic hair becomes sparse. Some women's skin thickens to a leathery consistency and becomes brown and splotched in color. The atrophic skin is thin and easily irritated. Minute breaks or cracks in the surface of the skin may occur, and these may be the site of a low-grade bacterial infection.

Symptoms

Itching, which may become quite intense, is the primary symptom. The itching leads, of course, to scratching, which only irritates the vulva more, creating sores and red, irritated areas. Intense scratching may cause the skin in the area to take on a whitish color.

Treatment

The simplest form of therapy is the best. The area should be kept cool, dry and clean. Cold compressions will help relieve the itching. Drying agents or lotions should be avoided, as they may aggravate the itching. A lubricating cream may be applied, and antibiotic creams may be used to combat infection.

If the condition persists or tends to recur, estrogen replacement therapy (ERT), either orally or as a locally applied cream, may be prescribed. ERT should, however, be used with caution, for it has been implicated in various forms of cancer.[2] Women should carefully weigh the risks and benefits of ERT before accepting this form of treatment.

Women should also be hesitant about accepting treatment over the telephone or without a thorough examination. Too many times the doctor just assumes the itching or sores are a manifestation of postmenopausal vulvitis, but these same symptoms may also be caused by vulvar cancer. In cases of persistent symptoms, this possibility must be ruled out by a vulvar biopsy. If a vulvar biopsy is required, be sure to read the discussion of vulvar biopsy given in the introduction to vulvar diseases.

VULVAR FOLLICULITIS

Types: folliculitis
furunculosis

Associated Terms: carbuncles, or boils

Vulvar folliculitis is an infection of the hair follicles of the vulva. Certain bacteria, usually staphyloccocus, are prone to attack the hair follicles in the vulvar region because it is difficult to keep this area dry. Depending on the depth of penetration, the woman may have either a superficial infection of the follicles—folliculitis—or a deep one—furunculosis. This type of infection is particularly common in women who have diabetes.

Symptoms and Treatment

If the infection is superficial, small pimples pierced by a shaft of hair are seen. These pimples tend to break and crust over. Simple soap and water cleansing and the application of antibiotic ointments are all that is needed to clear up these superficial infections.

If the infection is deep-seated, carbuncles, or boils, may be formed. Treatment involves hot salt packs to promote drainage of the infected follicules or, if necessary, incisions to drain the carbuncles and infected areas. Antibiotics are then given by mouth, rather than locally by ointment. Usually penicillin is given, although some doctors will examine the pus microscopically so that they can select a more specific antibiotic.

HIDRADENITIS

Types: acute hidradenitis
Fox-Fordyce disease or chronic hidradenitis

Hidradenitis is an infection of the aprocrine (sweat) glands, which are located around the nipples and in the underarm and vulvar areas. If the vulva is infected, these other areas are likely to be affected as well.

Symptoms and Treatment

The symptoms may cause considerable discomfort. There may be intolerable itching and pain, and there are generally a number of boils on the skin.

If treatment in the acute stage is not successful, the disease may progress to the chronic stage, which is known as Fox-Fordyce disease and is characterized by even more intense itching and pain. The vulva may be dotted with fine, slightly raised, pimplelike growths or large boils.

Oral contraceptives, which modify the secretions of the aprocrine glands, may be used to control the disease and cut down on recurrences. In some instances it may be necessary to remove the infected skin. In the most extreme cases, a vulvectomy—removal of all or part of the vulva—and plastic surgery involving skin grafting may be necessary.

BARTHOLINITIS

AKA: Bartholin's adenitis

Associated Terms: Bartholin's abscess, Bartholin's cyst

Bartholinitis is an infection of the Bartholin's glands (Illustration 38). These glands lie right inside the vaginal opening on either side and secrete a fluid that keeps the vagina moist. In most women they are not noticeable unless they become infected.

Most cases of bartholinitis are caused by gonococcus, the bacteria that causes gonorrhea, but other organisms can also cause this infection. The disease may be acute or it may progress to a chronic state, punctuated by occasional acute flare-ups.

Illustration 38   *Bartholin's Cyst*

Symptoms

The skin around the opening of the gland may be quite red and swollen. The opening to the gland may be partially or totally obstructed. If the gland is open, pus mixed with glandular secretions may ooze out or be milked out by gentle pressure. If the duct is closed up, a collection of pus known as a Bartholin's abscess may form. The abscess is usually hot, swollen and tender. As the infection progresses, the overlying skin and the tissues around the bottom of the gland may become involved, and the whole labia may become quite swollen.

A woman with bartholinitis is usually intensely miserable and has difficulty both sitting and walking. Surgical incision and drainage may be performed for relief, although sometimes spontaneous rupture of the abscess will occur.

The symptoms during the acute stage—the swelling and discomfort— are more local than general. The temperature may be only moderately elevated. After the pus is drained away, the symptoms promptly subside. Then the disease may enter the chronic stage. The gland itself is not usually too seriously injured by the acute infection, but the duct may be partially or totally obstructed by scarring. Thus, the gland's secretions cannot be released and one or two Bartholin's cysts, full of these retained secretions, may develop. These cysts vary in size and may even get as large as a hen's egg. The cysts, as opposed to the abscesses, are generally not painful. Depending on the size of the cyst, a woman may be completely unaware of the cyst or it may interfere with intercourse and become a nuisance.

Treatment

The treatment for acute bartholinitis usually consists of bed rest, sufficient painkillers to relieve the discomfort, ice packs or hot sitz baths and some form of antibiotic therapy. If an abscess has formed, antibiotics alone may not be enough and the doctor may have to cut and drain the abscess.

If Bartholin's cysts are large enough to cause bothersome symptoms, they will require treatment but not while there is active, acute infection. Some doctors will treat these cysts by cutting, draining and cauterizing (burning) with electricity or with chemicals; others will treat the problem by removing the contents of the cyst by needle and replacing them with a penicillin solution. Still others will cut open the cyst, drain its contents and keep the cut open until it starts to heal from the inside out, a process known as marsupialization that can usually be performed in the doctor's office. Still others will remove the entire cyst surgically, but not until the acute infection or flare-up has subsided. If large or recurring abscesses have formed, these may be treated in the same way. In some cases it may be necessary to drain a large abscess even though there is acute infection. However, draining is usually not enough, for these abscesses will tend to recur unless surgically removed.

SKENEITIS

AKA: infection of the Skene's glands

Types: acute skeneitis
       chronic skeneitis

The openings to the Skene's glands are two small slits located on either side of the opening of the urinary tract. These glands secrete a small amount of fluid that helps keep the urinary opening moist. The disease can be acute or chronic. If the disease-causing organisms retreat deep into the gland tissue or if infected areas become walled off by a hardened fibrous substance manufactured by the surrounding healthy tissue as a defense mechanism, then the organisms cannot be reached by antibodies and the disease becomes chronic. It may persist for months, with occasional acute flare-ups.

Cause

Acute skeneitis is often caused by gonococci, the organisms that cause gonorrhea; however, other organisms may also be responsible. Sometimes chronic skeneitis is the result of gonococci that have resisted treatment. In most cases the gonococci have been killed but have paved the way for other bacteria that are responsible for the chronic skeneitis. In the rare cases where gonococcus is responsible for chronic skeneitis, the woman may pass gonorrhea on to her sex partners even though she shows no laboratory evidence of gonorrhea.

Symptoms

Pus can often be seen oozing from the openings of the glands or can be milked from the glands by gentle pressure. The openings of the glands may be red, hard, swollen and tender. Abcesses—collections of pus—may form on one or both sides and may be quite swollen and painful.

Skeneitis is often associated with infections of the urethra, the tube that leads from the bladder to the urinary opening. Infection in the urethra spreads easily to these glands because of their proximity and vice versa. Thus, there may be a frequent and urgent need to urinate, and urination may be accompanied by pain and burning.

Treatment

If pus can be milked from the glands, it should be examined microscopically to determine what specific organism is causing the infection so that a specific antibiotic can be given. If no pus is present, a broad spectrum of antibiotics is given. However, if the disease has progressed to its chronic stage, often the only way to get rid of the infection is to destroy the glands by electric cautery.

CIRCULATORY DISEASE OF THE VULVA

AKA: varices, varicose veins

Circulatory diseases may occur anywhere in the body, including the vulva. The most common of the circulatory diseases affecting the vulva is varicose veins, or varices, which are swollen, twisted, enlarged veins.

Symptoms

Circulatory diseases of the vulva usually affect the outer lips and usually occur on only one side. Like varicose veins elsewhere in the body, veins here may swell up with blood, especially when the woman is standing, and tend to empty and become smaller when she is lying down. They may become extremely large, and although it is not common, they may even burst, causing bleeding. Usually, the dilated veins appear as a group of small, purplish elevations, although they may occur singly as well. Varices may be caused by pressure on the veins from pregnancy or a large tumor; however, no specific cause can be identified in most cases. Other circulatory diseases that may cause swelling of the vulva are usually secondary in nature (which means they are the result of or are associated with some other condition that already exists). Generally, the only time that varicose veins on the vulva become symptomatic is during pregnancy, when they cause burning and pain.

249

Treatment

There is no specific treatment other than resting in a prone position as necessary. The varices regress after pregnancy. In rare cases, surgery may be necessary.

CONGENITAL AND ACQUIRED ABNORMALITIES OF THE VULVAR ANATOMY

Types: imperforate hymen
absence of the hymen
double vulva
depigmentation, leukoderma or vitiligo
agglutination of the labia
clitoral hypertrophy
lacerations of the vulva

Associated Terms: hydrometrocolpos, hematocolpos, hematocolpometra, hematosalpinx

Abnormalities of the anatomy of the vulva may be either congenital (that is, birth defects) or acquired as a result of an injury or accident that occurred after birth.

Imperforate Hymen

Congenital abnormalities of the vulva are rare. Of the ones that do occur, the imperforate hymen is the most common. Normally, the hymen, the thin strip of tissue that surrounds the vaginal opening, has one or more openings through which vaginal, cervical and menstrual fluids may pass. If there are no openings, as is the case with imperforate hymen, these fluids cannot escape and are built up inside the body.

This condition may be discovered in infancy. Sometimes a mother's hormones are strong enough to activate the newborn's uterus and vagina, causing the infant to pass vaginal secretions and possibly a bit of blood. If this happens in a child whose hymen is imperforate, these secretions can't pass through and the hymen may be seen bulging at the vaginal opening. In some cases the backup of fluids will cause the infant's vagina and uterus to swell up and may be confused with the presence of a tumor.

Most of the time this condition is not discovered until failure to menstruate brings a young girl to the doctor. The girl may actually have started to menstruate and may have cyclic menstrual symptoms like cramps, pain in the lower abdomen, backache and so forth. Upon examining her, the doctor finds that she has indeed been menstruating, but has an imperforate hymen, so none of the blood has escaped. If she hasn't yet menstruated, there may still be a buildup of clear mucus.

There are a number of names for these conditions. A buildup of the watery mucus in the vagina and uterus is called a hydrometrocolpos. If blood has backed up in the vagina, the condition is called a hematocolpos, and if the uterus is also involved, it is called a hematocolpometra. If things really get filled up, then the tubes too distend with blood, a condition known as hematosalpinx. The doctor may be able to see a bulging hymen, which has a bluish tinge due to the accumulated blood. These conditions can cause swelling and pain, especially at the time of the menstrual period. It's amazing, though, how large an accumulation can build up with relatively little discomfort. In extreme cases, this blood may back up through the Fallopian tubes and spill into the pelvic cavity. Since the tissue that lines the pelvic cavity is extremely sensitive to blood, this can cause great irritation and pain. There may be associated pelvic endometriosis, a condition in which the menstrual tissue implants and grows on the ovaries and other abnormal locations, causing a variety of problems.

The treatment for an imperforate hymen involves making an incision in the hymen. If there is backed-up blood, this must be drained away. An antibiotic is usually given, since this old blood is a perfect environment in which infection can develop. In some extreme cases, where the retained menstrual blood has filled the vagina and uterus and has spilled into the pelvic cavity, causing great pain and irritation, the doctor may actually have to perform abdominal surgery to drain the blood from the cavity and the Fallopian tubes. Normally, though, simple incision and drainage will correct the problem.

Absence of the Hymen/Double Vulva

It should be noted that some girls are born without hymens, although this is so common as to hardly be considered an abnormality. Such a situation causes no diseases or medical problems of any kind. It is also possible, though incredibly rare, to be born with a double vulva, which is associated with certain congenital vaginal and uterine abnormalities.

Depigmentation

A pigment is a substance that imparts color. The pigment of our skins gives us our characteristic skin color; absence of pigment makes the skin white. Some people are born without pigment in certain areas of their body or with a condition that causes them to lose pigment at some point in their lives (usually in the late teens and early twenties). This congenital condition is referred to as leukoderma. The lack of pigmentation may also be acquired as the result of a chronic infection or an injury, for instance, scarring resulting from an X-ray burn. Acquired loss of pigmentation is referred to as vitiligo.

Both vitiligo and leukoderma can occur on the vulva and can produce white patches on the skin. The condition in and of itself is not serious, is not very common and doesn't usually require treatment. It is mentioned here because it can be the cause of a whitish appearance of the vulva that could be confused with the white patches that are symptoms of other, more serious vulvar problems.

Agglutination of the Labia

Although it is not a congenital abnormality, the condition known as agglutination of the labia is often discussed under this heading in medical textbooks. In this condition the lips—labia minora and/or labia majora—are fused or stuck together. This is very rare and much more likely to occur in children than in adults, although it is occasionally seen in adults with gonorrhea. The labia are fused together as a result of a mild childhood inflammatory process that may have been so mild that it passed unnoticed. Occasionally, the fusion is so great that it prevents normal urination. Treatment consists of surgical separation of the labia and the use of petroleum jelly or estrogen creams to prevent the labia from getting stuck together again.

Clitorial Hypertrophy

The labia may be fused together or other vulvar abnormalities may occur as a result of certain congenital abnormalities involving the chromosomes, as in hermaphroditism, a condition in which the sexual tissues and structures of both male and female are present in the same person. Abnormalities in the appearance of the external genitals might also include a clitoris that resembles the tip of a penis, a condition known as clitorial hypertrophy. This condition may be caused by certain types of hormone therapy in adults. These sorts of abnormalities may also be caused by hormones the mother took during pregnancy. Treatment for these vulvar abnormalities may include surgery and/or hormone therapy.

Abnormalities in the normal anatomy of the vulva may also result from injury. These are discussed under the heading Lacerations of the Vulva, Perineum, and Vulva.

VULVAR CYSTS

Types: endometrial cysts
Bartholin's duct cysts
sebaceous cysts
mucinous cysts
Wolffian duct cysts
cyst of the canal of Nuck

There are a number of varieties of benign (noncancerous) cysts that can appear on the vulva. They appear as soft, fluid-filled, bluish swellings or bumps. Two of these, the endometrial cyst and the Bartholin's cyst, are discussed elsewhere.

Sebaceous Cyst

One of the most common of these vulvar cysts is the sebaceous cyst, which is the result of the blockage of the sebaceous or oil-producing glands that dot the skin of the vulvar area. These cysts are filled with a cheesy, oily material. They are prone to infection and abcesses (collections of pus surrounded by inflammed tissue). If they are small and cause no symptoms, they don't require treatment. If they are large enough to be bothersome, they may need to be removed by simple surgery, using a local anesthetic.

Mucinous Cyst

Mucinous cysts occasionally appear near the urinary openings or on the inner surfaces of the small lips. They are probably the result of a displacement of cellular elements in the early stages of embryonic development. They develop in various sizes and may be pendunculated, that is, connected to the surrounding tissue by a pedicle, or stem of tissue. Some small cysts that appear at the vaginal opening and are classified as mucinous are probably related to the minor glands that exist in the vestibule, the smooth boat-shaped area between the small, or inner, lips. Again, these may not require treatment unless they are large enough to be bothersome or become infected.

Wolffian Duct Cysts and Cysts of the Canal of Nuck

Wolffian duct cysts, which are also the result of an early embryonic developmental problem, rarely appear on the vulva, but if they attain any size, they may protrude through the vaginal opening. Likewise, an even more uncommon cyst, the cyst of the canal of Nuck, which also results from abnormalities in the developing embryo, may appear on the vulva. They don't usually require treatment unless they become large enough to cause problems, in which case they are removed.

BENIGN SOLID TUMORS OF THE VULVA

Types: Fibroma, lipoma, lipoma fibrosum, fibrolipoma, myoma, leiomyoma, leiofibroma or leiomyofibroma
neuro fibroma
granular cell myoblastoma
angioma (hemangioma, senile hemangioma, lymphangioma, angiokeratoma)
hidradenoma
nevus (plural, nevi.), or mole

The vulva is subject to a number of lumps and bumps. The general medical word for such lumps and bumps—for any kind of localized swelling—is *tumor*. Such tumors may be cancerous or noncancerous. Noncancerous tumors are called benign tumors, and these may be either solid or cystic.

There are a number of solid benign tumors that can appear on the vulva. Some of them have the potential of becoming cancerous, so they must be watched carefully. Others, though benign, may mimic the appearance of cancer and so must be removed or biopsied and examined microscopically to rule out that possibility. Still others may be associated with one of the sexually transmitted diseases, and even if they go away, the disease itself will still need treatment. Some of the more common benign vulvar tumors are described below.

Fibromas

Fibromas, lipomas, fibrolipomas and leiomyofibromas are all tumors that can appear on the vulva as well as other parts of the body. Fibromas arise from fibrous tissue; lipomas, from fatty tissue; fibrolipomas, from a combination of the two; and leiomyofibromas, from smooth muscle and fibrous tissue. They are usually of small or moderate size and can be felt as firm to soft, movable lumps under the skin. They cannot be distinguished from one another except by microscopic examination. They are rarely noticed unless they grow large and become pedunculated, which means that they have grown a stem, or pedicle, by which they are attached to the surrounding tissue. On occasion, they may grow extremely large and become so pedunculated that they actually dangle between the legs. The fibroma, in particular, is a favorite of medical-textbook writers who, with the spirit of proud fishermen taking snapshots of their biggest catches, always include at least a half-page illustration of a Dr. Buckner's classic (1851) vulvar fibroma, which weighed 268 pounds.

In some cases the underlying skin may become ulcerated (form an open sore), and if this happens, the fibroma may be confused with vulvar cancer, perhaps necessitating a biopsy. Unless treated, fibromas usually continue to grow and may become a nuisance. Treatment consists of surgical removal.

Neurofibromas

Neurofibromas are tumors arising from certain tissues that sheath the nerve fibers. They may appear as small, single, flabby, brownish-red pedunculated tumors or as a number of brown spots. They are usually a local symptom of a central nervous system disease known as von Recklinghausen's disease. Since they do not produce symptoms or cause inconvenience because of their small size, they do not require removal unless they become so numerous that they are bothersome.

Granular Cell Myoblastoma

The granular cell myoblastoma appears as a nontender swelling of no great size in and around the vulva as well as on other parts of the body. Sometimes the surface of the lump ulcerates, mimicking the appearance of certain forms of cancer, so that it must be cut out and examined microscopically to rule out this possibility. The doctor will cut a wide margin of tissue, since it is not clearly separate from surrounding tissue.

Angiomas

Angiomas are tumors that involve dilation of the blood vessels (hemangioma) or lymph vessels (lymphangioma). They are often congenital and may appear as raised strawberry-colored birthmarks. Occasionally, these may be irritated in infants by diapers and urine, but they don't usually require treatment and usually regress as the child grows. Hemangiomas may appear as a cluster of little bumps of a deep purple color and may extend upward into the vaginal canal, causing considerable alteration in the normal anatomy, which can sometimes lead to problems. They can, for instance, cause maternal bleeding during delivery. If they are small and asymptomatic, no treatment is necessary, but if they are large and cause problems, they must be removed. Yet another form is the senile hemangiomata—darkish, red-blue, small nodules that are frequently seen in the vulvar area of postmenopausal women, although they may occur in other age groups as well. Sometimes these blood-filled tumors, because of their exposed position, may bleed, but this can easily be controlled by removing the hemangioma. Still another variety of angioma, the angiokeratoma, may appear on the vulva as single or multiple wartlike, reddish-brown (occasionally bluish-black) tumors. Sometimes they may leak a bit, producing bloody stains on the underwear. They may increase in size during pregnancy due to pressure on the veins. They are often misdiagnosed as moles, warts or hemangiomas. They may cause alarm when they swell during pregnancy or bleed, since this type of change in a wart-like growth is also associated with cancer. A biopsy may be necessary if these types of changes occur.

Hidradenoma

Hidradenomas are tumors of the vulvar sweat glands and often appear as pea-sized swellings on the vulvar area. In some cases the overlying skin may be red, grainy and sorelike, perhaps with slight bleeding. In such instances they may mimic the appearances of vulvar cancer. Most of the time there are no bothersome symptoms, but they may itch. Treatment consists of simple surgical removal because in rare cases they have become cancerous.

Nevus

The nevus is, in layman's terms, a mole. It may be flush with the skin or raised above it. It may be about the color of the surrounding skin, have a slightly tannish hue or be quite dark. If it has been present since birth, it may become darker around the time of puberty. Nevi are usually benign and don't produce any symptoms, but must be watched carefully, for moles anywhere on the body, and particularly those in the vulvar area, have the potential of becoming cancerous. If a nevus in the vulvar area shows any sign of change (increase in size, change in color or a tendency to bleed), then it should be biopsied, that is, cut out, along with a wide margin of surrounding tissue and examined microscopically. Fortunately, the wide cutting may also provide a cure should the nevus turn out to be cancerous.

Vulvar Dystrophy

VULVAR DYSTROPHY

Types: leukoplakia, leukoplakia vulvitis or leukoplakia vulvae
hyperplastic dystrophy
lichen sclerosus, lichen sclerosus et atrophicus
kraurosis vulvae
mixed dystrophy

The term "vulvar dystrophy" refers to a group of diseases that causes abnormal changes in the skin of the vulva. In the past, terms such as "leukoplakia," "kraurosis vulvae," "lichen sclerosus" and "lichen sclerosus et atrophicus" were used to refer to these diseases. Unfortunately, these terms caused a great deal of confusion, for they were frequently misused. Part of the confusion was due to the fact that these diseases can all cause itching and white patches on the vulvar skin, so that microscopic examination is usually necessary in order to differentiate between them. Moreover, doctors use the terms differently. A few years ago, in an effort to clarify things, the powers-that-be reclassified these diseases under the general term "dystrophy."[3] Dystrophies were broken down into three groups: 1. lichen sclerosus ("lichen" due to the similarity to lichens, the white patches that grow on rocks); 2. hyperplastic (used to describe an increase in the number of cells in a given area); and 3. mixed (including primarily lichen sclerosus, but also including hyperplastic areas). Knowing what kind you have is important, for a few types of dystrophy are precursors of cancer.

Incidence

Vulvar dystrophies usually appear in the postmenopausal woman; however, at times they may appear in younger women. Lichen sclerosus has even been found in young children.

Symptoms

The vulvar dystrophies may take on a wide variety of appearances. They may start out as a dry, thick, red, swollen area of skin, but as the disease progresses, the red color changes to an opaque white. Small white pimples may dot the surface of the skin. These pimples may group together to form white, raised patches. The layer of fat under the lips of the vulva may be lost, and the lips may flatten out. In the case of lichen sclerosus, the skin tends to have a dry, thin, whitish, parchment surface. In kraurosis vulvae, which most experts feel is not a separate disease but just a more advanced stage of lichen sclerosus, the skin may become thin and shiny; the lips and

257

clitoris may shrink, and the vaginal opening may become constricted. Not all women have bothersome symptoms, but the whitish areas do tend to crack and cause minute fissures, and if this happens, there is apt to be itching and subsequent burning sensations. Secondary infection may occur, the whole vulva may become swollen, and intercourse may be painful due to the narrowing of the vaginal opening.

Diagnosis

The diagnosis of vulvar dystrophies involves a vulvar biopsy, a simple office procedure that can be done under a local anesthetic. Many doctors will hospitalize a patient and use a general anesthetic. This is not really necessary in the vast majority of cases and involves needless risk and expense. The vulvar biopsy is discussed in greater detail in the general introduction to this section.

The biopsy is vitally important, for more serious conditions—like carcinoma in situ of the vulva and invasive cancer of the vulva—can both produce similar white patches. Moreover, there seems to be some relationship between cancer of the vulva and vulvar dystrophies, and the biopsy will help to determine if there are any cancerous or precancerous cells present.

Vulvar Dystrophy and Cancer

When the first studies of vulvar dystrophy were done, it was noted that many women who had vulvar cancer also had the white patches characteristic of vulvar dystrophy. Reports on how often the two conditions coexist varied widely. Figures ranged from 12 to 80 percent.[4] This variation was probably due to the confusion caused by misuse of the old terminology.

At any rate, since the initial studies had indicated that a high percentage of vulvar cancers were associated with white patches, it was decided on this basis that the white patches were a precursor to cancer. To prevent the later development of cancer, then, it became common practice to do a "skinning" vulvectomy, an operation that involves removing the outer layers of vulvar skin. Eventually the question was raised by some researchers as to whether these white patches were really precursors to cancer, or whether cancerous tissue wasn't just more conducive to their growth. Which came first, the cancer or the white patches? Further studies were done to evaluate this question and showed that although the white patches might be present in women with cancer, the vast majority of these white lesions did not go on to become cancerous.[5]

Under the revamped classifications, the category of hyperplastic and mixed dystrophies was broken down into two groupings, based on the results of a biopsy: those that have atypical cells and those that don't. The small number of cancers that do develop in women who have vulvar dystrophies are most likely to develop in women who have these atypical cells in their biopsy. Probably less than 5 percent of all vulvar dystrophies go on to become cancer, although some authorities will place this figure at 10 percent.[6] The experts in the field now feel that vulvectomy should be done only in those cases in which atypical cells are present in the biopsy. Unfortunately, it takes a while for this information to filter down from the experts. As one authority in the field, Dr. Raymond Kaufman, explains:

> ...frequently patients would be seen by their gynecologists with so-called white lesions of the vulva, and these patients would be treated rather radically by having their vulva removed to act as a prophylaxis [preventive measure] against the development of carcinoma. And I'd say to this day, this is still very commonly done and it's not uncommon at all that I'll receive a set of slides to review in a patient with lichen sclerosus, the game plan being to do a vulvectomy on this patient, to go ahead and cure the disease process. Well, first of all, it's not necessary. Second of all, it probably doesn't cure the disease process because these changes will generally recur even after vulvectomy in the vast majority of cases.[7]

Treatment

Vulvectomy, then, is no longer the treatment of choice for vulvar dystrophies, except in cases where biopsy has shown premalignant changes. There are now less radical treatments available. These treatments are also more effective, for, as Dr. Kaufman points out, many of the vulvar dystrophies, especially lichen sclerosus, tend to recur after vulvectomy.

First of all, contributing factors should be eliminated. If, for instance, a woman has a vaginal infection, uses certain powders, deodorants, perfumes or wears tight jeans or synthetic undergarments that keep moisture from evaporating or that contain irritating chemicals, these factors should be eliminated before treatment of the dystrophy. Eliminating these possible contributing factors will help alleviate the symptoms and changes in the vulva that are seen in dystrophies.

The symptoms should also be treated, not only so that the woman is more comfortable but also because any irritated lesion on the vulva has the potential of becoming malignant. If there is swelling in the area, the doctor may prescribe cold boral solutions to help reduce the swelling and also to relieve the itching. If a woman has hyperplastic dystrophy, the doctor may prescribe cortisone in the form of cream or lotion to be applied three to four times a day to relieve itching. Once the itching and consequently the scratching is stopped, the white patches will also subside in most cases. If a woman has lichen sclerosus, the doctor may prescribe testosterone propinate, an ointment that is frequently useful. This is applied two to three times a day to relieve the itching and the appearance of the white patches. If a woman has the white patches, but no distressing symptoms, treatment is usually not necessary as long as she remains symptom free.

If the treatments described above do not relieve the itching enough to stop the woman from scratching, the doctor will try more extreme forms of treatment. S/he might inject an alcohol solution into the skin of the vulva in several spots within the infected area. This may relieve the symptoms for several months, but it is rather a last-resort treatment, for it may be followed by sloughing of cells in the vulvar area. There is also another drastic treatment, which involves incisions or cuts in the area of the labia or lips to disrupt the sensory nerves. This treatment is employed only in cases where there is extremely severe itching.

Follow-up treatment for any woman with vulvar dystrophy consists of periodic biopsies every six months or every year, depending on the severity of her symptoms. This way the doctor can spot any atypical changes and detect any cancer that might occur right away.

PREINVASIVE CANCER OF THE VULVA*

AKA: noninvasive cancer, carcinoma in situ, intraepithelial cancer or Stage O carcinoma of the vulva

Types: Bowen's disease
Paget's disease
Erythroplasia of Queyrat

The diseases described here involve abnormal changes in the cells of the tissue that make up the skin of the vulva. The very early stages of these diseases are akin to cervical dysplasia, that is, they are considered the first step in a process of abnormal changes that may or may not lead to cancer. When the cells have all the characteristics of cancer, except that there is no evidence that they have invaded beyond the skin layer to involve the lower tissues, the terms "carcinoma in situ," "intraepithelial cancer," or "Stage O carcinoma of the vulva" are used to describe these conditions.

Types

The term "carcinoma in situ," which means "cancer that is in place," is often used synonomously with the term "Bowen's disease." Most

*The reader is also referred to the general discussion of cancer and to the following section on invasive cancer.

authorities classify another of these preinvasive diseases, which has the exotic name erythroplasia of Queyrat, as a specific type of carcinoma in situ. A third type of preinvasive disease, Paget's disease, is considered by some to be a separate category, while others lump all these conditions under the heading carcinoma in situ. Sometimes it is extremely difficult to distinguish among them, even under a microscope. There is a good deal of debate among pathologists as to the classification of these conditions, and different terminology may be used by different pathologists. This is another reason why good communication between the doctor and the pathologist, to ensure that they are both using the terms in the same way, is important.

Bowen's Disease

Bowen's disease is not peculiar to the vulva but may precede invasive skin cancers anywhere on the body. The disease tends to precede invasive cancer of the vulva and has a very slow growth rate. Women with Bowen's disease have an average age of 49 as compared to 63 for invasive vulvar cancer. Approximately one-third of the women with untreated carcinoma in situ will either develop or already have an invasive cancer.

The disease may show up as red, raised areas with a grainlike surface or as shallow, open sores. If the growth is softened by the moisture often present in the vulvar area, it may appear as a white patch. Itching is a common symptom.

It tends to occur in areas where vulvar dystrophies have developed and is more likely to develop when the vulvar dystrophies have extended into the vagina. Although the symptoms may appear in only one area, microscopic examination of tissue taken from other, nonsymptomatic areas of the vulva will often show evidence of the disease.

Erythroplasia of Queyrat

Erythroplasia of Queyrat is a rare condition, most often seen on the penis, but it may affect the vulva as well. It appears as a red, velvety patch, which may have a finely granular surface resembling the surface of a strawberry. Here again, itching is a frequent symptom. Under the microscope, it may look quite similar to Bowen's disease, but its appearance and the fact that it arises only on mucous membranes may help to distinguish it. It may appear in a single area, but like Bowen's disease it may also exist in other areas without obvious signs. The growth rate is slow, although it may be somewhat faster than in Bowen's disease.

Paget's Disease

Paget's disease is another rare precancerous growth that can occur on other parts of the body as well. It occurs in the apocrine (sweat) glands of the vulva. It usually appears in women in their 50s and 60s, rarely in younger women. About 25 percent of the cases are associated with underlying invasive cancer.

It appears as red, clearly separated areas interspersed with white patches. The red areas may be ulcerated (that is, have formed sores) and "weep." Occasionally, these weeping sores will crust over. There is often intense itching.

Since it is a rare disease, many times the biopsied material is misdiagnosed by the pathologist. It may be confused with Bowen's disease or with truly invasive forms of cancer. If there is no cancer in the underlying sweat-gland system, the disease does not spread, or metastasize. But it does tend to recur later, even when the tissue left behind has not shown any microscopic evidence of the disease.

Diagnosis

All of these diseases are diagnosed by vulvar biopsy, which is described in the general introduction on vulvar diseases. Vulvar biopsy is usually a simple office procedure involving a local anesthetic. If the doctor proposes hospitalization and a general anesthetic for the biopsy, be sure to read the introduction to this section carefully.

Treatment

There is some disagreement as to what is the best method of treatment to use once it has been established that one of these preinvasive conditions exists. Some doctors will merely remove the affected area and a wide area of surrounding tissue. Most experts, however, consider this an inadequte form of treatment, for the disease in most cases is multicentric, that is, although it appears to be confined to one area, there may be other microscopic diseased areas throughout the vulva. Thus, most doctors will do a "skinning" vulvectomy, an operation in which the outer layers of vulvar tissue are removed. They feel that the entire substructure of the vulvar skin has "gone wrong" and merely cutting off the affected areas is not sufficient, for the disease will only recur later. If the recurrence is not caught in time, it could become invasive cancer, and spread to adjacent tissue or regional lymph nodes, which then requires more extensive surgery—and may be fatal. Some doctors are experimenting with cryosurgery (freezing), but long-term results are not yet available.[8]

Other doctors have advocated chemotherapy instead of surgery for treatment of carcinoma in situ. However, the chemotherapy used to treat these conditions, which is given in the form of a cream called FU-5, is extremely painful and is associated with a high rate of recurrence and complications,[9] so most experts feel that surgical vulvectomy is preferable. Any woman whose doctor proposes chemotherapy would do well to seek a second opinion (see p. 226).

It should also be mentioned that in the case of pregnancy, the doctor may delay treatment until after delivery, for a few cases of carcinoma in situ of the vulva have been shown to spontaneously regress after pregnancy.[10]

Women who have had a preinvasive type of vulvar cancer will need to have careful follow-up for the rest of their lives.

INVASIVE CANCER OF THE VULVA*

Types: epidermoid carcinoma
basal cell carcinoma
malignant melanoma
adenocarcinoma or cancer of the Bartholin's gland

Invasive cancer of the vulva is uncommon, but occurs often enough to account for about 3 to 5 percent of all cancers of the female genital organs.[11] The vast majority of vulvar cancers involve a type of tissue known as epidermal tissue. More rarely, cancer of the vulva may be of a type known as basal cell cancer. Yet another rare type is melanoma of the vulva, which may arise from moles. Occasionally, cancer will arise in the Bartholin's glands.

Inciden⌐

Cancer of the vulva most often occurs in elderly women. The majority are in their 60s, but a third of the women are in their 70s.[12] The disease can, however, occur in younger women, and about 15 percent of the cases occur in women under 40 years of age.[13]

Causes

The cause of invasive cancer, like the cause of all cancers, is unknown. However, there seem to be certain predisposing factors.[14] Failure of the

*Anyone reading this section should first read the background information on cancer (see p. 661).

263

ovaries to produce estrogen as a result of natural, surgical or radiation-induced menopause is one such factor. Most women who have the disease are postmenopausal, and in younger ones who do develop it, there is usually a history of early ovarian failure. There seems to be some association with venereal diseases such as syphilis, lymphopathia venereum and granuloma inguinale, but this is not clearly established. Here again, the younger women who develop invasive vulvar cancer are more likely to have a history of such diseases. Vulvar dystrophy is also associated with vulvar cancer.

Symptoms

Although the symptoms may appear only on one side or area of the vulva, vulvar cancer is usually multicentric, that is, the cancer will generally exist in more than one area. The most common symptom is itching, although this is not universally present. There is often a lump that does not disappear. Less frequently, instead of a lump the tumor is a raised sore that does not heal. Most of the time, the lump or sore first appears on the inner or outer lips. Sometimes these tumors first appear on the clitoris or fourchette (the area, below the vaginal opening, where the lower edges of the vulvar lips meet), but in most cases these areas only become involved as the disease spreads. The lumps or sores may be solitary or multiple.

The skin covering the tumor almost always ulcerates (forms an open sore) as the cancer progresses; however, the lump may sometimes remain firm and hard, with an intact skin covering. If this occurs and the lump is located on the side of the vaginal opening, it may be mistaken for a chronically infected Bartholin's gland.

Once the tumor has ulcerated, the area may become tender and painful. The pain may be due to exposed nerve endings or to the infection that frequently affects the ulceration. Urination is likely to be accompanied by intense burning as the urine passes over the open sore. Vulvar cancer, incidentally, is one of the few types of cancer in which the cancer itself produces symptoms of pain and tenderness. The pain gets worse as the disease progresses. The ulcerated lump may also produce some bleeding, but this is usually rather slight. If the ulceration is extensive, there may be a bothersome discharge.

There may also be a good deal of swelling of the vulvar tissue. If the cancer is associated with one of the vulvar dystrophies, white patches and other symptoms associated with dystrophies may also be present.

The growth may spread up into the vagina. In very advanced cases, the urethra and the area between the anus and vaginal opening may also be ulcerated. When the disease spreads beyond the local area, it is usually via the lymph nodes, and these too may be swollen.

It should be noted that a certain rare type of vulvar cancer may develop from a mole. The mole may be dark or skin-colored, and the symptoms of this form of cancer, which tends to be more deadly, are itching and, sometimes, bleeding. Any change in the appearance of such moles should be considered a suspicious symptom.

Spread

Cancer of the vulva usually spreads by direct invasion and/or via the lymph system. In most cases the cancer spreads to the lymph nodes in the groin and from there to the pelvic lymph nodes. In rare instances, cancer is found in the more distant pelvic nodes even though none has been found in the lymph nodes in the groin. Some authorities feel that in these rare cases the woman actually did have cancer in the groin nodes, but the cancer was missed by the pathologist who examined the removed groin nodes.

Diagnosis

The early symptoms may be so slight—just itching and soreness—that the woman hesitates to see a doctor. Most growths are fairly large, four cm or more, before a woman consults the doctor. Then, too, the diagnosis is sometimes delayed by the doctor's failure to biopsy the lump or sore until the disease has progressed to a more extensive stage. The fact that the vulvar area is sensitive and tends to bleed freely may explain in part the doctor's reluctance to biopsy vulvar tissue. Moreover, doctors are taught that cancerous lumps and sores are painless. Even though vulvar cancer is an exception to this rule, many doctors have a sort of mental block that prevents them from doing biopsies on the often painful lump or sores of the vulva. This is especially true when the patient is younger and is therefore less likely to have vulvar cancer. Since vulvar cancer as well as any number of infections may produce lumps and bumps with a wide variety of appearances, it is a risky business for a doctor to decide on the basis of appearance alone that the lump isn't cancerous. Any vulvar ulceration or lump that doesn't disappear within three to four weeks should be biopsied.

The biopsy should, with rare exceptions, be an office procedure, requiring only a local anesthetic. See the discussion of vulvar biopsies in the general introduction to vulvar diseases if your doctor suggests hospitalization and/or general anesthetic.

Once the presence of cancer has been confirmed by biopsy, routine tests to detect metastasis (*see* p. 676) are done to rule out the possibility that the cancer has spread to other parts of the body.

Careful attention is also given to the lymph nodes. These will be carefully palpated (felt) by the doctor. If the doctor feels unusually enlarged lymph nodes and/or lymph nodes that are not freely movable, s/he will suspect that cancer has already spread to these areas, though infection can cause these symptoms too. Even in cases where the feel and appearance of the lymph nodes are not suspicious, cancer may be present. In addition to careful palpation, the doctor may do a lymphangiogram, an X-ray examination of the lymph nodes, in order to make a more accurate estimate of the possibility of cancer there, but this test is not entirely reliable and is only rarely used.

The visible cancerous area or areas will be carefully measured, for it is known that tumors over two cm in diameter have a much greater likelihood of lymph node involvement.

Staging

Table 5 outlines the staging scheme for vulvar cancer.[15] The size of the cancer is important in Stage I and II, as is the condition of the lymph nodes. The lymph nodes in the groin will be removed and examined by the pathologist at the time of operation, but the doctor's estimate of the possibility of groin node involvement prior to the operation may be important in decisions about how to treat the pelvic lymph nodes (see below). The doctor's physical exam and the results of tests to detect metastasis will help in classifying Stage III and IV cases.

Table 5
Staging Scheme for Cancer of the Vulva

Stage O:	Carcinoma in situ
Stage I:	Cancer confined to the vulva, two cm or less in diameter. No suspicious lymph nodes.
Stage II:	Same as above, only the cancer is larger than two cm in diameter. No suspicious lymph nodes.
Stage III:	Cancer of any size that has 1. spread to the urethra, all or part of the vagina, the area between the vaginal opening and the anus, and/or the anus itself; 2. and/or suspicious lymph nodes.
Stage IV, A and B:	Cancer of any size that has infiltrated A. the bladder and/or rectum; and/or B. cancer that is fixed to the bone and/or has metastasized to distant sites.

Treatment [16]

The treatment of Stage O vulvar cancer is discussed elsewhere. Here we are only concerned with invasive vulvar cancer—Stages I, II, III and IV. Since 90 to 95 percent of all vulvar cancers are of a type known as squamous cell cancers, the following discussion centers around treatment of this type of vulvar cancer. Other rare forms are mentioned only briefly.

The aim of treatment in these cases is to remove the actual tumor, the surrounding areas where microscopic cancer may be lurking and the lymph passageways and nodes that may be involved.

Vulvectomy

Simply removing the tumor itself would not suffice, for vulvar cancer tends to be multicentric, that is, to have many points of origin. The entire vulva must be removed, an operation known as a vulvectomy. To do anything less than a total vulvectomy would be taking too great a chance of leaving behind microscopic areas of cancer that could metastasize before they were discovered.

There is some debate about how extensive the total vulvectomy should be. Some doctors feel that it is acceptable in certain instances to do an operation that allows for what is known in surgical circles as "primary closure," in which enough skin remains to close over the operative wound. If primary closure is not possible, skin grafting (removing skin from other areas of the body and transplanting it to the wound area) must be done. Other doctors feel that doing a vulvectomy that allows for primary closure, while it offers better cosmetic results and superior healing, is too dangerous, since it is associated with higher rates of recurrence. This is one issue that women with vulvar cancer interviewing prospective doctors might wish to discuss, and to seek second opinions regarding.

Although radiation therapy could theoretically be effective in treating cancer in the immediate area of the vulva, this is generally not done, for tissues in this area are extremely sensitive to radiation. Doses of radiation high enough to destroy the cancer would cause too much damage to these tissues. In certain cases, where a woman is in such poor health that the general anesthesia required for surgery would pose too great a threat to her life, removal of the tumor alone under local anesthetic and/or radiation therapy may be used. Since this results in lower cure rates, surgery is done whenever possible. In certain cases, where the tumor is too large to be removed surgically, radiation treatment may be given prior to surgery, in order to reduce the tumor to the point where it can be removed surgically. Most of the time, however, the vulvar area is not radiated.

Another instance in which surgery might not be done is in Stage IV cases, when the disease has spread to the bones or other distant areas. In these cases the surgery will not improve a woman's chances of survival, so there is no point in subjecting her to the risks and discomforts of surgery. An exception would be the woman with Stage IV B disease who has intense itching and heavy discharge. In her case a partial vulvectomy may be helpful in relieving the symptoms and making her more comfortable.

Inguinal Lymphadenectomy

In most cases, the surgery will also involve removal of the lymph nodes in the groin, a procedure known as inguinal lymphadenectomy. Even if there is no suggestion that these lymph nodes are involved prior to surgery, they must be removed, for even in Stage I A cases there is a chance that microscopic areas of cancer may be lurking in these nodes. The only way to find out is to remove them and examine them microscopically.

There is a tendency among some doctors to do the vulvectomy and not to remove the lymph nodes as well if there are no symptoms of swelling, especially when, as is often the case, the woman is elderly. Such doctors may delay the treatment of the lymph nodes until the woman actually develops the swelling in the nodes that indicates that cancer may be present. This is considered a dangerous course of action by most experts, for cancer is sometimes present even though there is no swelling. By waiting for signs of swelling, the woman's best chance for a cure is lost. Sometimes, in women who have such poor general health that the more prolonged and taxing operation of lymph node removal would be too much of a strain, even the experts concede that the more radical surgery should not be done. However, most of these experts caution against this modification of surgery on the basis of age alone. While some surgeons argue that the elderly patient won't live long enough to justify subjecting her to the risks of extended surgery, most experts feel that the facts don't justify this line of thinking. They believe that it is unfair to do less than adequate surgery, which will jeopardize her long term chances of survival, just because she is elderly. Many times a team approach to surgery is used. One doctor does the vulvectomy, while the other removes the lymph nodes. This allows for a faster operation and less anesthesia time, and hence there is less risk.

There are certain specialized cases in which removal of the lymph nodes in the groin may be omitted. Carcinoma in situ and certain rare types of cancer, for instance one known as basal cell carcinoma, don't require removal, for the nodes are rarely, if ever, involved in the disease process. Many doctors feel that certain early invasive cancers in which the depth of invasion is less than five mm (some would say three mm) and in which the tumor cells are low grade (see p. 677) don't require lymph node removal.

It is possible to survive without lymph node surgery, but generally speaking, survival rates are improved when the lymph nodes in the groin are removed.

Pelvic Lymphadenectomy

The pelvic nodes may also be removed, via a procedure known as a pelvic lymphadenectomy. Here again, removal makes the operation more extensive, requiring longer anesthesia time, and therefore the risk is greater. The rate of complications is significantly higher as well. There has been a good deal of uncertainty about when it is worthwhile to remove these pelvic lymph nodes.

If the woman is a good enough surgical risk to allow for vulvectomy and removal of the lymph nodes in the groin, then the surgeon will send the removed groin nodes to the pathology lab for analysis via frozen section. If the pathologist sends back word that the groin nodes are cancer free, then most surgeons will not remove the pelvic nodes. While some doctors favor removal of the pelvic nodes even if the groin nodes are negative, the majority of doctors would consider this to be unnecessary and to involve too many extra risks and complications to be worthwhile.

If the pathologist's report indicates that the groin nodes are positive, the situation is a bit more complicated. Just because the groin nodes have cancer in them does not necessarily mean that the pelvic ones do. Although vulvar cancer spreads from the original site to the immediately adjacent groin lymph nodes relatively quickly, it then seems to slow down. It apparently remains in the groin nodes for some time before spreading to the pelvic nodes. It is thought that only about 16 percent of the women in whom the pathologist has found cancer in the groin nodes will have cancer in the pelvic nodes. It is estimated that 20 to 25 percent of the women with pelvic node metastases can be cured. But this means that only 20 to 25 percent of the 16 percent who have positive pelvic nodes, that is, only 3 to 4 percent of those women with cancerous groin nodes, would actually benefit from having their pelvic lymph nodes removed. To remove the pelvic lymph nodes in all women with negative groin nodes doesn't then seem justifiable to many doctors. Still, other doctors will remove these nodes routinely.

In recent years some authorities have adopted special criteria for deciding whether or not to remove the pelvic nodes. Some studies have shown that those women who, on the basis of the pathologist's report, were shown to have positive lymph nodes in the groin *and* who also have had suspicious-appearing nodes in the groin prior to surgery are the ones most likely to have positive pelvic nodes.[17] If the nodes did not appear suspicious prior to surgery and cancer was found only during the pathologist's microscopic examination, there is little chance that the pelvic nodes are involved. Sometimes, however, the pelvic nodes can be cancerous even if the groin nodes do not appear suspicious before surgery.

The groin lymph system narrows down to one specific node called Cloquet's node before branching out to the pelvic network of lymph passageways. This key node may be removed by the surgeon and subjected to frozen section analysis. If it tests positive, the woman may require removal of the pelvic nodes, regardless of the appearance of the groin nodes prior to surgery. Many doctors, then, will remove the pelvic nodes only if the woman has positive groin nodes both by frozen section analysis and by the doctor's clinical opinion preoperatively, and/or if the Cloquet's node is found to have cancer by frozen section analysis at the time of surgery.

The question of pelvic lymph node removal is a problematic one and opinions, even among experts, differ. Every woman has the right to a full discussion of her doctor's operative plans. She should know what nodes the doctor plans to remove, how these decisions will be made and on what basis. She should know, given her particular state of health, what the possible risks and complications of less extensive or more extensive surgery are. Second opinions (*see* p. 226) are, of course, in order.

Pelvic Exenteration

In certain advanced cases, a partial or total pelvic exenteration may be combined with vulvectomy and pelvic/inguinal lymphadenectomy. Total pelvic exenteration involves removal of the vulva, vagina, uterus, tubes, ovaries, supporting and connective tissue, urethra, bladder and/or rectum. Partial exenteration involves the removal of only some of these organs. If the bladder, urethra and/or rectum are removed, new openings are constructed surgically and waste products are collected in plastic bags. This is an extensive operation and can be done only in cases where the woman is in good health. It is not done in Stage IV B cases, where the disease has spread to distant sites in the body, for it would not result in improved survival. However, in women who are good candidates for this type of extensive surgery, 50 to 75 percent success rates in controlling the disease have been reported.[18] Even if it does not result in absolute cure, it can prolong life significantly.

Radiation Therapy

As discussed earlier, radiation therapy is not generally used to treat cancer in the vulvar area; however, in recent years, there has been a great deal of interest in using radiation instead of or in conjunction with lymphadenectomy to treat the groin and pelvic nodes. Since the vulvar area is not radiated directly, the problem of excessive damage to these radiation-sensitive tissues does not arise. Proponents of this form of therapy feel that there would be fewer risks and complications than with lymphadenectomy. At the present time, we simply do not know enough to say conclusively whether radiation would or would not be superior to lymphadenectomy.

Some doctors will use radiation therapy to treat women who refuse or are not candidates for pelvic exenteration. But, here again, there is the problem of radiation damage to the sensitive bladder and rectum. Radiation therapy may be used to treat recurrent cancer.

Radiation has also been used in palliation, that is, in treatment designed to relieve symptoms and make the woman more comfortable. This may be done in certain cases of distant metastases, but many doctors question palliative value in treating the vulvar area. They feel that the radiation does little to relieve symptoms, that it may actually shorten the woman's lifespan and that the aftereffects of the radiation cause so much pain and discomfort that it is not worthwhile to use it. Here again, women have the right to a full discussion of the benefits and risks of radiation therapy in their particular case and to second opinions or consultations as needed.

Chemotherapy

Chemotherapy is only used on an experimental basis. Although there have been a few reports of limited success in controlling vulvar cancer, most results have been disappointing.[19]

Recurrent Cancer and Follow-Up

All women with vulvar cancer must be followed for life in order to detect recurrences and the cancers that such women frequently develop in their other female organs.

Survival Rates

Surgery is only possible in about three-quarters of the women with vulvar cancer, and survival rates are lower for those who are inoperable. Table 6 gives survival statistics by stage.

Table 6
Five-Year Survival Rates for Squamous Cancer of the Vulva

Stage	Survival %
I	85
II	58
III	24
IV	0

SOURCE: Adapted from J.L. Benedet *et al.*, "Squamous Carcinoma of the Vulva: Results of Treatment 1930−1976, *American Journal of Obstetrics and Gynecology,* 134:2 (May 15, 1979), p. 201−7.

The Vagina

The anatomy of the vagina is described and illustrated in Chapter Two. The changes that occur in the vagina over the course of the menstrual cycle and during a woman's lifetime are discussed in Chapter Four. In this section we are concerned with vaginal diseases.

Vaginitis

The first several diseases discussed in this section of the book are forms of vaginitis. The term vaginitis is a broad one, used to refer to any inflammation of the vagina. The chief symptom of vaginitis is excessive vaginal discharge, which may smell badly and cause itching.

A certain amount of vaginal discharge is normal, for the vaginal discharge helps to cleanse the vagina and keep it healthy. The discharge is made up of secretions from the vaginal walls and cells shed from the uterus, cervix and walls of the vagina. The amount and character of this discharge changes over the course of the menstrual cycle and over the course of a woman's lifetime. It also varies from individual to individual. Most of the time the discharge is clear or milky white in color, moderate in quantity, thin or watery in consistency and has a mild odor. It may leave a slightly yellowish stain on underclothes. Women who practice self-exam and are familiar with their own discharges can detect abnormal discharges and seek treatment for vaginitis in the earliest stages of the disease when it is easiest to treat.

Vaginitis is associated with changes in the normal acid/alkaline balance of the vagina. Most of the time the vaginal secretions are rather acidic. Scientists measure acidity on a relative scale called the pH scale that looks like this:

The scale runs from 1 to 14 and 7 represents a neutral condition, that is, neither alkaline (sugary) nor acidic. The average pH of the vagina of a woman in her reproductive years is usually about 4.5 to 5. Most disease-causing organisms prefer a more alkaline environment. For instance, Trichomonads, the culprits responsible for trich, one of the most common forms of vaginitis, thrive best in a pH of 4.9 to 7.5. Monilia, the organisms responsible for yeast infections, prefer a pH of about 5.4. Gonococci, the bacteria that cause gonorrhea, and streptococci, other disease-causing organisms, do best at a pH of 7.4.

The protective, slightly acidic environment of the vagina is maintained by bacteria known as lactobacilli, or Doderlein's bacteria, that normally live in the vagina. Without them the vagina would be quite alkaline, for the cervical secretions and the cells that are constantly being shed from the vaginal walls are alkaline. The cells of the vaginal wall contain large amounts of a sugar known as glycogen. This sugar is derived from carbohydrates taken into the body when sugars and starches are eaten. As the cells of the vaginal wall are shed and break down, releasing their alkaline glycogen, the lactobacilli convert the sugar to a weak acid known as lactic acid.

The pH of the vagina changes over the course of the menstrual cycle. It is most alkaline at the time of ovulation, when levels of estrogen are highest. The cervical secretions are then more abundant, and there are greater numbers of sugar-rich vaginal cells. Symptoms of vaginitis, which are sometimes cyclical, appearing for a while and then subsiding, only to appear again, are apt to manifest themselves or to be particularly intense at the time of ovulation. The pH of the vagina also changes after menopause. Typically, the vagina of a postmenopausal woman has a pH of about 7. This change in pH, coupled with the fact that after menopause the vaginal walls become thinner and are easily irritated, a condition known as postmenopausal vaginitis, explains why postmenopausal women are so prone to vaginal infections.

There are a number of other things that can alter the vaginal pH, making the vagina more alkaline and more susceptible to infection. Sometimes antibiotics prescribed to combat infections elsewhere in the body also destroy the lactobacilli. Then, disease-causing organisms that may already have been present but were held in check by the acid environment of the vagina or that are introduced into the body at this time, thrive in the vaginal environment, which has become more alkaline without the lactobacilli. Women taking antibiotics are thus especially prone to yeast infections, for yeasts are frequently present in the vagina and antibiotics affect the lactobacilli but not yeasts. Some doctors prescribe yeast medication to be taken along with the antibiotic, especially if the woman has a history of yeast infections.

Yogurt, which contains lactobacilli, will help to maintain the acidity of the vagina, and is also effective in treating yeast infections and nonspecific vaginitis.[1] A spermicide or medicine applicator can be used to insert the yogurt into the vagina. Eating yogurt will help, but inserting a couple of applicators full of yogurt once or twice a day and again at bedtime during the course of antibiotic treatment will be even more helpful in preventing infections. Using a tampon to help keep the yogurt in the vagina or a sanitary napkin to catch the yogurt that may leak out is a good idea.

In order to be effective, the yogurt must contain live lactobacilli. Most of the yogurt sold in the grocery store has been pasteurized after the lactobacilli were added. Because the heat from the pasteurization process destroys the lactobacilli, it is important to find yogurt that has not been pasteurized or that was pasteurized prior to addition of the lactobacilli. Health food stores often carry this type of yogurt. It is also possible to purchase yogurt culture and make your own.

Birth control pills also alter vaginal chemistry. Not only do the extra hormones in the blood stream stimulate the cervical glands to produce more secretion, but the Pill also changes the chemical composition of the vaginal cells. This makes the vagina more alkaline and more susceptible to infection. This is especially true for women taking high-dose estrogen pills containing more than .05 mg of estrogen per pill. In fact, the Pill makes the vagina so alkaline that women who take the Pill have nearly a 100 percent chance of developing gonorrhea after a single act of intercourse with an infected partner as opposed to a 40 to 50 percent chance for women who are not on the Pill.

Pregnant women may also have more alkaline vaginas, for during pregnancy hormone levels are higher and the vaginal changes that result are similar to those created by birth control pills. It is often difficult for pregnant women to get rid of a vaginal infection.

Women with diabetes, a disease in which the body is not able to metabolize nutrients properly and which causes high levels of sugar in the body, also tend to have more alkaline vaginal environments. Their vaginal cells have high levels of glycogen and they are thus particularly susceptible to yeast infections.

Excessive douching can also alter the vaginal pH. Although the value of the douches that are sometimes prescribed as part of the treatment of vaginitis is not questioned, many doctors feel that douching as a routine hygiene measure is not a good idea since it can alter the acid/alkaline balance, making the woman more susceptible to infection. In addition, the chemicals used in many of the commercially available douche mixes may irritate the vagina. Most women who douche do so because they are concerned about odor. Sexual activity, emotional changes and the stage of the menstrual cycle can all cause changes in the composition and hence the odor of vaginal secretions, but genital odor usually emanates from the outer genital organs. Improper wiping with toilet tissue can trap urine and feces in the vulvar lips and cause odor. Hot weather and inadequate ventilation of the genital organs due to tight clothing or synthetic undergarments (which trap air and moisture) also contribute to the problem. Daily washing of the genitals with soap and water will usually eliminate any odors, and such routine hygiene is preferable to disturbing the pH balance of the vagina with commercial douche preparations.

Some doctors advise women who use tampons to douche at the end of their menstrual periods because leaving a tampon in for an extended period of time traps the menstrual blood and vaginal discharges, creating a breeding ground for infection. Women who use tampons should change them frequently to avoid this problem. Pregnant women should never douche, since the douche water could be forced up into the uterus and cause an infection, miscarriage or fetal death.

Women who do douche should not do so more than twice a week and should avoid commercial douche preparations. Two tablespoons of white vinegar diluted in a quart of warm water is a less expensive alternative and one that closely mimics the pH of the vagina. Bag-type douches are usually more effective than syringe-type douches (Illustration 39). Douching equipment should not be shared, because infection can be transmitted by a douche nozzle that has not been properly cleansed. Before douching, you should inspect the nozzle for cracks, which could injure the vaginal tissues or harbor infection. The nozzle should be washed thoroughly with soap and hot water but should not be boiled since the nozzles are usually made of plastic, which could melt at high temperatures.

To douche, lie on your back in the tub or shower with the douche bag about one foot above your hips. The higher the bag, the more forceful the flow of water into the vagina, but too much pressure could injure the vaginal tissues or force bacteria or other disease-causing organisms up into the normally sterile environment of the uterus.

Illustration 39   *Douching*

Prevention

Vaginitis is generally not serious in terms of general health, but it is often hard to get rid of and recurrences are common. Prevention is the best form of treatment. The following suggestions will help to prevent vaginitis:

☐ Take care of yourself! Being run down, not getting enough sleep and eating improperly make you more susceptible.

☐ Avoid eating sugars and starches and thereby creating an alkaline vaginal environment. Include yogurt in your diet, and if you are susceptible to infection or take birth control pills, apply yogurt to your vagina, especially at the time of ovulation, when your pH rises.

☐ Insert applicators full of yogurt into the vagina a couple of times a day if you are taking an antibiotic. If you have a history of yeast infections, ask the doctor to prescribe yeast medication to be taken along with the antibiotic.

☐ Avoid douching.

☐ Change tampons frequently.

☐ If you use a diaphragm, don't leave it in place longer than necessary, for this can cause vaginitis in some women.

276

☐ Use condoms if you have more than one sexual partner or are starting a sexual relationship with a new partner, as these two factors make you more prone to infections.

☐ Always wipe from the front to the back to avoid spreading bacteria from the bowel into the vagina.

☐ Wear cotton underpants; avoid synthetic undergarments, pantyhose and tight pants.

☐ Avoid using feminine hygiene sprays, bubble baths and other such products that can irritate the vulva and vaginal opening and also mask odors that are one of the signs of vaginitis.

Diagnosis and Treatment

Practicing self-exam regularly will make you familiar with your own discharge and help you to learn what is normal for you at various points in your menstrual cycle. Vaginitis can be detected in its earliest stages, before the infection has gotten to the point where the discharge is so profuse that it is leaking out of the vaginal opening and causing burning, itching and redness of the external genitals. Some women who are familiar with their own bodies use yogurt at the first sign of vaginitis and this often clears up the infection and avoids the expense and inconvenience of a doctor's visit and medications, but this could be a risky practice. Any women who does this must be absolutely positive that she has not been exposed to gonorrhea. We know of one woman who practiced self-exam and noticed an unusual discharge that looked like the classic yeast infection discharge. She had a long history of yeast infections, so she used yogurt for a week and her discharge returned to normal. As it turned out, the woman didn't have a yeast infection at all; she had gonorrhea. Gonorrhea is often asymptomatic in its early stages or there may be minimal symptoms, one of which is a slight vaginal discharge. These early symptoms may subside even though the infection has not gone away. This woman's discharge did subside, though it didn't do so because of the yogurt, for yogurt is not effective against gonorrhea. Luckily, this woman went to the doctor a couple of weeks later for her yearly checkup, which included a gonorrhea culture. Her gonorrhea was therefore detected and treated. If it had not been caught, it could have had serious consequences, including pelvic inflammatory disease, sterility, and perhaps even death. This woman had only one sexual partner, and her sexual partner was supposedly having sex only with her. He wasn't, and she got gonorrhea.

Any woman who is having heterosexual sex and notices an unusual discharge should consider the possibility that she has gonorrhea and should ask that a gonorrhea culture be done. Women should also insist that the doctor do a wet smear. A wet smear takes only a few minutes. With a speculum in place the doctor takes a sample of the discharge. The discharge is then smeared across a glass slide and viewed under a microscope.

The organisms responsible for most forms of vaginitis are easily identified via wet smear. Some doctors don't do a wet smear. They sometimes feel that they can diagnose the type of vaginitis just by looking at the discharge. While it is true that each form of discharge has its characteristic appearance and odor, it is easy to be fooled. For one thing, it is not at all unusual to have two infections at the same time. In these cases of mixed infections, the symptoms of one form of vaginitis may mask the symptoms of the other. Each type of vaginitis requires its own specific medication. If a woman had trich and yeast infection, the medication used to treat the trich wouldn't be effective against the yeast, and her yeast infection would persist. She would return to the doctor, who might assume her trich was still present and prescribe another round of medicine for it. A wet smear will avoid such confusion. But do not douche before going to the doctor, for this can alter the results of a wet smear or other tests.

With vaginitis, your sexual partner may need to be treated as well. And you should use condoms until the infection clears up or you will constantly reinfect each other, even if you are both taking the medication.

It is important to take all the medication that is prescribed. Too many times women will discontinue the medication as soon as the symptoms disappear, but the stronger organisms that have not yet succumbed to the medication remain. Eventually they will reproduce until their numbers are sufficient to produce symptoms. Then, you've got a recurrence of the infection that will be harder to cure since the new infection will be caused by the offspring of the stronger, more drug-resistant organisms.

Anatomical Abnormalities

Although vaginitis is the most common type of vaginal problem, there are other problems that can affect the vagina. One group of problems involves alterations of the normal anatomy of the vagina. The vaginal canal may become smaller and less elastic, a condition known as vaginal stenosis. The opening of the vaginal canal may be disturbed as a result of injury. This sort of problem is discussed under the heading Lacerations of the Vagina, Vulva and Perineum. Sometimes because of a muscle weakness or defect in the vaginal wall, the bladder or urethra may sag and bulge into the vaginal wall. If this happens, the woman has either a cystocele or urethrocele. Similarly, a portion of the rectum or intestines may bulge into the vagina, conditions known as rectocele or entrocele. A woman may also experience involuntary spasms of the vaginal muscles, a condition known as vaginismus. Another distortion in the normal vaginal anatomy is the fistula, a condition in which there are abnormal connections or passageways between the vagina and the urinary tract or the vagina and the rectum. A woman may also be born with a vagina whose anatomy is abnormal. This problem is discussed under the heading Congenital Abnormalities of the Vagina.

DES-Related Problems

One type of congenital abnormality of the vagina that has received considerable attention in recent years occurs in the daughters of women who took certain synthetic hormones during their pregnancies. This is discussed under the headings Vaginal Adenosis and Clear Cell Adenocarcinoma. Many DES daughters are not aware of the fact that they have been exposed. All women should read the discussion of DES.

Benign and Malignant Tumors

Lastly, the vagina may be the site of tumors, either benign or cancerous. Both benign and malignant tumors are discussed below.

TRICH

AKA: trichomonas vaginitis, trichomoniasis, trichomonosis, TV

Trich, or TV, is a form of vaginitis. Important information about the cause, diagnosis and treatment of vaginitis is given in the introduction to this section, so be sure to read that material as well as the information below.

Incidence

The exact incidence of TV is hard to determine since many women carry the organisms without having any symptoms. Various studies have reported that anywhere from 20 to 65 percent examined have the organisms in their vaginas even though they have no symptoms. It is estimated that 15 percent of these women will become symptomatic. TV is, then, a very widespread disease.

Cause and Transmission

TV is caused by a microscopic organism whose scientific name is *Trichomonas vaginalis*. This organism does not normally inhabit the vagina or any other area of the human body. Since the disease may be asymptomatic, it is possible for a woman to carry the organism for many years without ever knowing she has trichs in her body. Some doctors think that additional organisms, for instance, streptococci, must also be present in order to produce symptoms. Some authorities feel that emotional stress and strain may be responsible for a flare-up, persistence or recurrence of symptoms.

Trichs are usually introduced into the vagina by sexual intercourse. There is circumstantial evidence that the disease can be passed by nonsexual contact, as the organisms have been cultured from Bakelite toilet seats, wash cloths and the wooden benches of washroom at room temperature after 24 hours, but it has thus far been impossible to actually prove that the disease is transmitted in nonsexual ways. Most authorities feel that the majority of cases of TV are transmitted through sexual intercourse.

Anyone who gets TV is likely to wonder, "Who did I get it from?" Sometimes this question may be hard to answer. First there is the possibility, although it is probably a pretty remote one, that the transmission *was* nonsexual. Secondly, there is the possibility that a woman could have been harboring the trichs for some time, for years even, without knowing it. Emotional stress, a general lowered resistance or changes in the vaginal pH can cause the disease to suddenly become symptomatic. Even if a woman has had many wet smears done for other infections it is still possible that she may have had TV for quite some time. The wet smear would have shown the presence of the trichs, but there are some doctors who do not inform the woman of the fact that trichs are present unless she is symptomatic. The third possibility is that although the trichs were in her body for some time, the other organisms that some experts believe must also be present to produce symptoms may not have been there.

Symptoms

As mentioned above, many women are asymptomatic and it is also possible for the disease to be present for quite some time before the symptoms appear. Sometimes the symptoms are cyclical in nature, appearing for a few days and then disappearing for a month or even for many months. In the great majority of cases, it is thought that the symptoms appear within 4 to 28 days of the infected contact. The symptoms may be mild or very severe. Since other diseases, especially gonorrhea, yeast infections and hemophilus often occur along with trich, symptoms of these diseases may also be present.

In some cases, the only symptom may be a vaginal discharge. The discharge is usually yellowish white or green-yellow in color, but may be white or gray. The discharge is usually thin and watery, but in case of mixed infections, it may be thick and creamy. It tends to be frothy, that is, to have little bubbles in it (caused by fermentation of the trichs) and to smell bad.

The vaginal opening may be red and sore due to irritation from the discharge. There is apt to be itching and burning, especially on urination. Sexual intercourse may be painful. In extreme cases the whole vulvar area and even the inside of the thighs and/or the anus may be irritated.

The symptoms of TV are likely to be more severe just before and just after the menstrual period. This may be because the vagina is more alkaline (as opposed to acid) at this time and trichs thrive in an alkaline environment. Pregnant women, whose vaginal environments are also apt to be more alkaline, are particularly susceptible and may have more severe symptoms. The introduction to this section discussed acid/alkaline balance and vaginal infections in more detail.

On speculum exam, it may be possible to see a pool of the typical thin, greenish-yellow, bubbly discharge around the cervix. The walls of the vagina may be quite red. In severe cases the upper walls and cervix may be covered with strawberrylike red patches.

Men rarely suffer symptoms; however, some men may notice a burning after ejaculation or urination. There may be a slight moistness on the tip of the penis and some itching. Trichs do not survive well on the male sex organs, though on uncircumcized men the area under the foreskin may afford an environment conducive to the trichs. Such men may notice a discharge from this area.

Diagnosis

Sometimes the symptoms are so characteristic that the diagnosis is obvious. However, even if the classic symptoms are present, a woman should insist that the diagnosis be confirmed by a microscopic examination of the vaginal discharge—by a wet smear—for other diseases are frequently present along with TV, and the treatment for TV may not be effective against these other diseases. A wet smear precludes the problem of unnecessary or ineffective treatment.

Since the discharge may be heavy and tends to smell bad, many women douche before going to the doctor. This should not be done, for it may flush out a large number of trichs and cause a negative wet smear, even though trichs may still be present and will multiply, causing symptoms again later. Sometimes women who are familiar with their discharges will note a slight increase or an unpleasant odor in the early stages of TV. In very early cases, a doctor, seeing none of the signs of TV and not noticing an unusual odor or unusual discharge, might be reluctant to do a smear. One woman reported that her doctor told her, "Some vaginal odor is normal," in response to her complaint. When, at her insistence, he reluctantly did a wet smear, he found trichs. Women who notice unusual symptoms should insist on having appropriate tests done.

The smear is not always entirely accurate. Trichs may be present and yet be missed. In doubtful cases or when the symptoms lead the doctor to suspect that other diseases are present, it is possible to grow the trichs in a special culture, but this takes some time and is more costly, so the culture is not routinely used to diagnose TV. It is probably a good idea to have a gonorrhea culture done as well, since the two diseases often coexist.

Women should be aware of the fact that some doctors, finding trichs in routine wet smears, will not even bother to tell asymptomatic women. Such doctors also don't believe in treating the disease if it is asymptomatic. However, even if a woman isn't symptomatic, she is still liable to pass the trichs on through intercourse and, eventually, to cause TV in some other woman. It is important to communicate with your doctor on this issue and to make it clear that you want access to any information s/he has about your body. Other doctors feel that if a woman has a population of trichs in her vagina large enough to show up on a wet smear, she is likely to become symptomatic in the future and should be treated.

TV occasionally shows up as an incidental finding on a routine Pap smear. As long as a woman has no symptoms, the majority of doctors will not treat trich when it is only discovered as an incidental finding. The drug used to combat TV is a potent one, and they feel that if the trichs haven't shown up on a wet smear and aren't producing symptoms, it is better to rely on the body's own defenses to keep the problem in check.

It should be noted that TV can also cause an abnormal Pap smear. The pathologist's report will usually say that "inflammatory cells" are present. This is nothing to worry about, since the Pap will revert to normal once the TV is cleared up. However, on rare occasions TV will cause changes in the Pap smear that mimic dysplasia, a possibly precancerous condition. Occasionally a Pap smear indicating dysplasia in a woman with TV will revert to normal after the TV is treated, but usually when the Pap smear indicates dysplasia, the dysplasia will persist.

Treatment

In this country, TV is usually treated with metronidazole, which is sold under the brand name Flagyl. Flagyl can be used by most people and doesn't usually produce severe side effects; however, the drug is contraindicated (that is, should not be taken by) for certain people.[2] Obviously, anyone who has had a previous allergic reaction to Flagyl should not take the drug. People who have certain blood diseases cannot take it because it can cause a temporary decrease in white blood cell count. People taking certain types of anticoagulant drugs should not take Flagyl because the two drugs can interact in dangerous ways. People who have active disease in the central nervous system should not take it because there is some evidence that the drug may affect the central nervous system. The drug is officially contraindicated for women in the first three months of pregnancy, for it can cross the placental barrier and enter the fetal circulation system. Although Flagyl has not been shown to cause birth defects in either animal or human studies, there is not sufficient data available to rule out the possibility. Moreover, there is some evidence that Flagyl can cause both cancerous and noncancerous tumors (see below). Since it can produce tumors and affect the central nervous system, many doctors feel that it should not be used in pregnant women at all, regardless of the stage of pregnancy. Since the drug is secreted in breast milk, a nursing mother taking the drug must discontinue breastfeeding for a while.

Flagyl can cause adverse reactions in some people. Nausea, sometimes accompanied by headaches, loss of appetite, occasionally vomiting, diarrhea, abdominal cramping and constipation are the most common type of complaints. A person taking Flagyl should not drink alcohol, for drinking can aggravate these reaction.

A metallic taste in the mouth is not uncommon. A furry tongue, dryness of the mouth, vulva and vagina, nasal congestion, itching, hives, painful urination, painful intercourse, a sense of pelvic pressure, fever, decreased sex drive, pus in the urine, excessive urine, inability to control urine flow, inflammations of the bladder and the rectum, confusion, irritability, depression, weakness, insomnia, dizziness, lack of coordination and even convulsive seizures have been associated with Flagyl. Pain in the joints or numbness of the arms, legs and hands are important side effects since these sorts of effects have persisted even after the drug was discontinued in some people who had taken Flagyl for a long time. If any of these side effects appear in a person taking Flagyl, the medicine should be discontinued, the symptoms reported to the doctor and possible alternative treatments discussed.

Women taking Flagyl are more apt to get yeast infections because the acid/alkaline balance of the vagina is altered. Prevention of such yeast infections is discussed in the general introduction to vaginal diseases (*see* p. 276).

Although Searle, the company that sells Flagyl, has asserted over the years that Flagyl does not cause cancer, in 1972 an article in the *Journal of the National Cancer Institute (JNCI)* reported the results of an experiment in which a greater number of cancerous and noncancerous tumors appeared in a group of mice given Flagyl compared to a control group[3]. This lead to a reexamination of the data Searle had provided to the Food and Drug Administration. The reexamination was apparently necessary, for as it turned out, the original Searle rat data confirmed the *JNCI* findings.

Since that time, other studies have been done that showed an increase in the incidence of various tumors in rats, particularly breast tumors.[4] Two other studies done on hamsters, however, were reported as negative.[5] Moreover, the animal studies have been criticized because in some of them, the animals were given the drug every day for their entire lives. Even in the studies where the animals were given the Flagyl intermittently, critics point out that the dosages were rather high. More recently, studies of the urine excreted by people taking Flagyl have shown some evidence that the drug has the power to cause mutations in bacteria.[6] The implications this may hold for human cancer is not yet known.

Originally, the dosage was one 250 mg tablet, three times a day, for ten days; however, many people stopped taking the drug as soon as the symptoms cleared up, often after only two or three days. This led to a high rate of recurrence of the disease due to insufficient dosage, so shorter dosage schedules with higher dose tablets were tried. Currently, the Food and Drug Administration (FDA) has approved a schedule of one 250 mg pill three times a day for seven days; however, some doctors will give 500 mg two times a day for five days, while others feel that 250 mg three times a day for three days is sufficient. These two alternatives seem to work about as well, but are not officially approved by the FDA. Recently, there have been experiments in which Flagyl was given in a single eight tablet (two gram) dose or split into a double dose of four tablets each taken in the same day. Some researchers report cure rates as high as 90 percent while others report rates as low as 56 percent. It is unclear why there should be such a variance in rates. It has been suggested that the studies that yielded high cure rates may have had inadequate follow-up and recurrences may have been missed. At any rate, such dosages are experimental and there may be more intense side effects with these high-level doses. Indeed, in our experience, people taking this much Flagyl are apt to get quite sick and to vomit up the medication, thus necessitating another course of Flagyl.

Some cases of TV do not respond to Flagyl. There has been some suggestion in recent articles that Flagyl is not as effective as it once was. Whereas Flagyl provided a 97 percent cure rate in 1967, the results now being recorded are not as good and may be as low as 74 percent. This may be due to the development of a stronger strain of trichs or it may be that the bacteria that often accompany TV tend to inactivate Flagyl. If the latter proves to be true, an antibiotic may be given along with the Flagyl in the future. In either case, larger doses of Flagyl may someday be required.

Recently, a newer drug, nitrimidazone, which is sold in Great Britain under the brand names Naxogin and Minerazole and which is about as effective as Flagyl (indeed, possibly more effective in single-dose therapy), has been used to treat TV. It is not yet sold in this country, so information as to its possible side effects is not readily available; however, it would not be surprising if the drug were, in the not too distant future, available in the United States.

In about 25 percent of the people treated with Flagyl, there will be a recurrence of the disease. This may be due to reinfection or to failure of the drug to destroy all the trichs. If the Flagyl is taken a second time, there should be a waiting period of four to six weeks before the second course to allow the white blood cell count, which may be depressed by the Flagyl, to return to normal.

There are numerous other drugs that can be used to treat trich in pregnant women or others who cannot use the drug, but the cure rates for these are not as high as with Flagyl. Antibiotics in the form of triple sulfa cream applied to the vagina or Aureomycin and Terramycin given orally have met with some success. We personally prefer Betadine to sulfa cream, Aureomycin or Terramycin.

Douches of five tablespoons of ordinary vinegar to two quarts of water may be used in the treatment of TV. The douches will make the vagina more acid so that the trichs have trouble surviving. The douches often help to cut down on the symptoms; however, they are not likely to cure the disease, for it is virtually impossible to flush out all the trichs that may be lurking in the recesses of the vaginal folds and some may survive despite the acidity. Keeping the vulvar area dry, using cotton underpants instead of synthetic garments (which trap moisture) and avoiding the use of powders, ointments and sprays will also cut down on the severity of symptoms.

Some doctors prohibit intercourse during the treatment period; others allow intercourse as long as the male wears a condom. The point of prohibiting or protecting intercourse is to prevent the woman from being reinfected and the male from picking it up.

Still another debate centers around whether or not the male partners should be treated.[7] Some doctors will write out extra prescriptions for the women's sexual partners; others will not. Some will prescribe for one, two or even three partners, but they may be reluctant to write out a larger number of prescriptions. There are basically two schools of thought on the issue. Those who won't prescribe for the male partner say that since there are contraindications to the drug, they are reluctant to prescribe without interviewing the man concerning the possibility of his being at risk. They also point out that the man may not actually have the disease and that the drugs should be given only when disease is actually present, to prevent things like acquired resistance and side effects. Moreover, some doctors feel that the organisms do not survive well on the penis and will die out without treatment. Those who do prescribe it for the unseen male sexual partners do so because they fear that he, who is likely to be asymptomatic, may not bother to go to a doctor for diagnosis and may reinfect his partner and/or pass it on to another female. They question how quickly and thoroughly the organisms die out on the male and point to the high recurrence rate. Untreated males, they feel, are too often responsible for reinfection.

YEAST INFECTIONS

AKA: fungus infections, candidiasis, moniliasis, vaginal thrush, fungus vaginitis

Associated terms: *Monilia vaginitis, Candida vaginitis, Candida albicans, Monilia albicans*

Yeast infections, which are called by a number of different names, are not serious, but they can be very bothersome. They are often hard to get rid of and recurrences are common. In addition to the information given here, the general introduction to vaginal diseases (*see* p. 272) contains important information about yeast infections.

Incidence

Yeast infections are very common. They tend to occur more frequently in women during the menstrual years, when, under the influence of the monthly ebb and flow of hormones, the vagina provides a rich environment for their growth.

Cause and Transmission

Yeast infections are thought to be caused by a fungus of the yeast family known as *Candida albicans*. Some authorities feel that other, similar organisms may be responsible for the milder forms of the disease.

The organism may be passed through sexual intercourse. A man may give the disease to a woman; however, he is much more likely to get it from her than to give it to her. Nonsexual methods of transfer—douche nozzles, washcloths, etc.—may explain how the organism is originally introduced into the vagina. It is present in the feces of somewhere between 17 to 40 percent of all people, so, careless wiping may also explain how the organism gets into the vagina. *Candidae* are apparently normal inhabitants of the vagina in many women. They usually don't cause any problems. The mere presence of the organisms doesn't mean that there will be symptoms of infection. *Candidae* only seem to cause problems when the environment of the vagina is disturbed. They do not thrive in the normally acid vaginal environment, preferring a more alkaline environment. If, however, the vagina does become more alkaline, they will multiply. Taking antibiotics, douching, eating a lot of carbohydrates, having diabetes, being pregnant and using oral contraceptives may alter the normal acidic vaginal pH.

Chemotherapy or radiation therapy used to treat cancer may make a woman more susceptible, probably because they weaken the body's immunological system. Some women seem to have deficient immunological systems, which makes them more prone to yeast infections.

Symptoms

The symptoms vary somewhat from woman to woman and may be very similar to those of trich. There may be discharge, burning, itching, localized soreness and pain. Women with yeast infections often complain of a frequent need to urinate and of painful intercourse.

The most common symptom is a vaginal discharge, which tends to be less abundant than with trich. The characteristic discharge is whitish in color, thin and watery with thick, curdlike chunks of a white, cheesy substance that gives the discharge a cottage-cheese-like appearance. The discharge may have a disagreeable odor, which some women liken to fermenting yeast. The symptoms tend to be worse just before and after the menstrual period, when the vagina is usually more alkaline. On speculum exam, the walls of the vagina may appear red and swollen. There may be chunks of white discharge, which, in some cases, adhere firmly to the vaginal walls.

If the discharge is profuse, it can cause an itchy rash on the external genitals. The vulva can be affected as well and may be dry, red, swollen and tender to the touch. If the infection is widespread, the whole vulva may take on a whitish appearance. Itching, of course, can cause scratching, which makes the area even more irritated and swollen and can lead to a secondary infection. There may be soreness or pain in the whole genital area. As mentioned earlier, intercourse can become very painful. There may also be pain when urine passes over the red, raw tissues.

Diagnosis

Many times the symptoms alone will be enough to make an accurate diagnosis; however, the doctor should also do a wet smear, for in 35 percent of cases there is an associated infection.[8] Hemophilus and trich often go hand in hand with yeast infections. Moreover, the second infection may be masked by the symptoms of the yeast infection and will go undetected unless a microscopic examination is made. Many doctors ignore this vital step, but it is essential. If a woman is treated only for a yeast infection, she will not get rid of the second infection. If she comes back in a week complaining, the doctor may not bother to do another microscopic examination, and she may get treated for the yeast infection all over again. The second infection, when finally recognized, may require an antibiotic, which in turn could provoke another yeast flare-up. It's best, then, to take the medications simultaneously. Women should always insist on a wet smear before accepting treatment.

The diagnosis can also be made by growing a culture. This is done by spreading a bit of the discharge on a special substance that is favorable to the growth of *Candida*. In four or five days, patches of the fungus can be seen growing in the culture dish. Some doctors question the value of this since *Candida albicans* often exists in the vagina and will, therefore, "grow out" on the culture even in women who are not having problems. Other doctors feel that the extent of culture growth is indicative of a heavier than normal concentration of *Candidae*. The value of doing a culture is, then, debatable. Fortunately, most infections can be diagnosed accurately with a simple wet smear.

The culture that is done to diagnose gonorrhea will also tell the doctor whether or not a yeast infection is present. One danger in diagnosis is that a woman with a yeast infection will be diagnosed via wet smear and her doctor, assuming that the yeast infection alone is responsible for her discharge, will fail to investigate the possibility that the woman also needs a gonorrhea culture. This is especially likely to happen to middle-class women or other women who the doctor considers "nice girls," the theory being, of course, that "nice girls" don't get gonorrhea. Unfortunately, the gonococcus is not such a moralistic organism; it thrives as well in "nice girls" as it does in "wanton women." So if you have a discharge and have slept with someone who might possibly have given you gonorrhea (which means just about anybody), you should also have a gonorrhea culture.

Treatment

In the past, gentian violet, a rather messy purple staining medication, was used. The gentian violet was painted on the vagina and cervix. This was supplemented with gentian violet tablets or creams inserted into the vagina for home use. Although gentian violet is still used by some doctors, especially for recurrent cases, newer antifungal drugs sold under brand names like Mycostatin or Gyne-Lotrimin are more widely used now. They are taken in the form of a suppository or creams inserted into the vagina at bedtime. If reinfection occurs or if the doctor suspects that the gastrointestinal tract and the feces are also infected, medication may be given orally as well. Women who have had a recurrence after treatment with a suppository or a cream should ask their doctors about oral medication.

Many women feel uncomfortable having intercourse during treatment, and some doctors will tell patients to refrain from intercourse during this time because they feel it further irritates the area. Other doctors, especially in cases where the symptoms are mild, will simply suggest that the male use a condom to prevent the penis from becoming irritated or likewise infected. Men, though, are much less likely to have problems with fungus infections since their genitals don't provide the same kind of warm, wet environment conducive to growth of the fungus that the vagina does. Still, in cases where a woman has a stubborn case that is not responding to treatment, the doctor may suspect that the man is harboring the *Candidae* and is constantly reinfecting her, and s/he will want to check him as well.

It is sometimes very difficult to treat pregnant women because their alkaline vaginal environment is very conducive to fungus growth. Successful treatment may have to wait until after delivery. Some doctors think it's especially important to treat pregnant women who are about to deliver, even if they have little or nothing in the way of symptoms, so that the baby doesn't get the fungus infection (thrush) in his or her mouth and throat during delivery. Other doctors point out that thrush is fairly rare and is easily curable, so they don't treat asymptomatic pregnant women even if they find a lot of *Candidae*. Still others will treat such a woman because they feel she probably will become symptomatic.

Sometimes it is difficult to treat women using birth control pills. Use of the Pill may have to be discontinued while they are being treated.

Some doctors prescribe prophylactic (preventive) medication. For instance, women who have a history of yeast infections might be given yeast medication to take along with an antibiotic. This is discussed more fully in the introduction to this section (*see* p. 276). In women for whom recurrences are serious problems, some doctors will prescribe medication in advance. Then, at the first sign of a symptom, the woman can begin the course of medication. Thus, she is able to catch the infection in its earliest stages, when it is easiest to cure.

HEMOPHILUS

AKA: Hemophilus vaginitis, nonspecific vaginitis

Hemophilus is a common form of vaginal infection. In the past, hemophilus infections were called nonspecific vaginitis, but it is now known that many of these nonspecific cases are actually caused by *Hemophilus* bacteria. Indeed, some authorities argue that *all* cases of nonspecific vaginitis, at least during the reproductive years, are actually hemophilus infections.

Incidence

The exact incidence is hard to determine since some women may not have symptoms; however, it is generally agreed that *Hemophili* are a very common cause of vaginitis. Hemophilus infections don't usually occur in women before puberty or after menopause, for without estrogen stimulation of the vaginal tissues, the vaginal environment is not rich enough to support the growth of these organisms.

Cause and Transmission

The infection is caused by the organism *Hemophilus vaginalis,* which likes moist places and is killed by drying. The *Hemophilus* bacteria don't survive well in the normal vaginal environment. In order for them to thrive, the normal acid/alkaline balance of the vagina must be disturbed. This is discussed more fully in the introduction to this section (*see* p. 273). Although it is possible to acquire the infection from douche nozzles, toilet seats, washcloths and other, similar sources, the most common method of acquiring and transmitting the disease is through sexual intercourse.

Symptoms

As many as 75 percent of women will be without symptoms in the early stages of the disease. The most common symptom is an increase in vaginal discharge. Typically, the discharge looks like a thin flour paste and has a grayish hue. It tends to smell quite bad. There may be burning and itching of the external genitals, but this is less likely to happen with hemophilus than with TV or yeast infections.

Hemophilus may occur in conjunction with other forms of vaginitis, so symptoms of these diseases may also be present. For instance, about 25 percent of women with trich will also have hemophilus.[9]

Diagnosis

The diagnosis of hemophilus can be made with a wet smear or a culture. Since the wet smear is cheaper and quicker, it is routinely used; however, the culture may be used in questionable or stubborn diagnosis. As explained in the introduction to this section (*see* p. 277), specific diagnosis is important, particularly in mixed infections. For instance, if a woman also has trich and is treated only for the trich, her hemophilus will probably not be cured.* The persistence of the smelly discharge may be interpreted as a persistence of the trich infection. Another round of Flagyl, the drug used to treat trich, may then be given, again to no avail. Specific diagnosis, via wet smear, is therefore essential.

Treatment

Hemophilus responds well to vaginal suppositories of antibiotics. The milder forms react very quickly to sulfanilamide vaginal tablets or suppositories, which are marketed under names like Sultrin or Furacin. Since the use of antibiotics causes yeast infections in some women, susceptible women should take the precautions described in the introduction to this section of the book. In more severe cases, Terramycin vaginal tablets with polymyxin B or similar medications are used. Terramycin alone is effective, but it is notorious for its tendency to lead to yeast infections; polymyxin B is added to prevent this. In recurrent or stubborn cases, antibiotics like ampicillin may be given by mouth.

Sexual intercourse is either prohibited or a condom must be used. This prevents further irritation of the vagina and the possibility of passing the infection back and forth.

---

*Flagyl, the drug used to treat trich, has mild antibiotic effects and may be effective in early, mild cases of hemophilus.

291

NONSPECIFIC VAGINITIS

AKA: Hemophilus

There is some controversy about the use of the term "nonspecific vaginitis." Some doctors think that all nonspecific vaginitis that occurs during the reproductive years is caused by *Hemophilus* bacteria and that the term should be reserved for cases of vaginitis occurring in prepubescent girls and postmenopausal women. Others feel that other organisms besides *Hemophilus* may be responsible for nonspecific vaginitis. At any rate, the symptoms are generally the same as those of any form of vaginitis: increase in vaginal discharge, soreness, itching and burning. The diagnostic procedure is also the same: a wet smear or, in confusing or stubborn cases, a culture to rule out one of the specific forms of vaginitis like trich, yeast infection or hemophilus. Treatment consists of a broad-spectrum antibiotic, which may be given in the form of vaginal suppositories or, if the infection is more severe or recurs, orally.

POSTMENOPAUSAL VAGINITIS

AKA: senile atrophy of the vagina, atrophic vaginitis

Associated terms: adhesive vaginitis

After menopause, when the tissues of the vagina are no longer stimulated by estrogen from the ovaries, the walls of the vagina become smooth, dry, shiny and less elastic. The vaginal secretions are scant, so there is little lubrication. The entire vaginal canal shrinks in size. In some women the walls of the vagina may stick to each other, a condition known as adhesive vaginitis. Tiny sores may appear on the vaginal walls, causing a slightly blood-tinged discharge. There may be a burning or itching feeling or a general soreness in the vagina, and intercourse may be painful. The dried-out skin is prone to injury and minute cracks, which may become secondarily infected and cause nonspecific vaginitis. Postmenopausal vaginitis is often associated with postmenopausal vulvitis.

Treatment

If there is a secondary infection, this is cleared up with antibiotics. Estrogen, given either by mouth or as a locally applied cream, will usually return the vagina to its premenopausal state and eliminate symptoms; however, estrogen replacement therapy (*see* p. 763) has been implicated in the development of cancer, so it must be used with caution. Sometimes less drastic treatments such as vinegar douches and a well balanced diet, especially one rich in vitamin A and B complex, may help. Regular sexual activity will stimulate blood flow to the area, help keep these tissues supple, and help to prevent postmenopausal vaginitis. If adhesions form, they can usually be broken up quite easily by carefully dilating the vaginal canal. This is done by gently probing the vaginal canal with a finger or two and is best done by the woman herself, although the doctor can also do it.

VAGINAL STENOSIS

AKA: narrowing of the vaginal canal

The term "stenosis" means "a narrowing" or "stricture." In women with vaginal stenosis, the vaginal canal becomes smaller and narrower.

Causes

Sometimes vaginal stenosis is a natural part of the aging process. After menopause, the levels of estrogen are diminished. Without estrogen stimulation, the vaginal canal and opening become smaller. The vagina loses its elasticity as the blood supply to these tissues is diminished and the elastic tissue is replaced by fibrous tissue. The skin becomes thinner and drier. Vaginal stenosis also occurs in younger women whose ovaries have been surgically removed or irradiated, or in women who, for some other reason, have a premature menopause.

Radiation treatment for cancer can also cause vaginal stenosis, partly because the ovaries are often sterilized, which brings on premature menopause, and partly because there is damage and scarring from the radiation itself. Before abortion was legalized, it was not uncommon to find cases of vaginal stenosis in women who had put caustic substances such as lye into their vaginas in an attempt to abort themselves. Fortunately, thanks to liberalized abortion laws, this type of vaginal stenosis is a medical rarity today. Sometimes stenosis occurs after vaginal surgery; for example, a radical hysterectomy, in which the upper third of the vagina is removed along with the uterus, shortens the vagina and may leave scar tissue that further narrows the vaginal cavity. Lacerations of the vagina, that is, injuries received as a result of rape or accidents, can also cause scar tissue and vaginal stenosis.

Symptoms

Vaginal stenosis can cause pain or difficulty with intercourse. In women who have high doses of radiation therapy, the vagina may become so

293

stenotic that intercourse is extremely painful or downright impossible. The vagina is apt to be rather dry, a common problem for postmenopausal women, which can also cause painful intercourse. Postmenopausal women with bothersome stenosis may also have postmenopausal vaginitis. If minute cracks occur in the drier vaginal tissue, such women may also be susceptible to other forms of vaginitis, particularly nonspecific vaginitis.

Diagnosis

The diagnosis of vaginal stenosis is made on the basis of the symptoms and a physical examination and in light of a history that includes menopause (natural, surgical, or radiation-induced), radiation treatment, vaginal surgery, rape or injury.

Treatment

The type of treatment for vaginal stenosis depends on the cause and the severity of the condition. In mild cases the use of a vaginal lubricant like K-Y Lubricating Jelly, which is available without a prescription from pharmacies (and is also greaseless, water-soluble and nonstaining), will relieve the difficulties or discomfort associated with intercourse.

Extreme cases of postmenopausal stenosis can be effectively treated by giving estrogen replacement therapy, either orally or by locally applied creams. The estrogen will thicken the vaginal tissues and restore tissue elasticity; however, estrogen has been associated with an increased risk of certain types of cancer (*see* p. 421) and cannot be used by some women. We suggest that a woman try some of the alternative treatments for menopausal therapy (*see* p. 612) before resorting to estrogen.

Unfortunately, there is little that can be done for women who have stenosis as a result of radiation therapy. For those women who have had vaginal surgery or injury, it is often possible to create an adequate vagina using plastic surgery techniques, but after radiation therapy, the tissues are usually too thin and heal too poorly to allow for this.

LACERATIONS OF THE VAGINA, VULVA AND PERINEUM

AKA: tears or stretching of the vagina, vulva or perineum

Associated terms: relaxation of the vaginal outlet

Lacerations or tears of the vagina, vulva or perineum (the area between the vagina and anus) may be the result of surgery, accidental injuries, rape or insertion of an object into the vaginal canal with or without consent. For instance, a hymen may be torn as the result of rape and the tear may extend into the vaginal canal or perineum. A woman may also fall on a sharp object that projects into the vaginal canal. More often such lacerations are the result of difficult childbirth or abortion. Women who have exceptionally large children, rigid or unyielding tissues, small or unprepared vaginal canals, forceful spontaneous deliveries or complicated labors that require instruments are more likely to have lacerations.

Symptoms and Treatment

Bleeding may be profuse, and in rare instances fatal, but this is not usually the case. Such occurrences may result in a hematoma or a localized collection of blood, but generally these are reabsorbed by the body and seldom become infected or form abscesses. Treatment usually consists of the application of hot packs and sitz baths.

For the most part, lacerations of the perineum and vaginal wall heal quickly and do not require sewing or suturing; however, excessive bleeding must be controlled, and larger tears, especially those acquired in childbirth or abortion, should be repaired.

Sometimes the tear involves the underlying muscle structure; at other times, the lacerations may occur under the surface of the skin, in which case stretching is probably a better word to describe the situation.

Lacerations are generally not serious in and of themselves; however, over time they may contribute to muscle weakness and thereby contribute to relaxation of the vaginal outlet. The vaginal opening has been compared to the mouth, one being a horizontal and the other a vertical opening. Both have a fixed upper portion and a movable lower portion. If the muscles that control the movable portion are injured or grow weak with age, then the opening no longer closes snugly. Relaxation of the vaginal outlet is often associated with other forms of genital relaxation such as uterine prolapse, cystocele and rectocele.

If they are extensive, the tears may extend all the way from the vagina to anus, exposing the mucous lining of the rectum. If the muscles are torn or stretched to an extreme, it might become impossible for such a woman to control her bowel movements. In such cases, surgical repair may be required.

CYSTOCELE AND URETHROCELE

AKA: fallen, or prolapsed, bladder, or vesicocele; fallen, or prolapsed, urethra

Associated Terms: stress incontinence

A cystocele (Illustration 40) is a condition in which the bladder drops down from its normal position and bulges into the vagina. An urethrocele is similar, only it is the urethra, the tube that connects the bladder to the urinary opening, that is involved. These conditions are usually associated with a general relaxation of the muscles and tissues that support the pelvic organs. They may be a result of a congenital defect in the supportive tissue and muscle or of an injury, usually one connected with childbirth. Over time, what started as a weakness can become an actual defect. The muscle and tissue can become so stretched and thin that the fibers actually separate and a hole is created. The process is somewhat akin to wearing a hole through the heel of a sock. The bladder or urethra is no longer held firmly in its proper place, sags down next to the vagina and eventually bulges into the vaginal wall. These conditions occur most frequently in older women or in women who have had many children, which lends support to the theory that these conditions are caused by tears and injuries during childbirth. At times, though, they occur in women who have never had children, so it is thought that an inherited muscle weakness or some other type of injury may also be involved.

Symptoms

A woman with cystocele and/or urethrocele may not have any symptoms; however, she may complain of a sense of pelvic fullness or a discomfort when bearing down. It may feel as if her pelvic organs are dropping out. She may sense or feel a bulge in the wall of the vagina that is nearest to the bladder and urethra. She may actually see the bulge at the vaginal opening.

The symptoms are often aggravated by long hours of standing. If the cystocele or urethrocele is small, there is rarely more than minor discomfort, but if the descent of the bladder or urethra is extreme, it may be uncomfortable to sit down or difficult even to walk. If the cystocele or urethrocele is very large, it may even protrude through the vaginal opening. In rare instances, the tissue that covers the bladder or urethra may be stretched so thin that its exposure to the vaginal secretions will result in an ulcer, an irritated sore that produces a discharge or bleeding, but bleeding is only rarely a symptom.

If the back part of the bladder drops below the neck of the bladder, there may be mechanical difficulties in completely emptying the bladder. Urinary frequency due to the diminished capacity of the bladder may occur. The woman may feel she has to urinate even though she has just done so. The urine that stays in the bladder quickly stagnates and provides an excellent environment for bacteria. Thus, urinary infections with symptoms like painful and frequent urination may develop.

Illustration 40   *Cystocele: The bladder prolapses and bulges into the vagina (A). Urethrocele: The urethra, the tube that conducts urine, prolapses and bulges into the vagina (B).*

With the urethrocele, since the position of the bladder in relation to the bladder neck is altered, the muscle at the base of the bladder that controls the flow of urine may be disturbed. It may be difficult to control the urine, and sudden movements like coughs and sneezes may result in leaks of urine, a situation referred to as stress incontinence.

Diagnosis

In the majority of cases, these conditions are not difficult to diagnose. The doctor can feel or even see a round, soft, elastic bulge if the woman coughs or strains, especially if she is standing up. The bulge can easily be pushed back into its proper place. Occasionally, the cystocele may be so small as to be hidden, especially if the woman is lying down. If so, the doctor may ask her to strain downward as s/he presses against the area or to stand up for the exam. On rare occasions, the cystocele will be evident only when the woman is relaxed under anesthesia. Diagnosis is usually an easy matter, for

297

there are only a few rare vaginal cysts whose presence could be mistaken for a cystocele.

Treatment

If a cystocele or urethrocele is small, or even only moderately large, and a woman has little in the way of symptoms and no repeated bouts with cystitis or urinary infections, there is no rush for treatment. This is especially true if a woman is young and plans to have more children, since the surgical repair job is often destroyed by childbirth and subsequent repair jobs might not be as successful. But if a woman has distressing symptoms and recurring urinary tract infections or if the cystocele or urethrocele is becoming larger, the doctor will repair the defect surgically even if it is a small one. A larger one, even if it isn't producing symptoms, will require treatment, for chances are that it will eventually cause symptoms. Repairing it before the defect gets larger and the muscles weaker will result in better long-term results.

Sometimes surgery can be avoided. A series of exercises that involve alternately tightening and relaxing the muscles involved may be helpful in less severe cases. In order to know which muscles need exercise, a woman should practice stopping the flow of urine midstream. These are the same muscles that help support the pelvic organs. The exercise consists of tightening these muscles and holding for three seconds. (Don't push down as if making a bowel movement; rather, tighten and pull the genitals together). It should be done about 200 times over the course of the day (work up to this point gradually). It takes a couple of months to get results, but doing these exercises can help avoid discomfort and the need for surgery in future years.

Some doctors prescribe estrogen replacement therapy (ERT), which will thicken the lining of the vagina and the urinary tract. ERT will not cure the problem, but it may alleviate symptoms. ERT, however, has been implicated in cancer and must be used with caution.

The surgical repair of a cystocele or urethrocele is called vaginal repair, plastic surgery or cystocele repair. It is done via a vaginal incision. The bladder is pushed back into its normal position and sewn in place. The back wall of the vagina may also be repaired if the woman has a rectocele or if the tissue is so stretched and torn that a rectocele is likely to occur in the future.

The results of vaginal repair are reasonably good; however, the doctor cannot promise that it will relieve stress incontinence, which continues to be a problem for about 20 percent of the women who have the operation. If the stress incontinence is not cured and is creating serious problems, another operation, done through an abdominal incision, in which the surgeon changes the angle of the bladder opening may be undertaken. This involves more risks and complications. It is successful in about 50 percent of the cases.

RECTOCELE AND ENTEROCELE

AKA: prolapse of the rectum, prolapse of the small intestines

A rectocele (Illustration 41) is a condition in which part of the rectum bulges into the back wall of the vagina. An enterocele is a condition that involves a weakness higher up in the vagina in which part of the small intestine may bulge into the back wall of the vagina. Because the rectum is located below the small intestine, the rectocele is usually felt in the lower portion of the vaginal wall.

Illustration 41   *Rectocele: The rectum prolapses and bulges into the back wall of the vagina (A). Enterocele: Part of the small intestine prolapses and bulges into the vagina (B).*

Causes and Incidence

Both conditions are the result of a weakness in the tissues that support the organs and hold them in place. As the result of pregnancy and childbirth, especially prolonged and complicated labors and deliveries, the simple process of aging or, sometimes, a congenital on inherent weakness in the supportive tissues, the organs involved begin to sag. The organs slip down and press against the rear wall of the vagina. Slowly, over time, a defect or even an actual hole is opened in the vaginal wall and a section of the rectum or small intestines may bulge into the vaginal vault. These conditions are usually associated with a general relaxation of the pelvic organs and may occur together. It is rare to find only a rectocele; usually this condition is associated with a cystocele, lacerations of the vagina, vulva and the perineum, some degree of uterine prolapse and/or relaxation of the vaginal opening.

It is unusual to find either of these conditions in women who have never had children. When it does occur in such women, it is the result of a congenital defect in the vaginal wall or in the supporting tissues. It most often affects older, postmenopausal women.

Symptoms

The rectocele causes little discomfort. Women with this condition may, however, complain of some pain or discomfort when bearing down or be aware of a bulge in the vagina. If the rectocele is large, it may actually protrude through the vaginal opening. There may be difficulty in fully emptying the rectum when moving the bowels. In extreme cases, it might become necessary to press on the back wall of the vagina in order to fully empty the rectum and prevent constipation.

With the enterocele, a bulge may be felt in the vagina, but it is higher on the vaginal wall than with a rectocele. In some cases it can be seen or felt as a bulge immediately behind the cervix. It may expand and contract with breathing because of its connection with the abdominal cavity.

Diagnosis

Sometimes, these conditions are harder to detect when the patient is lying down. The doctor may need to do the examination with the patient in a standing position. The doctor will insert a finger into the rectum and into the vagina and ask the patient to bear down. Sometimes it is difficult to tell the difference between a high rectocele and an enterocele. It is important that the doctor make a correct diagnosis and determine whether a bulge is a rectocele or enterocele, since the operation for a rectocele will not correct an enterocele and the woman will have the same bulge after treatment. A doctor may shine a light into the rectum. If the bulge inside the vagina is not thereby illuminated the doctor will suspect an enterocele.

Treatment

Since a small rectocele causes little trouble, it doesn't usually require treatment and is ignored unless surgery is being done to correct some related condition, like prolapse of the uterus, a cystocele or urethrocele or a bothersome enterocele. If an abdominal hysterectomy is being done for some reason, it is a good idea to correct large rectoceles at the same time, even if they aren't causing problems, for many times, women who were previously unaware of the rectocele will start to have symptoms once the uterus has been removed. The larger rectoceles, especially those that cause problems with elimination should be repaired surgically.

The enterocele is somewhat more serious. The loop of intestine may swell and get caught in the bulge that protrudes into the vagina. If the blood supply of the intestinal loop is cut off, the hernia becomes strangulated, which may result in gangrene that could in turn lead to death. Prompt surgical attention and a proper repair job are necessary with all enteroceles.

VAGINISMUS

AKA: spasms of the vaginal muscles

Vaginismus is a condition characterized by involuntary contraction of the vaginal muscles. Most doctors feel the problem is a psychological one, but some cases may be due to congenital abnormalities of the vagina, imperforate hymen, vaginal stenosis or a particularly rigid and unyielding hymen. If one of these conditions is present, intercourse or the introduction of a speculum, a finger or, for that matter anything into the vaginal cavity will cause such pain that the muscles contract sharply. The muscles may spasm so tightly that intercourse is painful or downright impossible.

Diagnosis and Treatment

Diagnosis involves eliminating any of the physiological conditions that can cause the problem. If the problem seems to be psychological in origin,

301

there may be a history of rape, repression or a lack of education about sexual matters that has led to fear of intercourse. Psychological counseling may be in order, as well as basic sexual education. The woman is taught to explore her own genitals, gradually relaxing her vagina by inserting a finger or two. The woman's sexual partner may need education about sexual foreplay and the need for vaginal lubrication prior to insertion of the penis.

FISTULAS

AKA: genital fistula

Types: urinary fistula, bladder fistula, vesicovaginal
     fistula or vesicouterine fistula
urethra fistula or urethrovaginal fistula
ureter fistula or ureterovaginal fistula
rectal fistula, vaginal-fecal fistula or bowel fistula

A genital fistula is an abnormal passageway or connection between the genital organs and the urinary tract or intestinal tract. The vagina or, in some cases, the uterus may be involved. There are a number of different types of fistulas depending on exactly where the abnormal connection is located. A fistula between the bladder and vagina is a vesicovaginal fistula; between the uterus and bladder, a vesicouterine fistula; between the urethra (the tube that conducts urine from the bladder to the outside of the body) and the vagina, a urethrovaginal fistula; between a ureter (one of the tubes that conducts fluid from the kidneys to the bladder) and the vagina, a ureterovaginal fistula. When the intestinal tract and bowels are involved, it is called a rectal, bowel or vaginal-fecal fistula.

Cause

In the past, most fistulas were the result of prolonged and difficult childbirth or the improper use of forceps. As obstetrical care has improved, the incidence of childbirth-related fistulas has declined. However, increases in major surgery, more complex and risky procedures and the use of radiation for dealing with gynecological problems has led to a considerable increase in the incidence of surgically or radiation-induced genital fistulas. Fistulas may also be the result of the destruction of tissues by malignant tumors or ulcers (open sores) caused by foreign bodies, especially vaginal pessaries used to treat cystoceles and uterine prolapse. When the vagina and rectum are involved in the fistula, granuloma inguinale may be the cause.

302

Symptoms

The most common symptom of urinary fistulas, which involve the vagina and the organs of the urinary system, is leakage of urine from the vagina. With small fistulas, this may be only a slight dribble and may be more noticeable when the body is in certain positions. In other cases, the flow of urine may be constant and profuse. In fact, in extreme cases, all urine leaves the body through the vagina and none through the urethral meatus, the normal opening to the urinary tract. The vagina, vulva and surrounding areas may become irritated and there is often an unpleasant ammonialike odor. Unless very careful hygiene measures are taken, the fistula may become encrusted with mineral deposits, adding to the irritation. Fistulas that involve the rectum or bowels and vaginal canal may be so slight that only a small amount of fecal matter or gas gets into the vagina, and this may be a problem only when the stools are especially soft. If, however, such a fistula is large, there is bound to be considerable irritation as well as an offensive odor, not to mention possible infection.

Diagnosis

The diagnosis of a urinary fistula is usually fairly simple, although if it has occurred as the result of an operation, the usual postoperative vaginal discharge may confuse the issue. It is not, however, always easy to determine the exact nature and location of a fistula. Sometimes after an operation or childbirth, the muscle that controls the flow of urine becomes too weak and urine is leaked. At first glance, this can be mistaken for a fistula. In most cases, though, the doctor can see a fistula on speculum exam or feel it during a bimanual pelvic exam. Small, highly placed fistulas may require special diagnostic techniques involving colored water or air placed into the bladder. This will help the doctor decide whether the bladder or the tube that leads from the bladder to the opening is involved.

Treatment

Small urinary fistulas, unless they are the result of malignant disease may, on rare occasions, close up by themselves. Urinary antiseptics and the temporary use of a tube called a catheter to drain the urine from the body will sometimes help this natural healing process, but most of the time, surgical repair is necessary. Unfortunately, it is best to wait four to six months after the fistula has occurred, if it was surgically induced, to give the recently operated-upon tissues a chance to get back to normal. Since this delay can be very disturbing to a woman with a fistula, some doctors use cortisone to cut down on the waiting period. Antibiotics and local soothing treatments may also be given.

If there is a great deal of damage to the urinary tract, the doctor may have to perform a nephrostomy, an operation whereby a direct opening from the kidney to the outside of the body, bypassing the rest of the urinary system, is created. Although most of the time if this is done it is as a temporary solution to allow tissue to heal before attempting surgical repair, it is also done when surgical repair of the fistula is unsuccessful or impossible.

Like the urinary fistula, a fistula involving the bowels or rectum and vagina can usually be repaired surgically; but, in some cases, especially in ones caused by malignant disease or radiation, this is not possible. A colostomy, an operation that results in the contents of the bowels being emptied directly into a bag attached to the outside of the body, may then be necessary. Sometimes the colostomy is done as a temporary measure to allow the irritated tissues to heal before attempting surgery. Certain special X-ray techniques, such as a barium enema, may be used to pinpoint the exact location of a fecal-vaginal fistula. If the fistula is a "high" one involving the intestines, it must be treated promptly, without the usual waiting period, since the contents of the intestines could be pouring into the vagina.

CONGENITAL ABNORMALITIES OF THE VAGINA

Types: absence, or atresia, of the vagina
         transverse vaginal septum
         double, or septate, vagina, or vaginal partitioning
         vaginal adenosis
         vaginal ridges

The middle and upper vagina are formed from two tubelike organs in the developing embryo called Mullerian ducts. The lower portion of the vagina develops from the same embryonic tissue as the bladder. Sometimes there are irregularities in the normal process whereby these embryonic tissues grow and fuse together to become properly functioning organs. Some of these irregularities in development of the vagina are related to more serious situations, where sexual characteristics of both sexes appear in the same individual. These are discussed under the heading Congenital Abnormalities of the Ovary.

Certain vaginal abnormalities may occur in women whose mothers took hormones during pregnancy. These hormones may produce congenital abnormalities such as vaginal adenosis, a condition in which gland cells are present in the vagina, and raised ridges of tissue appear on the vaginal wall. These are discussed more fully under the headings Vaginal Adenosis and DES.

Symptoms and Diagnosis

Atresia, the most extreme form of congenital vaginal abnormality, is the partial or total absence of the vagina. The external genital organs, the vulvar lips, clitoris and so forth, may be quite normal in appearance. Sometimes the lower part of the vaginal canal is present, but usually only as a very shallow depression. In typical cases of atresia, the uterus, the mid- and upper portions of the vagina and sometimes the Fallopian tubes are missing. The ovaries are often entirely normal. There may be some rudimentary development of the uterus, and in some very rare cases, the uterus is actually present and functioning, which means its lining swells and is shed each month, which is a source of trouble since there is no opening through which the menstrual discharge can escape.

Another type of abnormality of the vagina is called a transverse vaginal septum. In this condition, there is a septum, or a wall of tissue, that runs crosswise through the vagina, usually at the junction of the middle and upper third of the vagina, although it can occur at other points. The transverse vaginal septum may be confused with partial absence of the vagina because the doctor can easily mistake the wall of tissue for the roof of a partial vagina. Sometimes this wall of tissue will have openings in it through which the menstrual blood and vaginal and cervical discharges can pass; at other times it will be solid, with no openings through which these secretions can pass.

There is also the double, or septate, vagina, which usually occurs with a double uterus. A double vagina may also occur with entirely normal uterus and tubes. There may also be a double vagina, double cervix and single uterus. The septum that divides the double vagina is longitudinal (going up and down) as opposed to transverse (going across). It may be partial or it may extend all the way to the vaginal opening. In some cases the wall of tissue may be off-center and fused to one of the vaginal walls, so that one side of the divided vagina is closed off.

Congenital absence, transverse septums and double vaginas are sometimes recognized in infancy, but usually it is not until a girl menstruates or attempts intercourse that these problems become apparent. Sometimes, these abnormalities become apparent in strange ways. A young woman might come to the doctor wondering why tampons don't seem to control her menstrual flow and she has to wear sanitary napkins. Upon investigation the doctor may find that she has a double vagina and therefore the tampon, which has, of course, been inserted into only one vagina, hasn't absorbed all the menstrual flow.

If there is a transverse vaginal septum without any openings, the menstrual blood will continue to collect. A young girl may seek medical attention because she has never menstruated. She may be having periodic menstrual symptoms, cramps, headaches and so forth, but no blood, and this may lead her to seek medical help. Or, the buildup of menstrual blood may lead to a swelling and pain in the abdomen. Again, this may bring her to a doctor.

A double, or septate, vagina may cause pain on intercourse because the penis hits the wall of tissue that separates the double vagina. In the case of a transverse septum, the same kind of pain on intercourse can occur. Or, if a woman has a transverse septum or partial atresia with some sort of lower vaginal opening, she may come to the doctor complaining of pain and difficulty on intercourse because the penis cannot penetrate her vagina. Sometimes, though, the double vagina will be constructed in such a way that the woman can have intercourse. Then, the abnormality may not be discovered unless she has a child, when it will usually become apparent during labor and delivery.

If the double vagina is off-center and fused so that one portion of it is closed off, vaginal secretions and menstrual blood may collect on the closed-off side, resulting in swelling and pain and possibly an infection due to the retained menstrual blood. For a description of the problems related to the retention of menstrual blood, see the information on imperforate hymen under the heading Congenital Abnormalities of the Vulva.

Treatment

Treatment of a double vagina or transverse vaginal septum that is causing symptoms or problems in childbirth is rather simple but bloody, consisting of surgical removal of the barrier. If menstrual blood has been retained, the doctor will usually prescribe an antibiotic to prevent infection following the operation. It is important to drain all the old retained blood since it is a perfect breeding ground for germs. In some rare cases, the old blood will have backed up into the uterus and spilled out the tubes into the pelvic cavity, causing such pain and irritation that abdominal surgery is necessary to drain off all the old blood. There may be associated endometriosis, a condition in which the tissue that lines the uterus is found in abnormal locations.

If a child is discovered to have an absent or partially absent vagina, this is usually not treated right away. If the child has normal ovaries and uterus, then at puberty a vagina can be created by plastic surgery so that the menstrual blood will be able to escape. If the uterus is absent, the plastic surgery may be delayed until the woman wants to have it done for purposes of intercourse. Since there's no need to worry about a buildup of menstrual discharge and since the surgically created vagina must be kept open by frequent intercourse or manual dilation, it's best to wait until a woman does intend to have intercourse.

BENIGN TUMORS OF THE VAGINA

Types: inclusion cysts
   Gartner duct cysts
   endometrial cysts
   condyloma acuminatum, genital warts or venereal warts
   fibroids

Associated terms: vaginal polyps

There are a number of benign tumors that can affect the vagina. In medicalese the term "tumor," in its broadest sense, simply means "swelling." "Benign," of course, means "noncancerous."

Benign tumors of the vagina fall into one of two categories: cystic or solid. The most common cystic tumors are inclusion and Gartner duct cysts. Endometriosis, a condition that can create blood-filled cysts, may also affect the vagina. Similarly, condyloma acuminata, fibroids and vaginal adenosis may form tumors or swellings in the vagina. Some of these tumors may take the form of polyps—teardrop-shaped growths on a stem. These polyps may also be formed as the result of the body's attempts to heal itself (see the section on Cervical Polyps for details). Generally, the benign tumors that affect the vagina can be treated by simple surgical removal. Most of these benign vaginal tumors are discussed in more detail under other headings, so only the most common benign vaginal cysts will be discussed here.

Inclusion Cysts

These cysts are found at the lower end of the vagina. They are caused by the inclusion of little tags of skin beneath the surface of the skin, usually as the result of imperfect healing of surgical scars or of tears or lacerations acquired during childbirth or through injury. Occasionally such cysts may be found at the top of the vagina near a hysterectomy scar. They are usually small, only a few centimeters in size, and the contents are usually rather cheeselike. If they are causing problems, they may be removed surgically, but if they are small and are not bothersome, no treatment is required.

Gartner Duct Cysts

These cysts arise from the remnants of an embryonic organ called the Gartner duct. They are the most common form of vaginal tumor. They may be small or they may become so large as to bulge from the vaginal outlet. They are treated in the same manner as inclusion cysts.

VAGINAL ADENOSIS

Associated Terms: cockscomb, pseudopolypoid, rim, collar or hooded cervix

Vaginal adenosis is a condition in which the glandular tissue that normally lines the inside of the cervical canal is found in the vaginal cavity—on the vaginal walls and vaginal portion of the cervix. In a sense, it is an advanced degree of cervical eversion, a condition in which this glandular tissue is found on the vaginal portion of the cervix but not on the vaginal walls. Having vaginal adenosis would be like having the tissue that lines the inside of the mouth growing out onto the lips and the face. Although the tissue might be healthy, it would be abnormally placed.

Cause

Most cases of vaginal adenosis are associated with certain hormones taken during pregnancy by the mothers of the girls and women who have this condition. Beginning in 1940, the synthetic hormone DES and DES-type drugs were given to millions of pregnant women in this country to help prevent miscarriage, premature birth and other pregnancy problems. It has since been shown that these drugs were of no use in preventing miscarriage or premature deliveries.[11] By 1971 the tragic consequences of this widespread, ill-advised use of hormones became apparent when a small number of the daughters of these women developed a rare form of vaginal cancer, clear cell adenocarcinoma.[12] Further investigation indicated that other, less serious cervical, vaginal and uterine abnormalities were also more common among DES daughters, that DES sons may also have problems[13] and that the mothers themselves may be at increased risk for certain types of cancer.[14] The whole DES problem is discussed in greater detail under the heading DES; here we are concerned with only one type of of DES-related abnormality, vaginal adenosis.

Sometime during the first 20 weeks of pregnancy the female fetal tissue undergoes changes that are critical to the subsequent development of the upper vagina, cervix, Fallopian tubes and uterus. If all goes well, the mature woman will have a vagina and outer cervix that are covered by pink tissue known as squamous cell tissue. The inner cervical canal will be composed of red columnar tissue that contains mucus-producing glands. The point where these two tissues meet, known as the transformation zone, or the squamocolumnar junction, will lie in the area of the cervical os, the opening to the cervical canal. In women who have vaginal adenosis, this orderly arrangement of tissue types is disturbed. The squamocolumnar junction is not located at the cervical os. Thus the columnar-type tissue, with its gland cells, extends out over the vaginal portion of the cervix (as in a cervical eversion) and, in many cases, well into the vagina, where it does not belong. In this manner, then, glandular tissue appears in the vagina in women with vaginal adenosis. The condition becomes obvious in the years before and during puberty, when the abnormal tissue is stimulated to new growth by the rising levels of estrogen.

It now appears that the dosage of the hormone given to the person's mother need not have been prolonged or excessive for the abnormality to occur. Indeed, abnormalities have appeared with dosages as low as 1.5 mg. In one known instance the drug was given for only a few days.[15]

Incidence

Vaginal adenosis is not a new disease. Reports of it have appeared in the medical literature since the late 1800s. It can occur even when there is no history of the mother's having taken a DES-type drug, but it is rather uncommon.

Studies of the daughters of DES mothers show that anywhere from 30 to 90 percent of them will have adenosis.[16] The wide variance in these percentages may be at least partially accounted for by the fact that the mothers took the drug at different times in their pregnancies. One study showed incidence rates for adenosis of 73 percent in daughters who had been exposed during the first eight weeks of pregnancy and 7 percent in those exposed later than 17 weeks.[17] Adenosis seems to result only when the hormone is administered prior to the fourth month of pregnancy.

Symptoms

Vaginal adenosis usually does not produce any obvious symptoms. Some women, however, do have an increase in vaginal discharge or irregular bleeding and some report having pain on intercourse. The vaginal discharge may be scant or quite profuse. Adenosis tends to occur in young girls, in whom bleeding patterns are often quite irregular. Thus, in girls of this age group, the irregular bleeding caused by adenosis may be mistaken for this more usual sort of menstrual irregularity.

The vaginal walls or cervix may have red patches that may feel sandy or rough and may bleed easily when touched. There may be ridges of tissue across the vagina or a wall of tissue that partially or totally divides the vagina, a condition known as a septate vagina. Cysts formed in the improperly located glands may give a nodular or lumpy feeling to the vaginal walls.

The cervix also may appear abnormal. Cervical erosions or eversions may be present. There may be transverse ridges of tissue running across the cervix. The cervix often has an unusual appearance, for which a wide variety of terms, including "hooded," "cockscomb," pseudopolypoid," "rim" and "collar," have been coined.

Recent studies have shown that DES daughters may have other abnormalities. Cervical abnormalities that result in cervical incompetence, which in turn causes miscarriages between the 18th and 32nd week of pregnancy, have been noted in DES daughters.[18] Uterine abnormalities, in particular a shortened or "T-shaped" uterus, have been attributed to DES exposure and may also occur with adenosis.[19] The ultimate effect of the abnormalities on the fertility of these women is not yet known, but very recent studies suggest that DES daughters are more likely to have difficulty getting pregnant and carrying a pregnancy to full-term live delivery.[20]

Vaginal Adenosis and Cancer

The biggest concern about vaginal adenosis is its relationship to cancer. Indeed, the whole controversy about DES began in 1970 when an alert physician, Dr. Arthur Herbst and his colleagues, reported seven cases of a rare form of vaginal cancer, clear cell adenocarcinoma, in women 15-22 years of age.[21] Until this time there had been only three reported cases of this rare cancer in women under the age of 35. After a year of careful investigation, the linkup between DES exposure and the cancers were made. This led to the establishment of a world-wide tumor registry to which such cancers could be reported. Some 300-400 cases have been recorded thus far. The overwhelming majority of the young women who developed the disease also had vaginal adenosis.[22]

The cancer findings led to attempts to screen females who were known to have been, or thought to have been, exposed to DES. As mentioned earlier, a number of these DES daughters were then found to have vaginal adenosis. Not all DES daughters have vaginal adenosis. Of those who do, only a small percentage have thus far developed cancer. Most experts feel that the risk of developing cancer in women definitely known to have been exposed is around 1 in 1,000.[23] But, the accuracy of this estimate is questionable; the actual risk may be much higher or much lower.

Those who argue that the estimate is too low feel that we are just seeing the tip of the iceberg, and that as time passes we will be seeing more of this type of cancer. Those who say the estimate is too high point to the fact that the peak incidence of clear cell adenocarcinoma in DES daughters occurs around the age of 19, and after that it seems to taper off.

Other experts fear that DES daughters with adenosis may be at increased risk for developing not just this rare form of vaginal cancer, but also for developing the more common cervical cancer.[24] Part of their concern comes from the fact that most cancers of the cervix arise in the region of the squamocolumnar junction. The simple fact that in DES women with adenosis this junction is not confined to the area of the os, but may extend over the surface of the cervix and down into the vagina, means that there is a wider transformation zone and thus a wider surface area of tissue with a potential for the development of cancer. The least serious of these cervical cancers, carcinoma in situ, most commonly occurs in women in their 30s and 40s. Again, some experts feel that enough time may not yet have elapsed for us to see the whole iceberg.[25]

Alarming recent studies have indicated that DES exposed women may have a higher incidence rate (as much as a fivefold increase) of a condition known as cervical dysplasia, an abnormality of the cells of the cervix that is thought by most experts to be the first step in a series of changes that eventually leads to cervical cancer.[26] However, other researchers have disputed this finding of an increase in cervical dysplasia.[27] They argue that the cell changes seen in these DES daughters are not due to cervical dysplasia, but to a totally noncancerous process known as squamous metaplasia. Squamous metaplasia is actually a developmental process in which the more differentiated, more sophisticated, misplaced glandular tissue in the vaginal walls is being replaced by the less differentiated, less sophisticated, glandless squamous cell tissue that belongs in the vaginal cavity. In other words, the cell changes being labeled cervical dysplasia are not abnormal, precancerous changes but are actually cell changes occurring as a result of a natural developmental process. In short, the vaginal adenosis is being healed spontaneously. These doctors point to studies that have shown that in women over 30, 80 percent of the adenosis was replaced with squamous tissue. From these findings, they postulate that the majority of women with adenosis will go on to spontaneous resolution of the adenosis in their 30s. They feel that only a small percentage will develop true cervical dysplasia, carcinoma in situ of the cervix or invasive cervical cancer in this process. Let's hope that they are right. At any rate, studies now being done should yield important information on this topic. One way to keep abreast of the research being done in this area is to join DES Action (*see* p. 778) and to read their excellent newsletter.

Diagnosis and Follow-Up

Careful diagnosis and follow-up of DES-exposed women, especially those with adenosis, is vitally important. This crucial diagnosis and follow-up should be done by doctors experienced in DES exposure who have access to the special equipment that may be required. The diagnostic procedures and follow-up programs are discussed in detail under the heading DES.

Since it is not known how often vaginal adenosis will progress to cancer and since many cases may spontaneously resolve themselves without treatment, most experts feel that the best treatment is careful follow-up, unless, of course, cancerous or precancerous changes are found, in which case treatment for the cancer is indicated.

When the news of the relationship between DES exposure, adenosis and cancer first broke, some doctors performed a rather radical form of preventive surgery—removal of the vagina, with, if possible, plastic surgery to provide a functional vagina. This type of operation, a vaginectomy, is now considered far too radical a treatment by the vast majority of experts. Any woman whose doctor proposes this treatment for noncancerous adenosis should definitely seek another medical opinion.

Some doctors will cut, freeze (cryosurgery) or burn (electric cautery) away the area of adenosis, a process that may require hospitalization. Laser treatment to destroy affected areas has also been advocated. In some instances the doctor may do the tissue removal in the office, and if the areas of adenosis are extensive, this may be done in gradual stages so that adhesions and scar tissue will not form. While some well-respected physicians advocate this form of treatment—removal of the adenosis—there has been a great deal of debate about it. The majority of doctors consider it unnecessary, the rare exception being made for the woman who has severe discharge and severe pain on intercourse.

There is some indication that the jellies used with diaphragms, which help make the vagina more acid, may have a healing effect on the adenosis. In addition, the problem of increased vaginal discharge, which affects some 15 percent of DES daughters, seems to respond favorably to these products; thus, some doctors prescribe spermicides or similar products for their patients.

Birth control pills that contain estrogen have been prescribed for DES daughters both for contraceptive purposes and to control menstrual irregularities, but many doctors question the wisdom of giving estrogen in any form to either DES daughters or mothers.

The general consensus of medical opinion at this time seems to be that DES daughters don't require specific treatment beyond careful follow-up. What constitutes careful follow-up is debatable, however. This issue is also discussed under the heading DES.

CLEAR CELL ADENOCARCINOMA*

AKA: DES-related cancer

Clear cell adenocarcinoma is a rare disease. Prior to 1970, the few cases of vaginal clear cell adenocarcinoma that were found occurred primarily in postmenopausal women; however, since that time, somewhere between 300 and 400 cases of clear cell adenocarcinoma have been reported, the majority of them occurring in young women and girls in their teens.[28] The upsurge in the disease is related to a synthetic hormone, DES, that was given to pregnant women in this country from 1940 until 1971.[29] The daughters of these women are at risk of developing this rare form of cancer.

Cause, Symptoms and Diagnosis

The cause of the disease, the symptoms it produces and the methods of diagnosis have been discussed in the section on vaginal adenosis. Related information is discussed in the section on DES.

Treatment

The types of treatment available and the considerations involved in deciding which is the best type of therapy for clear cell adenocarcinoma are basically the same as those for other forms of vaginal cancer; however, the fact that it strikes young women and that it may, with careful follow-up of DES daughters, be found at an earlier stage than most vaginal cancers influences the choice of treatment.

Most other cases of vaginal cancer are treated by radiation therapy. However, for a number of reasons most experts prefer to use surgery to treat clear cell adenocarcinoma, which generally occurs in younger women. First of all, though we know that exposure to radiation can cause cancer as

*See also the general discussion of cancer and the discussion of vaginal cancer.

well as cure it, radiation-caused cancer takes many years to develop. For women in their 60s and 70s, the possibility that the radiation therapy may actually cause cancer in another ten or twenty years is not so much of a consideration. But, for the younger woman, this possibility is much more threatening, since she has an expected lifespan of another 50 years.

Moreover, although radiation is preferred in older women because their general poor health and associated diseases may either prevent surgery altogether or at least cause much higher complication rates, younger women, whose general health is usually better, can expect fewer complications. Another factor is that surgery, even extensive surgery, allows for preservation of the ovaries. Here again, since most cases of vaginal cancer occur in older, postmenopausal women, the destruction of the ovaries is not a significant factor. But in younger women, destruction of the ovaries leads to premature menopause, which carries certain risks. The preservation of the vagina is a factor as well. Radiation will leave the vagina intact, but most of the time radiation, especially external radiation, will result in a vagina that is so dry and constricted that sexual intercourse is painful or impossible. In surgery, the vagina, as well as the uterus, cervix, lymph nodes and surrounding tissue may be removed, but, it is possible to reconstruct the vagina using skin grafts and specialized surgical techniques that will allow for intercourse and orgasm. However, once radiation has been given, it is not possible to perform plastic surgery and create a functioning vagina.

Little if any attention has been given to sexual response in women following this type of surgery. The personal reports we have received from a few individual DES daughters indicate a range of sexual responses. The clitoris remains intact, and orgasm is reported by many. Others feel so demoralized and shaken by their experience and the surgery that they cannot bring themselves to relate sexually; others find sex is difficult, painful and unsatisfying after the surgery.

Effectiveness of surgery versus radiation is, of course, an important factor. The survival rate for the small number of patients who have been treated thus far is about 75 percent, regardless of whether radiation or surgery was used.[30] But not enough time has elapsed to accurately compare survival rates. Since the survival rates for surgery versus radiation as treatment of adenocarcinoma are thus far the same, surgery, which allows for the creation of a functioning vagina as well as ovarian preservation, and doesn't involve long-term radiation risks, is the treatment of choice in most experts' minds.* However, as more time passes, this may change.

*For further information on therapy, see Note 31 in the references that appear at the end of the section on vaginal diseases.

The choices are difficult ones, and it may be some time before more information about the best treatment is available. Women who have clear cell adenocarcinoma of the cervix should be treated by experts and should have opinions from doctors who favor radiation as well as from those who favor surgery. One way to contact experts in the field is through the DESAD projects set up by the National Cancer Institute to monitor women exposed to DES-type drugs. They are listed in Table 27 (*see* p. 772). DES Action (*see* p. 778), a national organization of people concerned about DES, is also an excellent source of medical information.

CANCER OF THE VAGINA*

AKA: carcinoma of the vagina

Types: squamous cell cancer
adenocarcinoma
sarcoma
melanoma
sarcoma botryoides

Cancer of the vagina may originate in the vagina itself or it may appear as the result of direct extension of cancer of the adjacent organs, such as the cervix, vulva or uterus. It may also appear as the result of metastasis (spread) from a tumor growing at a distant site in the body. Sometimes, it is hard to tell whether the cancer is primary—originating in the vagina—or secondary—the result of direct invasion of metastases. We are concerned mainly with primary cancer in the following discussion.

Types

Most vaginal cancers are squamous cell cancers, arising from the squamous cell tissues of the vaginal walls. Occasionally, adenocarcinomas, cancer arising from gland tissue, will occur in the vagina. When these rare adenocarcinomas appear in young women, there is usually a history of their mothers' having taken synthetic hormones, like DES, during pregnancy. This unusual form of vaginal cancer is discussed under the heading Clear Cell Adenocarcinoma of the Vagina. Other rare forms of vaginal cancer include sarcoma, melanoma and sarcoma botryoides, which unlike other forms of vaginal cancer, usually affects children.

*Anyone reading this section should first read the general discussion of cancer and cancer terminology.

315

Incidence and Risk Factors

Primary vaginal cancer is a rare form of cancer accounting for only 1-2 percent of all female genital cancers.[32] It is estimated that for every case of vaginal cancer, there are 45 cases of cervical cancer and 3 cases of vulvar cancer.

Vaginal cancer is usually a disease of older women. Approximately 70 percent of the cases occur in women more than 50 years of age. The peak incidence occurs in women between the ages of 60 and 70; however, the disease has been reported in younger women, and even in infancy.[33] As noted above, a certain form of vaginal cancer related to DES exposure occurs in young women (7-29 years of age).

Risk factors such as those associated with cervical or breast cancer have not proven significant in vaginal cancer. Ethnic background, previous pregnancies and childbirth, marital status, sexual history, family history and genetic factors appear to be unimportant.

Cause

The cause of vaginal cancer, like the cause of all forms of cancer, is unknown.

Symptoms

Vaginal cancer may not produce any symptoms, especially in the early stages. Indeed, approximately 5 to 10 percent of those women diagnosed as having vaginal cancer, even some with cancer in advanced stages, are entirely asymptomatic.[34] When symptoms do occur, they may be so slight that they are hardly noticed. If symptoms do occur, the three most common ones are vaginal bleeding, vaginal discharge and pain.

The bleeding may take the form of slight bleeding or staining, prolonged or profuse menstrual periods, contact-type bleeding, or spotting, such as after intercourse or douching. About 60 percent of the women diagnosed as having vaginal cancer will have a history of one of these types of painless vaginal bleeding.

There may be an increase in vaginal discharge. It may be watery, brownish in color and may cause itching. About 20 percent of the women with vaginal cancer will have this symptom, either with or without the vaginal bleeding.[35]

Bladder pain, pain on urination and frequent need to urinate may be symptoms in the early stage but are more common in the later stages of the disease. Vaginal pain, pressure in the rectum, pain on moving the bowels and constipation may also occur. About 5 percent of women with the disease will first come to the doctor with symptoms of pain.[36] As the disease progresses and spreads to the bladder and rectum, pain and irregularities in bowel movements and urination are more common. Fistulas, openings or holes connecting the vagina and the bladder and/or rectum, are frequent complications.

A visible tumor or open sore can sometimes be seen on speculum exam, but usually only in the late stages of the disease. A lump or hardened area can sometimes be felt on the vaginal walls. The lymph nodes in the area may become swollen.

Diagnosis

Unfortunately, bothersome symptoms often fail to appear until the disease is fairly well advanced. Even though there may be symptoms of discharge, itching and bleeding, they are often not severe enough to cause the woman to seek medical help. Since the disease most often occurs in women who are no longer menstruating, the symptoms of bleeding between periods or prolonged, profuse menstrual periods are not relevant clues for most women who have this disease. All such women may notice is a slight staining after intercourse or douching. The doctor, too, is often to blame for the lack of prompt diagnosis. Since symptoms like itching or vaginal discharge are not uncommon in women in this age group and are more often caused by postmenopausal vaginitis, too often doctors prescribe for these symptoms over the telephone or without giving the woman a thorough examination. Women should insist on a complete physical and gynecological exam and not accept a telephone diagnosis or cursory examination.

Sometimes a routine Pap smear will detect vaginal cancer, but it is not as useful a tool in screening for vaginal cancer as it is in cervical cancer, for the usual Pap smear does not take cell samples from the entire vaginal cavity. A special four-quadrant Pap smear, which takes cell samples from the vaginal walls, may be done to detect vaginal cancer, but since this involves a considerably more involved laboratory analysis, this test is not done in routine examinations.

Determining the stage of the disease involves a careful bimanual pelvic exam and palpation (feeling) of the vagina, which may be done under a general anesthetic so that the woman is totally relaxed, allowing the doctor to feel the vaginal walls and pelvic area thoroughly. Generous biopsy specimens are taken from areas that appear suspicious when stained with a special dye. The vagina may be examined with a special magnifying instrument called a colposcope. Biopsy specimens may be taken from the cervix as well. In some cases, a cervical biopsy will be done to eliminate the possibility of cervical cancer. Such biopsies are done by conization, a process in which a central core of tissue is removed from the cervix. Endometrial biopsies or even a D&C may be done to eliminate the possibility of uterine cancer.

Cystourethroscopy, a procedure in which a special viewing instrument is used to examine the urinary tract, and proctosigmoidoscopy, a procedure in which a viewing instrument is used to examine the rectum, will usually be done while the woman is under anesthesia so that the doctor can decide about the possibility of bladder or rectal involvement and can stage the disease more accurately. In addition, other standard tests to assess local invasion and distant spread of the disease are done. The lymph nodes in the area are carefully felt, and suspicious ones are biopsied during surgery to determine whether or not they need to be treated.

Staging

Vaginal cancer can range from precancerous cell abnormalities called dysplasia to frankly invasive cancer that has spread to the lymph nodes, adjacent organs like the rectum and bladder or distant organs.

Because vaginal cancer is a rare disease, a clear-cut classification scheme on which to base treatment and compare the results of various therapies has been difficult to establish; however, the staging system outlined in Table 7 is now widely used.[37]

Table 7
Clinical Staging Scheme for Vaginal Cancer

Stage O:	Carcinoma in situ ("cancer that is in place") or intraepithelial carcinoma; cancer in which cancerous-type cells are present, but in which there is no evidence, microscopic or otherwise, to indicate invasion.
Stage I:	The cancer is limited to the vaginal wall.
Stage II:	The cancer has invaded the subvaginal tissues, but has not extended to the pelvic wall.
Stage III:	The cancer has extended to the pelvic wall.
Stage IVA:	The bladder and/or rectum is involved.
Stage IVB:	The cancer has spread beyond the pelvis, that is, there are distant metastases, or spread of the cancer to distant organs.

Treatment

The treatment of vaginal cancer is complicated by the fact that the vagina is located between the bladder and rectum. Since the bladder and rectum are extremely sensitive to radiation, massive doses of X-ray cannot be given. The fact that there is only a thin wall of tissue separating the organs means that surgical removal of the cancer along with adequate margins (cancer-free areas) of adjacent tissue may not be possible.

Treatment may be given by radiation, surgery or a combination of the two. A comparison of surgery and radiation therapy brings out some important differences. Except for a few instances when there are superficial cancers or small tumors in the upper vagina, or in certain cases of recurrent cancer, the surgery that must be done is quite extensive, requiring pelvic exenteration, an operation in which the uterus, tubes, ovaries, vagina, bladder and/or rectum are removed and urinary and/or bowel wastes are collected in plastic bags attached to the outside of the body. The age and physical condition of most women who have vaginal cancer and the loss of these organs makes this surgery impractical in many cases. Although serious complications may result from radiation therapy, it generally offers less overall risk and a better chance of preserving bladder, rectal and vaginal function.

Radiation Therapy

The great majority of women will be treated by radiation. Radiation is often effective in this area, for it can be administered through the vagina, which makes possible direct contact with the tumor, without having to pass through normal tissue to get at it.[38]

The radiation may be administered in a number of ways, depending upon the size of the tumor, its location and the extent of the spread:

- ☐ Radioactive implants, either in the form of intracavity implants—radiation sources placed in the vagina and possibly the uterus as well, for specified amounts of time—or interstitial radiation—needles filled with radioactive substances that are inserted directly into the tumor;
- ☐ External beam therapy—X-ray beams directed toward the vagina from outside the body; and
- ☐ Transvaginal cone therapy—an X-ray beam directed into the vagina.

When the cancer is located in the upper third of the vagina, the treatment plan closely resembles that used for cervical cancer. If the invasion of the vaginal tissue is less than one cm in depth, a single dose, applied by inserting the source of radiation into the vagina, may be all that is required. If it is deeper, external beam therapy is also required.

319

In most Stage I and II cases, both external beam therapy and internal radiation are used. External beam therapy is usually given first. This will shrink the vaginal tumor and make it more receptive to subsequent internal radiation. It is hoped that it will also succeed in killing any cancer that has spread beyond the vagina into the surrounding tissues and lymph nodes. External beam therapy that succeeds in shrinking the tumor is usually followed by implants in the vagina and the uterus. In some cases, particularly if the tumor has not been sufficiently reduced by the external beam therapy or has widely spread into the immediately adjacent tissues, interstitial radiation via needles may be used instead of intracavity implants.

If the cancer is located near the vaginal opening, external beam therapy will probably not be used because the vulva would also be radiated and vulvar tissues are easily destroyed by radiation. Instead, interstitial radiation or transvaginal cone therapy is generally used for early stage cancers in this location.

In Stage III, external therapy is more important, for the external beam can reach a wider area than the implants or needles, which are designed primarily to kill the central tumor and are not as effective in killing the cancer that has spread beyond the vagina into surrounding tissues and into the lymph nodes. Thus, a large external dose is given to the whole pelvic area over a period of weeks. This may be followed by lower external doses given directly over the tumor area or by interstitial radiation via needles planted directly in the tumor area.

Stage IV therapy is similar to Stage III; however, in cases where the rectum and/or bladder are bound by adhesions to the vagina or where the disease is too widespread for any hope of cure, lower doses of radiation are given in hopes of providing palliation, or relief of symptoms. Although the dose is not high enough to kill all the cancer cells, it may reduce the pain, lessen the discharge and help stop the bleeding. The dose is low enough to avoid radiation damage to the radiation-sensitive bladder and rectum.

Surgery

Sometimes surgery is used to treat vaginal cancer, either alone as primary treatment or in combination with radiation. If vaginal cancer recurs after a full course of radiation, surgery, usually pelvic exenteration, rather than reirradiation offers the best chance of a cure. In certain Stage IV cases where the vagina is bound by adhesions to the bladder and/or rectum, so that it is impossible to give high enough doses of radiation to kill all the cancer without undue damage to these organs, radical surgery—pelvic exenteration—sometimes in conjunction with lower-dose external beam therapy, may remove the central cancer and may be worth the risks involved and the unpleasant after-effects (the plastic bags for bodily wastes). This is one of those instances in which more than one medical opinion is of critical importance.

Other instances in which surgery might be used include small Stage I cancers (ones confined to the vaginal wall), Stage O cancers (carcinoma in situ) and certain Stage II cancers in which the tumor is in the upper third of the vagina. For small Stage I cancers, surgery can be as effective as radiation. If a Stage O or Stage I cancer is found after previous radiation treatment for cervical or uterine cancer, surgery rather than more irradiation is done. Surgery in these cases would include a radical hysterectomy, removal of the pelvic lymph nodes and total or partial vaginectomy (if the cancer is in only the upper third). If there hasn't been previous radiation treatment for cancer, some doctors prefer surgery in such cases, while others prefer radiation. Women should hear opinions from both sides, and here again, a team approach to treating cancer is of utmost importance.

Stage O

In the past few years, treatment of Stage O, carcinoma in situ, that is, cancer that is locally confined, has been reappraised because of evidence that the disease grows slowly and because it usually occurs in younger women in whom the sexual function is considered to be more important.*
Radical forms of surgery and extensive radiation both destroy the vagina, so less radical surgery and less extensive radiation are now used.

Cryosurgery, removal of the cancerous areas by freezing, or removal by excision (cutting away) have been tried.[39] Cryosurgery results appear to be good. There is none of the scarring or contracting of the vagina, a condition known as vaginal stenosis, that can occur with radiation or with surgery. However, these methods should not be used unless a staining and biopsy of suspicious areas have been done with the aid of a colposcope. A "blind" biopsy, one done without the aid of the colposcope, is not sufficient if cryosurgery or local incision is planned. The danger in this more conservative therapy lies in the fact that vaginal cancer tends to be multicentric—to have more than one point of origin. Other areas of cancer might exist that are not yet advanced enough to be recognized. The doctor must be satisfied that the cancer is clearly in situ (in place) and not invasive before these less radical methods can be attempted.

So far, treatment via cryosurgery seems to be quite effective; however, such cases have been followed for only about three years. More time is needed before the results can be accurately judged.

*This is not to say that preserving sexual function is not important to older women, just that the medical profession recognizes it to be more important in younger women.

Laser beam therapy has also been used in the treatment of Stage O cancer.[40] With laser therapy there is not the same degree of mutilating scar formation that there is with radiation therapy, and injury to the bladder and rectum can be avoided. Thus it is regarded by some as superior to radiation therapy as well as to cryosurgery or local incision for the treatment of this stage of cancer. Although several institutions are experimenting with laser surgery, the technique is not widely available. Too few cases have been followed for too short a period of time for an accurate assessment of its effectiveness.

Treatment of vaginal cancer must be highly individualized according to the size, type and location of the cancer, the age of the woman and the importance she attaches to preserving a functioning vagina. The basic principles in treatment have been outlined here, but these principles must be adapted to meet the specific situation. A doctor may recommend a treatment plan different from the ones outlined here, perhaps because of the particulars of the case or because new information has become available since the time of this writing. However, the material outlined here covers the usual therapy plans. If the doctor disagrees, the woman has the right to have his or her reasoning explained in language she can understand. She also has the right to seek other medical opinions (*see* page 226). Because of the rarity of vaginal cancer, it is especially important that women with this condition find specialists who have had experience with this particular form of cancer.

Chemotherapy

Experiments with chemotherapy have not produced any increase in survival rates. Any relief of symptoms provided by chemotherapy has unfortunately brought considerable risk to the patient. The dosage, in order to be effective, is too close to the lethal dose, and the side effects have so far negated any benefits obtained. However, new approaches to chemotherapy are constantly being developed, so at some time in the future, chemotherapy may become an important part of the treatment program.[41]

Survival Rates

Survival rates, of course, vary with the stage of the disease. Table 8 lists, stage by stage, the range of five-year survival rates reported for vaginal cancer treated by radiation.

Table 8
Five-Year Survival Rates for Vaginal Cancers Treated by Radiation*

Stage	Percent
I	69-83
II	41-68
III	27-40
IV	0-14
Overall	46-52

*SOURCE: Data for this table were condensed from survival data from three separate institutions: A. M. Anderson Hospital, Washington University and the University of Maryland. See Robert D. Hilgers, M. D., "Squamous Cell Carcinoma of the Vagina," *Surgical Clinics of North America*, vol. 58 (Feb. 1978), pp. 25-38.

The Cervix

The anatomy of the cervix is described in Chapter Two, and details about how it functions at various points in the menstrual cycle are discussed in Chapter Four. But in order to understand the disease processes that can take place in the cervix, it is necessary to understand the cellular makeup of this organ. The external portion of the cervix, the part that protrudes into the vaginal cavity, is covered by pink tissue known as squamous cell epithelium. The cervical canal, which leads into the uterus, is lined with red, columnar epithelium, which contains mucus-secreting glands. Normally, the squamous cell tissue and the columnar tissue meet at the cervical os, the opening to the cervical canal. The area where these two types of epithelial tissue meet is called the transformation zone, or the squamocolumnar junction.

Sometimes these two tissues do not meet at the cervical os. If the cervical canal becomes infected—a condition known as cervicitis—the columnar tissue may swell and protrude out of the cervical canal onto the vaginal portion of the cervix. This is known as cervical eversion and is discussed under the second heading in this section, along with cervical erosion, a condition in which the pink squamous tissue is eroded away by sores.

At other times, tears or injuries to the cervix can cause cervical eversion, and this is discussed under the heading Cervical Lacerations. About 20 percent of women are born with cervical eversions in which the squamous and columnar tissue meet somewhere other than the opening of the cervical os. This does not usually cause any problems; however, some women with congenital cervical eversion have the condition because their mothers took a synthetic hormone, such as DES during their pregnancy. This is discussed under the heading Congenital Abnormalities of the Cervix.

In addition to these disturbances in the normal cellular makeup of the cervix, the squamocolumnar junction may also be the site of more serious problems. Cancerous and precancerous conditions of the cervix often arise in the area of the squamocolumnar junction. Luckily, this junction is readily accessible, and a simple screening test known as the Pap smear, whereby cells from the cervix are collected and studied microscopically, can detect cancerous and precancerous conditions in their earliest stages. Every woman should have regular Pap smears.

Along with the conditions discussed above, this section also includes information on cervical cysts and cervical polyps, both of which may follow a case of cervicitis. Cervical stenosis, a blockage of the cervical canal that can be caused by cervical infections or other problems, is also discussed in the following pages. A description of a condition known as cervical incompetence, in which the cervix dilates prematurely during pregnancy, is also included.

CERVICITIS

AKA: inflammations of the cervix or cervical canal

Types: acute cervicitis
chronic cervicitis
endocervicitis

"Cervicitis" is the term used to describe a variety of inflammations of the cervix. The condition may be acute or chronic and may be caused in a variety of ways. In most cases it is associated with other, more general infections of the vaginal cavity or the female organs. For instance, pelvic inflammatory disease, especially when it involves the Fallopian tubes, is often accompanied by cervicitis. Any of the common vaginal infections can involve the cervix. Acute and chronic gonorrhea, as well as many of the other sexually transmitted diseases, can also affect the cervix. In some cases, however, only the cervix is affected, without involving the vagina or other pelvic organs.

Some authorities feel that many cases of cervicitis are the result of infections caused by tears or lacerations to the cervix, which can occur during childbirth. Other authorities feel that such injuries are only rarely associated with cervicitis. This confusion stems from the fact that after such injuries, the cervix may heal in such a way that it looks red, raw and irritated. But this irritated appearance may not be due to infection at all, but to the simple fact that on soft internal tissues like the cervix, scar tissue tends to have this unusual appearance. Some doctors upon seeing such scar tissue will do a culture or wet smear, find bacteria present and decide that a woman has a case of cervicitis. However, the bacteria found in many such instances are normal inhabitants of the vaginal cavity. Their presence does not necessarily mean that disease is present.

If such doctors also see what they consider to be an abnormal amount of cervical discharge, they consider this further evidence of infection. However, as any woman who practices regular self-exam knows, the amount and character of cervical discharge varies, depending on the phase of the menstrual cycle. It also varies from individual to individual. Thus a doctor who sees scar tissue from a cervical laceration that gives the impression of infection; what appears to be an abnormal amount of discharge (even though, in fact, for that woman, in that particular phase of her cycle, it may be quite normal); and test results showing bacteria—may decide that this is a case of cervicitis that needs treatment. Other doctors, aware of these confusions, do not consider such women to have cervicitis unless they complain of an unusual discharge.

In most bona-fide cases of cervicitis, when the external, vaginal part of the cervix is involved, the cervical canal—the passageway between the vaginal cavity and the uterus—is usually also infected. Sometimes, though, the cervical canal will be inflamed without any obvious problems on the external, vaginal portion of the canal, and this is known as endocervicitis.

Symptoms of Acute Cervicitis

The disease may be either acute or chronic. The chief symptom of acute cervicitis is a discharge from the cervical os. It may be quite abundant and pus-filled and may vary in color from clear to grayish, white or even yellow, depending on the type of infection. If the infection is due to gonoccocus, the cervical discharge is apt to be quite profuse, and usually the urinary tract, the Skene's glands and/or Bartholin's glands are also infected. If these other organs are involved, there may also be associated symptoms like urinary frequency and urgency and pain. If the cervicitis is associated with one of the common vaginal infections, the discharge is also apt to be quite profuse, and there may be burning and itching of the external genitals. On those rather rare occasions when the cervicitis is actually associated with lacerations and injury, and the only bacteria found are the normal vaginal inhabitants, the discharge is less heavy and irritation to the external genitals is likely to be minimal or altogether absent. Sometimes acute cervicitis will produce general systemic symptoms, such as fever, as a result of the white cells in the body attempting to fight off the infection, but this is not usually the case.

In acute cervicitis, the cervix may look quite abnormal. It may be quite swollen, with red, irritated-looking areas. If the cervicitis is associated with a vaginal infection or sexually transmitted disease, there may be other symptoms associated with these diseases. A syphilis chancre, for instance, may be present. In the case of trichomoniasis, the characteristic strawberrylike patches may cover the cervix. If moniliasis is the culprit, the cervix may be whitish in color. There may be a reddish ring or halo around the cervical opening or red sores on the surface of the cervix. These are called cervical erosions or eversions and may be associated with chronic cervicitis as well (see below).

Treatment of Acute Cervicitis

Since cervicitis may be caused by a number of different organisms, treatment will depend on identifying the specific organism and selecting an appropriate antibiotic or sulfa drug. Cauterizing (destroying the infected tissue by chemical or electrical means) or cryosurgery (destroying the tissue by freezing) should never be done in the case of acute cervicitis, for this could cause the disease to spread to other organs.

Care must be taken to keep the area clean so that the infection won't spread. Intercourse is prohibited. If the infection is severe and there are general systemic reactions such as fever or urinary problems, these should be treated as well and the woman should be confined to bed with plenty of fluids to drink.

Symptoms of Chronic Cervicitis

Acute cervicitis can become chronic. This frequently happens when the infecting organism is gonorrhea. It may not even be possible to detect any gonococci in a smear or culture, and such a woman may be an asymptomatic carrier of the disease. Chronic cervicitis may also be associated with lacerations or injuries caused during abortion, rape, childbirth or surgery. Here again, it may not be possible to detect any specific bacteria other than the normal vaginal bacteria. In such cases, cervicitis should be treated only when the woman herself feels that there is an abnormal discharge.

Chronic cervicitis doesn't look as extreme as acute cervicitis and does not look the same in all cases. In some instances, the cervix may appear to be quite normal on its vaginal surface, but the cervical canal is thickened and produces a whitish pus. Sometimes the entire cervix will become quite swollen and barrel-shaped.

In other cases the top layers of the tissues of the cervix have eroded away due to the irritation of the discharge. There will be a reddish area or sores, called erosions, around the os, just as in acute cervicitis. At times, these reddish areas will be slightly raised, with tiny nipplelike protrusions, and this is known as papillary cervical erosion.

If the chronic cervicitis is associated with lacerations due to injury during childbirth or, as is much more likely, due to an abortion, the cervix is likely to be quite swollen. Under such conditions, the infected and swollen mucous membrane lining of the canal often rolls out, much like the lining of a sleeve that is too long for the outer cloth. This is known as cervical eversion. The area around the os is quite red and angry-looking and is apt to be thicker and to cover a wider area than an erosion. Like an erosion, this sort of eversion may bleed easily upon the slightest contact.

In an attempt to heal and repair itself, the surrounding tissue proliferates and attempts to grow over the eroded or everted areas. In the course of this natural repair, the mucus glands in the inflamed tissue may be pinched off, forming Nabothian cysts. In other cases the overgrowth of the repair process may lead to the formation of teardrop-shaped growths known as cervical polyps.

In addition to these changes in the cervix, chronic cervicitis also produces a thick, gelatinlike, mucus discharge that may have quite a bit of pus in it and may be whitish or yellow in color. Often a mucus plug fills the cervical os and is difficult to dislodge.

There is apt to be a slight, irregular staining-type of contact bleeding, especially when polyps, erosions or eversions are present. There may be pain on intercourse if the penis pushes against the tense, rigid cervix. Backache is a common complaint because the disease-fighting lymph system for the cervix drains back along the rear supporting ligaments that hold the uterus in place, which may also explain the sense of pelvic heaviness that many women report. Urinary symptoms are not uncommon, since the bladder is so close by. Many cases of "honeymoon bladder" are probably the result of vigorous intercourse that has stirred up a low-grade infection in the cervix and bladder. Any attempt to treat the bladder problem without treating the cervix is unlikely to succeed.

Cervical infections have also been implicated in fertility problems. A thick discharge from an irritated cervix may affect the sperm or block its passage through the cervical canal. Long-standing cervical infection may affect the monthly ferning pattern of the cervical mucus (*see* p. 66), which creates pathways that aid the sperm in its passage to the uterus, thereby making conception impossible. The polyps associated with cervicitis may also cause problems with fertility if they mechanically block the passage of the sperm.

Diagnosis

Diagnosis of cervicitis will depend on a history of previous disease or injury, the presence of an irritating discharge and the particular appearance of the cervix. Cultures and wet smears must be done to identify the organism causing the cervicitis. Pap smears and biopsies may be in order to eliminate the possibility of cancer since the appearance of the cervix and the symptoms of cervicitis may mimic cervical cancer.

Treatment

Although antibiotics and sulfa drugs may be tried, they are often not successful in cases of chronic cervicitis. In such cases, then, the infected tissues must be destroyed by either electric cautery or, preferably, by cryosurgery. Cryosurgery is more comfortable and has fewer complications. Unfortunately, not all doctors have the equipment or skill to perform cryosurgery.

CERVICAL EROSION AND CERVICAL EVERSION

AKA: ectropion

Associated terms: congenital erosion, congenital eversion

Erosion and eversion (Illustration 42) are terms used to describe certain conditions of the cervix. The term "ectropion" is sometimes used instead of "eversion." There is a great deal of confusion about the terms and some medical writers use them differently. As if that weren't enough confusion, there is also a great deal of controversy about what causes these conditions, whether or not they need treatment and, if so, what exactly constitutes the proper treatment.

In the case of an eversion, the columnar tissue that lines the cervical canal is pushed to the outer, vaginal portion of the cervix. Just as the lining of a sleeve that is too long will hang out beyond the edge of the sleeve, so the angry-looking red columnar tissue will protrude beyond the os. There will usually be a ringlike shape to the eversion, or it at least seems to follow the contours of the os. Some women are born with this trait, in which case

329

Illustration 42   *Cervical Eversion (A) and Cervical Erosion (B)*

the term "congenital eversion" is used. Some writers use the term "congenital erosion" even though it is an eversion they are actually talking about. An infection of the cervical canal, endocervicitis, can also cause the swollen, irritated columnar tissue to pout out of the os, particularly when there are tears or lacerations of the cervix due to childbirth, abortion, rape or injury.

An erosion, as the name implies, means that some of the cells on the surface of the os have been worn away and the raw surface of the cervix exposed, just as happens when there is a graze on the skin of the outside of the body. Such sores look like dark pink or red spots on the cervix. It is estimated that about 95 percent of all women will have an erosion on the cervix sometime in their lives. An erosion may be associated with a white discharge that may have an unpleasant odor. If the erosion is infected, there may be a slightly blood-tinged discharge. Sometimes, especially in the case of cervicitis, the erosion too may seem to have a ring shape, forming a soft halo of redness around the os, and it may be mistaken for an eversion. At other times the erosion looks more like a separate little sore or graze on the skin and there is not a definite border between the redness and the normal pink tissue.

Causes

Some doctors believe that the Pill and the IUD string, as well as cervicitis, can cause these two conditions, but other doctors dispute this. It is thought that intercourse may also be a factor in erosions. Some women are born with eversions. Recently, it has been discovered that women whose mothers took certain hormones (see the section on DES) during pregnancy are apt to have congenital eversions. Using a natural sponge instead of a tampon during their periods has helped some women get rid of their erosions.*

Erosions and eversions don't usually produce much in the way of symptoms unless there is an associated infection. Then there may be contact-type bleeding during intercourse, speculum exam, or douching or even upon straining when going to the bathroom.

Diagnosis

Erosions and eversions are usually found on speculum examination. They can be quite scary-looking, because they alter the usual pink, healthy appearance of the cervix. The doctor should take a Pap smear to make sure that the process is a simple erosion or eversion and not something more serious, like cervical cancer.

Treatment

Some doctors treat erosions and eversions with drugs; however, unless there is an infection, such treatment doesn't really affect these conditions. Other doctors will destroy the eroded, everted tissue by means of electric cautery or by freezing the tissue off with cryosurgery. This too is of questionable value. Some doctors justify the expense, inconvenience and discomfort of such treatment by saying that they fear that erosions and eversions are related to cervical cancer. While it is true that cervical cancer often arises in conjunction with erosions, and less frequently with eversions, it is also true that the overwhelming majority of women with erosions and eversions never get cancer. It is our opinion, then, that any suspicious-looking sore or reddened area on the cervix should be examined by Pap smear and, possibly, a cervical biopsy. If such areas turn out to be benign, no treatment is needed.

CERVICAL POLYPS

AKA: growths in the cervical canal

Types: decidual polyps

Polyps (Illustration 43) are small protrusions that grow from a mucous membrane. Cervical polyps are tubular or tear-shaped growths with little

---

*Natural sponges may also cause problems; see the section on Toxic Shock Syndrome for details.

Illustration 43   *Cervical Polyp*

stems that grow from the mucous membranes of the cervical canal. In rare instances they may grow from the surface of the vaginal part of the cervix. Although polyps are abnormal growths, they are benign. Only in rare instances is cancer found in a polyp.

Causes

Cervical polyps are often the result of the body's attempt to heal itself after an infection of the cervix. The tissue around the infected area proliferates, growing new cells in an attempt to heal and cover over the raw, inflamed tissue. Sometimes the tissue may become so overgrown that clumps of excess tissue—polyps—are formed. In some cases the tissue irritates the cervical canal, which contracts in an effort to rid itself of the clumps of tissue. Thus, the tissue gets dislodged from its primary position and a stem, called a pedicule, is formed, with a tubular or tear-shaped clump of tissue at its end.

Polyps may also be formed during pregnancy, when hormonal excess provides too much stimulation and provokes a similar overgrowth of tissue. They are also found more frequently in women who take birth control pills.

Symptoms

Polyps are usually bright pink or red in color and somewhat spongy in texture; however, the rare varieties that grow on the vaginal portion of the cervix tend to be firmer and paler in color. They can occur singly or multiply and with speculum exam may be seen peeping through the cervical os. Generally, they are rather small, although they can grow to become as thick as a little finger and may become so elongated that they can be seen protruding from the opening of the vagina.

When they are small, they often don't cause symptoms; however, the larger ones, as a rule, usually do. The tip of the polyp may be subject to injury because of its exposed position and may therefore bleed on contact. Intercourse, douching, speculum examination, straining when going to the bathroom and the like may cause staining between periods or, in the case of larger polyps, more prolonged and heavier bleeding.

Pain is not usually associated with cervical polyps. The polyp may crowd the cervical canal, blocking it off so that sperm cannot pass through, thereby causing an infertility problem. Polyps may also be associated with an increase in mucus discharge from the cervix, perhaps because of irritation to the glands, perhaps because of associated infection. This too may affect fertility.

Diagnosis

In the rare instances in which polyps grow from the surface of the vaginal portion of the cervix, they are usually associated with sores called cervical erosions, which are described above. Sometimes the bleeding symptoms will lead a woman to seek medical care, but at other times the polyps are discovered only in the course of a routine physical exam. The doctor may feel them by manual exam or see them during speculum exam. The only real problem in diagnosis is that they may look like certain forms of cervical cancer and produce similar symptoms. A Pap smear and biopsy will determine the difference.

Treatment

The treatment of polyps is usually fairly easy and consists of removing them. Most of the time, this can be done in a doctor's office under a local anesthetic. The doctor twists off the polyp at its stem and may touch the base with an electric cautery point. The removed polyp is examined microscopically to rule out the possibility of cancer.

It is particularly important to remove the polyp right down to the base. Only rarely does cervical cancer appear in a polyp, but on those rare occasions when it does, the base is often involved. So the doctor must be sure that the polyp can be removed at the base before an office procedure is attempted.

Some polyps are too thick to remove in the office because of the danger of excessive bleeding. Likewise, if the polyps are multiple and the cervical canal is crowded, hospitalization might be required.

Polyps tend to reoccur, and if another polyp or significant bleeding occurs after initial treatment, the second attempt at treatment should be a dilation and curettage (D&C), done in a hospital. It should be mentioned that decidual polyps, overgrowths of the decidua (which is part of the rich lining of the pregnant uterus), are usually not treated during pregnancy, but are left alone because of the danger of excessive bleeding.

NABOTHIAN CYSTS

AKA: cysts on the cervix

Associated Terms: squamous metaplasia, epidermidalization

Nabothian cysts (Illustration 44) are cysts of the mucus-producing glands that are located in the cervical canal.

Causes

Most of the time the cysts are the result of natural healing processes known as squamous cell metaplasia or epidermidalization. As explained in the introduction of this section, the outside of the cervix is normally covered by squamous cell tissue, which is pinkish in color, while the inside

Illustration 44   *Nabothian Cysts*

of the cervical canal is lined with red, somewhat angry-looking tissue that contains mucus-producing glands and is known as columnar tissue. In most women, these two tissues meet at the cervical os, the opening of the cervical canal. In cases of chronic cervicitis, the squamous cell tissue attempts to grow over and cover up the raw, irritated areas of the infected cervix. In the process, the squamous cell tissue may pinch off the mucus-producing glands either by growing beyond its normal limits and into the cervical canal or because the glandular tissue itself is located beyond its normal boundary at the os and is growing on the surface of the cervix (a condition known as cervical eversion). In either case, cysts may be formed.

Nabothian cysts are also found in older women, who are no longer producing much estrogen. With the decline in estrogen levels, the tissue of the cervix thins and flattens out. As a result, the normal secretions, though more meager than those found in a younger woman, are trapped, again forming Nabothian cysts.

Symptoms

The cysts may be single or multiple and range in size from as small as a pinhead to the size of a grape or even larger. Usually, they are filled with the clear mucus-type fluid that makes up the cervical secretions, but if the cervix is infected, the contents of the cyst may be somewhat cloudy and pus-filled. The cysts generally do not cause any bothersome symptoms.

Treatment

The cysts do not become infected unless the entire cervix happens to become infected, as in cervicitis, so they do not usually require treatment. Nonetheless, some doctors will treat Nabothian cysts by electric cautery or cryosurgery, which involves expense, healing time and possible complications. But since Nabothian cysts produce no symptoms, cause no problems and are, in fact, just the aftermath of a healing process or part of a natural aging process, we do not feel that they need to be treated.

CERVICAL LACERATIONS

AKA: tears or stretching of the cervix

Cervical lacerations are tears in the cervix that are usually the result of injuries during childbirth or abortion. They may be slight or deep and may be associated with relaxation of the muscles of the vaginal opening. Writers of medical textbooks, who seem to relish the creation of new categories, classify cervical lacerations as unilateral, bilateral and stellate. But, as common sense will tell you, such tears may take all sorts of forms.

With improved medical care during childbirth and delivery, serious lacerations of this type are rare. Some amount of tearing during delivery is natural, and most of the tears that do occur do not require any surgical repair. Cervical lacerations that result from abortions are more likely to need treatment. This is especially true of late abortions that are done by saline or prostaglandins. In such abortions, the dead fetus is delivered through the cervix just as happens in normal deliveries, but, because the normal process by which the cervix dilates and is prepared for delivery does not take place during such an abortion, tears in the unprepared cervix may occur as the fetus is expelled. Since these sorts of lacerations tend to be more severe and do not usually heal naturally, the doctor will often have to suture or sew them up.

It is an important but often ignored procedure to check for lacerations of the cervix after late abortions, so ask your doctor about this problem if you have this type of abortion.

Untreated lacerations of this type will often result in cervical stenosis, a closing-up of the cervical canal. If the cervix is closed off, the menstrual debris cannot escape. There is a buildup of menstrual blood that can cause problems. Fistulas, abnormal connections between various genital organs—in this case, the cervical canal, vagina and uterus—can also result from such unrepaired lacerations. Cervical lacerations may also result in a condition known as cervical incompetence, which can cause miscarriages.

Lacerations are often associated with eversion, a condition in which the red glandular tissue that normally lies inside the cervical canal prolapses, or falls, and pouts out of the cervical os onto the normally pink tissue that covers the surface of the cervix. Lacerations due to late abortion may also be associated with cervical infections.

According to some authorities, lacerations due to childbirth are similarly associated with infections of the cervix; however, there is some controversy here. Sometimes lacerations from childbirth heal up in such a way that they leave no sign except for long fibrous scars. However, there is considerable debate about whether or not any given cervical laceration is healed or not. The traditional textbook explanation of events goes something like this: The tear or laceration occurs during delivery, and there is usually a subsequent infection. This is due to the fact that the bacteria that are normally present in the vagina in limited numbers blossom in the pregnant vagina as a result of the hormones involved in pregnancy, which create an alkaline environment conducive to their growth. The laceration and the presence of this bacteria combine to produce cervical infection, so that the inflamed tissue must be treated with drugs; if this is unsuccessful, as it often is in cervical infections, then the infected tissue must be cut, burned or frozen off.

However, in our experience, and that of many of our colleagues, it is extremely rare for cervical lacerations from childbirth to become infected or for the actual symptoms of cervicitis—a bothersome discharge—to develop. In the rare cases where there is a discharge so heavy that it becomes an annoyance to the woman herself, we of course treat it. But in the vast majority of cases, cervical lacerations from childbirth don't need treatment and don't become infected. Part of the confusion here is due to the nature of the tissue that makes up the cervix. It is soft, internal tissue, and what may look like an inflamed or irritated area is really just the way scar tissue manifests itself on this type of tissue. It is always possible to pick up some bacteria in the vagina. Thus, this angry-looking scar tissue and the presence of bacteria may be interpreted as an infection, when it is not really a pathologic situation. Therefore, what a doctor who treats cervical lacerations is really doing is simply removing scar tissue from the cervix, a bit of cosmetic surgery. No woman is vain enough to care whether the appearance of her cervix is flawed by scar tissue, so the process of freezing, burning or cutting away such tissue is obviously unnecessary—and may be uncomfortable and expensive as well.

INCOMPETENT CERVIX

AKA: premature dilation of the cervix during pregnancy

Some women have what is called an incompetent cervix, a condition that should probably be renamed, as the term sounds rather like a putdown of a woman with this condition. Normally, the cervix does not open up until a woman is actually in labor. Then it dilates until it is opened wide enough to permit the baby to pass through. In the case of an incompetent cervix, the cervix opens up long before it should and the woman has a miscarriage. Typically, this occurs during the 18th to 32nd week of pregnancy, even though there may *not* have been any prior problems, such as cramps or bleeding, during the pregnancy. Usually, the duration of each successive pregnancy is lessened. This sort of history will help the doctor make the diagnosis. Ultrasound techniques, methods of visualizing internal tissue via high-frequency sound waves, may also help in diagnosis.

Causes

In some cases the woman with an incompetent cervix will have a prior history of therapeutic abortions or difficult childbirth that has resulted in tears or lacerations of the cervix. In other cases there is no such history and the defect is thought to be congenital (that is, a birth defect). Recently there has been some evidence suggesting that women whose mothers took synthetic hormones such as DES during their pregnancies are more likely to have this congenital defect.

It used to be that women with incompetent cervixes were confined to bed for their entire pregnancies. Nowadays, however, the Schirodkar procedure, whereby the cervix is tied closed, usually during the 12th to 16th week of pregnancy, permits such women to have a normal pregnancy. Usually, the tie is cut prior to labor and a vaginal delivery rather than the riskier Caesarean section can take place.

Sometimes the cervix is tied off before the pregnancy takes place, a procedure called an internal trachelorrhaphy. There is some controversy about whether the cervix should be tied off before or after the pregnancy is established. The interval trachelorrhaphy will not prevent pregnancy, but some doctors are concerned because there is a 20 percent spontaneous abortion rate in all pregnancies and the uterus, if tied shut, will not be able to spontaneously abort. On the other hand, the process, no matter when it is done, is not always successful, and waiting to place the suture until the greatest risk of spontaneous abortion has passed—the 12th week—means cutting it pretty close to the wire, for some incompetent cervixes will open up on or before the 12th week. Each case must be decided on its own merits, and a woman has a right to a full discussion with her doctor of the pros and cons of each method for her particular case.

CERVICAL STENOSIS

AKA: partial or total obstruction of the vaginal canal

Types: acquired stenosis
          congenital stenosis

Associated terms: hematosalpinx, hydrometra

Cervical stenosis refers to a condition in which the cervical canal is partially or totally blocked.

Causes

It may result from a variety of causes. In some cases, the problem is congenital, that is, the blockage is present at birth. Due to disturbances in embryonic development, the canal never opens properly, is absent altogether or is obstructed by a wall of tissue (see Congenital Abnormalities of the Uterus and Congenital Abnormalities of the Vagina, for a more complete discussion). Sometimes the closure of the canal is the result of a mechanical blockage. Thus, abnormal growths like cervical polyps, endometrial polyps and certain fibroid tumors of the uterus and cervix may be the source of the obstruction. Scar tissue from conization or cauterization, especially in the hands of an unskilled, inexperienced doctor, can cause cervical stenosis as well. In fact, any surgical procedures involving the cervix, including biopsies and curettage, or scraping, of the cervical canal, can result in such a blockage. Infections in the cervix may result in adhesions—hardened bands of fibrous tissue produced by healthy tissue to wall off infections and prevent their spread—and these adhesions may cause blockage. Similar types of obstructing adhesions may occur after menopause and may also cause blockage.

Symptoms and Complications

A number of symptoms and complications can result from partial or total blockage of the cervix. First, there may be pain. Anything that obstructs the easy passage of menstrual blood may cause a bearing-down pain, painful uterine contractions and backache. If the obstruction is only partial, the menstrual blood will flow, but is likely to be dark brown or almost black in color.

If the obstruction is total, this prevents passage of the menstrual blood altogether. In a young girl with a congenital blockage, the problem may not be discovered until the expected time of menarche. She may seek help about her failure to menstruate. Sometimes such girls will actually have started to menstruate and may have monthly menstrual symptoms but no external bleeding. The blood has backed up in her uterus, a condition known as hematometra that can cause abnormal swelling and pain, especially at the time of menstruation. If the process continues untreated for long enough, the Fallopian tubes as well as the uterus may fill up with menstrual blood, a condition known as hematosalpinx. The blood may even back up through the tubes and spill out into the pelvic cavity. Since the lining of the pelvic cavity is very sensitive to blood, this can cause a great deal of irritation and pain and the formation of pelvic adhesions. There may even be associated pelvic endometriosis, a condition in which bits of uterine lining tissue are found growing on the ovaries and other abnormal locations. The same things can happen in a woman who has already begun to menstruate; however, they are less likely to go that far since her failure to menstruate will usually prompt her to seek medical attention.

When the blockage occurs in a young girl or a woman after menopause, there may be a buildup of watery and mucousy cervical secretions, a condition known as hydrometra. This is less likely to happen in a postmenopausal woman, since her cervical secretions are diminished. If

339

the blockage is associated with infection, there may be a backup of fluid and pus, a condition known as pyometra.

There may also be a fertility problem associated with the blockage because it may be impossible for sperm to nagivate the blocked canal. Even partial blockage may cause such problems.

Treatment

Treatment consists of removing the blockage surgically and may involve one or more follow-up dilations of the canal to prevent it from closing up again. This can be done in the doctor's office with a local anesthetic. If there has been a backup of fluids, they must be drained. Antibiotics are often given to prevent an infection from subsequently arising from the accumulated fluids, which, especially in the case of blood, tend to be a fertile breeding ground for bacteria.

CONGENITAL ABNORMALITIES OF THE CERVIX

AKA: cervical birth defects

Types: incompetent cervix
cervical stenosis
cervical eversion or ectropion
cervical agenesis
double cervix
septate cervix
transverse cervical ridges
hooded, rim, cockscomb, pseudopolypoid, or collar cervix

We have already discussed incompetent cervix, cervical stenosis and cervical eversion in this section. These conditions may be either congenital—present since birth—or acquired as the result of injury, infection, or something else that has happened since birth. There are several additional congenital cervical abnormalities. These include a complete absence of the cervix, called cervical agenesis, and a double cervix, called a septate cervix, in which the cervix is divided down the center by a wall of tissue. These conditions are discussed under the heading Congenital Abnormalities of the Vagina and Congenital Abnormalities of the Uterus and Tubes.

A special category of congenital cervical abnormalities includes transverse cervical ridges, which are ridges or ripples running across the surface of the cervix much as ridges of sand may form on a stretch of desert, and the hooded cervix, in which a flap of skin covers the top of the cervix. The terms "rim," "collar," "cockscomb" or "pseudopolypoid cervix" may also be used to describe the latter condition. The vast majority of birth defects in this category occur in women whose mothers took synthetic hormones, such as DES, during their pregnancy. These defects in and of themselves may not be serious; however, other more disturbing defects may occur along with these. This topic is discussed more fully under the heading DES.

LEUKOPLAKIA OF THE CERVIX

AKA: white patches on the cervix

Leukoplakia of the cervix is manifested as single or multiple white patches on the cervix that usually appear in women over the age of 40 and may be associated with vaginal discharge or bleeding. It is caused by an irregularity in cell growth and is thought by some to be precancerous.

While it is certainly true that leukoplakia and cancer often coexist, it is not entirely clear whether this is because malignant tissue is conducive to the development of leukoplakia or because leukoplakia is precancerous. A sort of which came first, the chicken or the egg, situation exists. Certainly not all women with leukoplakia develop cancer. However, even though the answers are not yet in, the fact that it is possible for an area of leukoplakia to mask a cancer growing beneath it means that the usual treatment involves excision (cutting out) of the areas of leukoplakia.

The leukoplakia may be discovered because the woman has symptoms and seeks medical attention or it may be discovered in the course of a routine gynecological exam with a speculum.

CERVICAL DYSPLASIA *

AKA: cervical intraepithelial neoplasia (CIN), grades I & II

Types: CIN grade I, basal cell hyperplasia, mild dysplasia, or moderate dysplasia
CIN grade II, or severe dysplasia

The term "dysplasia" means abnormal cell development; cervical dysplasia, then, is an abnormal condition of the cells of the cervix. It doesn't as a rule produce any obvious symptoms, nor in most cases can it be seen with the naked eye. The only way that most women know they have it is as a result of a Pap smear.

There is a good deal of controversy and confusion about dysplasia, especially about its relationship to cancer. Sometimes the cell abnormalities seen in cervical dysplasia become progressively more abnormal

*Important background information is given in the section on the Pap smear.

and the woman develops cervical cancer, but not all women with dysplasia do develop cervical cancer. Some 30-50 percent will, however, develop cervical cancer over a period of some years if the condition is not treated. Most authorities therefore consider dysplasia a precancerous condition.

Today there is a tendency to view dysplasia not as a separate entity but as the first step in a continuum of abnormal cell changes that progress in a few years to carcinoma in situ, which in turn progresses in about five to ten years to invasive cancer. Thus, the term "cervical intraepithelial neoplasia" (CIN) has been coined.

CIN is divided into three grades. Grade I includes mild and moderate dysplasia. In mild dysplasia, also known as basal cell hyperplasia, the cells in the bottom third or less of the tissue that covers the cervix (the cervical epithelium) are abnormal. Moderate dysplasia involves one-third to two-thirds of the cervical epithelium. Grade II is severe dysplasia, meaning that at least two-thirds but not the entire epithelial membrane is involved. Grade III, which is also known as carcinoma in situ, involves the full thickness of the cervical epithelium. Grades I and II are discussed here; Grade III is discussed under the heading Carcinoma in Situ.

Incidence and Cause

Cervical dysplasia is most frequently found in women aged 25 to 35 years old, but can also occur in women in their teens or early 20s and in older women as well. The cause of cervical dysplasia, like the cause of any precancerous or cancerous condition is unknown; however, studies of the women that are at high risk for developing such conditions have indicated some possible causes. Risk factors and possible causes are discussed under the heading Cervical Cancer.

Diagnosis

The first step is the Pap smear. If the Pap smear indicates mild, moderate or severe dysplasia, most doctors feel that the next step should be a biopsy. The biopsy must be done to confirm the Pap smear, for Pap smears can be wrong. They may be falsely negative or falsely positive. Moreover, Pap smears are, not infrequently, "off" by one class. A woman whose Pap smear indicates dysplasia could, in reality, have carcinoma in situ. The Pap smear may even be off by more than one class, so that a woman with a smear indicating dysplasia could actually have invasive cancer. A biopsy, which involves taking an actual tissue sample, is more accurate. The Pap smear provides the pathologist only with isolated cells; the biopsy allows him or her to study the architecture of the cells' relationship to each other and thus to make a more accurate diagnosis.

Not all doctors perform a biopsy when a woman's Pap smear indicates that she has dysplasia. Some doctors will merely tell her that her smear has indicated some abnormality and that another smear should be done in anywhere from three to six months. Their reasoning goes like this: Not all cases of dysplasia become cancer; some revert to normal on their own. Moreover, cancer of the cervix is usually a slowly progressing disease. Since the Pap smear indicates only the possibility of a precancerous condition, there is no great hurry. They maintain that, because these conditions progress so slowly, waiting will do no harm. Repeating the smear right away won't do any good, they say, because a lapse of at least a few months is necessary to give the condition enough time to progress, if indeed it is going to progress, to a more serious stage. Since the abnormal Pap smear may regress to normal by the time of the next smear, they argue that there is no need to subject a woman to a needless biopsy.

This wait-and-see approach should be taken only if the doctor cannot see or feel any irregularity on the cervix. If there is a visible abnormality, this approach should NEVER be used. A woman familiar with the appearance of her cervix can double-check her doctor on this. If the cervix looks different to her, she should insist on a biopsy, no matter what her doctor says. Likewise, the wait-and-see approach should be discontinued if the woman experiences any pain or intermenstrual bleeding. In such cases, a biopsy *must* be done.

If at the time of the second smear the dysplasia gets worse, or even if it has merely persisted, a biopsy should be done. The waiting should not be continued, for a smear that persists as positive is not very likely to return to normal. Even if the second smear *is* negative, the woman must have follow-up smears every three to six months for the next two years. This is necessary because the follow-up smears may be incorrect. As pointed out earlier, it is not unusual for a smear to be either one class more or one class less serious than the pathologist's report. Thus, a follow-up smear with a report of no dysplasia does not absolutely guarantee that the dysplasia is gone, but merely that the cells collected in that particular smear and analyzed by that particular pathologist are not judged to be dysplastic.

Many women and many doctors question the whole wisdom of a wait-and-see approach. First of all, most authorities now feel that true dysplasia usually does not regress to normal.[1] Many women object to the mental anguish of waiting three to six months to find out if they have a precancerous or cancerous condition. There is also the risk in delaying treatment. Although it is true that cancer of the cervix is usually a slowly progressing condition, there are exceptions. An approach that delays a diagnosis could, then, be dangerous.

Most experts feel that there should be no delay in cases of severe dysplasia. No one knows for sure whether severe dysplasia always goes through a carcinoma in situ stage or whether some progress directly to invasive cancer, a much more serious condition. Moreover, since it is known that Pap smears are often inaccurate, the reported severe dysplasia may in reality already be carcinoma in situ or even invasive cancer.

It is our recommendation that women with dysplasia insist on biopsies and not accept a wait-and-see approach, even if it means finding another doctor or traveling to another town for medical care.

The biopsy may be done in one of two ways. In the first approach, the cervix is stained with a special solution and any areas that do not take the stain are biopsied. The cervical canal must be also scraped, a procedure known as endocervical curettage, for the inside of the canal cannot be seen and yet that is where the cancerous or precancerous problem may lie. If the staining doesn't show any suspicious area or only a few such areas, biopsy specimens are taken from several locations on the cervix where studies have shown that these sorts of problems are most likely to occur. This is known as a blind biopsy.

The second way of doing the biopsy is to use a colposcope. The colposcope is a magnifying instrument, a sort of microscope on a stand. With a speculum in place, a beam of light from the colposcope is directed at the cervix. The doctor can often tell how serious the dysplasia is and can see suspicious areas not visible to the naked eye. In fact, the colposcope may detect suspicious areas even before cells that could be picked up on a Pap smear are shed. The interior of the canal still can't be seen, so it must be scraped. A special stain is also used in conjunction with the colposcope. The use of the colposcope means that numerous blind biopsies need not be taken.

The colposcope-directed biopsy is much more accurate. Even in the best of hands, the first method of biopsy is accurate in only 80 percent of the cases. The colposcope is more than 95 percent accurate. The problem is that not all doctors have colposcopes and not all are well trained in their use. If your doctor doesn't have a colposcope, ask to be referred to a clinic or doctor who does. Again, we recommend that women insist on cervical biopsies done with a colposcope, even if it means they have to travel to another city or town.

Sometimes it is necessary to do a conization, a procedure whereby a cone of tissue is removed from the center of the cervix. Conization requires hospitalization and a general anesthetic. It may involve complications such as excessive bleeding, scar-tissue blockage of the cervical canal and infertility due to destruction of the mucus-producing glands in the cervical canal. Because of this, a biopsy is preferred over conization. But if there is reason to suspect that the abnormality is in the cervical canal, a conization is necessary, for the scrapings from the cervical canal, like the Pap smear, provide only isolated cells. An actual biopsy of the canal—a conization—is necessary in the following instances:

☐ If the squamocolumnar junction, the area where the squamous cells of the vaginal portion of the cervix and the columnar cells of the canal meet and where most cancers of the cervix originate, is not visible.

☐ If the staining and colposcopic exam don't reveal any abnormalities on the surface of the cervix.

☐ If the cells obtained by scraping the cervical canal are abnormal.

☐ If the abnormal areas detected by staining or colposcopy lead into the canal.

☐ If the Pap smear indicated severe dysplasia but the biopsy indicated only mild dysplasia, the colposcopic-directed biopsy should be repeated. If the inconsistency between the Pap and the biopsy persists, conizations should be done.

Women should not agree to conization unless a colposcopic exam has been done first, for it can discover abnormalities that a mere staining of the cervix may miss. If your doctor suggests conization, make sure you understand his or her reasoning. If you get one of those because-I'm-the-doctor-and-I-say-so replies or you are not satisfied with the explanation, seek a second opinion (*see* p. 226).

Treatment[2]

Treatment for dysplasia ranges from hysterectomy to conization to electric cautery or cryosurgery to merely following the condition closely (see above).

Although hysterectomy is done for dysplasia, it is considered by most to be overtreatment, no matter what the age of the woman. The risks and complications involved are too high a price to pay now that effective, less radical treatment is available. If your doctor proposes to do a hysterectomy for dysplasia, read the section on hysterectomy carefully and get a second medical opinion before undergoing surgery.

If a conization has already been done as part of the diagnostic process, this may constitute treatment as well, as long as the cone was done properly and all suspicious areas seen by the colposcope were removed. However, a dysplasia will recur in 13-15 percent of the cases treated by conization. Because of this recurrence rate and because conization is a surgical procedure requiring hospitalization and an anesthetic, and is known to have complications, it is not a good treatment choice, particularly for women who have future childbearing plans.

Cautery, either electrocautery (heat) or cryosurgery (freezing) can also be used to treat dysplasia. The dysplastic areas are destroyed, thereby allowing normal, unaffected tissue to grow back in its place. Most doctors favor cryosurgery because it goes deeper and destroys more possibly dysplastic tissue. Another big factor in favor of cryosurgery is that it is essentially painless. Moreover, complications such as closing of the cervical canal and infertility may be associated with electric cautery but not with cryosurgery.

Follow-up is important, even when a hysterectomy has been done, for the vaginal tissue may develop cancer as well. Follow-up Pap smears and colposcopic exams are especially important in the less radical forms of treatment.

CARCINOMA IN SITU*

AKA: intraepithelial carcinoma, preinvasive cancer, precancerous anaplasia, non-invasive carcinoma, Bowen's disease of the cervix, cervical intraepithelial neoplasia (CIN) grade III, Stage O of cervical cancer

Carcinoma in situ means "cancer that is in place," or cancer that has not invaded the surrounding tissue. It is a condition in which cells that have all the characteristics of cancer are found but only the top layers of cervical tissue are involved, and there is no sign of the invasion of the surrounding tissue that characterizes true invasive cancer. Whether all carcinoma in situ of the cervix eventually progresses to invasive cancer is not yet known, largely because no one is willing to leave it untreated and risk the chance that it will become invasive.

At this time, the generally accepted view is that carcinoma in situ arises from a background of severe dysplasia and is part of a continuum of disease that leads to invasive cancer. Working from this assumption, one expert has coined the term "cervical intraepithelial neoplasm" (CIN) or Stage O of cervical cancer. CIN is further divided into three types, or stages, grades I and II, which encompass the various degrees of dysplasia, and grade III, which is carcinoma in situ, or Stage O of cervical cancer.

Carcinoma in situ most often arises in the area of the cervix known as the squamocolumnar junction. This is the point at which the pink, squamous tissue that covers the vagina and the vaginal portion of the cervix meets the red columnar tissue that lines the cervical canal. In the majority of women this junction lies just inside the cervical os (opening).

*See the general section on cancer and the section on the Pap smear for background information.

Incidence

Carcinoma in situ of the cervix is most frequently found in women in their 30s who have borne one or more children, as opposed to invasive cancer of the cervix, which is most often found in women in their 40s. Recently, however, carcinoma in situ is being found with increasing frequency in women in the 20- to 30-year-old age group. For a discussion of the reasons for this increase in incidence in younger women, see the section on Cervical Cancer.

Cause and Risk Factors

The cause of carcinoma in situ, like the cause for all cancers, is unknown. However, certain women seem more likely to develop this condition than others. For a discussion of causes and risk factors, see Cervical Cancer.

Symptoms

Carcinoma in situ of the cervix has no characteristic symptoms. While it is true that 85 percent of the women with this condition will have some sort of abnormality in the appearance of the cervix, this is not surprising since most of them have borne children. Cervical lacerations, erosions and eversions are common among such women and are not necessarily related to cancer. In other words, although most women with carcinoma in situ have these conditions, that does not mean that most of the women who have them will develop cancer.

Bleeding between menstrual periods or after intercourse occurs in about a third of the women who are diagnosed as having cervical carcinoma in situ. However, although some women will show a history of such irregular bleeding and may even have cervixes that bleed on the slightest contact, most women with this condition do not.

Cervical carcinoma in situ frequently occurs without any abnormality in the appearance of the cervix, particularly when it is located inside the cervical canal and when there is no bleeding. Luckily, even in the absence of symptoms or of abnormalities in the cervix, a routine Pap smear can detect carcinoma in situ.

Diagnosis

The Pap smear is the first step in diagnosis. If the smear shows carcinoma in situ, the next step is a biopsy, preferably a colposcopic biopsy, as described in the preceding section on cervical dysplasia. In certain cases a conization may be necessary. This too is described in the preceding section on dysplasia. A D&C may be done to rule out the possibility of invasive cancer.

Treatment[3]

Carcinoma in situ may be treated by hysterectomy, conization, electric cautery or cryosurgery (freezing).

Hysterectomy offers a 100 percent cure and is usually recommended for postmenopausal women and premenopausal women who don't have future childbearing plans. In the past, women adamant about preserving their ability to bear children were sometimes treated by conization. Unfortunately, conization often has an effect on fertility. Only about 65 percent of women treated by conization are able to get pregnant, and of these, approximately 25 percent will have miscarriages. Today, a newer form of therapy, cryosurgery, which destroys the affected tissue by freezing, is available. Conization may still be done for women whose carcinoma in situ is located in the cervical canal, but for most women who want to preserve their childbearing capabilities, cryosurgery is the best choice.

Women who are treated by cryosurgery must commit themselves to a lifelong follow-up program that includes Pap smears every three months, regular colposcopic exams and a yearly endocervical curettage, that is, a scraping of cells from the inside of the cervical canal. This follow-up program is essential, for in 7-11 percent of cases the cryosurgery will not be effective and the carcinoma in situ will recur. Without a careful follow-up program, the recurrent carcinoma in situ might be missed and progress to frankly invasive cancer before being detected, which would greatly reduce a woman's chances of survival. If recurrent carcinoma in situ is discovered in follow-up, a second cryosurgery treatment or a hysterectomy may be done.

Most doctors feel that cryosurgery is an acceptable alternative to hysterectomy for women anxious to retain their ability to bear children. Even though they have no future childbearing plans, some women anxious to avoid the risk and expense of hysterectomy are choosing cryotherapy over hysterectomy.

Women who choose cryotherapy are taking a certain risk. Theoretically, even if a woman were to report faithfully for her follow-up visits, there is a small chance that a recurrence could be missed. The cancer could recur high up inside the cervical canal where it could not be seen with a colposcope. The Pap smear might fail to detect a recurrence. False negative rates (that is, failure to detect cancer that is actually there) of 1.4-30 percent have been reported in studies of Pap smears. The generally accepted false negative rate is 11-22 percent. It is highly unlikely that a woman who is having four Pap smears a year would be unlucky enough to have a false negative reading each time, but it is possible. It is also possible, although unlikely, that the yearly endocervical curettage could fail to detect a recurrence in the cervical canal. However, even if a recurrence were missed one year, it would probably be caught the next year, and since carcinoma in situ usually takes seven years to progress to invasive cancer, missing it one year would not be too serious.

The other risk involves the problem of misdiagnosis. It is possible that the woman might really have invasive cancer, and not carcinoma in situ, but that a mistake was made in the diagnostic work-up. If treated by hysterectomy, this misdiagnosis would probably not present a problem, for the cervix and uterus would have been removed. If, on the other hand, the woman is treated only with cryosurgery, she would not be cured of the invasive cancer.

Cryosurgery has not been used on a large enough group of women for a long enough period of time for anyone to say with absolute certainty that it is as safe as hysterectomy or to precisely define the magnitude of the risks involved. The studies done so far are encouraging, however, and we personally feel comfortable with this form of treatment.

Cautery—destroying the tissues by burning—has also been used, but cautery involves more discomfort and complications that may affect fertility, so most doctors prefer cryosurgery.

CERVICAL CANCER

AKA: carcinoma of the cervix

Although the incidence of cervical cancer is on the rise, the death rate is declining. This is because the disease, thanks to widespread use of the Pap smear, is being detected in its earlier stages, when it is virtually 100 percent curable. The Pap smear, then, is an invaluable tool and should be part of every routine physical exam.

Incidence and Risk Factors

Cancer of the cervix is the third most common cancer occurring in women. The average age of the diagnosis of invasive cervical cancer is 48, but the disease may affect both younger and older women. The annual incidence rate in this country is 14.9 cases per 100,000 women, but cases of cervical cancer are not randomly distributed throughout the population. In other words, not everyone is equally likely to get the disease; some women are definitely at higher risk of developing the disease than others. A number of factors come into play: Incidence rates vary according to ethnic group, for instance, with rates having been reported of 3.6 cases per 100,000 for Jewish women, 13.5 per 100,000 for non-Jewish white women, 47.8 per 100,000 for black women and a high of 97.6 per 100,000 for Puerto Rican women. It is also known that of the women with cervical cancer, 97 percent have had children. Women who marry at an early age and whose first child is born when they are still young also have higher incidence rates. Women with three or more husbands have higher rates, as do prostitutes. Numerous studies with results along these lines have been done.[4] It has not always been entirely clear what all this information means. At one time it was thought that having children at an early age or frequent sex put a woman at higher risk. At the present time, however, most authorities feel that having sexual intercourse at an early age and multiple sex partners are the two factors most likely to increase a woman's chance of developing cervical cancer.[5] Some authorities question the accuracy of this. They point out that there are unproved assumptions behind the reasoning that earlier sex and multiple partners account for the high incidence among poor women. It has long been a popular piece of social folklore that the poor are more promiscuous, but there is no scientific evidence to substantiate this and as one middle-class friend of ours says, "You couldn't prove it by me."

Still, there is other evidence to suggest that these two factors put a woman at higher risk of developing cervical cancer. Women with these sexual patterns may want to have more frequent Pap smears.

Cause

The role of heredity is not considered to be very important in cervical cancer. Cervical cancer does not seem to run in families, and the different incidence rates in various ethnic and economic groups is not thought to be the result of an inherited trait but of socioeconomic factors, since certain ethnic groups and women in low-income groups tend to marry earlier and have their children at an early age.

The fact that nuns never get cervical cancer, while prostitutes have high incidence rates, and that women who have sex at an early age or have multiple sex partners seem to be at greater risk, while women who use diaphragms (which presumably protect the cervix from sperm) are at lesser risk, first led to the suspicion that cervical cancer may be caused by some sort of agent—possibly a virus—passed during sexual intercourse. It is known that the cervical tissue is still maturing in a woman in her teens, and this maturation process may not be complete in some women until about the age of 20. It has been theorized, then, that the introduction of some sexually transmitted agent into the immature cervical tissue causes changes that only become apparent years later.

The evidence linking one agent known to be sexually transmitted, the herpes virus (*see* p. 548), to cervical cancer is quite strong. Over the past ten years there has been a growing body of evidence suggesting a relationship between herpes virus and cervical cancer.[6] Studies that showed that herpes is found much more frequently in women with cervical cancer than in women without the disease were the first indication that herpes might be a factor in cervical cancer. A number of other studies further advance the case for a connection between herpes and cervical cancer.

A which-came-first-the-chicken-or-the-egg? sort of question comes up in evaluating the relationship between herpes and cancer. Does herpes infection cause, or at least predispose a woman to, cancer, or does herpes just happen to find cancerous or precancerous tissue a more conducive environment in which to grow? Perhaps the cancerous or precancerous changes in the cervix make it more susceptible to herpes infection. However, the fact that the mean age of women with herpes is 20 years of age, that with cervical dysplasia it's 25, that with carcinoma in situ it's 31, and that with invasive cancer it's 48, does suggest that herpes may be the first step in a series that leads over the years to the development of cervical cancer. Moreover, studies that have followed women with herpes over a period of years have shown that such women are up to eight times more likely to subsequently develop some form of cervical cancer. But that may be because of precancerous changes that occur in the cervix years before the actual cancer is diagnosed and that also happen to make the cervix more susceptible to herpes infection. These sorts of data do not finally answer the chicken/egg question.

Still there is other laboratory evidence that doesn't look good for women with herpes. Herpes virus has been implicated in the development of tumors in laboratory animals. More to the point, herpes-associated substances have been found in cervical cancer tumors in humans. The laboratory evidence is again not conclusive, but there are persuasive indications that herpes is either a cause or a factor in the sequence of causative factors that leads to cervical cancer. While the link between herpes and cervical cancer isn't strong enough to be called conclusive in the strictest medical sense, it is firm enough to suggest that any woman with a history of herpes should have an annual, perhaps even biannual, Pap smear.

Another causative factor in cervical cancer may be DES-type hormones, taken during pregnancy by the mothers of the women with these conditions. This topic is discussed in greater detail elsewhere in this text.

There has also been some evidence that the use of birth control pills is associated with certain precancerous changes in the cervix, that is, cervical dysplasia, and may therefore play a role in the development of cervical cancer.[7]

Symptoms

The symptoms of cervical cancer include vaginal bleeding, discharge and an abnormal appearance of the cervix. In the later states there may be pain, weight loss and possibly urinary and bowel problems. Not all of these symptoms are always present. In fact, the disease is often asymptomatic in the early stages. Approximately 70 percent of the women with Stage IA, or microinvasive, cancer have no unusual bleeding, and in 60 percent the cervix appears perfectly normal. Only 20 percent of these women will have both symptoms.

Since the menstrual cycle is not disturbed, bleeding, when it does occur, is of the intermenstrual, or between periods, type. Except in advanced cases of this disease, the bleeding is rarely of the gushing type, and in most cases the bleeding is slight. Spotting may occur after intercourse or douching. A woman may notice a slight vaginal bleeding while straining to make a bowel movement or after exercise, intercourse or even riding in a car. The bleeding may be so slight that it doesn't even require a sanitary pad. It is not necessarily constant and tends to come and go. Several days may go by with no bleeding at all. Unfortunately, invasive cancer of the cervix tends to appear in women around the time of menopause and therefore such bleeding irregularities are often attributed to the menopause.

Bleeding is much more likely to appear in more advanced cases and is apt to be more profuse. However, even in these cases, it may never be excessive, especially in the postmenopausal woman. Still, bleeding is one of the causes of death in the terminal cases of cervical cancer.

In the earlier stages of the disease, vaginal discharge tends to be constant but of such a slight amount that it is rarely enough to alarm a woman. The discharge is usually odorless, thin and watery. Only rarely does the discharge precede the bleeding; sometimes the two symptoms coexist. The color of the discharge varies from yellow to brown, depending on the amount of associated bleeding. The vaginal discharge tends to become more profuse and to smell bad in the advanced cases.

Pain combined with discharge and bleeding is the most frequent combination of symptoms in women with advanced disease. The pain varies in severity. It is usually a vague lower back pain that may spread to the hip and down the side. It is usually worse at night and is not relieved by lying down. If the bladder and rectum are involved, there is often pain when voiding or moving the bowels. There may also be constipation or retention of the urine.

The appearance of the cervix in invasive cancer varies considerably. About one-third of the women with this disease will have cervixes that appear perfectly normal. Others, in the early stages, will have what appear to be cervical erosions or even slighter abnormalities. For example, there may be an area of the cervix that merely seems a bit more red, darker or less shiny than another, a condition that has been described as a "tomato blush."

In the more advanced stages, the appearance of the cervix is more apt to be abnormal. If the disease is on the surface of the cervix, or growing from the canal outward, there may be a large sore or a bulky cauliflower-type growth. If the tumor is in the canal or tends to grow inward, the entire cervix may be increased in bulk, and although its surface may appear normal, the cervix takes on a barrel shape and extends lower into the vagina.

Recurrent cancer, that is, cancer that occurs even after the initial treatment, doesn't produce much in the way of symptoms in its early stages either; approximately 10 percent of such women will have some vaginal bleeding. As the disease becomes more extensive, there is usually pain in the lower back radiating down the thighs. There may be swelling of the legs. If the bladder or ureters (the tubes that conduct urine from the kidney to the bladder) are affected, the woman may have associated urinary and kidney problems.[8]

Diagnosis and Staging

The first step in diagnosing cervical cancer is the Pap smear. Sometimes a woman will come to the doctor complaining of one of the symptoms described earlier, and, in the course of investigating the cause of the symptom, a Pap smear will be done. Often, however, there are no symptoms and the abnormalities are discovered only in the course of a routine Pap smear. It is important, then, that all women have a Pap smear once a year. Biannual Pap smears might be a good idea for those women who are at high risk because of a particular history of sexual activity (see above), a history of herpes infections or exposure to DES-type drugs or who are in the 40-50-year-old age group and thus are more likely to develop such cancer.

However, the Pap smear is only a screening test. Although it is 95 percent accurate in detecting cancer, it is not always accurate in indicating the seriousness of the disease. It is possible that the smear will show carcinoma in situ or the even less serious cervical dysplasia when, in fact, invasive cancer is present. It is important, then, that the Pap smear be followed by a cervical biopsy. The Pap smear contains only isolated cells, but the biopsy provides an actual tissue specimen, which allows the pathologist to study the architecture of the cells. By studying the cells in relation to one another, the pathologist can make a more accurate diagnosis.

Scrapings may also be taken from the cervical canal in order to help the doctor determine whether the disease has spread to this area. Certain cases will require conization, in which the central core of the cervix is removed, a process somewhat akin to removing the core from an apple. The reasons for doing a conization, as well as important information about cervical biopsies, are discussed under the heading Cervical Dysplasia. In addition, a conization is always done in cases where the biopsy has indicated that the woman has microinvasive cancer (see below). *No woman should accept a diagnosis of or treatment for microinvasive cancer unless a surgical cone has been done.* A simple biopsy does not provide enough tissue to allow for an accurate diagnosis of microinvasion; tissue samples from the more extensive conization procedure are necessary, for only three-quarters of the cases diagnosed as microinvasive on biopsy will turn out to be so when a surgical cone is done.[9]

Moreover, it is essential that a number of different sections of the cone be examined, for studies have shown that in busy labs, where only one section was studied, errors have run as high as 17 percent. Women should make sure that a board-certified pathologist (*see* p. 674) has examined her tissue slides.

Once the diagnosis of invasive cervical cancer has been confirmed by biopsy or, if necessary, by conization, the next step is staging the disease.

Staging is made prior to operation and is based on the doctor's estimate of how far the disease has spread. Table 9 outlines the most widely used staging scheme for cervical cancer. Recently, TNM classifications, as outlined in Table 10, have been used as well.[10]

The first step in staging is a careful palpation of the cervix, vagina, bladder, uterus, rectum, pelvic lymph nodes and abdomen. This helps the doctor determine the size and spread of the cancer. Knowing the size is important because smaller cancers are much less likely to have spread beyond the cervix and therefore will require less aggressive treatment.

Obviously, the skill and experience of the doctor will affect the accuracy of the staging. But in some cases, even the best doctors will not be able to make an accurate pretreatment estimate of the spread of the disease. Scar tissue from previous pelvic diseases may lead the doctor to believe that cancer is present in areas where, in fact, there is no malignant disease. Similarly, lymph nodes may be swollen as a result of infection and this swelling may be mistaken for the presence of cancer. On the other hand, the cancer may have spread to the surrounding tissue but may be too small or too inaccessibly placed to be felt, or the lymph nodes may contain cancer cells without being noticeably swollen. Then, too, not all nodes may be involved, and those that are may be too deeply placed to be felt.

Certain tests can help the doctor in making his or her estimate. Routine blood and urine tests may be of help. Chest X-rays are also done, to rule out the possibility that the disease has already spread to the lungs. X-ray studies may be done to assess kidney, bowel and liver function. Specialized viewing instruments may be used to examine the bladder, lower colon and rectum.

Table 9
Staging Scheme for Cervical Cancer

Stage O: Carcinoma in situ, also called intraepithelial carcinoma grade III, in which the cancer is limited to the outer skin (epithelial) layer of cervical tissue.

Stage I: Cancer strictly limited to the cervix.

    Stage IA: Microinvasion, also called early stromal invasion. The cancer has penetrated deeper than the epithelial level described in Stage O, but the penetration into the lower tissue is limited to a depth of not more than five mm (some authorities use three mm as the cutoff point).

    Stage IB: The cancer is still limited to the cervix, but the penetration is more than five mm.

Stage II: The cancer has extended beyond the cervix, but has not extended to the pelvic wall.

    Stage IIA: The cancer has extended down into the vagina and all or part of the upper third of the vagina is involved, though the parametrium, the connective tissue surrounding and supporting the cervix, is not.

    Stage IIB: Same as above, only the parametrial tissues are involved, but not all the way to the pelvic wall.

Stage III: The disease has now invaded the side wall of the pelvis and/or the lower third of the vagina.

    Stage IIIA: The cancer has invaded the lower half of the vagina, but has not reached the pelvic wall.

    Stage IIIB: The cancer has reached the pelvic wall.

Stage IV: The cancer has extended beyond the pelvis and/or has involved the bladder or rectum.

    Stage IVA: The bladder and/or rectum are involved.

    Stage IVB: Distant metastases.

Table 10
TNM Classifications for Cervical Cancer

T = Primary Tumor

T1S: Carcinoma in situ

T1:   Tumor confined to the cervix

    T1a: Microinvasive tumor

    T1b: Tumor beyond microinvasion, but still confined to the cervix

T2:   Tumor extending beyond the cervix, but not reaching the pelvic wall, or cancer involving the vagina, but not the lower third

    T2a: Tumor has not infiltrated the tissues adjacent to the uterus and cervix

    T2b: Tumor has infiltrated beyond just the tissues adjacent to the uterus and cervix

T3:   Tumor involving either the lower third of the vagina or reaching the pelvic wall

T4:   Tumor involving the bladder and/or rectum or extending beyond the pelvis

    T4a: Tumor involving the bladder and/or rectum
    T4b: Distant metastases

N = Lymph Nodes

NX: Not possible to examine the nodes

N0:   No clinically obvious nodal involvement

N1:   Nodes involved as shown by diagnostic tests

N2:   Nodes involved

M = Metastasis

M0:   No evidence of metastases

M1:   Distant metastases

Stage/TNM Correlations*

Stage O:	T1S		
Stage I-A:	T1a	NX	M0
Stage I-B:	T1b	NX	M0
Stage II-A:	T2a	NX	M0
Stage II-B:	T2b	NX	M0

356

Table 10
TNM Classifications for Cervical Cancer

Stage III:	T3	NX	MO
	T1b	N2	MO
	T2a	N2	MO
	T2b	N2	MO
Stage IV-A:	T4	NX	MO
	T4	N2	MO
Stage IV-B:			Any M1

*NO and N1 are not taken into account in Stage grouping.

All of the information gained from the palpation and tests to detect metastases (*see* p. 677) is used to stage the disease and to decide upon the proper treatment. Unfortunately, this preoperative diagnosis or staging process is frequently in error. Indeed, in some 30 percent of the cases, the estimate of disease spread is incorrect. Because of this high rate of error, researchers have long sought other, more accurate methods of staging.

One of these is lymphangiography, which involves injecting a substance into the lymph system that will show up on X-ray film. Unfortunately, studies have shown that the estimates of lymph node involvement based on the lymphangiogram are wrong in more than 50 percent of cases. Too many times the lymphangiograph completely misses the cancer. The process is, nonetheless, of some value. When correlated with the results of palpation, it may provide important clues. Moreover, a dye added to the injected substance will stain the nodes, and if surgery is the treatment of choice, this will make it easier for the surgeon to locate and remove them. The lymphangiogram can also act as a map for the radiotherapist if irradiation is the choice of treatment.

Another pretreatment method used by many doctors is an exploratory operation called a staging laparotomy. The doctor makes an incision in the abdomen that allows for direct inspection of all the pelvic organs and the lymph nodes for signs of disease. Suspicious lymph nodes are biopsied. The staging laparotomy can help in making a more accurate estimate of disease spread and allows for removal of lymph nodes that may be too large to be cured by radiation therapy. The staging laparotomy also allows for biopsy of certain lymph nodes, known as the para-aortic nodes, that are located higher in the body, roughly at the level of the belly button. These nodes are not necessarily included in the field of radiation when treatment is given. Thus, if cancer is present in these nodes, it will not be destroyed

357

by the usual therapy. Anywhere from 30-50 percent of women with Stage III and Stage IV disease may have cancer in these para-aortic lymph nodes.[11] Unfortunately, the biopsy of the para-aortic nodes may not always indicate the cancer. The staging laparotomy is not, then, 100 percent accurate. And it's much more useful at the later stages of cancer. For instance, in Stage IB only 7 percent of the women show positive nodes; 93 percent do not.[12] For the vast majority of these women, then, the operation would not be beneficial. Moreover, the complications, which include death, may outweigh the benefits. Some lives have definitely been saved by prestaging laparotomy, but because of the risks, it is presently a controversial procedure. Most experts agree that if it is done, it should be done only on patients thought to have at least Stage IIB disease who are otherwise in good health and are therefore good operative risks.[13] This issue should be thoroughly discussed prior to surgery by the woman and her doctor.

Treatment

The treatment of cancer is always a complex subject. In some ways the treatment of cervical cancer, which usually involves either surgery or radiation therapy, or, in some cases, a combination of the two, is especially complex because there is such a variety of treatment programs. Indeed, there are more than ten different surgical procedures that may be used in the treatment of this form of cancer. In another sense, though, the treatment of cervical cancer is a fairly simple, straightforward subject, for although there are many different treatment options, the decision as to which form of treatment should be given is fairly well defined—or at least more so than with other forms of cancer. In contrast to breast cancer, where the same woman might be treated in radically different ways depending on the personal philosophy of the doctor doing the treatment, a woman with cervical cancer is apt to get pretty much the same treatment regardless of whom she sees. One surgeon or radiation therapist may be better or more skilled than another, but the same basic treatment approach will be used. There are exceptions to this generalization, however, especially in Stage IA, where there is some controversy, and to a lesser degree, in Stages IB and IIA, where there is a choice between radiation and surgery. Moreover, although Stage IV cases are generally treated by radiation, certain Stage IVA cases may be treated surgically.

In Stage IB and IIA, where there is a choice between surgery and radiation, it is especially important that women with cervical cancer have opinions from both a radiologist and a surgeon. Human nature being what it is, specialists tend to think that if a choice of treatments exists, their specialty should be that choice. Thus, as a general rule, surgeons will recommend surgery and radiologists will favor radiation therapy. At larger cancer centers, a team approach, involving experts from each specialty in the treatment decision-making process, is standard. At other places, these routine consultations among experts may not automatically take place and a woman should then ask for second opinions or consultations (*see* p. 226) with board-certified doctors from each specialty. In cases where there is a difference of opinion as to the type of surgery, as there is in Stage IA, women should seek second opinions or consultations from various surgeons.

The basic aim of treatment, whether it's surgical or radiation therapy, is to destroy the cancer that is in the cervix, the adjacent tissues to which it may have spread and, in most cases, in the lymph nodes in the area. The type of treatment chosen will depend largely on the extent of the disease and the age and the general health of the woman.

Radiation Therapy

Radiation therapy is given in one of two ways:

External Beam Therapy: This type of radiation is delivered from outside the body by means of a beam of radiation generated by a machine and directed at an area of the body. With cervical cancer, the beam of radiation is directed at the pelvic area and is designed to destroy cancer both in the tissues adjacent to the cervix and uterus and in the pelvic lymph nodes. In some cases the area radiated is more extensive and includes the para-aortic lymph nodes, which are located at about the level of the navel. In advanced cases, Stages III and IV, some doctors routinely radiate this area in all their patients receiving curative radiation therapy; however, radiation to this area involves a significantly greater number of complications, some of which may be fatal.[14] Some doctors do the prestaging laparotomy discussed earlier and make the decision about radiation to the para-aortic nodes on this basis. The question of how to treat the para-aortic nodes is controversial. Women should discuss this issue as it applies to their cases with their doctors.

Often, external beam therapy is given first because it will shrink the tumor, making it more susceptible to radiation implants. At other times, implants are used prior to external beam therapy. In cases where the woman is in such poor health that she cannot withstand the anesthesia required for implants, external beam therapy is used alone, but the chances of a cure are usually reduced if the two methods of delivering radiation cannot be combined.

Intracavity Implants: This form of therapy is designed to destroy the cancer in the cervix, as well as any cancer in the uterus and vagina. Special

359

containers are inserted into the vagina and the uterus, loaded with a radioactive material, and left in place until the specified dose of radiation has been achieved. In certain cases, hollow tubes or needles inserted into the tumor are used.

In some cases internal implants cannot be used. If, for instance, the woman has had previous pelvic surgery or pelvic inflammatory disease, there may be too much scar tissue in the pelvis. Older women whose vaginas and uterus are smaller, inelastic and distorted in shape may be poor candidates for internal implants because their anatomy will not permit the insertion of containers large enough to deliver an evenly spread dose of sufficient quantity to destroy the cancer.

Surgery

As mentioned earlier, there are a number of different surgical procedures used to treat cervical cancer. The most commonly used forms are described below:

Radical Hysterectomy and Pelvic Lymphadenectomy: This operation involves removal of the uterus, tubes, the tissues immediately adjacent to the uterus and cervix and the upper third of the vagina. The ovaries are usually removed as well, although in younger women the ovaries may be preserved in order to avoid a premature menopause. The pelvic lymph nodes are also removed.

Pelvic Exenteration: This operation removes all of the pelvic organs including the uterus, tubes, ovaries, adjacent pelvic tissues, the vagina, the bladder and/or the rectum. In some cases a partial exenteration procedure in which either the bladder or the rectum is preserved may be done. If the bladder is removed but the rectum is preserved, the urinary tract may be diverted to the bowels. If the rectum and/or the bladder are removed, new openings must be created on the outside of the body and waste products collected in plastic bags.

Stage by Stage Treatment Programs

Many different factors will affect the choice of treatment. Stage by stage treatment programs are outlined below. Treatment for cervical cancer is not standardized but is highly individualized, and each case must be considered on its own merits. If the treatment recommended by your doctor differs from the treatment outlined below, this certainly does not mean that your doctor's recommendations are wrong; however, every woman has the right to know what type of therapy is planned and why. The following information is intended to provide a *general* understanding of the types of therapy available and the reasons for their use, so that you will have enough information to know the right questions to ask and to be able to evaluate your doctor's treatment recommendations.

Stage IA

The treatment of Stage IA, or microinvasive, cancer is somewhat controversial.[15] There is general agreement that it should be treated by some form of surgery (unless, of course, the woman is in such poor health that surgery is out of the question. Such women are treated by radiation).

However, there is considerable disagreement as to how extensive the surgery should be. There are a few doctors who believe that a simple conization will suffice. Other doctors feel that a radical hysterectomy and pelvic lymphadenectomy is necessary. In between these two extremes are the doctors who recommend either simple hysterectomy (removal of just the uterus and cervix), the somewhat more extensive radical hysterectomy, without the pelvic lymphadenectomy, or the Schauta procedure (also called the radical vaginal hysterectomy), which however, is rarely done anymore.

One reason that there is such disagreement about the extent of the surgery needed to treat microinvasive cancer is that no one is quite sure how this form of cancer behaves. We know that in more extensive cancer, like Stage IB, even though the cancer appears to be confined to the cervix, there is a significant chance that cancer cells are lurking in the supportive tissues immediately adjacent to the cervix and uterus or in the pelvic lymph nodes, so that these areas must be dealt with in planning treatment for Stage IB. Obviously, those who favor the radical hysterectomy and pelvic lymphadenectomy for Stage IA feel that there is a chance, although a small one, that the adjacent tissues and pelvic lymph nodes are harboring unsuspected cancer despite the microinvasive diagnosis. Those who favor the Schauta procedure or radical abdominal hysterectomy feel that Stage IA cancers may be accompanied by unsuspected cancer in the supportive tissues adjacent to the cervix, though not in the lymph nodes. Those who favor a simple hysterectomy feel that neither the adjacent tissues nor the pelvic lymph nodes are harboring cancer cells and that removal of these tissues is therefore not necessary.

Even though they don't sound much different on paper, the radical hysterectomy and the pelvic lymphadenectomy involve significantly higher complication and mortality rates than the simple hysterectomy. For one thing, the ureters, the tubes that conduct urine from the kidney to the bladder, may be damaged and a fistula, a hole, may be created. If this happens, the woman may have to have an operation whereby a new opening for urinary wastes is made and the urine then collected in a plastic

361

bag attached to the outside of the body. Then, too, there is a higher death rate for radical operations than for a simple hysterectomy. All of this must be balanced against the chances that doing less than a radical hysterectomy will leave microscopic areas of cancer behind.

A few doctors will argue that conization is sufficient, but most doctors believe that this form of surgery is inadequate for Stage IA cases. Even if the tissue removed via conization encompasses the entire microinvasive area, they feel that the chances are too great that cancerous or precancerous cells may be lurking in the remaining portions of the cervix. Since some areas of the cervix have already "gone bad"—have developed invasive cancer—they feel that there may be some basic fault in the cervical tissue that will eventually produce more cancer, which, if not detected in time, could become truly invasive cancer. If this happened, the woman's chances of surviving would be significantly reduced. Therefore, the vast majority of doctors do not advocate conization for Stage IA. Women whose doctors do suggest that conization is adequate treatment would be wise to seek a second opinion.

One reason that no one is quite sure how microinvasive cancer behaves, that is, whether or not the tissues adjacent to the cervix and the pelvic lymph nodes are ever involved, is that definitions of microinvasion differ. Basically microinvasive cancer is a carcinoma cancer that is "in place," that has begun to invade, but the invasion is in its very early stages. In fact, the invasion is microscopic. Some authorities are very conservative and define microinvasion as penetration of three mm or less; others use five mm as the cut-off point. Still others feel that it is the total volume of the cancer that is significant. Most doctors feel that evidence of invasion of the blood or lymph vessels excludes a diagnosis of microinvasion.

Because the definitions of microinvasion differ, it is difficult to compare the results of studies that attempt to find out whether microinvasion does or does not involve these adjacent tissues and lymph nodes. Studies in which radical hysterectomies and pelvic lymphadenectomies were done on women diagnosed as having microinvasive cancer and in which the removed lymph nodes were examined microscopically have reported between 0-5 percent incidence of lymph node involvement.[16] The trouble is that the authors of these studies have used different definitions of microinvasion. However, it seems fairly certain that microinvasive cases in which the penetration is less than 3 mm and the width less than 2.5 cm, and in which there is no sign of blood or lymph vessel penetration, don't involve the pelvic lymph nodes or adjacent tissue. A simple hysterectomy will therefore suffice in these cases.[17] Women with microinvasive cancer should discuss the various treatment options as they relate to their particular cases and should seek second opinions before deciding on a course of treatment.

Stages IB and IIA[18]

In these cases it is necessary to treat the cervix, uterus, upper third of the vagina and the pelvic lymph nodes, for even when there is no obvious sign of involvement of these areas, there is a high likelihood that they are involved in the disease process.

Two forms of treatment, surgery or radiation therapy, are used to treat Stage IB and IIA. In certain instances they may be used in combination. Both forms of treatment have been shown to be about equally effective in terms of survival rates. Generally speaking, if the woman is in good health, a radical hysterectomy and pelvic lymphadenectomy will be done, for this allows for better vaginal function. Radiation therapy causes a narrowing of the vaginal canal, a condition known as vaginal stenosis, which can make intercourse painful or downright impossible. Even though the upper portion of the vagina is removed surgically, and the vaginal canal is therefore shortened, intercourse is usually still possible.

Moreover, radiation destroys the ovaries, whereas surgery can sometimes allow for preservation of the ovaries. This is important in younger women, for destruction of the ovaries can cause premature menopause, which is apt to be more severe than a natural menopause. Even if the ovaries must be removed surgically, the operation is preferable to radiation, for there is some evidence that radiation-induced menopause puts a woman at higher risk for hypertension than a surgical or natural menopause.

Moreover, it is known that radiation can cause as well as cure cancer. By having surgical treatment the woman can avoid exposure to dangerous radiation. For older women this may not be as important a consideration as it is for younger women, since it may take 15-20 years for the radiation-induced cancer to develop.

If, after microscopic examination of the tissues removed surgically, cancer is found in the lymph nodes or at the outermost edges of the removed tissue, external beam therapy is given postoperatively. Postoperative radiation is also given if the cancer turns out to be more advanced than was originally thought, if there is any sign of ovarian involvement or if the tumor turns out to be too widespread for complete surgical removal. Radiation therapy is also used in cases where the woman's health will not permit surgery. External beam therapy is generally given first, before internal radiation. This shrinks the tumor and makes it easier to insert the containers for the radioactive implants. One advantage that radiation has over surgery in these cases is that should the woman treated with surgery require postoperative radiation, her complication rates are much higher. If she had been treated with radiation in the first place, she would have had fewer problems. Of course, the assumption in these Stage IB and IIA cases is that the woman will not require postoperative radiation, but as explained above, pretreatment estimates of the disease are frequently wrong. Upon operation the disease may turn out to be more serious, requiring postoperative radiation.

In certain instances, external beam therapy may be followed by surgery in the form of a hysterectomy. This is done when the woman has a tumor that is large and has caused the cervix to assume a bulky, barrel shape and protrude into the vagina. Such tumors are difficult to treat with radiation implants because of their size and because they distort the anatomy so much that the proper containers can't be inserted.

Stages IIB and IIIA and B[18]

The treatment choice in these cases is limited, for the disease has spread so widely that surgical removal is not feasible. The complication and fatality rates would simply be too high, so radiation is the treatment of choice. Generally, external beam therapy is given first, followed by radiation implants. In certain cases interstitial radiation, which involves inserting needles directly into the tumor, may be used.

Stage IV[18]

Most of these cases are treated with radiation therapy; however, in certain instances, surgery may be the treatment of choice. For example, if a woman has Stage IVA disease, in which the bladder and/or rectum is involved, but there is no evidence that the tissues adjacent to the uterus are involved, partial or total pelvic exenteration may be done, for the bladder and rectum are extremely sensitive to radiation and doses sufficient to kill the tumor would destroy these organs. In other Stage IV cases, radiation therapy may be used. Sometimes, when the disease has spread to distant points in the body, lower doses of radiation may be given in hopes of providing relief of symptoms even if it is not possible to cure the disease.

Follow-Up and Recurrent Cancer[18]

Women who have been treated for cervical cancer will need lifelong follow-up. The nature of the follow-up program will depend on the extent of the initial disease. Many cases of recurrent cancer are asymptomatic and may be discovered only when a Pap smear is made. If a woman has been treated by radiation therapy, however, there may be problems in diagnosing recurrent cancer, for radiation can alter the character of the cells and the Pap smear may be hard to read. Needle biopsies or conization may then be necessary.

Although many cases of recurrent cancer are asymptomatic, there is a classic triad of symptoms that is often present, which includes swelling of the legs, pain in the lower back and urinary problems.

Treatment of recurrent cancer will depend on what type of therapy was used initially. If radiation was used to treat the original cancer, surgery must be used to treat the recurrent cancer, for, assuming that the woman was treated properly in the first place, the tissues in the area will already have had the maximum dose of radiation they can tolerate.

If the recurrent cancer is limited to the cervix, a radical hysterectomy and pelvic lymphadenectomy may suffice. But most recurrent cancer has already spread beyond the cervix and will require a partial or total pelvic exenteration. Not all women with recurrent cancer are in good enough health to allow for this radical form of surgery. For those who are, there is a 20—30 percent five-year survival rate following pelvic exenteration,[19] so the operation may well be worth the risks. Several factors affect a woman's chances of surviving following radical surgery for recurrent cancer, including the presence or absence of obvious symptoms, the location and extent of the recurrence, the time between the primary treatment and the diagnosis of recurrent cancer and the results of special X-ray studies known as intravenous pyelograms. Each woman should discuss the exenteration procedure and survival rates as they apply to her case before deciding about this procedure.

If the woman was initially treated by surgery, the recurrent cancer is generally treated by radiation therapy. But in cases where the initial surgery was minimal, it may be possible to do more extensive surgery for recurrent cancer.

Survival Rates

Survival rates for cervical cancer are generally given in terms of five years. Table 11 reflects typical survival rates.

Table 11
Five-Year Survival Rates For Cervical Cancer*

Stage	Percent
I	79.2
II	58.1
III	32.5
IV	8.2

*SOURCE: Juan A. del Regado and Harlan J. Spjot, *Cancer,* 5th ed. (St. Louis: C. V. Mosby Co., 1977), p. 789.

The Uterus and the Fallopian Tubes

The anatomy of the uterus and the Fallopian tubes is described and illustrated in Chapter Two. The uterus has two parts, the body, or fundus, and the neck, or cervix. In this section, we are concerned only with diseases that affect the Fallopian tubes and the body of the uterus; cervical diseases are discussed in a separate section.

In some cases, though, the uterus and tubes are just the focal point for more widespread pelvic diseases. For instance, the first disease in this section, pelvic inflammatory disease, may involve only the Fallopian tubes, or less frequently, only the endometrial lining of the uterus; however, the infection in the tubes may spill out into the pelvic cavity, causing a more generalized infection. In a similar vein, endometriosis, described under the second heading in this section, is a condition that can affect the entire pelvic cavity. In endometriosis the endometrial tissue, which is normally found only on the inside of the uterus, grows on the ovaries or other organs in the abdominal cavity. Adenomyosis, the third condition discussed in this section, is basically the same as endometriosis, the only differences being that adenomyosis is usually diagnosed in older women and that the misplaced endometrial tissue is not spread throughout the pelvic cavity but is confined to the muscular tissue of the uterine walls.

Another set of problems that may involve the uterus and tubes are conditions that cause distortions of the normal anatomy. A woman may have congenital abnormalities and may be born with a uterus or tubes that are malformed or absent altogether. The uterus may not lie in the usual anatomical location. It may be tipped forward or backward. It may fall, or prolapse, to a lower position that normal. The anatomy of the uterus may also be disturbed by a condition known as Asherman's syndrome, in which the walls of the endometrial cavity are partially or totally stuck together.

Abnormal growths may be found in the uterus and/or the Fallopian tubes. These may be noncancerous, like fibroid tumors, endometrial polyps and benign tumors of the tube, or they may be malignant, as in cancer of the uterus or cancer of the Fallopian tube. Sometimes the endometrial lining of the uterus grows too thick, a condition known as hyperplasia, which, in some instances, may be the first step on the road to cancer.

Many of the conditions described in this chapter will cause abnormal uterine bleeding or irregular menstrual periods; however, a separate section, Menstrual Problems, is devoted to these topics.

PELVIC INFLAMMATORY DISEASE

AKA: PID

Types: subacute pelvic inflammatory disease
acute pelvic inflammatory disease
chronic pelvic inflammatory disease

Associated terms: genital tuberculosis; endometritis; paraendometritis; salpingitis; oophoritis; peritonitis; pelvic cellulitis; tubal occlusion; tubal, tubo-ovarian, or pelvic abscess; tubo-ovarian cyst; pyosalpinx, hydrosalpinx, or pyohydrosalpinx; thrombophlebitis; blood poisoning, or septicemia

Pelvic inflammatory disease (PID) is a catch-all phrase that refers to inflammations of the pelvic organs. The disease may be subacute, acute or chronic. Subacute is the least severe and most common type. It is slow in its onset, and mild or moderate symptoms may persist for a week or two before a woman seeks treatment. Acute PID refers to an infection that is more sudden in its onset and more severe. The woman is apt to experience a sudden onset of pain, weakness and fever or chills. Chronic PID is a low-grade infection that may persist for a week or months, and in some women it never seems to go away completely. There may be constant mild, moderate or even severe pain, or the chronic infection may flare up occasionally, causing acute attacks.

Cause

PID is caused by germs that migrate from the vagina through the cervical opening into the upper organs. Any number of organisms may be responsible for PID. Gonococcus, the organism that causes gonorrhea and that gets into the vagina during sexual intercourse, is frequently the culprit. *E. coli*, a bacteria that lives in the rectum, may make its way into the vagina and past the cervix. Other types of bacteria, some of which are normal inhabitants of the vagina, may move past the cervix into the normally germfree uterus and tubes and cause infection. Some doctors think that the organisms that cause some of the common vaginal infections may, at times, be responsible for PID, but most doctors feel that these organisms are rarely, if ever, the cause of PID. A few cases of PID may be the result of tuberculosis bacteria. Cases of genital TB are, however, rare in this country. When it does occur it is usually secondary to tuberculosis somewhere else in the body (usually the lungs), which has traveled via the bloodstream to the pelvic organs. It can also be transmitted sexually through intercourse with an infected partner, but this is quite rare.

Most of the time, the cervix forms a natural barrier that prevents the bacteria that normally live in the vagina from moving upward into the sterile uterus or tubes; however, at certain times the cervical canal is dilated (opened up); thus, the germs may spread beyond this natural barrier. For example, the opening to the cervical canal is slightly dilated during a woman's period to allow for the passage of menstrual blood. Gonococci, in particular, seem to thrive on menstrual blood, and symptoms of gonorrheal PID often make their first appearance after a menstrual period.

The cervix is also dilated after childbirth, abortion, miscarriage and various types of pelvic operations, such as a D&C. Similarly, inserting an intrauterine device (IUD) involves dilating the cervix, so infections can occur after insertion. Some doctors feel this type of infection occurs only rarely; others feel it is a relatively common occurrence. At any rate, whether it's common or rare, IUD-related PID certainly does exist (*see* p. 123).

Spread of the Disease and Possible Complications

Different types of organisms will have different ways of spreading. With some bacteria, gonococcus in particular, the disease may pass the cervical barrier and the endometrial lining of the uterus may become infected, a condition known as endometritis. The endometrial lining is, however, shed each month and has a particularly strong immunological response to defend it from bacteria, so infections of the endometrial lining are often self-limiting. It is also possible for the uterine muscles as well as the lining to become infected, a condition known as endoparametritis. These deeper infections are not self-limiting.

The blood-rich endometrial lining provides a nourishing environment for disease-causing organisms, so that even though the endometrial lining is shed each month, ridding the uterus of superficial infections, bacteria may thrive and quickly spread to the Fallopian tubes. By the time the menstrual flow washes the infection out of the uterine lining, it may have already spread to the tubes. When the infection involves the tubes, the term salpingitis is used. In the past, most cases of PID involved both tubes; today, however, we are seeing IUD-related PID, which often involves only one tube, with increasing frequency.

From this point, the infection may spread along the length of the tubes and spill out the ends, infecting the ovaries. Infection of the ovaries is called oophoritis. It may also spill into the pelvic cavity, causing an infection of the peritoneum, the layer of tissue that coats the inside of the pelvic cavity. This condition is called peritonitis. The term "peritonitis," is not, however, exclusively associated with PID, for a number of different conditions, including a burst appendix, a ruptured ovarian cyst and endometriosis, can also cause this condition.

Rather than following this path along the mucous membranes, through the uterus, into the Fallopian tubes and possibly the ovaries and pelvic cavity, some organisms tend to spread through lymph or blood systems, causing a generalized pelvic infection. The term "pelvic cellulitis" may be used in such cases.

Sometimes, infections spreading through the tubes will cause a good deal of pus, distending the tubes. Adhesions (bands of scar tissue) may be formed within the tube as the body tries to defend itself against infection. The ends of the tube may seal themselves off, either partially or totally. In this manner, tubal occlusions (blockages), tubal abscesses or a hydropyosalpinx (localized collections of pus) may be formed. If the ovary is involved in the abscess, the term "tubo-ovarian abscess" or "tubo-ovarian inflammatory cyst" may be used. If the infection spills into the pelvic cavity, adhesions or abscesses called pelvic abscesses may be formed. Any of these abscesses may rupture, destroying the tubes or creating extensive adhesions that can restrict the movement of the tubes and other pelvic organs. Infertility or sterility may result from cases of PID involving tubal blockages, abscesses and extensive adhesions.

If the disease spreads through the blood system, infection in the veins may cause the formation of blood clots, a condition referred to as thrombophlebitis, or blood poisoning, a condition referred to as septicemia. Both of these conditions can be serious and, in some cases, fatal.

Symptoms

The kinds of symptoms produced by PID and their severity will depend on the type of germ causing the infection, the strength of the particular strain

369

of bacteria, the organs that are affected as the disease spreads and the woman's own resistance to disease.

The symptoms, which may be mild, moderate or severe, may develop gradually or come on suddenly. Any of the following symptoms may occur with acute PID: pelvic pain or tenderness, low back pain, pain during or after intercourse, persistent cramps, fever, chills, abnormal vaginal discharge, abnormal menstrual periods, bleeding between periods, urinary frequency and urgency, abdominal pain with bowel movements or urination, fatigue or weakness, cramping or rigidity of the abdominal muscles, swelling of the lymph nodes, nausea, vomiting or a rapid pulse.

Chronic PID may cause some of the same symptoms. The pain in chronic PID may range from a mild bearing-down discomfort to a nagging discomfort in the lower abdomen to severe, sharp pains. The pain may be constant or may come and go. Characteristically, the pain symptoms are worse just before or during the menstrual period.

Diagnosis

Sometimes diagnosing PID is a fairly straightforward matter. A history of recent gonorrheal infection, childbirth, abortion, IUD insertion or other situations causing cervical dilation, plus the symptoms mentioned above, will make the doctor suspicious. Bimanual exam, which may be quite painful, may reveal tubal enlargement and the presence of tubal, tubo-ovarian or pelvic abscesses, which may feel quite hot and be extremely tender. Speculum exam may show pus dripping from the cervix, and the doctor will take a sample of the discharge and run a culture and sensitivity (C&S) test. This may indicate what type of organism is causing the disease and help the doctor to select an appropriate antibiotic. Unfortunately, culture and sensitivity tests are not always accurate in determining the cause of PID. Even when pus is coming out of the uterus, the C&S test may be inaccurate, for a different organism may be at work in the tubes and ovaries than in the uterus.

The diagnosis of PID is not always an easy task. Both chronic and acute PID may be mistaken for a number of different conditions, including appendicitis, rupture or torsion of an ovarian cyst, ectopic pregnancy, or pelvic endometriosis. Sometimes the only way to make a definite diagnosis is through laparoscopic or culdoscopic examinations, in which specialized viewing instruments are inserted into the pelvic cavity through surgical incisions. In certain cases, ultrasound or X-ray exams may be used in diagnosis.

Diagnosis can be a real problem in mild cases with subtle symptoms. One of the insidious things about PID is that a subtle, smoldering infection can cause infertility and lead to recurrent attacks of severe pain in the future. So if you have one of the symptoms described above, especially if you have recently given birth, had a miscarriage, abortion or surgery or have an IUD, be sure to consult a doctor.

Treatment

Oral antibiotics are almost always used to treat PID. As soon as the diagnosis is made, treatment is begun with one of the broad-spectrum antibiotics, such as ampicillin or tetracycline, which are effective against a wide variety of bacteria. If the final results of the culture and sensitivity test indicate that another, more specific type of antibiotic would be more effective, the medication may be changed. The antibiotic may be given for a period of one or two weeks, at which time the woman is reexamined. If the disease has subsided, another week's worth of antibiotics may be given to prevent a recurrence.

Many women are justifiably hesitant about taking antibiotics; however, PID is one of the instances in which antibiotics are vitally important. Attempting home remedies can be dangerous in treating acute or subacute PID. It is important to treat the disease as early and as effectively as possible in order to prevent adhesions and abscesses, which can lead to infertility, sterility, chronic pain, surgical removal of the pelvic organs or, in extreme cases, death. All the prescribed medications should be taken, even if the symptoms have subsided, for an incomplete course of medication can lead to recurrences.

In addition to antibiotics, bed rest and plenty of fluids to flush out the body are *vitally* important. Bed rest will prevent jarring of the uterus and tubes, which might aggravate the inflammation and slow down the healing process. Ideally, the woman should stay in bed until the pain is gone and her temperature has returned to normal, getting up only to use the bathroom or to eat. Vaginal or anal intercourse, which can move the pelvic organs, should be avoided because it could spread pus from one part of the tube to the other or even cause pus to spill out into the pelvic cavity.

Heat is helpful in treating PID, for the blood flow to the tubes may be severely restricted and heat will increase the blood flow to the area. It will also help in relieving the pain. Hot sitz baths three or four times a day will bring heat to the pelvic area. Hot-water bottles and heating pads are less efficient but still effective.

If the first course of antibiotics doesn't clear up the infection, a second and possibly a third course may be prescribed. If the infection doesn't improve or if it gets worse, particularly if there is a temperature over 102°, persistent vomiting, diarrhea or pain, the woman may be hospitalized and given intravenous (IV) antiobiotics. Administering antibiotics directly into a vein allows for higher, more effective doses than can be absorbed through the stomach when the drugs are given orally. A week of IV antibiotics and complete bed rest often cures PID.

If a woman has PID and has an intrauterine device, it may be necessary to remove the IUD. If the symptoms of PID do not subside within the first several days of treatment, or perhaps sooner if the symptoms are severe, the IUD must be removed. Unfortunately, some doctors are not conscientious about this. Leaving an IUD in could aggravate the PID and lead to some of the serious complications described earlier, so if you have an IUD be sure to discuss removal with your doctor.

Sometimes the disease will become chronic. Tissues may have been so damaged by the infection that they never heal properly, making a woman vulnerable to repeated infection, or the bacteria may become walled off by adhesions or become buried in pelvic abscesses where antibiotics cannot reach them. Thus, the woman may have a low-grade infection and chronic pain that may flare up in acute attacks of PID from time to time.

There are a number of treatment options with chronic PID. If oral antibiotics have failed, IV antibiotic treatment, as outlined above, may be tried. If, however, there are pelvic abscesses, even IV antibiotics may not work. In such cases, it is sometimes possible to operate and drain the abscesses with a needle.

If a woman has tubo-ovarian abscesses, it is necessary to operate to make sure that the ovarian enlargement is not due to a benign or malignant ovarian tumor. Moreover, the abscesses could rupture and cause acute peritonitis or blood poisoning. In some cases, it is possible to drain these abscesses.

Sometimes a hysterectomy is the only way for a woman to get relief from chronic pain; however, women should ask their doctors if IV antibiotics or drainage can be attempted before consenting to a hysterectomy. If the PID is not too severe, some women choose to live with their symptoms or to explore alternative therapies like acupuncture rather than having a hysterectomy. In certain cases it is possible to remove the uterus and obtain relief from chronic PID and yet spare at least one ovary, thereby preventing premature menopause. Women who are anxious to obtain relief but who are reluctant to have a premature menopause should investigate this possibility with their doctors.

Prevention

Women can minimize their chances of getting PID by being very careful anytime the cervix becomes dilated. For two to three weeks after having an abortion, a D&C or miscarriage, nothing should be put into the vagina. This means no intercourse, tampons, fingers or douche nozzles. Nor should they take a bath, swim or douche. (Showers or sponge baths are all right). After childbirth the same precautions should apply, but for a period of six weeks.

If a woman wants to minimize her chances of getting PID or has a history of pelvic infections, she should probably not use an IUD. Women should also know that taking birth control pills not only increases their chances of getting infections such as gonorrhea, but also increases the chances that the infection will progress to PID should they get gonorrhea. Wiping from front to back after a bowel movement will help prevent rectal bacteria from entering the vagina. Prompt treatment of vaginal infections may also help to prevent PID. Routine gonorrhea cultures are also an important part of PID prevention.

ENDOMETRIOSIS

Associated terms: chocolate cysts

The uterus is lined with a special type of tissue, the endometrium, which, in response to stimulation by the female hormones, swells and thickens each month in preparation for the possibility of pregnancy. If there is no pregnancy, this blood-rich lining is no longer needed. It then breaks down, begins to shed and the menstrual flow starts. Normally, this type of hormone-responsive tissue is found only inside the uterus; hence the name, endometrial—*endo* ("inside") and *metrial* ("uterus") tissue.

With endometriosis, it's a case of the right thing in the wrong place, for endometriosis is a condition in which the endometrial tissue is found growing outside the uterus. It may, for instance, be found on the ovaries or on the peritoneum, the layer of tissue that coats the surfaces of the organs and the interior walls of the pelvic cavity. In some rare cases it has even been found in such remote locations as the forearm and the lungs. Even though the endometrial tissue has wound up in some abnormal location, it continues to thicken, break down and shed each month, which, as we shall see, can cause pain and other problems.

Incidence

Since the condition is related to hormone production, it is not surprising that it is most commonly reported in women whose hormones are active, that is, women between the ages of puberty and menopause. Seventy-five percent of the cases are reported in women who are 25 to 45 years old. It has, however, been found both in adolescents and in older women who have passed menopause and are no longer menstruating. Some doctors think that pregnancy has a preventive or curative effect on endometriosis.

Cause

No one is certain what causes this condition. There are basically three theories, all of which may be correct. One theory is that tiny shreds of endometrial tissue find their way into the pelvic cavity through the Fallopian tubes during menstruation. In other words, it's a sort of backup problem (please excuse the plumbing analogy). Instead of being shed through the cervical os into the vagina and onto a sanitary napkin or tampon, some bits of menstrual tissue and blood may float up through the tubes, spill out the ends and float around the pelvic cavity until they attach themselves to the ovaries or to one of the other organs in the area.*

Another theory is based on the fact that for the most part, the tissue that makes up the organs in the female pelvis is the same basic tissue with various modifications. It all develops from the same fetal tissue. As the fetus grows, this tissue is modified. The simplest modifications of this basic tissue form one kind of organ; with a few more modifications, there is another variety of tissue that becomes another sort of organ, and so on, until a very fancy material, the endometrial tissue, develops that can do all sorts of wonderful tricks and is complete with such options as the ability to respond to hormonal messages by growing rich and thick or breaking down and to feed the developing fetus in the case of pregnancy. In a sense, the other pelvic tissues are just endometrial tissues that didn't continue developing and get all these extra options. With all this unrealized growth potential in these other tissues, it's not surprising, according to this theory, that here and there are nests of tissue that, perhaps in response to hormone stimulation, haven't stopped modifying. Thus, this tissue goes on to get the extra options, even though they aren't necessary for the job it's supposed to be doing.

The third theory suggests that endometriosis may be spread through the blood or lymph systems, which would explain the presence, though rare, of endometriosis in some bizarre locations, such as the lungs, underarms and thighs.

*Vaginal tampons cannot *cause* the menstrual flow to back up. In fact, tampons actually act as a wick to draw the blood out of the uterus.

Symptoms

Endometriosis can occur almost anywhere in the pelvic cavity. It will look and behave somewhat differently depending on where the endometrial tissue is located.

On the ovaries, which are involved in about 60 percent of the cases, there may be single or multiple areas of endometriosis. The areas may be as small as a pinhead and are rarely larger than an orange. The smaller ones look like blood blisters and may be bluish, dusty red or brownish black in color, depending on how much fresh or old blood is present. Typically, both ovaries are affected.

The ovarian tissue may protect itself from this foreign endometrial tissue by growing a sort of lid of tissue over the implant, forming what is called an endometrial cyst. Since the misplaced endometrial tissue can respond to hormones just as the normal tissue within the uterus does, it may bleed cyclically, at the time of menstruation. Thus, the cysts swell with menstrual blood. Over time, this blood takes on a thick, tarry texture and a dark brown color; hence, the term "chocolate cysts" that is sometimes used in reference to endometriosis.

The periodic swelling may cause the cyst to rupture, usually just before or immediately after menstruation. When the cyst breaks, the contents are spilled into the pelvic cavity. This is one way in which bits of endometrial tissue may be spread to other parts of the pelvic cavity.

This swelling and rupture also explain much of the pain that is associated with endometriosis. The old blood from the cyst is highly irritating to the lining of the pelvic cavity and causes inflammation and pain. In some cases, the pain may be so severe that emergency surgery is necessary.

In response to this inflammation, the cells in the rest of the area secrete bands of fibrous material that solidify and, typically, seal over the ruptured cyst. These fibrous adhesions can literally plaster the ovary to the broad ligament, the wall of supportive tissue that extends from the side of the uterus to the wall of the pelvic cavity. Repeated spillage from ruptured cysts can produce adhesions that bind the organs together, so that the pelvic organs become one large immovable mass. Then the pelvis can no longer yield to pressure. Movement of the cervix due to intercourse or a doctor's exam or any sort of pressure on this unyielding pelvis can produce severe pain and backache.

Endometriosis may also be present in other locations in the body, either in conjunction with endometriosis on the ovary or independently. If endometriosis is present on the lining of the pelvic cavity or on the supportive tissues that hold the uterus in place, it may look and behave somewhat differently. In most cases it appears as a varying number of small blueberrylike spots. These may group together to form solid, knobby bumps. These areas of endometriosis may also menstruate at first, but as the disease progresses, so much scar tissue is formed that the endometrial tissue is compressed and can no longer menstruate. Thus, there will often be puckered, clawlike areas of endometriosis that are no longer active. The damage may be considerable before this inactive stage is reached, for the scarring draws more tissue and adjacent organs inward as it progresses. The endometrial tissue, even though it is no longer menstruating, may continue to swell somewhat each month. Since the scar tissue is firm and unyielding, this can result in a considerable amount of pain.

Endometriosis can also affect the large and small intestines. On the large intestine it may look just like cancer, but unlike cancer, endometriosis, except in rare instances, will not cause bleeding from the rectum. In the rare case where such bleeding is associated with endometriosis, it occurs only at the time of menstruation. In both the large and small intestine, the endometrial implants can cause obstruction. In the large bowel this may cause increasing constipation, which gets worse at the time of menstruation and is often accompanied by a sharp cramp and the urgent need to go to the bathroom even though little urine or feces is eliminated. In the small intestine this endometrial blockage may be associated with lower abdominal pain, abdominal swelling and vomiting. These symptoms may also be aggravated at the time of menstruation, but not as noticeably as in the large intestine.

If the endometriosis is extensive, it may involve the rectum, vagina and vulva. In the vagina it can be seen on speculum examination as firm, bluish domelike bulges. These may cause considerable pain on intercourse if located near the top of the vagina. Less often, these bluish bulges may be seen on the vulva. If the rectum is involved, there may be severe intestinal cramps and pain when moving the bowels, especially at the time of the menstrual period.

Infrequently, endometriosis affects the bladder and the urethra, the tube that runs from the bladder to the urinary opening. When this does happen, it can cause pain on urination, urinary retention, urinary frequency, very occasionally blood in the urine (particularly on or at the time of menstruation) and pain in the flanks radiating toward the groin.

Single nodules of endometrial tissue called endometriomas may be found in scars from operations and childbirth. Although such growths have appeared as long as sixteen years later, most appear in less than two years. Similarly, these endometriomas may appear in the region of the belly button even if there has not been an operation. They may appear as blue-colored bulges and occasionally will break through the skin and cause bleeding. In rare cases, endometriomas have even been found in lungs, thighs, forearms and underarms. Edometriomas are firm, even hard, vary considerably in size and are painful and tender to the touch, especially when they swell as menstruation approaches.

In general, pelvic pain associated with the menstrual cycle is the earliest and most common symptom associated with endometriosis. The pain is usually one of two types. The first type of pain, associated with the menstrual period, typically occurs in women who have previously had relatively painfree periods. It is usually steady and dull as opposed to cramplike and becomes progressively worse with each subsequent menstrual period. In contrast to this type of pain, the second type is a lower abdominal pain that begins just before the period. It varies according to the location and extent of the endometriosis. In certain locations there is no pain. In fact, about 25 percent of the women afflicted have no pain at all. In the early stages there is usually less pain, but it gets progressively worse.

One curious thing is that women with relatively little endometriosis may have a lot more pain than women who have fairly widespread implants. It is not entirely clear why this happens, but it is probably related to the amount of scar tissue, where it occurs and how often the cysts rupture. For example, women with large ovarian cysts may not ovulate, while those who have endometriosis only on the lining of the pelvic cavity often do. Absence of ovulation seems to cause the disease to regress, and thereby minimizes pain.

Women who have endometriosis frequently have abnormal menstrual bleeding. About a half to two-thirds of all patients with endometriosis have such problems. However, it is not clear that the irregular bleeding is caused by the endometriosis. The disease is often accompanied by associated problems, such as fibroids and uterine polyps. The bleeding may actually be due to these associated diseases. If women with associated fibroids and/or polyps are eliminated, only about 20 percent of the women with endometriosis will complain of menstrual irregularities.

Infertility is also common to women who have endometriosis; however, about 20 percent of the women involved already have one or more children. Often, such women will be unable to add another child to their families no matter how hard they try. No one is sure just why such women are infertile. Perhaps the adhesions around the ovary and Fallopian tube interfere with the normal process of ovulation. The pain associated with intercourse may have some relationship to the low fertility rate as well.

Diagnosis

At times, the diagnosis of endometriosis is a simple matter, but other times it can be very tricky, especially when the endometriosis is minimal. The symptoms may alert the doctor to the possibility, but 25 percent of the women with endometriosis will be asymptomatic. Moreover, many times the symptoms that are present could be caused by a number of other diseases. Sometimes a careful bimanual exam will help the doctor make the diagnosis. If, for instance, the doctor can feel knobby endometrial growths in certain areas, it may clear up the confusion that often exists between endometriosis and chronic pelvic inflammatory disease. But sometimes the areas of endometriosis are too small to be felt or too inaccessibly placed to be reached by the examining doctor's fingers. Sometimes the doctor's palpation (feeling) will identify swollen areas that might be endometriosis but could also be other things. For instance, chocolate cysts on the ovaries may be large enough to be felt, but it may not be clear whether these are ovarian tumors or endometrial tissue.

It is often impossible, then, to make a definite diagnosis of endometriosis without actually taking a look at the pelvic organs by means of a laparoscopic examination, which involves making a small incision in the abdomen and inserting a lighted viewing instrument into the abdominal cavity. Sometimes a culdoscopic examination, which involves inserting a similar viewing instrument into the pelvic cavity through an incision in the upper vagina, will be useful.

Because a definite diagnosis can be obtained only by laparoscopic or culdoscopic examination, both of which involve the risks of surgery, in certain cases a woman might decide to try hormone therapy (described below) even though her doctor cannot be sure that she actually has endometriosis without these examinations. (This choice, however, cannot be made if the woman has ovarian enlargement, for reasons explained under Treatment.) However, since diagnoses made without benefit of laparoscopic or culdoscopic evaluation are wrong in more than 40 percent of cases, accepting treatment on the basis of a presumptive rather than a definite diagnosis may very likely mean that the woman is subjecting herself to unnecessary treatment. If a woman decides to accept treatment on the basis of the presumptive diagnosis, she should be convinced that the risks and expense of laparoscopy outweigh the risks and expense of undergoing possibly unnecessary hormone therapy.

Treatment

Treatment of endometriosis is a complex subject. The type of treatment suggested will depend on many factors, including the age of the woman, the severity of the symptoms, the location and extent of the endometriosis and future childbearing plans. In certain cases there is general agreement among doctors about treatment of the condition, but in other cases there is considerable debate. Since there is such controversy, women with endometriosis should familiarize themselves with the various treatments available.

If the symptoms are not severe and the endometriosis is not widespread, a wait-and-see approach may be appropriate. Women nearing menopause may decide to avoid the risks and expense of treatment and to use painkillers or live with their symptoms, since, with the diminished output of ovarian hormones at menopause, the condition often regresses. Younger women with mild symptoms may make this same sort of decision, especially if they don't have an associated infertility problem or future childbearing plans. Even women in their 20s who *do* plan to have children in the future will sometimes decide to forego treatment, at least temporarily, for a number of women with endometriosis do achieve pregnancy without treatment. Indeed, spontaneous cures of endometriosis sometimes occur. But it should be mentioned that many doctors recommend that women with endometriosis begin their childbearing earlier than they may have otherwise intended since the disease generally tends to become progressively worse and may impair fertility. Delaying pregnancy may make it difficult or even impossible for such women to get pregnant.

In cases where there are large areas of endometriosis on the ovaries, a wait-and-see approach is not appropriate even if the symptoms are minimal. This is true for a number of reasons. First of all, the enlargement of the ovaries may be due to cancerous or noncancerous ovarian growths. Since this possibility exists, any persistent ovarian enlargement deserves investigation. Secondly, the possibility also exists that the ovarian endometrial cyst will rupture, necessitating emergency surgery. Rupture could also spread disease to other areas of the pelvic cavity, causing more severe symptoms and necessitating more radical surgery later on. Moreover, the endometrial cyst may continue to grow larger, progressively displacing the ovarian tissue and impairing ovarian function, which could bring on premature menopause or result in infertility.

When there are large areas of ovarian endometriosis, severe symptoms or an infertility problem that cannot be traced to another cause and that the woman is anxious to overcome, the wait-and-see approach must be abandoned. Two types of treatment are then available—hormone therapy or surgery.

Hormone Therapy

The idea of using hormones to treat endometriosis stemmed from the observations of early researchers that pregnancy, a time of high hormonal levels and suppression of ovulation, often resulted in cures, or at least nine symptomfree months. Some researchers have since disputed this observation, claiming that as many cases of endometriosis progressed as regressed during pregnancy. The traditional recommendation that a woman have her first child at an early age and space her children every few years in order to prevent or cure endometriosis is therefore losing credibility, perhaps because women decided the "cure" (that is, having a large family) was more limiting than the disease. At any rate, aside from the question of whether or not the original observations about pregnancy and regression of endometriosis were valid, the fact remains that hormone therapy has worked for many women.

Over the years a variety of different hormone therapies have been used. All of these treatments have one thing in common: They stop a woman from having her period. Stopping the process during which the thickened endometrial lining inside the uterus breaks down and is shed means that the misplaced endometrial lining won't thicken or shed either, and that the symptoms of endometriosis, which are aggravated by this thickening and shedding process, are therefore relieved. Sometimes stopping menstruation for a while also seems to "dry up" existing disease, resulting in a cure. In the past, male-type androgen hormones in the form of methyltestosterone, sold under brand names like Metandren and Oreton, were used, but these often caused masculinizing side effects, like male hair-growth patterns, decrease in breast size, clitoral enlargement and deepening of the voice, some of which were not reversible once drug use was discontinued. Moreover, since this type of hormone therapy did not always suppress ovulation, there was a chance that the woman might get pregnant, and if so, there was the very real risk that the child would have abnormalities. Thus, this type of therapy is rarely used today and any woman whose doctor suggests it should question the reasoning behind this type of therapy. She should also seek a second opinion (*see* p. 226) before accepting such treatment.

High doses of estrogen were also used in the past; however, this also produced a high rate of side effects, of the type associated with any overabundance of estrogen (nausea, breast tenderness and weight gain). Moreover, the use of estrogen, particularly in high doses, has been associated with serious, even fatal complications, so that it too has fallen out of favor.

Today, a new drug, danazol, sold under the brand name Danocrin, is the preferred medical treatment for moderate and severe cases of endometriosis. It stops ovulation, preventing the egg from bursting out of its follicular sac. Without a burst follicle, no progesterone can be produced. Thus, there is no shedding of endometrial tissue, which in turn means relief from symptoms. In addition, danazol seems to work directly on the endometriosis, "drying" it up. It also works faster than the other types of hormone treatments, often providing relief of pain during the first menstrual period after treatment is begun. Moreover, women taking danazol, unlike those taking progesterone-type drugs (see below), whose menstrual cycles may take many months or even years to return to normal after treatment is stopped, resume normal menstrual cycles within, at most, three months after the drug is discontinued. Thus, the drug is particularly appropriate for women who have future childbearing plans. Then, too, while on the drug a woman reportedly cannot get pregnant, so the chances of hormone-induced birth defects are eliminated. Pregnant women should not, however, take danazol, for the possibility of birth defects does exist.

Danazol also has less severe side effects than many of the other hormone treatments. This is not to say that danazol doesn't have side effects; it does. It can cause weight gain, bloating, bleeding between periods, acne, growth of facial and chest hair, decrease in breast size, deepening of the voice, increased skin and hair oiliness, enlargement of the clitoris, and symptoms associated with diminished estrogen, such as hot flashes, postmenopausal vaginitis and postmenopausal vulvitis. The larger the dose, the greater the incidence of side effects. The original researchers testing danazol used 800 mg doses, but many doctors today feel that 600 or 400 mg will work as well. These lower doses significantly reduce side effects. Women taking danazol should discuss dosage levels with their doctors, for some of the masculinizing kinds of side effects may not be reversible once the drug is stopped.

Another advantage that danazol enthusiasts point out is that unlike other hormone treatments, danazol does not lead to a softening of ovarian endometrial growths, which has lead to rupture of these growths in some women on other hormone therapies. However, other doctors have reported that this problem does exist in patients on danazol, so this point is still being debated.

Despite all its advantages in comparison to other hormone therapies, danazol is not the only type of hormone therapy recommended by experts, for it has a big drawback in terms of cost. Danazol is quite expensive. Each 200-mg pill costs anywhere from $1 to $1.50. Treatment, depending on the dosage prescribed, costs anywhere from $2 to $6 a day! Minimally, the treatment takes three to four months and, in a number of cases, requires nine months. Treatment, then, could cost anywhere from $180 to $1,600, and this figure includes only the cost of the drug. Office visits for checkups during the treatment period would, of course, add to the cost of treatment. Some insurance companies, realizing that use of danazol may preclude the necessity of even more costly surgery, will cover this expense; others, however, will not. Medicaid programs may not cover the cost of danazol either; however, if the doctor is willing to write a letter explaining the need for this drug, payment can often be authorized.

Some women—those with certain heart and kidney conditions, those who are pregnant or breastfeeding, or those in whom side effects are too pronounced—cannot use danazol. If, for whatever reasons, danazol cannot be used, the second choice for hormonal treatment of moderate or severe endometriosis is a progesterone-type drug. Continual progesterone stimulation will stop the menstrual period. The progesterone drug used by many doctors is Provera. Provera is less expensive than Danocrin but also less effective. It carries the same risks and may cause the same side effects as the progesterone used in birth control pills, as well as estrogen-deprivation symptoms. It may soften ovarian endometrial implants, which could result in rupture and the spillage of the irritating contents into the pelvic cavity, causing pain, scar tissue (which could cause infertility) and further spread of the disease. Moreover, although it is unlikely, women on Provera can become pregnant. Pregnancy while on such hormones may result in birth defects.

The biggest problem with Provera is that it disrupts normal hormonal processes so thoroughly that it may take some time before normal menstrual cycles are resumed. Women who are using the injectable form of the drug, Depo-Provera (*see* p. 761) may become permanently infertile. Even with oral forms, subsequent pregnancy rates are low and disease-recurrence rates high. The drug, then, to put it mildly, has serious drawbacks for a woman with future childbearing plans.

In mild cases of endometriosis, it may not be necessary to use either danazol or Provera. Such cases may respond to treatment by low-dose oral contraceptives. Some doctors will merely put women with this problem on birth control pills. Preventing ovulation in this fashion, even though there may be withdrawal bleeding, can be effective in relieving symptoms in mild cases. More often, it will be necessary to use the birth control pills continuously, rather than in the usual off/on cyclical dosage pattern followed when the pills are used for contraception. However, after a while, in order to prevent breakthrough bleeding it may become necessary to take four to eight birth control pills a day, and the side effects from taking this many pills may be so severe that the woman has to discontinue treatment. Some doctors will stop the treatment for a week once dosage gets this high and then start again. The problems of softening and possible rupture also exist. This type of treatment is generally considered to control rather than cure the condition and is often followed by a recurrence of the endometriosis. It also prevents conception for the treatment period, which may be as long as one-and-a-half years, and defeats the purpose of a woman who is seeking prompt treatment for endometriosis-related nnnnnnnuertility. Many doctors have abandoned this form of treatment.

It should be noted that most doctors don't like to prescribe hormone therapy without first confirming the diagnosis of endometriosis by laparoscopy. As noted earlier, diagnoses made on the basis of physical exam are frequently wrong. Thus, there is a good possibility that the woman may have a condition that won't benefit from hormone therapy. It may even get worse. Moreover, the laparoscopic exam will reveal whether or not adhesions, which could be causing infertility, are present. If such adhesions are present, hormone therapy will not solve the infertility problem. Some doctors are strongly against giving hormone therapy without laparoscopic confirmation. They feel that before beginning treatment of this magnitude, they want a laparoscopic exam to be sure the diagnosis is correct.

Other doctors are willing to try the less drastic forms of hormone therapy first, especially if they are fairly confident of their diagnosis. They point out that even laparoscopy done under a local anesthetic carries risk. Five out of every 1,000 women will have complications; about half of those complications will be serious ones.[2] If a general anesthetic is used, the risk as well as the cost is increased.

Certain characteristic signs may make the doctor more sure that s/he is actually dealing with endometriosis. If the doctor feels nodules or thickenings on the uterosacral ligaments, the bands of supporting tissue that hold the uterus in place, or in the cul-de-sac, the area behind the uterus and in between it and the bowels, this increases the likelihood that the woman actually has endometriosis. If these signs are present and the woman has the classical symptoms of endometriosis, coupled with a family history of the disease, she may feel more comfortable about the doctor's diagnosis and thus, may be willing to forego laparoscopy. But this is one of those areas in which there are no clear-cut medical answers, and each woman must, with the aid of the medical opinions she gathers, make her own decisions.

No type of hormone treatment is 100 percent effective. Approximately 30-40 percent of the women using the most effective treatment, danazol, will have a recurrence of the disease within three years.[3] The treatment can, however, be repeated. No hormone therapy is effective in cases where there is marked ovarian enlargement. Still, most doctors feel that hormone therapy, in the absence of marked ovarian enlargement, should be tried before resorting to surgery. There is some debate about the wisdom of trying hormone therapy before attempting surgery in women in their late 20s or early 30s who are anxious to have children, but before unraveling that issue, the types of surgery used to treat endometriosis will be reviewed.

Surgery

The surgery may range from conservative—removal of the areas of endometriosis—to radical—removal of the uterus, ovaries and tubes.

In conservative surgery, which usually requires a general anesthetic, the doctor will remove as much of the endometriosis as possible by either cutting or burning with electric cautery, depending on where the endometriosis is located. If there are cysts on the ovary, these will be removed, leaving as much normal tissue as possible. Even if only a small nub of normal tissue is left, the ovary can often still function normally.

Some doctors will also do procedures known as presacral and uterosacral neurectomy, in which the nerves that transmit pain to the brain are cut. Even if the woman has not had pain as a symptom, some doctors will do this in order to prevent pain should the endometriosis reoccur. This procedure will also prevent involuntary contractions or spasms of the uterus thought by some doctors to be a factor in the backup through the tubes of endometrial tissues that causes the condition in the first place. Other doctors are less inclined to do this procedure, fearing that it will cause scar tissue reactions that could reduce fertility, one of the problems that they are often trying to avoid. It is important for women who have this procedure done to know that they may not have any pain in the first stages of labor, and thus may not head toward the hospital until the middle of giving birth. (The occasional woman may not make it to the hospital.) Women who have future childbearing plans and whose doctors suggest this procedure should seek a second opinion before making a decision.

If there are adhesions around the Fallopian tubes or binding the pelvic organs together, these will also be cut. If the uterus has been pulled back toward the spine by adhesions, these are also cut. The doctor will then perform a uterine suspension, a procedure that tightens the uterine supports and lifts the uterus.

The problem with conservative surgery is that it doesn't always work. In a fair number of cases, the disease will reoccur, requiring further surgery. A younger woman, with hopes of future pregnancy, may decide that the time she buys by conservative surgery is worth the risk of needing a second surgery, for she has a fair chance of achieving pregnancy. A woman who doesn't have future childbearing plans may decide that something more extensive than the conservative surgery described above is preferable. More radical surgery may be necessary when the disease is so extensive that there is no choice but to remove the uterus, ovaries and tubes, regardless of the woman's desire to have children. However, in some women, the question of preserving the ovaries comes up. This is probably not a serious question when the woman is approaching or has passed menopause, but with younger women, removing the ovaries as well as the uterus will cause premature menopause, which may result in distressing problems and possibly increase her risk of certain serious diseases. Some doctors will simply do a hysterectomy in younger women with extensive disease in whom ovarian preservation is possible. They remove all the visible endometrial implants as well as the uterus. They point out that even though the ovaries are still there to produce the hormones that aggravate the disease, removing the uterus eliminates the menstrual pain and bleeding problems, much of the abdominal pain and pain on intercourse and "quiets the pelvis down." Although the recurrence rate is somewhat higher in women whose ovaries remain and continue to put out estrogen, which of course could aggravate any remaining disease, premature menopause is avoided. Other doctors, less concerned about ovarian preservation, point out that leaving the ovaries in means that the disease will not be cured. They also point out that the recurrence rate is higher when the ovaries remain. Here again, women have to balance the risks and problems of premature menopause against the likelihood of recurrence of the disease, which might then require a second surgery.

Hormones vs. Surgery

One of the great debates in gynecology is whether to treat endometriosis in those women in their late 20s and 30s who are anxious to get pregnant with hormones or with surgery. A woman's fertility declines significantly after the age of thirty. Since hormone therapy often suppresses the menstrual period for six to nine months or more, and on top of that, it often takes some time for the menstrual cycle to resume its normal rhythm after the therapy, sometimes as long as a year, depending on the type of hormones administered, a woman on hormone therapy may thereby lose a year or two of fertility. If she is over 30, her statistical chances of achieving pregnancy are all the while declining. Some doctors feel that such a woman has a better chance of achieving pregnancy if her endometriosis is treated by surgery instead of hormone treatments. A woman in this situation owes it to herself to get opinions from doctors on both sides of this debate.

Endometriosis can recur after any form of therapy, but is most likely to happen with the hormone treatments. Recurrence rates after conservative surgery vary, depending on whether the woman got pregnant after surgery. In about 4 percent of those who get pregnant following conservative surgery, there will be a recurrence, but the figure may be as high as 40 percent in those who don't become pregnant.[4]

The recurrence rates after hysterectomy, regardless of whether or not the ovaries are removed, is low. If there is a recurrence, it is generally treated with danazol; however, at times a second or even third conservative operation may be done, and removal of the ovaries may eventually be necessary in some rare cases.

Sometimes, after surgical treatment in cases where there have been widely scattered small implants, danazol may be given to clear up any endometriosis that was missed. In the past, hormones were given before surgery to soften up the pelvis, making surgery easier, and to enlarge the endometriosis so the surgeon will be less likely to miss it. However, this approach has now been discredited and any doctor who suggests it may be a bit behind the times.

Radiation Therapy

It should also be noted that X-ray treatment is never appropriate for endometriosis, the exception being cases of ovarian endometriosis in which the surgeon wasn't able to remove all the fragments of ovarian tissue. Low doses of radiation therapy may be used, but this would be a rare case.

ADENOMYOSIS

AKA: internal endometriosis, endometriosis interna

Adenomyosis is a condition in which the endometrial tissue that lines the inside of the uterus (and which is shed each month during the period) is found growing into the muscle wall of the uterus. It is thought that the endometrial lining grows down into the muscle due to some weakness in the muscle wall. Sometimes the surrounding muscle tissue will "pinch off" the invading endometrial tissue, creating islands of endometrial tissue within the muscle. At other times the invading tissue is still connected to the normal endometrial lining inside the uterine cavity. In still other cases, the endometrial tissue will grow all the way through the muscle wall to the outer surface of the uterus.

At one time this condition was called internal endometriosis, since both adenomyosis and endometriosis, the condition described above, involve endometrial tissue in abnormal locations. In adenomyosis, however, the endometrial tissue is confined to the muscle wall, whereas in endometriosis it is found growing on the ovaries and other pelvic organs entirely separate from the uterus. Moreover, adenomyosis is usually diagnosed in women who are in their 40s and 50s and who have borne children, while endometriosis is most commonly found in younger women who have not borne children.

According to some authorities, the two conditions frequently coexist, while others say this is true in only a minority of cases. It is now thought that the two conditions are separate and distinct, so the term "internal endometriosis" (or "endometriosis interna") is no longer used.

Incidence and Cause

There is some debate about how frequently this condition occurs. Many women, even though they have a considerable amount of disease, are symptomless. The disease may not, then, be discovered until the uterus is removed for some other reason and examined microscopically. These reported incidence rates range from 10 to 60 percent. The wide variation is due to different definitions of exactly what constitutes adenomyosis; i.e. experts do not agree on how much endometrial tissue, how far down in the muscle tissue it should be and exactly what type of cells have to be present before adenomyosis is diagnosed. The method of sampling (that is, single samples or multiple samples) also has an effect on incidence rates, since adenomyosis may exist in one tissue sample while another sample from another location may be disease-free.

As mentioned, most women treated for adenomyosis are in their late 40s and 50s and have had one or two children. It is uncommon to find the disease in much younger women or in women who have never borne children. This lends credence to the theory that adenomyosis results from bits of endometrial tissue getting more or less "caught" in the muscle tissue in a process known as involution, during which the uterus returns to its normal size after pregnancy. Some doctors think of adenomyosis as a sort of endometrial hernia, which has poked through weak spots in the muscle wall—weak spots that were perhaps the result of repeated pregnancies. There are, however, other (somewhat less plausible) theories, and the actual mechanism by which the endometrial tissue invades the muscle wall is not entirely clear.

Symptoms

The two chief symptoms of adenomyosis are abnormal menstrual bleeding and menstrual pain, although for some unknown reason, about 25 percent of those with the disease are entirely free of symptoms. Adenomyosis is characterized by excessively profuse or prolonged periods. This occurs in about two-thirds of the cases. Frequently, the bleeding is so excessive that the woman is actually hemorrhaging. The severity of the bleeding seems to be related more to how widespread the condition is within the uterus than to how deep the penetrations are. This abnormal bleeding suggests a hormonal imbalance. It is suspected that adenomyosis may also be related to excessive hormone production.

About a third of the women treated for adenomyosis will have severe, sometimes incapacitating pain with their menstrual periods. One explanation for the pain is that the ingrown endometrial tissue continues to develop and swell each month in response to the monthly ebb and flow of hormones. Since the muscle walls of the uterus are unyielding and do not permit expansion, pain results. However, there is some question about whether or not the ingrown tissue always continues to respond to hormones. Another explanation is that the increase in the blood vessels in the area that usually accompanies this disease causes the walls of the uterus to become swollen with blood. This swelling, along with the scarring within the walls where the endometrial tissue has invaded, interferes with the normal contractibility of the muscle walls, causing pain. In any case, the degree of pain seems to be related to the depth of penetration into the muscle wall. It is interesting that although bleeding and pain are the two common symptoms, they occur together in only 20 percent of the women with adenomyosis.

Diagnosis

Upon physical examination the doctor will usually find a uterus that is rather firm and diffusely enlarged, but the enlargement rarely exceeds three times its normal size. This, in addition to the symptoms mentioned above, may make the doctor suspect adenomyosis, but a definite diagnosis is difficult because there are many diseases that coexist with adenomyosis. Often the diagnosis is impossible short of an actual operation and dissection of the uterus.

Moreover, sometimes it is hard to distinguish between adenomyosis and certain other diseases. Some types of uterine fibroids, for example, produce excessive bleeding, although in adenomyosis there is less tendency toward the gushing-type flow associated with these fibroids. Certain fibroids also produce a symmetrical enlargement of the uterus, but generally a uterus with adenomyosis feels firmer. The chief point of difference between these types of fibroids and adenomyosis is pain. The fibroids, although they may produce pain, are less likely to do so than adenomyosis. Adenomyosis will be suspected in a woman who has borne children when there is a diffusely enlarged uterus with symptoms of cramplike uterine pain that persists through the entire period, becoming worse as menopause approaches. During the rest of the cycle, the adenomyosis is relatively pain-free, which distinguishes it from endometriosis.

Treatment

When adenomyosis is accompanied by only moderate degrees of uterine enlargement, the woman is frequently treated for dysfunctional bleeding with hormones or by dilation and curettage (D&C), a scraping of the uterine cavity, neither of which will be successful. Indeed, the hormones may make the situation worse.

Since the disease is related to estrogen, and its chief symptoms—

menstrual pain and excessive menstrual bleeding—diminish once menopause occurs, a woman near menopausal age with only minimal symptoms can just be given treatment to relieve or minimize the symptoms. Such women should, however, have a D&C to rule out uterine cancer, which could also produce these symptoms.

If, however, the symptoms are extreme, surgery—in the form of a hysterectomy, removal of the uterus and possibly the tubes and ovaries— may be necessary. If a hysterectomy is performed, the fate of the ovaries will be decided on the basis of such factors as the personal judgment of the surgeon, the age of the patient and the presence or absence of associated diseases. Any woman whose doctor suggests a hysterectomy for adenomyosis should carefully weigh the decision. Are the symptoms that severe? Is menopause—and relief— just around the corner? The risks of hysterectomy must be weighed against the severity of the adenomyosis.

CONGENITAL ABNORMALITIES OF THE UTERUS AND FALLOPIAN TUBES*

Types: congenital absence of the uterus
unicornuate, unicornus, or unicorn uterus
rudimentary uterine horn, uterus bicornis unicollis or blind uterine horn
double uterus, double symmetrical uterus, uterus didelphys, uterus duplex, uterus bicornis bicollis, bicornuate uterus
septate uterus, subseptate uterus, uterine partioning
arcuate uterus
immature, or undeveloped uterus
T-shaped uterus

Back when we were all developing embryos in our mothers' wombs, certain masses of tissue with specific functions began to develop and differentiate themselves from the surrounding tissue. In females, two tubelike embryonic structures known as Mullerian ducts fuse together to form what will become the uterus, the Fallopian tubes and the mid- and upper portions of the vagina, at some time prior to the eighth week. Sometimes, however, this normal process of development and fusion is distributed, causing a wide variety of congenital abnormalities (Illustration 45).

*The position of the uterus within the pelvic cavity may also be unusual, and sometimes this is due to congenital problems; however, these are discussed separately under the headings Tipped Uterus and Prolapse of the Uterus and Cervix.

Illustration 45 *Congenital Abnormalities of the Uterus: (A) Normal, (B) Unicornus, (C) Rudimentary Uterine Horn, (D) Rudimentary Uterine Horn (with cavities connecting). (E) Bicornuate, (F) Septate and (G) Didelphys.*

Types

Different doctors use different categories to classify and describe the various types of congenital abnormalities of the uterus and tubes. We have found the following ones useful:

Congenital Absence of the Uterus

Sometimes there are no Mullerian ducts at all, so there is a total failure of development. Or both ducts fail to develop properly and cannot fuse. Such women, then, have no uterus at all. This absence is almost always accompanied by an absence of the vagina. Absence of the uterus may also be associated with certain congenital abnormalities of the ovary.

Unicorn Uterus

If only one of the Mullerian ducts fails to develop, the uterus and the Fallopian tube may be formed from the other duct. This condition may cause fewer problems than the other uterine abnormalities. It is known also as unicornuate uterus or unicornous uterus.

Rudimentary Uterine Horn

When the development of one Mullerian duct is normal but the other is abnormal or underdeveloped, varying degrees of what is called a rudimentary uterine horn will result. The term "uterus bicornis unicollis" is used to describe certain types of rudimentary horns. In some instances of rudimentary horns there is some fusion between the underdeveloped duct and the normal uterus that has developed from the other duct. In such cases the rudimentary horn and the uterus are said to "communicate," meaning that there is a passageway between them. If so, pregnancy can occur in the underdeveloped portion, which, as we shall see, can cause problems. More often, however, the underdeveloped duct does not communicate, but is merely attached to the uterus by a band of connecting tissue. In some of these attached horns the endometrial lining, which normally covers the inside of the uterus and bleeds, or menstruates, each month, is not functional. But in other cases the lining of the horn behaves just like normal uterine lining, swelling and shedding blood each month. However, since the horn is closed off, there is no place for the menstrual debris to go, which can lead to problems.

Blind Uterine Horn

If the two embryonic Mullerian ducts develop about equally well but one fails to "communicate" with the other or with the cervix, a condition referred to as a blind uterine horn results. It differs from the rudimentary horn in that it is fully or almost fully developed. But, like some types of rudimentary horns, it has no passageway to the other, normally developed uterus or to the cervix. Since the blilnd horn is sufficiently developed to menstruate but has no outlet for the menstrual debris, once again there are apt to be problems.

Double Uterus

When the two Mullerian ducts develop fully, so that there are two uterine cavities, two tubes, two cervixes and two vaginas, but there is no passageway or communication between them, this is referred to as a double, or double symmetrical, uterus, or uterus didelphys. There are a number of variations. A single vagina with all other structures duplicated is a uterus duplex, or a uterus bicornis bicollis. If both the vagina and cervix are single, the term for this is "uterus bicornis unicollis," or "bicornuate uterus."

Septate Uterus

Sometimes the double uterus does not consist of two totally separate systems. On the outside it may feel like a single uterus. There may just be a septum, or wall of tissue, inside the uterus that separates it into two cavities. If this wall of tissue runs from the top to the bottom of the interior cavity, it is called a septate uterus, and if the wall of tissue is only partial, it is known as a subseptate uterus.

Arcuate Uterus

Sometimes there is a single vagina, a single cervix and two Fallopian tubes, and the uterine cavity is almost normal, except for a slight depression at the top of the uterus caused by an incomplete fusion. This results in a sort of heart-shaped interior cavity and is referred to as an arcuate uterus.

Underdeveloped Uterus

Some doctors recognize yet another type of uterine abnormality, which they call an underdeveloped, or immature, uterus. Such uteri are smaller than average. Many times these sorts of uteri are associated with other abnormalities, such as hermaphroditism or polycystic ovarian disease. Sometimes these so-called underdeveloped uteri will cause difficulties in getting pregnant, in carrying a baby to term or in delivery, but this is usually only in association with other conditions. Some doctors attempt to stimulate the growth of an underdeveloped uterus with hormones, but it is not usually successful, nor is it necessary. Unless a woman actually has some underlying disease, there is no reason to do anything about a small uterus. We don't worry whether a woman is six foot two inches or four foot nine inches tall when she has a baby, and it is our experience that the size of the uterus is equally irrelevant.

T-Shaped Uterus

Recently, another type of uterine abnormality, called a T-shaped uterus, has been discovered in some of the daughters of the mothers who took the synthetic hormone DES during their pregnancies. No one knows yet how widespread this is, nor how it will affect the fertility of DES daughters.

Incidence and Cause

No one knows exactly what causes these abnormalities, nor how frequently they occur. Many of these defects don't cause any symptoms and don't interfere with fertility or pregnancy, so they are not discovered unless there is an autopsy at death or they are found in the course of another operation.

Symptoms, Complications and Diagnosis

Many women have no symptoms. For those who do, pain is a common complaint. Women with certain of these abnormalities may experience severe pain with their menstrual periods. There may also be irregularities in the menstrual bleeding pattern. The bleeding is apt to be very heavy and may last for many days, especially in double uterus, where there is more endometrial tissue and hence more bleeding. The periods are likely to be delayed. If there is a double vagina or if one of the horns of the uterus is in an inappropriate position, there may be pain associated with intercourse.

Infertility is often associated with uterine abnormalities. In cases where there is a complete absence of the uterus or vagina, the reason for this infertility is obvious. However, with other types of uterine abnormalities, the cause of difficulty in achieving pregnancy is unclear. Perhaps there is a problem in implantation due to lack of space in the malformed uterus. The consensus of opinion is that uterine abnormalities are not usually the cause, per se, of a woman's inability to get pregnant, although abnormalities that are related may be. The presence of uterine abnormalities does not mean that a woman cannot get pregnant, for many women—probably the majority—do, but it certainly doesn't increase the chances. However, once a woman with a congenital abnormality of the uterus does become pregnant, she is apt to have problems. Miscarriage is not uncommon.

Many times these uterine abnormalities are not diagnosed until a woman comes to the doctor because she is unable to get pregnant or because she has some of the symptoms described above. Careful examination with a speculum will reveal the abnormality if it is one that involves a double vagina or cervix. Or the doctor may be able to feel an abnormality in shape when a bimanual exam is done.

A history of repeated miscarriages will also help the doctor in diagnosis, for if a woman with a congenital abnormality of the uterus does conceive, there are likely to be problems. Generally, such women have only about a 50 percent chance of carrying the pregnancy for a full nine months, as compared to the normal rate of 85 percent. This is probably due to lack of sufficient space to allow the fetus to develop properly. Certain types of abnormalities are especially likely to result in spontaneous abortions. For instance, approximately 33 percent of all pregnancies occurring in a septate uterus will result in miscarriage in the third or sixth month of pregnancy.

Pregnancy in one horn of a double uterus may proceed to term, where it produces its own particular problems, but miscarriages are also frequent. If a woman with a double uterus becomes pregnant, she may continue to bleed cyclically from the other, nonpregnant uterus. Pregnancy in a rudimentary horn can be very difficult to recognize and is often mistaken for a fibroid tumor. Of course, the rudimentary horn is too underdeveloped to sustain a pregnancy. Such a pregnancy involves the same dangers as an ectopic pregnancy. As the fetus grows, the rudimentary horn ruptures, or bursts open, and this can result in the death of the fetus and the mother.

Even when a woman with uterine abnormalities does manage to get pregnant and carry her baby to term, there are likely to be problems. If the woman has a unicorn uterus, there may not be so many problems, but most abnormalities result in difficult deliveries and a much reduced chance of having a normal baby; 93 percent of the babies born from normal uteri are healthy, as compared to 64 percent born from abnormal uteri. It depends somewhat on the extent of the malformation, but even the only slightly abnormal arcuate uterus results in a high number of complications, including premature or postmature delivery, prolonged labor, sudden fetal death and breech or transverse presentations, in which the baby is born feet first or sideways.

Another serious complication of uterine abnormalities involves the buildup of menstrual blood. If a woman has a blind uterine horn or a rudimentary horn that does not communicate with the normal uterus, but does bleed, there is no place for the menstrual blood to go. It builds up over time and forms a collection of blood known as a hematometra. This can cause abdominal swelling, especially at the time of the menstrual period, and pain. If there is a Fallopian tube, this too may fill up with blood (hematosalpinx). These conditions are discussed more fully in relation to a condition known as imperforate hymen. Pelvic endometriosis, a condition in which menstrual debris backs up through the Fallopian tubes, spills into the pelvic cavity and starts growing on the ovaries or in other abnormal locations, where it can cause serious problems, is also associated with these types of uterine abnormalities. In addition to these complications, women with uterine abnormalities often have associated abnormalities of the urinary system, for the tissues from which these two structures evolve are very closely related.

Treatment

Generally, a doctor will not operate to correct a uterine abnormality unless a woman has a history of repeated miscarriages, long and complicated labors or infertility in which all other causes have been ruled out. Then, the partition between the double uterus or the abnormal portions of the uterus may be removed. Obviously, if there is no uterus, it is impossible to create one; however, it is possible to use plastic surgery procedures to create a vagina, if necessary.

In some cases, where delivery could be particularly dangerous to the mother, the doctor may suggest sterilization, but though the fetal death rate is nearly ten times higher in the malformed uterus, the maternal mortality rate is approximately normal, so only in rare cases is sterilization an appropriate option.

TIPPED UTERUS

AKA: displaced uterus

Types: anteflexed uterus
   retroflexed uterus
   retroverted uterus

Associated terms: pelvic passive congestion syndrome, Masters-Allen syndrome

A woman's uterus may be located in an unusual position in the pelvis (Illustration 46). Basically, the uterus can be located forward (ante) or backward (retro). (It may also be lower; lowered uteri are discussed separately under the heading Prolapse of the Uterus, Vagina and Cervix.) The terminology used to describe the various forward and backward positions may be slightly confusing.

In most women the uterus is tilted forward, almost forming a right angle to the vagina and resting on the bladder. In some women the cervix and the body of the uterus are at a more acute angle than usual, that is, the uterus is bent at the neck. The term "anteflexion" is used to describe such uteri. About 20-25 percent of all women have a uterus that is retrodisplaced, that is, one that is tipped backward, away from the bladder. The term "retroflexion" is used to describe this situation. If the uterus is tipped backward and is bent at the neck, the term "retrocession" may be used. The term "tipped uteri" is a general one, used to refer to anteflexion, retroflexion and retrocession.

Cause

A woman's uterus may become tipped in one of three ways. First, the problem may be congenital. As mentioned, 20-25 percent of all women are born with retrodisplaced uteri. Second, the uterus may become retrodisplaced if the ligaments that normally hold it in a forward position become stretched as a result of childbirth. And third, diseases such as pelvic inflammatory disease and endometriosis may cause adhesions— bands of scar tissue—that may fix the uterus in an abnormal position. A large ovarian tumor or fibroid tumor may push the uterus out of its normal position.

Symptoms

The vast majority of women who are either born with a tipped uterus or develop one after childbirth don't have any symptoms. Occasionally, a severely tipped uterus that is lying right next to the end of the vagina will cause pain on intercourse, but this is not generally the case.

A uterus that is fixed or forced into retrodisplacement due to some pelvic disease may produce symptoms. If, in such cases, the uterus is immovable and cannot yield to pressure, there may be pain on intercourse or a constant dull pain in the pelvis and lower back. Menstrual bleeding may be irregular, and there may be pain associated with it. These symptoms, however, are not due to the position of the uterus but to the fact that it is fixed in place.

In the past, gynecologists attributed a multitude of symptoms to the

TYPICAL

A

ANTEFLEXION

B

RETROCESSION

C

RETROFLEXION

D

Illustration 46 *Tipped Uterus*

tipped uterus. Since the tipped uterus and backache were such common, everyday conditions, putting the two together gave doctors a seemingly logical explanation for the pain (and also a quick and lucrative method of treating it). However, more discerning gynecologists began to realize that the vast majority of women with tipped uteri did not have any symptoms, and that treatment didn't usually relieve the backache. Indeed, it is now realized that less than 1 percent of all backache is related to uterine problems.

Still, misunderstanding about the tipped uterus persists today among both women and doctors. There are some women who have chronic pelvic pain, and the term "chronic pelvic passive congestion syndrome" is sometimes used to describe the condition. Usually, it is associated with a retrodisplaced uterus that is congested with blood. There is some question as to whether this condition really exists or not. Another similarly vague condition is the so-called Masters-Allen syndrome. In this condition, the broad ligaments that help support the uterus have tears or holes, thought to be the result of trauma during delivery, and therefore are not able to hold the uterus firmly in place.

Diagnosis

The diagnosis is made by bimanual pelvic exam. Some doctors will not mention the fact that the woman's uterus is displaced unless it's causing problems because they don't want to alarm her or because they feel that she might invent symptoms once she knows she has this condition. We, of course, feel that a woman has a right to any information a doctor may have about her body.

Treatment

At one time, it was quite the fashion to treat a tipped uterus by inserting a pessary, a ringlike support device, to hold the uterus in the usual position or by performing an operation known as a uterine suspension, in which an incision is made in the abdomen and the ligaments that hold the uterus forward are shortened, which pulls the uterus back into position. But, the vast majority of women with tipped uteri do not require treatment of any kind.

It is fortunate that the use of the pessary has fallen out of favor, for it almost invariably causes infections and sores. Besides, if the pessary can push the uterus forward easily, there is no need for one, and if there are adhesions present, there is no pessary in the world that can move the uterus. It has been jokingly said that some gynecologists have gotten wealthy inserting pessaries and that others have gotten wealthy removing them. (This is funny?) A woman whose doctor proposes the use of a pessary for her tipped uterus should pass on this "joke" and seek a second opinion (*see* p. 226).

Sometimes a woman will seek medical help because she is unable to get pregnant, but the doctor won't be able to discover any reason for her infertility. If such a woman has a displaced uterus, the doctor may suspect that uterine displacement and the resulting displacement of the cervix is the problem. The cervix may be at such a weird angle that it does not lie in the pool of seminal fluid, and thus the sperm cannot easily move up the cervical os into the uterus. Some doctors will treat this problem surgically, with a uterine suspension operation, resuspending the uterus and sewing it back into its so-called proper place. In our opinion, this is unnecessary, a case of overtreatment somewhat akin to using an elephant gun to kill a chicken. In the rare case where infertility is actually related to uterine displacement, there are much simpler solutions. First, during and for half an hour or so after intercourse, the woman should lie on her back, with her hips elevated. Or she may lie on her stomach and the man enters from the rear. In extreme cases, a vaginal pessary may be used on a temporary basis; however, women whose doctors suggest a uterine suspension for infertility should seek a second opinion.

The doctor may also suggest a uterine suspension for the relief of chronic backache; however, this too is of questionable value. Any woman whose doctor proposes the use of a pessary, uterine suspension operation or, heaven forbid, a hysterectomy for the relief of back pain should realize that such treatment is not likely to relieve the pain. She should, by all means, seek a second opinion.

PROLAPSE OF UTERUS, VAGINA AND CERVIX

AKA: decensus uteri, uterine descent or fallen uterus, fallen vagina or cervix

Types: first-degree prolapse
second-degree prolapse
third-degree prolapse, complete prolapse or procidentia uteri

Prolapse of the uterus (Illustration 47) refers to a condition in which the uterus "falls," or is displaced from its normal position. Prolapses are classified in three categories, depending on the degree of the displacement. In first-degree prolapse, the uterus has fallen into the vaginal cavity but does not actually protrude through the vaginal opening. In such cases the uterus has usually fallen or flopped backward so that it is not in its normal

399

position, resting on the bladder, but instead lies closer to the rectum. This is called retrodisplacement. This position usually prevents further prolapse. In second-degree prolapse, the uterus has fallen so far that all or part of the cervix protrudes through the vaginal opening. In such cases part of the vaginal vault may also have fallen or collapsed in upon itself. In third-degree prolapse, there is a complete descent of the entire uterus, with inversion of the entire vaginal canal. Third-degree prolapse is also called complete prolapse, or procidentia.

Prolapse of the uterus is usually associated with prolapse of other organs, such as the bladder (cystocele), the urethra (urethrocele) and the rectum (rectocele).

Cause

The underlying cause of prolapse is some sort of injury to the support tissues, usually during childbirth. However, since many women have traumatic deliveries and never have prolapse, and since in some cases, women who have never had children have prolapse, it is thought that some sort of congenital or inherent weakness in the support structures is also a factor. Although the initial injury may occur during childbirth, it usually takes years for the signs and symptoms of uterine prolapse to develop, and it appears most often in women over the age of 40.

In some rare cases there may be prolapse of the vagina after the surgical removal of the uterus, and this may be very difficult to repair if a functioning vagina is to be preserved.

Symptoms

A minimal degree of prolapse may not cause any symptoms at all. But as the uterus falls lower, many women have a heavy, bearing-down sensation in the vagina. Others, particularly when they stand, may have a feeling that something is falling out of their vaginas. These symptoms are apt to be worse if the woman has been standing on her feet all day. If the cervix or the entire uterus is protruding from the vagina, sores and other irritants may develop, due to its exposed position.

Diagnosis

The diagnosis of uterine prolapse is fairly easy, although when a woman is lying down it may not be as obvious. The doctor may ask the woman to bear down, may pull at the cervix gently with an instrument or may ask her

Illustration 47   *Prolapse of the Uterus*

to stand up in order to make a diagnosis. The doctor should be careful to make sure that it is not a case of an elongated or swollen cervix due to cervicitis or cervical cancer and that the uterus is actually descended. If there have been associated urinary tract infections, a tube may be inserted and urine extracted and examined microscopically for signs of infection.

Treatment

Treatment of uterine prolapse will depend on the age of the woman, whether or not she desires to have children, the severity of the symptoms and the extent of the prolapse. If a woman has only first-degree prolapse with no bothersome symptoms, it is usually not treated and is examined on a yearly basis. When the discomfort is intense and the prolapse is severe, the treatment of choice in women who have completed their families is a hysterectomy. Prolapse is often accompanied by a cystocele, urethrocele or rectocele and these can be repaired at the same time that the hysterectomy is done.

If the prolapse is severe or if a woman is having symptoms but wishes to avoid a hysterectomy or is unable to have surgery due to health problems or advanced age, then the doctor may prescribe a device known as a vaginal pessary to help alleviate the symptoms. The pessary comes in various shapes and sizes and is made of rubber. It fits up around the cervix at the top of the vaginal vault and helps prop up the prolapsed organs. Although a pessary won't cure the prolapse, it will prevent it from becoming worse. There are, however, problems with the pessary. It has to be removed (by either a doctor or the woman) and cleaned and replaced each month. Sometimes, despite daily douches, the rubber sets up an irritation that produces an annoying vaginal discharge. This may even cause open sores or ulcers to develop, perhaps with bleeding, making it necessary to remove the pessary. If the pessary is too large, it may press against the urethra, the tube through which urine is eliminated, causing urinary retention. If it is too small, it may cause sores or slip out. Sometimes a woman's particular anatomy precludes a proper fit with any of the standard pessaries available. Then, too, over the years the pessary may lose its effectiveness.

ASHERMAN'S SYNDROME

AKA: Asherman's disease, uterine synechia, sclerosis of the uterus

Asherman's syndrome is a condition in which the walls of the uterus are partially stuck together by bridges of scar tissue (synechiae) or in which the front and back walls of the uterus are totally adherent.

Cause

The condition is caused by too vigorous a scraping of the uterine walls during a D&C or, more rarely, by genital tuberculosis. Sometimes a suction curettage can also result in Asherman's disease.

Symptoms

One symptom associated with Asherman's syndrome is infrequent menstrual periods. If the scarring is too great, the endometrial layer may be too thin to build up enough thickness to allow any menstruation at all. There is also infertility, because the fertilized egg cannot implant in the uterine wall or because the embryo cannot develop properly in the constricted uterus. Only about 33 percent of women with Asherman's syndrome will be able to get pregnant, and to carry full term is even less likely.

Diagnosis

A history of curettage for gynecological problems, along with the symptoms mentioned above, will suggest the possibility of Asherman's syndrome. The doctor may explore the uterine cavity with a curette and biopsy any obstruction encountered. A hysteroscope, an instrument used to view the inside of the uterus, or special X-ray studies of the uterus, called hysterograms, may also be used to diagnose Asherman's syndrome.

Treatment

Sometimes the insertion of an IUD will succeed in separating the uterine walls enough so that the endometrial lining is restored. Sometimes hormone treatment will also succeed in building up the endometrial lining so that menstrual bleeding can be resumed.

UTERINE FIBROIDS

AKA: leiomyomata uteri, fibroleiomyomata or fibromyomata of the uterus, myomas, leiomyomas, fibroid tumors of the uterus

Types: intramural, or interstitial, fibroids
subserous, or subperitoneal, fibroids
submucous fibroids
cervical fibroids

Associated terms: fibroid polyp

Uterine fibroids (Illustration 48) are noncancerous tumors of the uterus. They grow in the thick muscular wall of the uterus and vary greatly in size from microscopic to mammoth. Although freak tumors of immense proportions are lavishly illustrated in grotesque detail in gynecological textbooks, such tumors are rarities. Obviously, most women seek treatment before the tumors get that large.

Incidence

No one knows exactly how common fibroids are since many of these tumors produce no bothersome symptoms and are too small or too inaccessibly placed to be felt by the doctor. It has been estimated that one out of every five women over the age of 30 has a fibroid. Next to pregnancy, it is the most common cause of an enlarged uterus.

Fibroids are only very rarely seen before puberty and they don't usually develop or grow larger after menopause. They are most frequently found in women who are in their middle and late menstrual years. In black women, who, for unknown reasons, seem to be particularly susceptible, the peak incidence occurs at slightly earlier years.

Illustration 48 *Uterine Fibroids*

Cause

The cause of uterine fibroids is unknown, but it does appear that they are related to the production of the hormone estrogen. They are prevalent in women who are in their reproductive years and are producing a monthly ebb and flow of estrogen. In pregnant women and women on birth control pills, both of whom have higher levels of estrogen, the normally slow growth rate of fibroids is accelerated. Moreover, fibroids rarely develop, and indeed often shrink in size, after menopause, when the level of estrogen is diminished.

Symptoms

Not all fibroids cause bothersome symptoms. A woman may have small single or multiple tumors, or even a fairly large one, without troublesome symptoms. She may not even be aware of the fibroid until her doctor happens to discover it in the course of a routine pelvic examination. A fibroid tumor may also be present for many years before it begins to produce symptoms.

If there are symptoms, their nature will depend in great part on exactly where in the uterus the fibroid is located. The tumors usually begin as small seedlings in the thick muscle wall of the uterus. They are well separated from the surrounding tissue by a capsule and may be single or multiple. Most fibroids stay confined within the muscle wall, and these are referred to as intramural, or interstitial, fibroids. They may grow large and expand in the direction of the outer surface of the uterus, in which case, they are called subserous, or subperitoneal, fibroids. Less often, they may grow toward the interior uterine cavity, in which case they are called submucous fibroids. In some rare cases fibroids may appear in the lower, cervical portion of the uterus and these are called cervical fibroids.

Frequently, there are small multiple tumors scattered throughout the muscular wall of the uterus, and the uterus is symmetrically enlarged due to the presence of the tumors and the swelling they produce in the surrounding tissue. If the tumors grow in the direction of the outer surface of the uterus, the fibroids may be felt as irregular bumps, or nodules, on the surface of the uterus. They may continue to grow larger and in an outward direction. Then they may become pedunculated, which means that they grow a stalk or stem, called a pedicle, by which they are attached to the uterus. In this instance, they are more mobile and may move to various locations within the pelvis. The pedicle may be broad and provide an adequate blood supply to nourish further growth or it may become very thin. A large tumor supported by a thin pedicle is subject to twisting of the

405

stem, an event which is known as "torsion of the pedicle" in medical circles. If this happens, there may be a good deal of pain. Also, the blood supply to the tumor may be cut off, which results in necrosis, or death, of all or part of the tissue that makes up the fibroid. If necrosis occurs, the dying tissues may swell up, causing pressure on the outer capsule of the fibroid and pain. If the tumor grows out toward the bladder or becomes pedunculated and moves into a position that causes pressure on the bladder, it may cause pain and disturbances in urination. A cervical fibroid growing out toward the bladder can also cause these sorts of disturbances. Sometimes the cervical fibroid will remain within the wall of the cervix and cause distortion and elongation of the cervix, pushing it down into the vaginal cavity. In extreme cases the fibroid may even protrude through the vaginal opening.

Less frequently, a fibroid will grow in the direction of the interior cavity of the uterus. These are most often single tumors and may fill the entire uterine cavity, which becomes increasingly larger as the fibroid grows. Usually, the uterus enlarges symmetrically, and the tumor cannot be felt as a separate growth. The uterus does not tolerate these submucous type of fibroids and reacts, as it does to any foreign body, by contracting in an effort to expel it with each menstrual period. Severe menstrual pain that continues throughout the menstrual flow is common in women with submucous fibroids. As a result of the continued uterine contractions, these tumors may also become pedunculated. They may even dilate the cervix and protrude into the vagina, in which case they are called fibroid polyps. Then, the blood supply to the tumor may be affected, resulting in necrosis of some of the tissue. If the fibroid protrudes through the cervix, it is subject to injury and infection.

These submucous fibroids may bleed as a result of the tissue death, injury and/or infection. They also tend to produce excessive menstrual bleeding of the gushing or flooding type, probably because they distort the endometrial lining of the uterine cavity and because they interfere with the normal contractions of the uterine muscle that aid in slowing down blood loss during menstruation. Even small submucous fibroids can produce excessive bleeding. Other types of fibroids may interfere with these normal contractions. If they grow large enough, they, too, can distort the endometrial lining and produce menstrual irregularities. But it is usually only the submucous ones that are responsible for heavy, prolonged menstruation and for the shortening of intervals between periods that sometimes occurs.

These submucous fibroids sometimes produce a vaginal discharge, which, if present, is usually rather mucuslike. If the fibroid becomes infected, the discharge may also include pus and may be tinged with blood.

If portions of the tissue that makes up the tumor die, the discharge may become thin, watery and brownish and have a bad odor.

Pain, as we have said, may accompany the fibroid. The exact nature of this pain will depend on the location of the fibroid. Intramural (within the wall) fibroids are apt to produce a pain that comes on suddenly over a localized area in the lower abdomen. The initial pain may be severe, gradually subsiding into a dull, pelvic "toothache." A pedunculated tumor that has twisted on its stem may produce pain that is apt to be sudden, colicky and severe.

If there is inflammation associated with the fibroid, adhesions (thick banks of fibrous tissue formed by the surrounding tissues to protect themselves) may be created. These adhesions may cement the organs in the area together, causing a constant back or lower abdominal pain that may get worse at menstruation. Submucous fibroids may produce a cramplike uterine pain that may become almost as intense as labor pains as the uterus tries to expel the fibroid through the cervix. Subserous tumors, since they may have veins stretched over their surface, can produce pain if an abdominal injury results in rupture of the veins, causing bleeding into the pelvic cavity, which is very sensitive to blood. However, this is a rather rare occurrence.

The fibroids may also produce discomfort through pressure on nearby organs or tissue. Usually such pain is felt in the back, the lower portion of the abdomen or the thighs. Prolonged standing, particularly at the time of the period, exaggerates this discomfort. A large tumor may produce pressure on the stomach or diaphragm, causing gastric or respiration disturbances. Similarly, pressure on the veins may result in swollen, distended veins in the legs, a condition known as varicose veins, or in hemorrhoids.

The bladder or ureter (the tube that leads from kidney to bladder) may be compressed, producing pain in the flank and kidney area on the affected side, as well as urinary symptoms. There may be urinary retention, which may be chronic and only partial or sudden and total, requiring catheterization (insertion of a tube through the urinary opening to the bladder). This sudden blockage is most likely to occur at the time of menstruation, when the pelvis is congested with blood, which results in swelling of the fibroid. If the bladder is constantly distended, incontinence (lack of control of urine flow) may result as the urine in the bladder spills over. Such overdistention and retention of urine lead to infection, since stagnant urine is a perfect breeding ground for bacteria. This infection may in turn cause pain on urination.

Infertility is often associated with fibroids, though sometimes the fibroid itself is not to blame. For instance, the infertility may actually be due to endometriosis, a condition in which uterine tissue grows outside the uterus, or salpingitis, an infection of the Fallopian tubes, either of which frequently coexists with uterine fibroids. However, in other cases the fibroid itself may be the culprit. If the normally blood-rich lining of the womb is thinned out over a protruding fibroid, the implanted egg will have difficulty surviving, due to the faulty blood supply. Miscarriage may also be a problem for women with fibroids; however, many women get pregnant and have no trouble with their pregnancy despite the presence of fibroids.

Diagnosis

Fibroids are diagnosed by abdominal palpation (feeling) and bimanual pelvic exam. They are usually felt as one or more firm, nontender bumps on the uterus. Sometimes it is quite easy to make a diagnosis of fibroids, but not always. If the fibroid is growing from the side of the uterus, it may be difficult to distinguish it from a solid ovarian tumor. If portions of the fibroid have broken down and become liquefied, so that the tumor takes on a soft feel, it may then be very hard to distinguish from an ovarian cyst. Ultrasound, a method of visualizing the internal organs by means of sound waves, may be reliable in distinguishing between fibroids and ovarian growths.

Another problem in diagnosis is the confusion between a soft enlarged uterus caused by a fibroid, particularly one that has undergone cystic degeneration, and one caused by pregnancy. A pregnancy test will clear up the confusion.

A submucous fibroid may not cause uterine enlargement or irregularities that can be felt by physical exam, and yet it may produce troublesome bleeding. These fibroids are usually diagnosed by a dilation and curettage, D&C, a procedure in which the cervix is dilated and the uterine lining is scraped. During the D&C the doctor feels inside the uterus with an instrument known as a curette. If the doctor feels a lump that is too firm to be removed, s/he knows that it is probably a submucous fibroid rather than a uterine polyp.

A special X-ray examination, known as a hysterosalpingogram, in which a special fluid that will show up on X-ray film is injected into the uterus, will sometimes reveal the presence of a submucous fibroid.

Treatment

Not all fibroids will require treatment. A wait-and-see approach in which the woman is carefully followed at regular intervals may suffice, particularly if the woman is near menopause, after which fibroids tend to regress. If, however, the tumor grows larger, treatment becomes necessary, for the possibility exists that this is not a fibroid at all, but uterine cancer.

A fibroid tumor larger than the size of a 12-14 week pregnancy also requires treatment even if it isn't producing symptoms, for large tumors can create serious surgical problems. Large tumors are also subject to necrosis, cystic degeneration and other complications. Moreover, in all likelihood they will begin to produce symptoms sooner or later. It is best then to remove them before they grow large or complications occur and they begin to produce symptoms.

The wait-and-see approach may have to be abandoned if the fibroid arises in or near the cervix, for such fibroids frequently cause urinary problems. Moreover, they may also cause infertility or create problems during childbirth.

In the face of severe symptoms, the wait-and-see approach doesn't make sense, particularly if there is bleeding with severe blood loss. Some doctors will try to control such bleeding with hormone therapy by giving birth control pills. This treatment is not usually successful, but it may be worth a try, particularly in a woman approaching menopause for whom it may thus be possible to avoid surgery.

If surgical treatment is necessary, it may be possible on rare occasions to remove a pedunculated submucous fibroid with a D&C. A cervical or submucous fibroid that protrudes from the uterine wall can occasionally be removed during a D&C as well. However, most fibroids require at least a myomectomy (Illustration 49). A myomectomy involves simply removing the fibroids and leaving the uterus intact. In some cases myomectomy is a simple operation. If the fibroid is attached to the outside of the uterus by a pedicle, removal might be quite easy, but if the fibroids are multiple and scattered through the uterus, the operation is hard or sometimes impossible. The myomectomy has a slightly higher mortality rate and a much higher complication rate than the hysterectomy. The uterus is a very muscular organ, with a rich blood supply. Thus, shelling out the tumors can lead to bleeding complications. It may also leave scars and cause adhesions, or hardened bands of connective tissue, that could bind the uterus to the other pelvic organs. This could lead to pain on intercourse, backaches and abnormal uterine bleeding. Moreover, in about 10 percent of cases, the fibroids will recur, for some of the seedlings within the uterine wall may have been missed and the basic underlying cause of the fibroids won't have been dealt with. Usually only women who are particularly anxious to have children should have a myomectomy. Although the uterine wall is weakened by myomectomy, women in whom the operation can be done have about a 50 percent chance of subsequently

Illustration 49   *Myomectomy: Sometimes fibroids on the surface of the uterus can be removed by an operation known as myomectomy.*

getting pregnant. Even some women who have had more than one myomectomy have been able to have a normal pregnancy.

Prior to operation, there is usually no way of telling for sure whether or not a myomectomy is possible. Women who are particularly anxious for pregnancy should make the doctor aware of their desires. Since myomectomies are only rarely done, it is hard to find an experienced doctor, but experience is important, for it cuts down on complications. Don't hesitate to question your doctor about his or her experience in doing myomectomies and to seek out another doctor with more experience if necessary.

Because of the high levels of estrogen in pregnancy, some asymptomatic fibroids will flare up at that time, growing larger and creating such severe symptoms that myomectomy is required. Unfortunately, many times a myomectomy in a pregnant woman will result in a miscarriage so it should not be attempted unless absolutely necessary.

In women whose condition precludes myomectomy, who do not wish to have children or who are older, a hysterectomy is done. The hysterectomy can be done by a vaginal or abdominal approach. If the tumor is small, the vaginal approach is often used. The vaginal approach is a less serious operation, requires a substantially shorter recovery time and allows for any vaginal repair for prolapse or cyctocele to be done at the same time. Some doctors will use the vaginal approach even for a fairly large fibroid, but this involves what is known as a morcellation procedure, whereby the tumor is cut into small pieces before vaginal removal. This procedure requires a great deal of skill, so most doctors prefer an abdominal route for large fibroids. The vaginal route also cannot be used when there is a question as to whether the tumor is ovarian or uterine in origin, for it does not allow adequate visualization. Even if an abdominal approach is used, vaginal repair can still be done prior to making the abdominal incision. The pros and cons of vaginal versus abdominal hysterectomy are discussed in more detail under the heading Hysterectomy.

If surgery is not possible because a woman has serious heart, lung or kidney disease and is a poor surgical risk, radiation therapy of the type used in cancer treatment may be used. Radiation therapy destroys the ovary, ending the production of hormones, and shrinks the endometrial lining, thus stopping the troublesome bleeding. It may also shrink the fibroid. However, sometimes it fails to shrink large fibroids and causes necrosis and infections; increased bleeding may then result in some of these large or submucus fibroids. Radiation therapy cannot be used if the fibroid is adherent to the rectum, which is highly sensitive to radiation. Moreover, there is much controversy about whether a radiation-induced menopause may incite endometrial cancer. Some researchers have found an increase in pelvic-cancer deaths in women who have had radiation-induced menopauses. Radiotherapy is, then, only rarely used to treat fibroids.

Although some doctors will prescribe birth control pills, women with fibroids should probably not use them because there is a risk of increasing the size of the fibroid and thus perhaps necessitating a hysterectomy. If a woman with fibroids does take the Pill, she should be monitored closely and examined every three or four months to make sure the fibroids are not growing larger.

ENDOMETRIAL POLYPS

AKA: uterine polyps

An endometrial polyp is a soft outgrowth of the endometrial lining. The term "polyp" is used to describe any growth that is attached by means of a stem, or pedicle. Endometrial polyps are generally small, although they may grow large enough to fill the entire uterine cavity. They may be single or multiple.

Incidence and Cause

Endometrial polyps can affect any age group, but are most commonly found in women who are at the age of menopause. Since hormone levels fluctuate in women in this age group, this suggests that they may be caused by some sort of hormone imbalance. The exact incidence, however, is hard to determine, for polyps may be removed piecemeal during a D&C, a procedure in which the cervix is dilated and the uterine lining removed, and may, therefore, be unrecognizable.

Symptoms

Sometimes the polyp doesn't produce any symptoms and is discovered only in the course of an operation done for some other reason.

The most common symptom is abnormal bleeding. This may take the form of bleeding in between periods of premenopausal women. The bleeding is not usually profuse, although on occasion a polyp may cause heavy bleeding.

At times the polyp may protrude through the cervical opening. It may cause some cramping as it dilates the cervical opening. The polyp may even grow such a long stem that it actually protrudes through the vaginal opening. These protruding polyps may become injured, due to their exposed position. Large ones may outgrow their blood supply, causing portions of the tissue to die. Similarly, the polyp may become twisted on its stem, causing disruption of the blood supply and tissue death. If any of these things occur, the polyp may become infected. There may be a foul-smelling vaginal discharge. Occasionally, a woman's infertility problem can be traced to an endometrial polyp.

Diagnosis

Polyps that protrude through the cervical or vaginal opening are readily diagnosed, although in such cases they may be confused with a cervical polyp. More commonly they don't protrude and are discovered only during the course of a D&C, although, as mentioned before, they may be unrecognizable. Occasionally a polyp will be located high up inside the uterus and may be missed during a D&C.

Treatment

Treatment of a protruding polyp is removal with a D&C. If the polyp's presence has been discovered during a D&C, then cure has already been effected. Infrequently, a hysterectomy, or removal of the uterus, may be in order. The polyp is, by and large, a benign condition. Cancerous polyps are extremely rare, and those that occur are usually found in women in their 60s. A hysterectomy would be in order only if the polyp found showed cancerous or precancerous changes. If, for instance, the polyp showed changes resembling those found in adenomatous hyperplasia, then treatment similar to the one used for that condition would be in order.

BENIGN TUMORS OF THE FALLOPIAN TUBES

AKA: fibroid tumors
paraovarian cysts
tubo-ovarian inflammatory cysts
endometrial cysts
noncancerous tumors of the tubes

Types: adenomatoid tumors
salpingitis isthmica nodosa

"Tumor," in the broadest medical sense of the term, means simply a "swelling." "Benign," of course, means "noncancerous." There are a number of different benign tumors that can affect the Fallopian tubes as well as the broad ligaments and uterosacral ligaments (the bands of tissue that support the uterus and other pelvic organs).

Generally, these tumors are small and don't cause any symptoms, although on occasion they are thought to play a role in causing infertility or ectopic pregnancy. If they become large, they may lead to torsion, or twisting, of the Fallopian tube, which can cause a great deal of pain, not unlike that associated with an ovarian tumor that has undergone torsion. Since they are generally small and don't cause symptoms, however, they are usually not discovered unless surgery is done for some other reason.

Types

Many of these benign tumors of the tubes have been discussed in more detail elsewhere in this book. For instance, fibroid tumors of the type found in the uterus can affect the tubes and the ligaments, but fibroids are less common in these areas than in the uterus. Paraovarian cysts and tubo-ovarian inflammatory cysts, which are discussed under the section on the ovary, are all associated with the tubes as well. Endometriosis can also affect the tubes and ligaments.

Although they are relatively rare, the two most common types of tumors of the tube are adenomatoid tumors and salpingitis isthmica nodosa. The adenomatoid tumors are frequently associated with salpingitis, inflammations of the Fallopian tubes. They are sometimes mistaken for cancer.

Salpingitis isthmica nodosa are tumors that are also associated with salpingitis. The condition has a number of different names, including diverticulosis of the tube, adenosalpingitis and adenomyosis of the tube. These tumors may occur at any age. They tend to be small and rather firm; their presence may stimulate the formation of scar tissue and adhesions.

Treatment

Most of these benign tumors don't require treatment unless they produce pain or there is an associated fertility problem. If fertility is a problem, it is sometimes possible to remove the affected section of the tube and to rejoin the remaining healthy portion of the tube to the uterus.

ENDOMETRIAL HYPERPLASIA

Types: cystic hyperplasia
adenomatous hyperplasia
carcinoma in situ or Stage O uterine cancer

Endometrial hyperplasia is an abnormal condition in which the endometrial lining has grown too thick. The term "hyperplasia" means "overgrowth." "Endometrial" refers to the endometrium, the specialized tissue that lines the inside of the uterus, thickening each month in preparation for pregnancy and breaking down and shedding during menstruation if pregnancy does not occur. The endometrium is normally rather thin, and about half its thickness is lost each month during menstruation.

Most of the time, hyperplasia is not too serious. It is usually a benign disease that may not even require treatment in a young girl. At other times, however, it may be the first step on the road to endometrial cancer.

Types

Basically, there are two types of hyperplasia: cystic hyperplasia and adenomatous hyperplasia. The only way to tell the difference between the two is to examine the endometrial tissue under a microscope. It is possible for both types to exist in the same woman, and either type may coexist with endometrial cancer.

414

The majority of cases of hyperplasia do not lead to cancer. Cystic hyperplasia is less likely to lead to cancer than adenomatous hyperplasia. The age at which the hyperplasia occurs is an important factor. Hyperplasia in the young girl is less serious than hyperplasia in the older woman. Some studies have indicated that as many as 30 percent of the postmenopausal women with adenomatous hyperplasia will develop endometrial cancer, usually within three to six years.[5] Because of the precancerous nature of adenomatous hyperplasia, some doctors use the term "carcinoma in situ" or "Stage O endometrial carcinoma" to describe this condition.

Cause

Hyperplasia is caused by continual estrogen stimulation of the uterine lining without the counterbalancing effect of progesterone. During the first half of the menstrual cycle, the hormone estrogen stimulates the endometrial lining of the uterus, causing it to thicken and grow. After the ripe egg bursts from its follicle on the surface of the ovary, the hormone progesterone, which is produced by the remnants of the burst follicle, further stimulates the uterine lining, so that it will be able to nourish a fertilized egg. If the egg is not fertilized, then the endometrial lining is no longer needed. Progesterone plays a role in the breakdown and shedding of the endometrial lining. If, for a variety of possible reasons, the egg does not burst from the surface of the ovary, no progesterone is produced. The estrogen continues to stimulate the lining, which grows thicker and thicker without the progesterone to help it break down and shed.

In postmenopausal women, estrogen replacement therapy may cause hyperplasia. However, hyperplasia can also occur in postmenopausal women who are not taking estrogen. Hyperplasia may also occur in women with functioning ovarian tumors or polycystic ovaries.

Incidence

Hyperplasia most often occurs at the beginning and the end of menstrual life, just after puberty or during the menopausal years, when irregularities in the process of ovulation most frequently occur, as the monthly cycle gears up or slows down.

Symptoms

Hyperplasia causes irregular menstrual bleeding. At first, there may be a period of amenorrhea (absence of menstruation) as the estrogen continually stimulates the endometrial lining. Eventually, though, the estrogen cannot support the overgrowth it has stimulated and portions of it break down and shed. This may start as minimal spotting but may progress to profuse and prolonged periods.

Diagnosis and Treatment

Endometrial hyperplasia may be diagnosed by a D&C, a procedure in which the endometrial lining is removed. The lining is then examined microscopically to rule out the presence of cancer and to determine which type of hyperplasia is present. Endometrial biopsies may also indicate the presence of hyperplasia, but they may not tell the doctor what type of hyperplasia is present or whether cancer is also present.

The treatment of hyperplasia will depend on the age of the woman, the severity of her symptoms and her childbearing plans, as well as on the microscopic analysis of the tissue. Sometimes a D&C will cure the problem. Hormone therapy may be used, but sometimes a hysterectomy is needed.

In a young woman in her teens, it is often a wise idea to try to avoid a D&C. There is little point in subjecting her to one, for the problem often corrects itself with time. Using birth control pills for a few months may "prime" her ovaries and bring on regular ovulation, eliminating the hyperplasia problem.

In women past their teens, however, the D&C is important. First, it will rule out the possibility of cancer and allow the doctor to determine the type of hyperplasia. Secondly, unlike teenagers, women in the older age group are not likely to experience a spontaneous cure. Moreover, a D&C often provides a cure for the hyperplasia.

If the pathologist's microscopic examination of the tissue removed by D&C indicates *cystic* hyperplasia, further treatment may not be necessary, for, as noted, the D&C often cures the problem. If symptoms do persist, a second or even a third D&C may be done. If the woman is premenopausal, some form of progesterone, perhaps oral Provera, may be given instead of a repeat D&C. Within two weeks of stopping the drug, all of the progesterone is excreted from the body. The drop in the body's level of progesterone causes the endometrial lining to break down and shed, thus eliminating the hyperplasia and the irregular bleeding. The therapy may be continued for several months and then discontinued to allow the woman's body to resume its natural functioning.

If the microscopic examination of the tissue removed by D&C indicates *adenomatous* hyperplasia, more drastic treatment is necessary because of the relationship between adenomatous hyperplasia and endometrial cancer. The treatment of choice is a hysterectomy, removal of the uterus. Depending on age and other factors, the hysterectomy may be accompanied by removal of the ovaries and tubes, a procedure known as bilaterial oophorectomy. An alternative form of treatment uses progesterone therapy. Although this type of therapy is often used for cystic hyperplasia, its use in adenomatous hyperplasia is controversial. It has been used with apparent success, but there have been no long-term studies of its effectiveness. The progesterone can apparently cause the abnormal condition of the endometrium to regress to normal. But, even if a woman's symptoms subside, she should have a repeat D&C in three to four months to check for cancer. She must then continue the progesterone therapy and must be followed regularly with endometrial biopsies. The problem is that endometrial biopsies sample only a small portion of the endometrial tissue. Cancer could be lurking in another part of the uterine lining. The woman could conceivably be followed-up with D&Cs on a regular basis, which would rule out the possibility that cancer was present elsewhere in the lining. But the effect on a woman's body and uterus of frequent D&Cs, not to mention the expense and risk involved in such frequent surgery, make this impractical.

Even if a woman with adenomatous hyperplasia who is treated with progesterone is followed carefully, there is still the possibility that cancer could develop in between her follow-ups or be missed by the endometrial biopsy. If the cancer should become invasive before being discovered, it might require more extensive surgery and/or radiation therapy, and the woman's chance of survival would be significantly affected. Perhaps in the future, more data will be available on this alternative form of therapy, but until then, women with adenomatous hyperplasia who are anxious to retain their childbearing capacity or to avoid hysterectomy and who elect to try this therapy should realize that they are taking a calculated risk. No one should attempt this form of therapy unless they are willing to commit themselves to a lifelong follow-up program including frequent endometrial biopsies (which, not incidentally, can be quite painful).

Another important issue in endometrial hyperplasia involves the use of terminology. Different doctors use different terminology. Some will call a precancerous growth pattern "adenomatous hyperplasia," while others will use the term "atypical hyperplasia" to refer to the same growth pattern. Some doctors will refer to both cystic hyperplasia and adenomatous hyperplasia as "benign" unless the condition is definitely cancerous.

Over the years, there has been some confusion and controversy about endometrial hyperplasia. Some doctors felt it was basically a benign condition; others thought it represented the early stage of cancer. Perhaps this confusion was due to the lack of standardized terminology and a failure to distinguish between the different types of hyperplasia. Today, most gynecologists think of adenomatous hyperplasia as the first step on the road to uterine cancer, even though not all cases will necessarily progress to cancer.

This confusion about hyperplasia has filtered down to general surgeons and family doctors, who may not understand the seriousness of adenomatous hyperplasia. Postmenopausal women will require a hysterectomy, and younger women who are treated with progesterone will need a repeat D&C, even in the absence of symptoms.

After performing the D&C on such women, the family doctor or general surgeon may get back a pathology report that says "endometrial hyperplasia" or merely "hyperplasia" and will then assure the woman that there was no sign of cancer and that everything is fine. Women should be sure to ask the doctor what type of hyperplasia is present—cystic or adenomatous. If a woman's D&C was done by a family doctor or general surgeon, she would be wise to seek a second opinion (see p. 226). Second pathology opinions (see p. 674) are also a good idea, especially for women who have been operated on in small, rural hospitals where only one pathologist is available.

UTERINE CANCER

AKA: carcinoma of the uterine corpus

Types: endometrial cancer
sarcoma of the uterus

The uterus is made up of the body, or corpus, and the cervix, or neck. Cancer of the cervix is discussed elsewhere. Here we are concerned only with cancers that affect the corpus.

Most cancers of the uterus involve the endometrium, the uterine lining. There are, however, other forms of uterine cancer. Sarcomas, tumors that arise from connective and muscle tissue, may develop in the uterus, but these account for less than 1 percent of uterine malignancies and are mentioned only briefly at the end of this section.

Incidence

It is thought that the incidence of endometrial cancer is increasing.[6] For reasons that are not entirely clear, white women seem to develop the disease more frequently than black women. The incidence rates for endometrial cancer in white women are 21.6 per 100,000, while for black women the incidence rate is said to be 12.2 per 100,000.[7]

Cause

The cause of endometrial cancer, like the cause of all cancer, is unknown; however, there is strong if not conclusive evidence indicating a link between endometrial cancer and the hormone estrogen.

Women whose bodies are subject to a certain type of estrogen influence known as unopposed estrogen are more likely to get endometrial cancer. Women with a history of menstrual irregularities who ovulate only infrequently and therefore don't get the relief from constant estrogen stimulation normally provided by the hormone progesterone (which is produced following ovulation) are subject to unopposed estrogen. Overweight women who produce higher levels of estrogen in their excess fat tissue are also at higher risk, as are women who have a late menopause and therefore have more years of estrogen stimulation.[8]

Unopposed estrogen in certain birth control pills has also been associated with increased rates of endometrial cancer. Sequential birth control pills, which relied on unopposed estrogen, were withdrawn from the market for this reason.[9] The use of estrogen replacement therapy (ERT), frequently given to menopausal women for relief of menopausal problems, has been associated with an increased risk of endometrial cancer.[10]

Risk Factors

Certain women are more likely to develop endometrial cancer than others. The following risk factors have been identified.[11]

Obesity

Extreme obesity is a strong risk factor, especially in the postmenopausal years. About one-half of the women with endometrial cancer are extremely overweight.

Childlessness

Women who have never borne children have an incidence rate about twice as high as those who have children and three times as high as those with five or more children. About one-half of women with this form of cancer have not borne children.

Late Menopause

The average age at menopause for women with the disease is higher. The risk of developing endometrial cancer is approximately two times greater for women whose menopause occurs after the age of 50 than for those whose menopause occurs before the age of 49.

Diabetes Mellitus

It is thought that women with diabetes, a disease of the pancreas gland, are at increased risk. Some authorities have placed the relative risk at slightly better than twofold for the development of endometrial cancer in a woman with a history of diabetes.

Hypertension

Hypertension, a condition characterized by high blood pressure, has not been as consistent a characteristic as the other factors listed here. It is not surprising to find high blood pressure in overweight women of this age group with diabetes. So, although many women with endometrial cancer have this condition, it is not clear that high blood pressure is in and of itself a risk factor.

Ovarian Disorders

Both Stein-Leventhal syndrome and granulosa cell tumors of the ovary have been associated with increased risk for endometrial cancer.

Cancer of Other Sites

There are increased rates of endometrial cancer in women with breast and ovarian cancer. This may be due to the fact that all of these cancers have some common cause or that women with these cancers have some common factor in their makeup or background that makes them susceptible to all three diseases. Cancer of the bowel has also been associated with increased risk.

Radiation Exposure

Exposure to radiation therapy, used to control postmenopausal bleeding (a form of treatment that has been discontinued), is associated with increased risk for this form of cancer. Some researchers feel this is one of the best-documented examples of radiation-induced cancer; others suspect that the woman treated in this manner who subsequently developed cancer may actually have had cancer at the time of the radiation treatment.

Use of Estrogens

In several studies the use of estrogens has been observed to be associated with a four- to sevenfold (or greater) increase in the risk of endometrial cancer. This is discussed in detail under the heading Estrogen Replacement Therapy.

Menstrual Irregularities

Almost 80 percent of women with endometrial cancer have a history of menstrual irregularities. One of the major symptoms of the disease is irregular menstrual bleeding due to the disease itself; however, for many of these women, the abnormal bleeding patterns date back as far as menarche, the first menstrual period. It is not entirely clear whether menstrual irregularities in and of themselves are risk factors or whether the women have menstrual irregularities because they have certain other risk factors, such as diabetes and ovarian problems, that are associated with menstrual irregularities.

Inherited Characteristics

Somewhere between 12 and 20 percent of women with endometrial cancer will have a family history of the disease. Here again, it is not entirely clear whether there is an inherited tendency to develop the disease itself or merely an inherited tendency to develop diabetes, obesity, polycystic ovaries, menstrual irregularities and other risk factors.

Women who are at high risk should discuss their medical situations with their doctors. In some instances, it may be wise for women at high risk to have routine endometrial biopsies so that any cancer that might develop could be detected while still in its early stages.

Symptoms

The most common symptom is vaginal bleeding, which appears in over 90 percent of cases. In premenopausal women, the bleeding may take the form of a prolonged menstrual period, a sudden flow of blood between periods or a slight staining between periods or after going to the bathroom. In rare cases this type of bleeding may occur after douching or intercourse. These types of abnormal uterine bleeding may be due to many other causes. The presence of vaginal bleeding in premenopausal women is more likely the result of some other factor, but continued abnormal bleeding should be brought to the attention of a doctor.

In the menopausal woman, skipping menstrual periods and gradually "tapering off" is not uncommon, so abnormal vaginal bleeding due to uterine cancer may be misinterpreted as normal menopausal bleeding. If the menstrual periods stop for six months to a year and then start up again, however, this should be investigated (see below).

Of the postmenopausal women who experience vaginal bleeding, about one-third will have cancer, one-third will be bleeding due to some benign condition and one-third will be bleeding for unknown reasons. The bleeding may be nothing more than intermittent spotting; however, it may be constant and may even be quite heavy. Any postmenopausal bleeding deserves investigation. Too often, women taking estrogen replacement therapy (ERT) for menopausal symptoms and their doctors are apt to blame the bleeding on the drug, but we know that women on ERT are at increased risk, so it is particulary important that their bleeding symptoms be investigated.

Vaginal discharge is another symptom of uterine cancer, but here again, this symptom may be caused by a number of other factors. The discharge may precede the bleeding. A clear, watery discharge is particularly significant, especially when it comes in bursts after heavy exertion or after straining while going to the bathroom. If the cervical canal is partially closed, as it often is in older women, there may be cramplike pain as the uterus tries to expel the discharge through a blocked cervical canal. This is particularly true if there is an associated pyometra, a condition in which a collection of pus and fluid is built up inside the uterus, either due to the cancer or some benign condition. The discharge may then become brownish or blood-tinged. If portions of the tumor begin to break down, the discharge may begin to smell bad.

Pain is sometimes present, but the significance of the pain is hard to evaluate. Pain in women with cancer is often a sign of advanced or incurable disease, but this is not always true with this form of cancer. Fibroids, endometrial polyps, pyometra and other benign conditions frequently coexist with endometrial cancer and may be the source of the pain.

Diagnosis

There is no simple painless screening test like the Pap smear, used to screen for cervical cancer, available for uterine cancer. Nor is the Pap smear reliable in detecting uterine cancer. It simply fails to detect the cancer too many times. For high-risk women, an office procedure known as an endometrial biopsy may be done. This, however, is a painful procedure and is not entirely accurate, so it is not a practical solution for mass screening.

Abnormal bleeding is a critical symptom, since it may be the only one. Once a woman comes to the doctor with abnormal bleeding, she may be given either an endometrial biopsy or a more involved hospital procedure known as a dilation and curettage (D&C), a procedure in which the cervix is opened and the lining of the endometrial cavity is removed. If the woman is menopausal or postmenopausal, an endometrial biopsy is usually done first. If it indicates that cancer is present, then the doctor can proceed to treat her without subjecting her to the additional expense and risk of a D&C. If the biopsy is negative, a D&C must still be done because the endometrial biopsy is not 100 percent accurate.

If, however, the woman is still in her menstrual years, it is much more likely that her abnormal uterine bleeding is due to some less serious problem. Many of these more common causes of abnormal bleeding will be cured by the D&C. So, in this age group, the D&C, which will rule out cancer and may also be curative, rather than an endometrial biopsy, is generally done.

If the D&C is done, tissue samples from the cervix are taken separately to rule out the possibility that the disease has spread to the cervix. If a D&C is not done, cervical samples may be done at the time of surgery. The uterus is always measured, either during the D&C or upon operation. This is an important step, for an enlarged uterus is generally a sign that a larger volume of cancer is present, which will require more aggressive treatment.

The tissue samples are sent to the pathology laboratory for analysis. The pathologist's report will tell the doctor whether or not cancer is present. It will also tell the doctor what grade (*see* p. 677) of cancer the woman has. The grade of the cancer is particularly important, for if the cancer is a low-grade one, this means that the cells are less abnormal and that the cancer is a less serious one. This will affect the treatment that is given.

Any of the standard preoperative tests to detect metastasis (*see* p. 676) may also be done as part of the diagnostic workup. Once the doctor actually operates, the abdominal cavity is carefully inspected for signs of cancer. The lymph nodes are carefully examined. Tissue samples from various locations within the abdominal cavity and, in particular, from certain lymph nodes may be taken in order to help the doctor detect microscopic spread of the disease.

Staging

The results of the pathologist's analysis of the cell and tissue samples and the doctor's measurement of the uterus and careful inspection of the abdominal cavity, along with the results of tests to detect metastasis, will be used to estimate the spread of the disease, that is, to stage the disease.

Table 12 outlines the official staging scheme for uterine cancer.[12] The grade of the tumor cell is of particular importance in Stage I. The grade refers to how well-differentiated or mature the cells are. The less mature the cells, the higher the grade, and the higher the grade, the more serious the disease. Grade, as we shall see, can influence decisions about treatment.

Although it is not included in the official treatment scheme, the depth to which the cancer has penetrated the uterine wall will also affect treatment. The length of the uterus is also important, for experience has proved that the larger the uterus, the more likely it is that microscopic cancer has already spread to the adjacent tissues and lymph nodes.

Once the cancer has spread to the cervix (Stage II), the likelihood of involvement of the surrounding tissues and lymph network again increases and treatment must include the areas adjacent to the cervix as well. Once the cancer has spread outside the uterus itself, the situation becomes more serious. In Stage III, this spread has begun and the adjacent tissues are obviously involved. Stage IV involves the bladder or rectum and/or spread to distant organs, frequently the lungs.

Table 12
Classification and Staging of Uterine Cancer

Stage I: The cancer is confined to the body of the uterus

    Stage I A: The length of the uterine cavity is eight cm or less

    Stage I B: The length of the uterine cavity is more than eight cm

    Stage I A and I B cases are subgrouped according to grade:
    G1:   Highly differentiated
    G2:   Highly differentiated with undifferentiated areas
    G3:   Predominantly or entirely undifferentiated

Stage II: The cancer has involved the body of the uterus and the cervix, but has not extended outside the uterus

Stage III: The cancer has extended outside the uterus to the adjacent tissues

Stage IV: The cancer has involved the bladder or rectum

    Stage IV A: Direct spread to adjacent organs

    Stage IV B: Spread to distant organs

Treatment

Most of the time, the treatment of endometrial cancer involves surgery and some form of radiation therapy. In certain cases one or the other form of treatment may be used alone, but generally speaking, the combination of the two offers the best chance for a cure.

Surgical Procedures

A variety of surgical procedures may be used in treatment of uterine cancer.

Hysterectomy: At a minimum the surgery will include removal of the uterus. A vaginal cuff, a small portion of the upper vagina that adjoins the cervix, is also removed.

Bilateral Salpingo-Oophorectomy: In this procedure the tubes and ovaries are removed as well.

Lymphadenectomy: This operation involves removing the lymph nodes in the area. There are a number of lymph passageways to which the cancer might spread. Cancer located high in the uterus might spread to one set, while cancer near the cervix typically spreads to other lymph nodes. The location of the cancer will be a factor in determining which nodes are removed. At the time of operation, certain key nodes may be biopsied using frozen section to help determine which nodes should be treated.

Radical Hysterectomy: Sometimes this more extensive type of hysterectomy, in which the uterus, tubes, ovaries, upper one-third of the vagina and the connective tissues adjacent to the uterus and cervix are removed, is done.

Pelvic Exenteration: In a few cases this very radical form of surgery is used. It involves removal of the uterus, tubes, ovaries, vagina, bladder, connective tissues, urethra and rectum. In certain instances a partial exenteration, in which either the rectum or the bladder and urethra are preserved, can be done. If the bladder and/or rectum are removed, the urinary and bowel tracts must be diverted and new openings created on the outside of the body so that waste products can be collected in plastic bags.

Radiation Therapy

Two types of radiation therapy are commonly used to treat uterine cancer: radioactive implants and external beam therapy.

Radioactive Implants: This involves inserting containers, or holders, into the woman's uterus and/or vagina. Once the containers are in the proper position, they are loaded with a radioactive material and left in place until the specified dose of radiation has been achieved. The implants will kill or disable the tumor cells in the uterus or vagina.

External Beam Therapy: This type of radiation is administered from outside the body by directing a beam from an X-ray machine at the cancerous area. It is used to treat cancer that has spread to the adjacent tissues and lymph nodes.

Radiation therapy is generally given prior to surgery for several reasons. First of all, it is thought that the radiation will alter the cancer cells in a manner that makes it impossible for the cells to implant elsewhere. Secondly, radiation causes scarring of the blood vessels and lymph nodes in the area. Thus, by giving radiation prior to surgical treatment, the chances of spreading tumor cells to other areas of the body during surgery are supposedly reduced.[13]

Radiation is not always used preoperatively. In cases where a radical hysterectomy and lymphadenectomy are done, some experts feel that preop radiation is not as important, for a large area of tissue is removed, pretty much in one piece; thus, they argue, the danger of spilling cancer cells onto adjacent tissues or into the lymph system is not as great a problem.[14] Moreover, preoperative radiation delays surgery for anywhere from one to six weeks (depending on how much radiation is given), makes subsequent surgery more difficult, complicates healing due to the radiation damage and makes it difficult—sometimes impossible—to tell how deeply the cancer has invaded the uterine wall. The depth of invasion is sometimes a critical factor. In certain cases where the cancer has not invaded the uterine wall or the invasion is limited to the upper one-third of the wall, radiation may not be required.[15] Avoiding preop radiation in these cases allows for a more accurate analysis of depth of invasion and makes it possible to avoid unnecessary radiation in some cases. There are, then, instances when radiation is not given preoperatively or is not used at all.

Similarly, surgery is not used in some cases or is done in only a limited fashion. The extent of the surgery that is done will depend on many factors. The stage of the disease and the grade of the cancer cells are important factors. The low-grade cancers are less likely to spread to the adjacent tissues and lymph system and will require less radical treatment.

Many times the extent of the surgery is limited by the woman's general health. Since many of these women are obese and have associated medical problems like high blood pressure, they are often poor surgical risks. The more extensive the surgery, the longer the anesthesia time required and the greater the potential for complications. Sometimes only a simple hysterectomy can be done because the longer anesthesia time required for a radical hysterectomy or a pelvic examination procedure would pose too great a risk to the woman's life. Sometimes surgery cannot be done at all. Although the survival rates are lower when only radiation therapy is used, sometimes radiation therapy alone is used. Even radioactive implants require some form of anesthetic. An occasional woman is in such poor health that only external beam therapy is used.

The woman's general health, the location and extent of the disease and the grade of the tumor cells will all influence the type of treatment given. The same woman might be treated differently by different doctors. A doctor may advocate a particular therapy program over another simply because s/he was trained that way or because in his or her experience that particular mode of therapy seems to yield superior results.

While there are differences among doctors regarding treatment of endometrial cancer, there is not the sort of controversy that surrounds treatment of breast cancer. There are studies being conducted that should yield more precise information as to optimum treatment, but medical professionals don't expect these studies to reveal dramatic differences in survival rates.

Although, from the medical point of view, the results of these studies won't be all that significant, they may well be from the woman's point of view. If two plans of treatment are shown to be equally effective, but one causes the woman subsequent pain and difficulty with sexual relations, or makes sex altogether impossible, while the other one doesn't, then many women would consider this a rather significant difference. Doctors tend to measure things more in terms of cure rates. Moreover, many of the women with endometrial cancer are in the older age group. Despite obvious and unrefuted evidence to the contrary, many doctors persist in thinking that older women don't have sex lives and that, therefore, preservation of, say, vaginal function need not be a major concern. It is true that for some women, having a functioning vagina may not be of great importance in their sex lives. The clitoris is generally of more physiologic importance in sexual pleasure. But for other women, retaining a functioning vagina may be very important. Since the doctor may not consider these issues when planning treatment, it is important that women bring these subjects up and discuss their personal attitudes and priorities with their doctors.

Treatment Plans According to Stage and Grade

The treatment of uterine cancer, like the treatment of any form of cancer, is a complex subject. Descriptions of what is done and explanations of why it is done in the treatment of various stages and grades are outlined below, but these are only generalizations. Treatment is individualized according to the particulars of a woman's case. If your doctor recommends a treatment plan different from the one outlined here, this certainly does not mean that the recommendation is wrong. The information given here is intended to provide basic information, so that women will understand the issues and know enough to ask the right questions. Remember, every woman has the right to a full explanation of what the doctor plans to do and why. Second opinions (*see* p. 226) are, of course, always in order, and they are especially important in cancer.

Stage IA, Grade 1

These cases are usually treated by surgical removal of the uterus, tubes, ovaries and vaginal cuff. The uterus is then examined by the pathologist. If the cancer is indeed Stage IA, Grade 1, and has not penetrated beyond the first third of the uterine wall, some doctors do not recommend any further treatment.[16] If, however, there is deeper penetration, postoperative radiation may be given, for there is a greater likelihood that the cancer has spread to the adjacent tissues and lymph nodes.

There are some doctors who use preoperative radiation in these cases.[17] There are also some who use postoperative radiation regardless of the depth of penetration.[18] Those who advocate preoperative radiation point out that there is a chance, albeit a small one, of recurrence of cancer in the top of the vagina that can be prevented by preoperative radiation. Those who oppose it feel that the risks and complications of radiation outweigh the benefits. In fact, some doctors don't think that radiation has any effect on survival in these cases.[19] Also, radiation therapy usually makes for poor vaginal function, so that intercourse becomes painful or sometimes impossible. Rather than treating everyone, some doctors prefer to follow these women carefully, and to treat only those who do have recurrences. If a woman is conscientious about follow-up, vaginal recurrences are easy to detect.

Those who use postoperative radiation regardless of the depth of the invasion also do so in order to prevent vaginal recurrences. They point out that postoperative radiation is more comfortable and does not delay surgery. No one knows for certain which type of therapy is best, so decisions are based on the particulars of a woman's case and the doctor's personal experience and treatment preferences. Women with Stage IA, Grade I endometrial cancer, particularly those who are concerned about preserving vaginal function, will want to discuss these issues with their doctors and should certainly get multiple opinions before deciding on therapy.

Stage IA, Grade 2 and 3; Stage IB; Stage II [20]

These cases may be treated in a number of different ways. Generally, radiation is given preoperatively. Implants may be given, followed in a week or two by hysterectomy and bilateral salpingo-oophorectomy, or in some cases a radical hysterectomy may be done. Depending on the pathologist's estimate of the depth of invasion, subsequent external beam therapy may then be used. Sometimes both implants and external beam therapy are used, followed by hysterectomy and bilateral salpingo-oophorectomy in four to six weeks (greater doses of preop radiation mean a longer delay to allow for healing of radiation damage before surgery). Sometimes a radical hysterectomy and lymphadenectomy will be done first. This "surgery-first" treatment plan allows for a good pathological evaluation of the depth of penetration of the uterine wall and of the lymph nodes. In some cases no further treatment may be required. In other cases, where there is deep invasion in certain areas, subsequent external beam therapy may have to include the para-aortic as well as the pelvic nodes.

These cases represent one of those instances in which each of the available treatments has its advantages and drawbacks. For example, if radical surgery is done first, it may be possible in some cases to avoid subsequent radiation. Even though the upper one-third of the vagina is removed surgically, this usually permits better vaginal function than radiation therapy, which causes such severe vaginal scarring that intercourse may be painful or even impossible. However, doing surgery first means a delay in administering radiation therapy in those women who require it. If only implants rather than implants *and* external beam therapy are used, better vaginal function is possible.

Sometimes the particulars of a woman's case will dictate the choice of treatment plan. For example, a woman may be too poor a surgical risk for radical surgery and a pelvic lymphadenectomy to be done, so radiation followed by less radical surgery may be the treatment of choice for her. Or, if a woman has a high-grade tumor or a Stage II tumor, which means the cancer is more likely to have spread to adjacent tissues and lymph nodes, the doctor may use both implants and external beam radiation prior to surgery to increase the chances of disabling these more lethal high-grade cells so that they won't implant, should they be spilled during surgery.

These again are instances in which the decision about which treatment plan to use is not clear-cut. Although studies are being done to compare these options, it may be years before the results are available. Some doctors are reluctant to use the surgery-first type of treatment because, based on their personal experience, they believe it to be less effective or simply because they have been trained to give preoperative radiation. Here again, women, particularly those who are concerned about preservation of vaginal function, should discuss the pros and cons of the various treatment options with their doctors and seek second opinions from doctors who are advocates of the various different treatment plans that are possible options in their cases.

Stages III and IV [21]

Treatment of Stage III and IV cases is highly individualized and will depend on the extent of the disease spread, its location and the general health of the woman. External beam therapy and implants are generally used. Surgery may also be done, and if it is done, it generally includes removal of the uterus, tubes and ovaries. More extensive surgery is done in some cases, but this is generally not possible due to the extent of the spread and the generally poor health of these women. In a few cases, surgery as radical as pelvic exenteration may be done. In one study involving 33 women with Stage IV disease who were given pelvic exenteration, 6 survived more than five years. Such surgery can, then, be worthwhile in certain cases.

Chemotherapy and hormone therapy may also be used in the treatment of these advanced cases. Generally, some form of the hormone progesterone is used. This is particularly valuable in Stage IVB cases, where there is metastasis to the lung. The progesterone will be effective in about one-third of these cases. It is also effective in treating metastases in other locations as well as local spread in the pelvis. Currently, there are a number of studies evaluating other forms of chemotherapy for advanced and recurrent uterine cancer. Having a doctor who is up-to-date on the latest developments is of prime importance.

Recurrent Cancer [22]

The treatment program for recurrent cancer will depend on the location and size of the tumor and what type of therapy was used in the treatment of the initial cancer. If it recurs locally, for instance in the vagina or nearby tissues, this may be treated by external beam therapy if only radioactive implants were used in the initial treatment; however, if both external beam therapy and implants were used initially, further radiation therapy cannot be given, for the maximum dose of radiation will have been given during the initial therapy. Further radiation would damage the healthy tissue so much that the woman would die. If the maximum radiation has already been given, then in some cases pelvic exenteration may be done. Although this has been effective, it is rarely done, for the woman's health usually won't permit such radical surgery. If the disease recurs in some distant location and/or locally, chemotherapy of the type described above may be used.

Follow-Up [23]

Follow-up is important if recurrences are to be detected early. In the first year, the woman will see the doctor at least every three months or so. Most recurrences happen within the first two or three years following treatment. By the fifth year, women are generally seen only once a year, unless problems occur.

The extent of the follow-up will depend on the extent of the disease.

More advanced cancers are more likely to recur and therefore require more elaborate follow-up. At a minimum the doctor will do a Pap smear, bimanual examination, a thorough visual exam with a speculum, a careful palpation of the abdomen and liver and a complete physical. The abdomen may be measured and tapped to check for any accumulations of fluid. Symptoms like a cough or chest pain are important. Chest X-rays are often done routinely even if no symptoms are present since the lungs are a frequent site of recurrence. The bones may also be a site of metastasis, so any pain in the bones calls for a bone scan. The liver is another frequent site of recurrent endometrial cancer. So, in advanced cases, liver scans as well as IVPs may be done. The exact nature of the follow-up program will depend on the seriousness of the original disease.

Sometimes women who have been treated for endometrial cancer don't visit the doctor for follow-up. If they had low-grade, Stage I cancer, they may think their problems are over, but recurrences happen even in the best of circumstances. Follow-up of women with early stages is especially important, for they have the best chance of cure should the cancer recur. Some women get lax about follow-up as the years go by. Although it is true that most recurrences are detected within the first three years following treatment, some don't appear for many years. Still, many women neglect follow-up because they have been so drained by the recovery from surgery or the side effects of radiation therapy that in one woman's words, "It just took the fight out of me." Or they may feel that there is no hope for them should the cancer recur. While it is true that those women whose disease was less serious in the first place, and hence required less extensive and physically draining therapy, have a better chance of survival if there is a recurrence, even women with late-stage cancers have been cured by subsequent therapy. Even though the cure rate for recurrent cancer is only 10 percent, treatment may succeed in prolonging life and in making the remaining time more comfortable.

Follow-up is important for all women. A woman's best chance of being the one in ten who will survive recurrent cancer depends on early detection of the recurrence.

Sarcomas

Sarcomas, another form of uterine cancer, are often not detected until the cancer is in a fairly advanced stage. Treatment usually includes a hysterectomy and bilateral salpingo-oophorectomy. For certain types of sarcomas, treatment may involve radical hysterectomy and lymphadenectomy. In some cases radiation therapy may prove helpful. Chemotherapy is frequently used. Overall survival rates are around 20 to 30 percent but in early stages may run as high as 80 percent.

Survival

The survival rates for endometrial cancer vary with the stage of the disease, the grade of the tumor cells and other factors including whether or not the woman's health was good enough to allow for optimum treatment. Table 13 lists survival rates by stage and also breaks down survival rates for Stage I according to grade.

Table 13
Five-Year Survival Rates for Endometrial Cancer by Stage*

Stage	Percent
IA	80
IB	65
II	41
III	17
IV	2

Five-Year Survival Rates for Stage I Endometrial Cancer by Grade

Grade	Percent
1	91
2	74
3	48

*SOURCE: Adapted from Boutselis, John, "Endometrial Carcinoma," *Surgical Clinics of North America,* Vol. 58, No. 1, February 1978.

CANCER OF THE FALLOPIAN TUBE*

AKA: carcinoma of the Fallopian tube

Associated terms: hematosalpinx, or hydrosalpinx; torsion of the tube, hydrops tubae profluens, or hemohydrops tubae perfluens

Cancer of the Fallopian tube very rarely occurs. The disease may be primary, that is, it may originate in the tubes, or secondary, the result of

*See also the general discussion of cancer.

direct extension of cancer of the uterus or the ovary or of distant metastasis. It is sometimes difficult to tell whether the disease is primary or secondary.

Cause and Incidence

The cause of cancer of the Fallopian tube is unknown. It is extremely rare, accounting for somewhere between .3 and 1.1 percent of all gynecological cancers.[24] Even those cancer specialists who treat only patients referred to them by other doctors are unlikely to see more than one patient a year with cancer of the Fallopian tube.

Symptoms

Over 90 percent of the women with this disease will have symptoms. But the symptoms are often inconsistent, that is, they vary from case to case, are nonspecific (can be caused by many other diseases) and are so slight, at least in the early stages, that the symptoms are often ignored or misinterpreted.

Abnormal vaginal bleeding, spasmlike pain, heavy vaginal discharge that tends to be watery and mucus-filled or tinged with blood and abdominal distention are all possible symptoms of Fallopian tube cancer.

Diagnosis

Most of the time this disease is found unexpectedly in the course of exploratory surgery or surgery done for some other reason. Less than 5 percent of cases are diagnosed preoperatively.

Spread and Staging

Decisions about how far the disease has spread are usually made at the time of the operation. Cancer of the Fallopian tube most often spreads by direct invasion of the cancer into the surrounding organs. The disease may also be spread by the lymph or blood systems. Since the disease is so rare, no official staging scheme has been developed. The staging schemes used are similar to the ones used for ovarian cancer.

Treatment

The same principles that apply to the treatment of ovarian cancer apply to this disease. The treatment is primarily surgical and consists of total hysterectomy, that is, the removal of the tubes, uterus and ovaries.

Postoperative radiation in the form of external beam therapy may be given, though there is some debate about the effectiveness of such radiation.[26] Recently, chemotherapy has proven to be of some limited value. Despite the lack of spectacular results, chemotherapy is frequently used in the treatment of this disease.

Survival Rates

The overall five-year survival rate for this disease is 38 percent.[27] The stage of the disease is, of course, a significant factor in the survival rates. Five-year survival rates as high as 60 percent have been reported for Stage I.[28] Most deaths occur in the first two years after diagnosis.

The Ovaries

The anatomy and the function of the ovary, which is illustrated in Chapter Two and is discussed in Chapter Four, may be disrupted by a variety of disease processes. Basically, though, there are four kinds of things that can go wrong with the ovary.

Ovarian Infections

First of all, the ovary can become infected. Infections of the ovary alone, which are known in medical circles as oophoritis, are rare. When the ovary is infected, it is usually a part of a more widespread infection involving the Fallopian tubes and other pelvic organs. When these widespread infections occur, collections of pus, known as tubo-ovarian abcesses or cysts, may be formed. These infectious processes are discussed elsewhere in this book under the heading Pelvic Inflammatory Disease.

Birth Defects

Secondly, the ovary can be abnormal as a result of congenital problems, that is, due to birth defects. For instance, a woman may be born without any ovaries or even with extra ones. Her ovaries may not have the proper amount of eggs, causing her to have a premature menopause. A woman may have both ovaries and the male counterpart, testes, or may have testes instead of ovaries. Fortunately, these sorts of problems are rather rare and are discussed only briefly under the first heading in this section, Congenital Abnormalities of the Ovary.

Ovulation Problems

There may be disturbances in the process by which an egg is matured and released from the ovary each month. The follicular sac, inside of which the ripening egg develops, may not behave properly and may swell up, creating a follicular cyst. The corpus luteum, which is formed from the remnants of the follide after it has burst open and released its egg, may also function improperly, creating a luteum cyst. These are called physiologic cysts. Another type of ovarian problem associated with abnormal ovulation is a condition known as polycystic (meaning "many cyst") disease.

Ovarian Tumors

The fourth group of problems that can affect the ovary are ovarian tumors. The word "tumor" is a scary one that conjures up associations with cancer for most of us. But in the widest medical sense of the word, the term "tumor" merely means a "swelling." A pimple, for instance, would be a tumor in medical jargon. The luteum and follicular cysts mentioned above are also considered tumors in the medical sense of the term, but they are generally not serious problems. Indeed, physiologic cysts usually do not even require treatment, for they generally disappear all by themselves. These physiologic cysts, the cysts associated with polycystic disease and the tubo-ovarian cysts mentioned above, as well as another type of ovarian cyst known as an endometrial cyst, are all nonneoplastic tumors, which means that they are *not* ("non") *new* ("neo") *growths* ("plastic").

All of the other tumors of the ovary are neoplastic, or new growths. There are quite a few different types of neoplastic tumors that can occur in the ovary, for the ovary is a complex organ containing many types of tissue. Moreover, the ovary contains the ova, the female egg cells, which have the potential, if fertilized, to produce hair, skin, bone—indeed, all of the different types of tissue present in the adult human. Therefore, it is not surprising that a wide variety of tumors, including some rather bizarre ones that contain hair, teeth and bits of bone, can arise from the ovary.

These new growths may be cystic (fluid-filled), solid, semisolid or semicystic. They may be unilateral, affecting only one ovary, or bilateral, involving both ovaries. Most importantly, they may be either benign or malignant. Certain types of tumors are always benign, like the ovarian

436

fibroma; others like the cystadenocarcinomas, are, by definition, cancerous. Oftentimes, there is not a clear dividing line between cancerous and noncancerous ovarian tumors, and these are called borderline tumors.

The new growths of the ovary are divided into two major groups: the benign tumors and the cancerous ones. We have also included a third group, known as the functioning ovarian tumors. They are referred to as functioning tumors because they are capable of producing hormones. Some produce male hormones, causing the woman to grow chest hair and a beard and to develop other masculine characteristics. Some produce the female hormone estrogen and can cause irregular bleeding. Some of these functioning tumors are benign and some are borderline or clearly cancerous.

Unfortunately, there is usually no way to tell whether an ovarian tumor is benign or malignant short of actually operating, removing the tumor and examining it under a microscope. The woman's age, and the feel of the tumor and its location may give the doctor some clues as to whether an ovarian tumor is benign or malignant. Solid tumors, for instance, are more likely to be malignant, as are bilateral tumors. If the woman is in her reproductive years, she probably has a benign tumor. If the woman is past menopause, the situation is more serious, for 50 percent of the ovarian tumors in these women will be cancerous.[1] If the doctor can feel a suspicious enlargement in the pelvis of a young girl, the situation is less serious than it would be in the postmenopausal woman. But it is more serious than in a woman who is in her reproductive years, for although ovarian cancer is rare in young girls, any type of ovarian enlargement in young girls is rare. Statistically speaking, the chances are that the young girl's suspicious enlargement is the result of some benign condition. Perhaps it is not even an ovarian enlargement, for it is sometimes hard for the doctor to determine by simply feeling a young girl's pelvis exactly where the enlargement is located. However, the doctor will always suspect cancer in a young girl who has a pelvic mass.

Exploratory Surgery for Ovarian Masses

But these signs are only clues. Cancer can occur in any age group, regardless of whether the tumor is unilateral or bilateral, cystic or solid; therefore, any time the doctor feels a suspicious mass that might be ovarian in origin, prompt exploratory surgery is in order. This may be hard for some of us to accept, especially if the mass is small and not causing any symptoms. Such surgery may seem needless—why have an operation when it's not causing any problems?

The answer is twofold. First, there is the chance that it might be a cancerous tumor. Secondly, the tumor, even if it is benign, will continue to grow larger, eventually producing symptoms and possibly causing serious complications. Moreover, in women who have future childbearing plans or who are anxious to preserve their ovaries in order to avoid premature menopause and all its attendant problems, it is necessary to remove the tumor before it completely destroys the rest of the ovary.

There is one important exception to this prompt-surgery-for-ovarian-tumors rule. If a woman is in her reproductive years, is not using birth control pills and has a small, soft mass, chances are that she has a luteum or follicular cyst. Since these usually disappear spontaneously within one or two menstrual cycles, waiting for a few weeks before doing surgery will often allow a woman to avoid unnecessary surgery. If you fall into this category, don't allow yourself to be rushed into surgery, as too often happens. If your doctor suggests immediate surgery, discuss this issue with him or her and consider getting a second opinion (see p. 226) before consenting to surgery.

If you are scheduled for surgery for a possible ovarian tumor, you should read the sections on physiologic cysts, benign ovarian tumors, and ovarian cancer. There are many considerations. If the tumor turns out to be benign, do you want the doctor to remove your ovaries or try to conserve as much ovarian tissue as possible? Some doctors will routinely remove both ovaries in women over 35 who have completed their families. Others will go to great lengths to save the ovaries, even if the woman is 45. A woman who has a family history of ovarian cancer might decide to have hers removed regardless of her age. Another woman who is at high risk for developing hypertension, a condition characterized by high blood pressure that can have serious, even fatal, consequences, might decide to try and save her ovaries if possible, for premature menopause might increase her risk of developing hypertension. There are many factors involved, and each woman must make the decision for herself. Unfortunately, many doctors won't even present these alternatives to their patients or will present them in a biased fashion, pushing their own point of view.

There are other questions to be considered as well. If your tumor is benign and only an ovary needs to be removed, do you want the doctor to remove your uterus as well? If it turns out to be a certain type of cancer, there may be different treatment options and decisions you may want to have a voice in making. There are also certain things you should check out prior to operation. Is the pathologist top-notch? Will there be more than one pathologist reviewing your slides? These questions and other information that you, as a consumer of medical services, have a need to know are discussed in the following pages. Read and study them carefully, and then, armed with enough knowledge to enable you to ask the right questions, discuss these issues with your doctor, seeking second opinions wherever you feel the need.

CONGENITAL ABNORMALITIES OF THE OVARY

AKA: birth defects involving the ovary

Types: testicular feminization syndrome
true hermaphroditism
female hermaphroditism, pseudohermaphroditism, congenital adrenal
hyperplasia and adrenogenital syndrome
Turner's syndrome, gonadal dysgenesis, or gonadal agenesis
accessory ovaries
supernumerary ovaries
congenital absence of one ovary and Fallopian tube

Many, but not all, of the congenital abnormalities (birth defects) of the ovary are caused by abnormalities in the chromosomes, which are microscopic substances in the center of a cell that govern the cell's behavior. These are called developmental abnormalities. There may also be associated congenital abnormalities of the vulva. These conditions vary in their severity. One of the less serious ones, testicular feminization syndrome, is a condition in which a woman, normal in every other way, is born without a uterus and with organs that more closely resemble testes than ovaries. This is not as bizarre as it sounds, for testes and ovaries are actually rather similar and develop from the same fetal tissue. Such women have breast development and female secondary sex characteristics and function as normal women except that they do not have ovaries or a uterus and cannot, therefore, have children. The condition is generally diagnosed because the girl fails to start menstruating. It is difficult to distinguish between this syndrome and congenital absence of the uterus, but it is important to do so since the abnormal ovarian/testicular tissue must be removed, as it is subject to the development of cancer. The diagnosis and treatment of this syndrome is discussed under the heading Amenorrhea. Interestingly enough, women with this syndrome are often quite striking. They tend to be tall, with long graceful arms and legs.

True hermaphroditism is another developmental abnormality. It is a condition in which the person has male and female organs, both internally and externally. There may be both an ovary and testis on each side or an ovary on one side and a testis on the other. The condition is again due to a defect in the chromosomes and is often associated with mental retardation. The external genital organs may appear normal, although usually they are also deformed. At puberty, the development may be along male or female lines, depending on whether ovarian or testicular tissue predominates. Treatment may include hormone therapy and plastic surgery.

Female pseudohermaphroditism, congenital adrenal hyperplasia and adrenogenital syndrome are conditions in which masculine traits appear in a genetic female. They may be detected at birth if the external genitals are

439

abnormal. The clitoris may, for instance, be enlarged and may look more like a penis than a clitoris. Otherwise, they may not show up until puberty, when the child has rapid growth, a muscular, male body-type, early development of male hair patterns on the face and chest, acne and failure to have menstrual periods. These conditions are caused by an overproduction of hormones by the adrenal glands. In pseudohermaphroditism this overproduction is due to a chromosomal abnormality. Adrenogenital syndrome, on the other hand, may not be a birth defect at all, but may be caused by a tumor of the adrenal gland. The symptoms may be quite obvious or rather subtle. In some cases these conditions are diagnosed only because the girl fails to menstruate at the normal age. Diagnosis, which is made by certain laboratory tests, is discussed more fully under the heading Amenorrhea. Treatment may include surgery to correct abnormalities of the genitals, and hormone therapy to stimulate secondary sex characteristics. Other forms of pseudohermaphroditism, both male and female, can occur and require similar treatment.

Another type of developmental abnormality is Turner's syndrome, also called gonadal dysgenesis or gonadal agenesis. It is caused by abnormalities in the chromosomes of the genes. Since the ovaries are undeveloped or absent altogether, the hormones that stimulate growth and sexual development are also absent. The condition varies in its severity. It may be diagnosed at birth or may not become obvious until puberty or later. Children with this syndrome may have a webbed neck, a certain bone condition known as osteoporosis, widely spaced nipples, a low hair line, small jaw and short stature. The genitals do not develop properly, nor do the breasts. Such women have minimal sexual hair or sometimes none, do not menstruate and are infertile. The ovaries are absent or under-developed. The physical appearance and other symptoms will suggest the diagnosis and it can be confirmed by special tests. Treatment may involve estrogen therapy to stimulate secondary sex characteristics, but such therapy carries certain risks. These are discussed under the heading Estrogen Replacement Therapy. Plastic surgery may be done to create a normal vagina and external genital organs. Turner's syndrome is used to refer to a specific type of chromosomal abnormality. There are other, similar conditions whose symptoms may vary slightly. For instance, the woman may be tall rather than short, but similar treatment is used.

Some congenital abnormalities of the ovary are thought to be the result of faulty development in the ovary rather than chromosomal abnormalities. These include: an extremely rare condition known as accessory ovaries, in which excess ovarian tissue is found, usually located near or attached to the normal ovary; supernumerary ovaries, in which three or more ovaries are present; and the absence of one ovary and Fallopian tube, which may be associated with certain congenital abnormalities of the uterus. These conditions are fortunately rather rare.

PHYSIOLOGIC CYSTS

AKA: ovarian cysts, functional cysts*

Types: follicle, or follicular, cysts
       luteum cysts

Associated terms: corpus luteum hematoma, follicular hematoma

There are two types of physiologic cysts, luteum and follicle cysts. Follicle cysts occur quite frequently, for they are really just exaggerations of a normal process that occurs cyclically in the mature female. Each month a number of ova (eggs) resting inside sacs called follicles deep within the ovary are stimulated by hormones to develop and move toward the surface of the ovary. As they develop, specialized cells that line the interior cavity of the follicular sac secrete fluids that nourish the developing ovum, and these fluids cause the follicle to swell. Normally only one of these swelling follicles is chosen to mature fully, reach the surface and release its egg at ovulation. Countless others fail and disintegrate into microscopic specks of scar tissue.

Sometimes this normal process goes awry. Either the chosen follicle fails to release its egg and continues to grow larger or one or more of the competing follicles doesn't disintegrate and continues to swell with fluid. If either of these things happens, one or more cysts, that is, encapsulated collections of fluid, known as follicular cysts are formed.

Just as follicle cysts are the result of a distortion of the process of ovulation, so luteum cysts are an irregularity in the normal course of events. After the follicle bursts, releasing its egg at ovulation, the remnants of the burst follicle become the corpus luteum, which starts producing the hormone progesterone. This hormone helps the uterus get ready for a possible pregnancy by stimulating the uterine lining to grow rich and thick, so that the egg, if fertilized, will be well nourished. If a fertilized egg does not implant in the lining of the uterus, the corpus luteum normally stops producing progesterone and disintegrates. Without the progesterone to support its growth, the rich lining begins to disintegrate and is shed during the monthly period. In the case of a luteum cyst, the corpus luteum does not disintegrate as it should, but swells with fluid and persists on the surface of the ovary as a cyst. There is normally a small amount of bleeding into the corpus luteum after the follicle bursts. Sometimes this can become excessive, and the cyst fills up with blood. This is called a corpus luteum hematoma. Similarly, blood may fill a follicular cyst in which case the name follicular hematoma is used.

*These cysts are sometimes called functional cysts because they develop from normal ovarian process or functions. This is not to be confused with the term "functioning cysts."

Symptoms

These cysts are generally rather small, for the pressure of the fluid on the cyst wall prevents the further production of fluid and greater enlargement.

They may produce the same symptoms as any other ovarian cyst (*see* p. 448); however, since they are usually small, they are less likely to produce severe symptoms. If, however, they grow large, there may be a dull ache on the affected side.

They may affect the menstrual cycle. The luteum cyst, which affects progesterone production, is more apt to alter the menstrual cycle. The continued stimulation of the uterine lining by the progesterone may delay the period. When menstrual flow does start, the bleeding may be rather scant since much of the lining may be retained because of the effect of the progesterone.

Physiologic cysts generally don't become pedunculated, that is, they don't grow stems, or pedicles, as so many other ovarian tumors do. If, however, they grow large, they may develop pedicles, in which case they are subject to the same complications and may produce the same symptoms as any other pedunculated ovarian cyst.

These cysts may rupture spontaneously or as a result of some physical exertion. If a follicle cyst ruptures, there is generally little pain, for the fluid that spills into the pelvic cavity is not irritating. If blood has seeped into the follicle cyst and the cyst then ruptures, there may be some discomfort, but this usually passes away and rarely reaches the emergency proportions that rupture of other types of ovarian cysts can cause.

The luteum cyst is less prone to rupture; however, should it rupture, it is more likely to cause pain since it is more apt to contain larger amounts of blood, and blood is highly irritating to the pelvic cavity. A ruptured corpus luteum cyst can produce symptoms similar to those of a ruptured ectopic pregnancy. Laparoscopic exam may be the only way to distinguish between the two.

Diagnosis

These cysts are often diagnosed when bothersome symptoms of pelvic pressure or pain bring the woman to the doctor, or they may be discovered in the course of a routine pelvic exam. The diagnostic procedures are the same as those used for any other type of ovarian tumor (*see* p. 453).

Treatment

As explained in the introduction to this section, ovarian cysts generally require prompt surgery because of the possibility that they may be cancerous, but younger women with small cystic masses should not allow themselves to be rushed into surgery, as too often happens. In all likelihood such a woman will have a follicular or luteum cyst that will rupture spontaneously or be reabsorbed by the body within one or two menstrual cycles. Waiting a few weeks can prevent unnecessary surgery. We generally wait one menstrual cycle in these cases. Some doctors will wait for two cycles, since some of these physiologic cysts take that long to disappear. This is certainly acceptable medical practice; however, we are a bit more conservative about this and will recommend an operation if a cyst persists for more than one cycle because of the possibility that this could be ovarian cancer, a very serious disease. While this is our personal philosophy, many doctors feel that waiting for two cycles is justified.

If, however, the woman is past menopause or is using birth control pills, she is not ovulating and therefore could not have a physiologic cyst. In these women, surgery cannot be delayed. Chances are that she has a benign cyst, but follicular and luteum cysts are the only cysts that will disappear spontaneously, so there is nothing to be gained by delaying surgery in these women. Also, if a woman's cyst is larger than five cm, surgery should not be delayed, for cysts of this size rarely regress on their own.

If an operation is done and a follicular cyst is discovered, the ovary should not be removed, as is sometimes done. The contents of a smaller cyst can be aspirated with a needle, which will cause the cyst to collapse. The larger ones can be shelled out, leaving much of the normal ovary intact. If a luteum cyst is discovered, it is usually not removed or aspirated, unless it is large or is leaking blood into the pelvic cavity. The corpus luteum normally continues to function in the early stages of pregnancy to support the developing embryo. The woman might have an undiagnosed pregnancy and removing the corpus luteum could terminate the pregnancy.

A newer treatment, known as ovarian cyst fenestration, may be recommended to women suspected of having physiologic cysts. However, as explained elsewhere (*see* p. 456), we feel this procedure is too risky and do not recommend it.

POLYCYSTIC OVARIES

AKA: polycystic disease, or syndrome; Stein-Leventhal disease, or syndrome

Polycystic ovaries are another type of disturbance of the process of ovulation. In the normal monthly course of events follicles deep within the ovaries that contain unripe eggs are stimulated to grow, develop and move toward the surface of the ovary, where one of these follicles matures, bursts open and releases its egg. This process of stimulating eggs and their follicles is governed by hormones from the pituitary gland. After the egg is released at ovulation, the remnants of the burst follicle become the corpus luteum, which produces the hormone progesterone. The primary effect of this hormone is to stimulate the lining of the uterus to grow rich and thick in case it needs to support a fertilized egg. The rising levels of progesterone also affect the pituitary, which has been busily sending out its hormones to stimulate the eggs to develop. In effect the progesterone tells the pituitary: "Stop stimulating eggs, ovulation has occurred."

In patients with polycystic disease, this normal progression of events doesn't take place. The follicles with the unripe eggs never get to the surface of the ovary. Instead, they just sit there, literally stuck beneath the surface of the ovary. Since there is no egg, there is no burst follicle. Therefore, no corpus luteum is formed and there are no rising levels of progesterone, which means that no "turn-off" message is sent to the pituitary. The pituitary therefore continues to send out its hormones, which stimulate more and more follicles.

These follicles continue to get trapped just below the surface of the ovary. After a while both ovaries become studded with multiple small cysts just below the surface. Even though these individual cysts may measure only a fraction of an inch, all together they can cause the ovary to enlarge to as much as two or three times its normal size. There is a sort of thickened capsule surrounding the ovary. It is unclear whether this thickened capsule is actually a result of the presence of many follicle cysts or is perhaps the cause of them. Occasionally, some women with polycystic disease have a successful ovulation, but most of the time, no ripened eggs are released.

Polycystic disease is also called Stein-Leventhal disease after Dr. Irving Stein who defined the characteristic group of associated symptoms. Not all patients with polycystic ovaries have all the symptoms Dr. Stein identified. Some doctors don't use the term Stein-Leventhal in such cases, but most doctors use the two terms interchangeably.

Incidence and Cause

This disease is usually found in women between the ages of 17 and 30. The cause of the disease is unknown, but heredity seems to be a factor.

Symptoms

The symptoms include irregular or absent menstrual periods, infertility (due to lack of ovulation), pain, abnormal hair growth and excessive weight gain.

444

The most outstanding symptom is irregularity or absence of menstrual bleeding. This symptom usually occurs shortly after a young woman begins to menstruate for the first time, but it can also occur in women who have been menstruating normally for quite some time. At first there may be heavy, erratic bleeding, interspersed with fairly regular periods. After a while though, the bleeding becomes more scanty and less frequent and stops altogether. Because these women do not ovulate they are, of course, infertile.

Because of the thickened capsule surrounding the ovary, the follicles cannot develop normally, so that women with polycystic disease may have lower abdominal pain due to pressure as the follicles push against the capsule. About 40 percent of the women with Stein-Leventhal syndrome are overweight. Approximately 70 percent of women with polycystic ovaries have a condition known as hirsutism, which means that they grow extra facial and body hair. This is probably a result of the fact that polycystic ovaries produce more androgens than normal ovaries do. The body converts androgens into testosterone, the so-called male hormone (so-called because all normal women have some testosterone in their bodies). Although there may be male-type body hair patterns, most women with this disease don't have the more drastic masculinization effects, such as decrease in breast size or balding. Some women do, however, have some enlargement of the clitoris, due to an excess of male hormones. It should be noted that polycystic ovaries are not the only cause of hirsutism. Unless the appearance of this excess hair is sudden, it is more likely that excessive body hair is the result of racial and individual genetic heritage.

Diagnosis

In addition to these symptoms, the doctor will probably be able to feel an enlargement of the ovaries. Usually both ovaries are equally enlarged, although in some rare cases in the very early stages of the disease, one ovary may be enlarged slightly more than the other. The uterus in Stein-Leventhal women is sometimes smaller than normal. It may in fact be about the same size as the enlarged ovaries, so that on bimanual exam the doctor feels three masses of about the same size.

These symptoms and signs are not enough to allow for a definite diagnosis of Stein-Leventhal disease. The doctor can also make certain hormone tests since patients with polycystic disease generally have certain characteristic differences in their hormone levels. These tests are described more fully under the heading, Amenorrhea. Diagnosis may include some form of visual examination of the ovaries either by culdoscopy or laparoscopy, procedures in which a special viewing instrument is inserted into the body through a small incision either in the vagina or the abdomen. The characteristic appearance of the ovaries and the absence of any corpus luteum (although, as mentioned before, in some cases there may be evidence of occasional ovulation) will help to establish the diagnosis.

Treatment

Once the diagnosis has been established, precise treatment can be given. The ultimate aim of treatment is to establish regular menstrual cycles, for if the lining of the uterus doesn't build up and shed in the usual cyclical fashion, precancerous conditions like endometrial hyperplasia or actual cancer of the uterine lining may occur. Some studies indicate that the rate of uterine cancer is quite high in Stein-Leventhal patients, although Stein himself reported very few cases.

In the past, ovarian surgery was the preferred treatment, but in the last few years, hormone therapy has proven more effective. If a woman wants to become pregnant, fertility drugs may be used.

In women not concerned with pregnancy, a progesterone compound, such as Provera, taken orally, is given once a month, usually for about 5 days. Within 24 hours this drug will cause the lining to thicken and swell, and once the drug is eliminated from the body the endometrial lining, deprived of the progesterone, will break down and shed. It may not be necessary to use progesterone each month. Most doctors feel that every two or three months is sufficient to prevent hyperplasia or endometrial cancer.

Some doctors will prescribe birth control pills instead of progesterone therapy for women with polycystic disease. The progesterone in the pill suppresses the pituitary hormones that keep stimulating all those follicles, thus stopping the continual cystic enlargement of the ovaries. Using the pill cyclically, three weeks on and one week off, will allow the uterine lining to be shed. The Pill will also cut down on the amount of testosterone being produced and may solve hirsutism problems. In most cases, though, hormone therapy won't make the excess hair growth that has already taken place disappear.

We prefer to use progesterone therapy rather than birth control pills, for the Pill also contains estrogen, which can have serious side effects and complications. Although synthetic progesterones can also cause problems, these are not thought to be as serious as estrogen's side effects and complications.

Progesterone treatment won't cause a woman to ovulate. If a woman

Illustration 50 *Wedge Resection: A wedge-shaped portion of the ovary is removed (A). The edges of the ovary are sutured (B) and the ovary is closed back up (C).*

wishes to get pregnant, she must, of course, ovulate. In order to stimulate ovulation, fertility drugs, like Clomid, may be used. Some doctors will use Clomid to treat a woman with polycystic disease even if she doesn't want to become pregnant; however, the use of Clomid involves certain risks and we feel it should be used only if pregnancy is desired.

If Clomid and other fertility drugs are not successful, surgery may be done. A procedure called a bilateral wedge resection (Illustration 50) cures menstrual irregularity in 85 percent of the cases and produces pregnancy in 75 percent of the polycystic patients who desire it. This form of surgery involves reducing the bulk of the ovaries, and although there are a couple of theories, no one is quite sure exactly how it works. If ovulation doesn't occur after surgery, the use of Clomid may prove effective even if it has been ineffective prior to surgery.

BENIGN OVARIAN TUMORS

AKA: noncancerous tumors of the ovary

Associated terms: Meigs' syndrome

Types: serous and mucinous cystadenomas
fibromas
dermoid cysts
teratomas
paraovarian cysts
Brenner tumors
germinal inclusion cysts

There are many different types of ovarian tumors, and no one knows what causes them. Since all benign tumors require the same type of treatment, produce pretty much the same symptoms and require the same diagnostic procedures, they are all considered here.

Symptoms and Complications

Ovarian tumors may not produce any symptoms at all when they are small. Some women, however, experience pain on intercourse, and as the tumors grow larger, they may produce swelling of the abdomen and a feeling of fullness or bearing-down discomfort in the abdomen or pelvis. If, due to their size or location, they put pressure on adjacent organs like the bladder or rectum, they may cause irregularities in bowel movement or urination. If they block the blood or lymph channels, they can cause varicose veins, hemorrhoids and swelling of the legs or vulva. If they grow large enough, they may displace the uterus, moving it to one side or another. Ovarian tumors can also cause irregularities in the menstrual cycle or, in postmenopausal or prepubertal women, abnormal uterine bleeding. Certain ovarian tumors are capable of producing male or female hormones. These tumors often create menstrual problems as well as other symptoms related to hormone imbalance, such as excessive facial hair, deepening of the voice, flattening of the breasts, and premature breast development and other symptoms of precocious puberty, depending on whether male or female hormones are produced by the tumor. These symptoms most often occur with these tumors, called functioning ovarian tumors, but can occur with other types of ovarian tumors as well.

There is generally little pain from the tumor itself, but these tumors, especially the cystic ones, are subject to certain complications that can produce pain. Some of these complications arise from the fact that these tumors may be pedunculated, which means that they are attached to the ovary by means of a stem or stalk, called a pedicle, through which the blood and lymph supply to the tumor circulates.

If the tumor is not blocked by scar tissue from previous pelvic infections and is light enough, and the pedicle is long enough, the tumor may rise upward in the pelvic cavity, floating like a helium balloon attached to a string and moving freely to different locations. They are then subject to twisting of the stem, an event known as torsion of the pedicle. This, of course, is much more likely to happen with the lighter, fluid-filled cystic tumors than with the heavier, solid ones.

Once the pedicle is twisted, a number of things may happen, producing a variety of symptoms. The severity of the symptoms will depend on how much twisting there is and on how rapidly the twisting takes place. If the twisting is only partial, there may be little in the way of symptoms. Even if the twisting is complete, the symptoms may not be too severe provided that the twisting has occurred slowly. In fact, the cyst may untwist itself. On rare occasions it may twist itself completely off.

The pain associated with torsion of the pedicle may be sharp and persistent, or it may be only moderately severe and transitory. Not infrequently, however, it is sudden and excruciating. There may be nausea, vomiting, an accelerated pulse and a rise in temperature. If the ovary on the right side is affected, the doctor may think the woman has appendicitis. Severe symptoms like these may require emergency surgery.

If the twisting is only partial, the arteries that provide the blood supply to the ovary are not usually affected, but the veins that carry the blood away from the tumor may then become enlarged and swollen. They may break and cause bleeding into the tumor, which in turn causes the tumor to swell up, producing pain due to pressure on the walls of the tumor.

The blood supply to the tumor may be cut off if this swelling becomes too severe or if the pedicle is completely twisted. Without the nourishment

449

provided by the blood flowing into the tumor, portions of it may die. Tumors that grow too large for their blood supply also tend to break down in their centers. This dying tissue can also cause the tumor to swell and may also produce pain due to pressure on the tumor walls. These dying areas of the tumor are a perfect breeding ground for infection, again causing swelling and pain. Secondary infection of an ovarian cyst may produce symptoms similar to those produced by acute pelvic inflammatory disease.

On rare occasions, the bleeding, tissue death or infection produces so much swelling that the tumor breaks open and the irritating contents of the tumor either leak or spill into the abdominal cavity.

Spontaneous rupture of cystic tumors can occur even though the stem is not twisted and the tumor has a completely adequate blood supply. Cysts have been known to rupture after intercourse, a fall, a direct blow to the abdomen or childbirth, or when they are being removed surgically. The symptoms produced by a ruptured cyst will depend on how irritating its contents are. There is bound to be some pain, but certain cysts contain fluids that don't irritate the abdominal cavity much while others contain much more irritating contents. However, as long as the contents are not infected, the reaction is usually not overwhelming. The contents tend to collect in certain areas. In defense, the neighboring tissue produces a fibrous substance that hardens into bands of tissue called adhesions, which wall off the irritating contents. These collections of cyst contents are usually tender to the touch and may cause pain upon exertion or intercourse.

If, however, the rupture is accompanied by bleeding into the pelvic cavity, the symptoms of pain, nausea, vomiting and faintness may be severe. If a blood vessel has been broken, the bleeding may even be fatal. Such extreme bleeding is rare, however, for in the majority of cases cysts are made up of little separate compartments and only one is involved in the rupture. The initial pain and other symptoms may therefore subside after a few hours, although for a few days there may be tenderness and rigidity in the lower abdomen, with moderate fever. This may be confused with a ruptured ectopic pregnancy.

Sometimes ovarian tumors will be accompanied by the production of ascites, that is, they will leak fluid into the abdominal cavity. Ascites is more likely to occur with malignant tumors than with benign ones; however, it does happen even with benign tumors. Sometimes, the fluid produced by the tumor will affect the area around the lungs as well. When an ovarian tumor is accompanied by ascites and this type of lung-cavity involvement, the term Meigs' syndrome is used. Again, this can happen with either benign or malignant tumors.

Types

There are many different types of benign ovarian tumors. Some of the more common ones are discussed below.

Serous and Mucinous Cystadenomas

These are the most common of the cystic tumors of the ovary. They may be filled with a thin, watery serous fluid or a thick, sticky mucinous fluid. They are noted for their unusually large size. Sometimes they reach incredible proportions, weighing many pounds and completely filling the abdominal cavity. The mucinous varieties tend to be larger than the serous ones. Doctors apparently love to take pictures of them and no medical textbook is considered complete without at least a couple of photos of a 200-pounder.

They are often pedunculated and are subject to the types of problems that can occur with any pedunculated ovarian tumor, including rupture. If they do break down and spill their contents into the pelvic cavity, the mucinous cysts are more likely to cause pain and adhesions than the serous ones, for the gluelike contents of the mucinous cysts are highly irritating to the lining of the pelvic cavity.

Fibromas

Fibromas are the most common of the solid benign ovarian tumors. These tumors are composed of fibrous connective tissue. Sometimes, there are other types of tissue, such as bone or cartilage, in the tumor as well. They are usually solid, although they may contain one large or several small, soft, fluid-filled, cystic areas. Certain varieties sometimes produce estrogen, just like the functioning ovarian tumors, and thus may cause some of the same symptoms associated with these tumors.

Dermoid Cyst

The dermoid cyst, one of the more bizarre types of ovarian cysts, is filled with an oily fluid and may contain hair and even teeth, bits of bone and cartilage. The dermoid belongs to a class of tumors that arise from the germ cells of the ovary, the cells which produce the egg, or ovum. Despite the fact that it has not been fertilized, the egg tissue can start to develop in an unstructured way and produce a dermoid tumor.

Dermoid cysts are the most common ovarian tumor in women younger than 20 and also the most common ovarian tumor occurring in pregnant women. They vary in size, but are rarely large and tend to be unilateral (affecting only one ovary), although in 25 percent of the cases they are bilateral. They are often attached to the ovary by a stem, or pedicle, and are thus subject to the usual complications. They rarely rupture; however, if they do spill their contents into the pelvic cavity, they may cause extremely acute symptoms, for the contents of these tumors are highly irritating to the pelvic cavity.

Paraovarian Cysts

Paraovarian cysts are soft, fluid-filled, benign tumors that take their name from the location in which they are found, the paraovarium, an area adjacent to the main body of the ovary. They are usually unilateral and are relatively common in women in their 30s and 40s. Most of the time they are small and don't produce symptoms, so they are generally found only in the course of an operation done for some other reason. They can, however, grow rather large, but even then they rarely reach the size of the cysts that affect the main body of the ovary. They don't have stems, or pedicles, so they are not subject to the complications that can occur with other ovarian cysts; however, if they are large, they may push the uterus to one side.

Brenner Tumors of the Ovary

Brenner tumors of the ovary are usually benign; however, in the past ten years, a small number of malignant Brenner tumors have been reported. They too are generally unilateral and small, but on occasion, tumors of considerable size, weighing many pounds, have been reported. They are mostly found in postmenopausal women but can occur in any age group; however, they are only rarely seen in women under 30 years of age. Sometimes these tumors produce excessive menstrual flow.

Germinal Inclusion Cysts

These cysts are microscopic in size, cause no symptoms, are entirely benign, require no treatment and, therefore, deserve only brief mention. They are found in middle-aged and older women and are part of the normal process of aging. They may be mentioned in a pathology report if the ovary has been biopsied or removed for some other reason. We only mention them since a woman reading the pathology report may be concerned about their significance (none, relax!).

Diagnosis and Treatment

An ovarian tumor may be discovered because bothersome symptoms bring the woman to the doctor or because a mass is found in the course of a routine pelvic exam.

One problem in diagnosing ovarian tumors is determining whether the mass is actually on the ovary or on some other pelvic organ. Sometimes it will be obvious that the suspicious mass is ovarian in origin; at other times it is not so easy to determine the origin. For instance, it is sometimes difficult to distinguish between a pedunculated fibroid tumor of the uterus and an ovarian tumor. In a woman in her 30s, it is often hard to tell the difference between endometriosis, pelvic inflammatory disease, and an ovarian tumor. Indeed, there is a wide variety of diseases, from various bowel diseases to congenital abnormalities of the uterus to ectopic pregnancy, that can be confused with ovarian tumors. Even a full bladder may be confused with a pelvic mass—possibly an ovarian tumor—so the pelvic examination should be done only after the bladder is emptied. It is important not to ignore this step, for women have been operated on, only to have it found that the suspicious mass was merely a swollen bladder.

If the doctor is not certain whether or not a mass is ovarian in origin, s/he may perform certain diagnostic tests. Sonograms, pictures of internal organs taken by means of high frequency sound waves, may be done; or laparoscopic or culdoscopic exams, procedures in which the ovaries are examined by means of special viewing instruments, may be done.

Another problem in diagnosing ovarian tumors centers around determining whether the tumor is benign or malignant. Generally, this cannot be done short of actually operating on the woman, removing the tumor and examining it microscopically. On rare occasions, a cancerous ovarian tumor will be detected by a Pap smear, but the Pap smear is not reliable in detecting ovarian cancer.

Definite diagnosis requires an operation. Special X-ray tests, including possibly an intravenous pyelogram (IVP) or a barium enema, may be done preoperatively. In addition, special viewing instruments, the cystoscope and the proctosigmoidoscope, may be used to examine the bladder and the small bowel.

Once the doctor has made the surgical incision, s/he removes all of the tumor, or at least as much as possible. In some cases it may be necessary to remove the entire tube and ovary. If the tumor is a fluid-filled cyst, great care must be taken to remove it without spilling its contents, for if the cyst is cancerous, spillage of its contents could spread the cancer to other parts of the abdominal cavity. The tumor or the portions of it that have been removed are then sent to the pathology lab for analysis via frozen section.

453

It is particularly important that the pathologist be top-notch and up-to-date. New information has necessitated frequent changes in the terminology used to describe various types of ovarian tumors, but it takes time for these changes to percolate through the ranks of pathologists. Those pathologists who have not kept up with these changes may be providing out-of-date diagnoses to surgeons. It is also important that the surgeon and the pathologist have good communication so that they are sure they are both using the same terms to mean the same thing. Mistakes do happen. Consider the case of a 19-year woman who was operated on for an ovarian tumor.[2] The pathologist reported that the woman had a cancerous tumor, on the basis of her frozen section. The permanent section, according to this pathologist, confirmed the diagnosis of cancer. Luckily for this woman, because of some technical problems at the time of operation the surgeon removed only the ovary and referred her to an ovarian cancer specialist. A review of the pathology of her tumor revealed that she did not have cancer at all. She had what is known as a papillary serous cystadenoma, a benign tumor. Thus, her other ovary and her childbearing capacity were preserved. The mistake was made because this woman's tumor had small papillary (nipple-shaped) protrusions. While it is true that most papillary serous growths are malignant, this is not always the case.

Women should find out ahead of time whether or not the pathologist is board-certified (*see* p. 223) and how many pathologists will be available to review her slides. The importance of having a high-caliber pathologist is discussed in greater detail in the section on cancer, along with more information about how to investigate the pathology situation before the operation.

While the surgeon carefully examines the rest of the pelvic organs, the pathologist examines the tissue and sends back a report to the surgeon. If the report indicates that the tumor is malignant or is borderline, appropriate therapy as described under the heading Ovarian Cancer is done.

If the pathologist's report indicates that the tumor is benign, it nonetheless needs to be removed. Not only will it continue to grow larger, possibly creating the complications described above and destroying the healthy ovarian tissue, but with certain types of tumors there is the danger of malignant degeneration—of the tumor's becoming cancerous.

Sometimes it is possible to remove the tumor and to save the rest of the ovary (Illustration 51). Even a small nubbin of ovarian tissue may be capable of functioning normally, and women with such an ovary not only continue to produce ovarian hormones but are, surprisingly, fertile. At other times, the tumor will have destroyed so much ovarian tissue that the

Illustration 51 *Ovarian Cyst Removal: Sometimes a cyst or tumor on the ovary can simply be removed and the wound sutured back together.*

entire ovary must be removed. If there are tumors on both ovaries, sometimes both or at least one of the ovaries or some portion of ovarian tissue can be saved. In some cases it may be necessary to remove both ovaries.

In young women desirous of having children, the doctor will make every effort to save all or some portion of the ovary. Even if the younger woman has completed her family, an effort is usually made to conserve the ovaries, for this will usually prevent premature menopause, which carries certain risks, including increased risk of getting hypertension or having a fatal heart attack, as well as other problems.

In older women the question of whether or not to conserve the ovary becomes more controversial. Some doctors advocate removal of both ovaries and the uterus as well in all women over 35; others use 40 or 45 as the cutoff point. The pros and cons of removing the ovaries and uterus are discussed in more detail under the heading Hysterectomy.

Another controversy revolves around the treatment of the woman who, although she has no future childbearing plans, wants to preserve her ovarian tissue if possible. If such a woman needs to have only one ovary removed, the question of what to do with her uterus arises. Some doctors feel it should be removed since the woman does not want to have children. Other doctors (and we lean toward this viewpoint) feel that since hysterectomy is a major surgical procedure, it should not be done unless necessary. We are reluctant to remove a healthy uterus. If birth control is a concern for the woman, we would recommend one of the barrier methods, or, if she were adamant about sterilization, tubal ligation. The decision, of course, rests with the individual woman.

Women faced with ovarian tumor surgery should read the appropriate sections indicated in the text and discuss these issues in detail with their doctors prior to operation, seeking a second opinion (*see* p. 226) where necessary. It's better to find out that your doctor is from the ovaries-out-at-age-35 school of thought prior to operation than afterward.

Mention should also be made of a new approach to treating ovarian tumors that is being done in some hospitals. It is called ovarian cyst fenestration.[3] This technique uses a laparoscope to locate the cyst. The fluid is aspirated from the cyst with a needle, and a tissue sample is taken from the cyst wall and sent to the pathology lab for analysis. Assuming the lab report indicates a benign tumor, then the cyst wall is destroyed by electric current, a technique known as electric cautery. This technique can only be used in certain cases: The woman must be under 35, and the tumor must be soft, smooth, unilateral and less than four to eight cm in size. The physical exam, laparoscopic inspection of the tumor and all other signs must indicate that this is actually a benign cyst. Ovarian cyst fenestration has been done extensively in Europe, and its proponents in this country point out that it avoids more extensive surgery and a larger incision; however, most doctors are very skeptical about this form of treatment. Even though the vast majority of women under 35 who meet the criteria outlined above will have benign tumors, many doctors have had the experience of operating on such a woman, who turned out to have cancer. Puncturing a cancerous cyst could cause spillage of cancerous cells and spread of the disease, greatly reducing the woman's chances of survival. Given the fact that ovarian cancer, especially once it has spread, offers very poor survival rates, most doctors are reluctant to take even a small chance. Women whose doctors suggest this procedure should consider the risks seriously before consenting and should definitely seek a second opinion before undergoing the procedure.

Having just spent the last several pages explaining the necessity for surgery in women with ovarian enlargements, we are now going to say something that may seem like a contradiction. As explained in the introduction to this section, a younger woman with a small (less than five cm), soft, unilateral, smooth tumor should not allow herself to be rushed into surgery, as often happens. The odds are that she has only a luteum or follicular cyst, which tends to disappear all by itself. Waiting for one menstrual cycle (some doctors will wait for two or even three, but we feel that that is taking too much of a chance) can prevent unnecessary surgery.

If, however, the younger woman is on birth control pills, waiting is riskier, for women on the Pill are unlikely to have physiologic cysts. If the cyst is larger than five cm, waiting is not recommended, for even if she has a physiologic cyst, a cyst of that size is displacing normal ovarian tissue and needs to be removed. Moreover, if the cyst is solid or grows larger during the waiting period, prompt surgery will be required, for even though it is still likely that she has a benign and not a cancerous growth, there is no way of telling for sure, short of operation.

FUNCTIONING OVARIAN TUMORS

AKA: hormone-producing tumors

Types: masculinizing tumors
      feminizing tumors
        granulosa cell tumors
        theca cell tumors
        dysgerminomas

Functioning ovarian tumors are tumors that are capable of producing hormones. There are many different types of functioning ovarian tumors, but they all have this hormone-producing ability in common. This is not to say that they always *do* so, but some of them do, and when this occurs, there are apt to be hormone-related symptoms.

Functioning ovarian tumors may be broken down into two subgroups: the masculinizing tumors and the more common feminizing tumors. They are considered here separately.

Masculinizing Ovarian Tumors

These tumors occur only rarely. They are usually small to moderate in size, although occasionally they grow quite large. They are usually unilateral and occur most frequently in women in their early 20s and 30s. They are all capable of producing male hormones, which can produce symptoms such as absence of the menstrual period, decrease in the size of breasts, loss of the rounded contours of the female figure, change to male body-type, facial and chest hair, an enlarged clitoris and a deepening of the voice. All of these symptoms, except for the change in the voice, generally disappear

457

once the tumor is removed. Occasionally, for reasons that are not clear, these tumors will produce the type of symptoms usually associated with female hormones, such as excessive menstrual bleeding, and if this happens, there may be associated endometrial hyperplasia or endometrial cancer of the uterus.

If these tumors are hormonally active, the masculinizing symptoms they produce will help in the diagnosis; however, if the tumor is too small to be felt, there may be some question about diagnosis, for other conditions can cause these symptoms. The doctor will do certain laboratory tests and X-ray examinations to rule out other possibilities. The same sorts of diagnostic procedures used with other ovarian tumors and the same considerations involved in the treatment of benign ovarian tumors (see above) apply to benign masculinizing tumors. Treatment of malignant tumors is considered in the discussion of ovarian cancer.

Feminizing Ovarian Tumors

There are a number of different types of feminizing tumors. The most common are the granulosa cell and theca cell tumors. Occasionally, these tumors may leak fluid (ascites) and the fluid may even involve the area around the lungs, a condition known as Meigs' syndrome. They vary considerably in size from very small to very large, averaging five to ten cm in diameter. There seems to be little direct correlation between the size of the tumor and the hormone output, for very small tumors can produce excessive amounts of hormone while very large tumors may be hormonally inactive.

The symptoms that these tumors can cause are the same as those of any ovarian tumor (*see* p. 448). The larger tumors are prone to break down, and if this occurs, there is often blood in the fluid of the cystic areas. If such cysts rupture, their contents are apt to be highly irritating. In addition to the usual symptoms, tumors that are hormonally active can produce symptoms related to excessive hormone production. In young girls, they may cause precocious puberty, a condition characterized by the early onset of menstruation and the early development of breasts, body hair and other secondary sexual characteristics. Although such symptoms as breast enlargement do not occur in women who are past the age of puberty, the menstrual cycle can be reactivated in postmenopausal women.

Abnormal uterine bleeding is the most distinctive hormone-related symptom. In some cases, there may be an absence of menstruation, sometimes lasting for quite some time, followed by excessive vaginal bleeding. In other cases, there may be irregularly spaced, excessively profuse periods.

Women with these tumors may still ovulate and get pregnant. The uterus may be enlarged to as much as twice its normal size. Part of this enlargement is due to excessive hormonal stimulation, but some of it can be explained by the fact that women with these tumors often have associated benign fibroid tumors of the uterus. The continuous estrogen stimulation may also account for the fact that 15-25 percent of women with feminizing ovarian tumors also have cancer of the uterus, for such cancer is related to the overproduction of estrogen. The older a woman with a feminizing tumor, the greater the chances that she will have associated uterine cancer. Since younger women are less likely to have uterine cancer anyhow (it is a disease that generally affects older women), it is not surprising that they are less likely to have uterine cancer along with their feminizing tumors. Nonetheless, the possibility does exist. As many as 70-80 percent of women with feminizing tumors may have endometrial hyperplasia, a condition that can, in some cases, lead to uterine cancer.

The distinctive, hormonal-induced symptoms of these tumors in prepubertal girls and postmenopausal women, coupled with the presence of a solid ovarian mass, may lead the doctor to strongly suspect the presence of some type of feminizing ovarian tumor. However, at times the tumor may be too small to be felt. Diagnosis and treatment involve the same problems and procedures as with other ovarian tumors (*see* p. 453). However, if the tumors are malignant, they may require special therapy (see the section on ovarian cancer).

Dysgerminomas are another type of functioning tumor. They aren't feminizing tumors in the usual sense of the word, for they produce hormones associated with pregnancy rather than female hormones. They are often hormonally inactive, although on occasion they are active and may produce a positive pregnancy test. They may be associated with an enlarged uterus and an absence of menstrual periods. They are often malignant and may require special treatment (see the section on Ovarian Cancer below).

OVARIAN CANCER

Types: epithelial cell tumors
      serous cystadenocarcinoma
      mucinous cystadenocarcinoma
      endometroid carcinoma
      clear cell, or mesonephroid, carcinoma
      Brenner tumors
      mixed tumors
      other metastatic or rare tumors

germ cell tumors
   dysgerminoma
   embryonal tumors
   endodermal sinus tumors
   choriocarcinomas
   immature teratomas
   cancer arising inside a benign dermoid cyst
   mixed tumors
   other rare tumors
sex cord stromal tumors
   granulosa cell tumors
   other functioning ovarian tumors
   other rare tumors

Ovarian cancer is a relatively rare form of cancer, accounting for about 5 percent of all gynecologic cancers, but it is the fourth leading cause of cancer deaths in American women.[4] Nearly three-quarters of the women who get the disease die from it. The ovary is not an accessible organ in the way that the vulva, vagina and cervix are. Since it is not possible to get at the ovary easily in order to take cell samples or perform other screening tests to detect cancer early, ovarian cancer is generally not detected until it is in a fairly advanced stage.

Incidence and Risk Factors

There are approximately 14 new cases of ovarian cancer each year per 100,000 women of all ages.[5] The disease occurs most often in postmenopausal women, but beyond this, risk factors that could tell us which women are more likely to develop ovarian cancer have not yet been clearly defined. We do know that for women who have breast cancer, the risk of developing ovarian cancer increases twofold and vice versa.[6] Women who have an initial cancer of the intestine or rectum are also at increased risk.

Types

As explained in the introduction to this section, a wide variety of different types of tumors are found in the ovary. About 85 percent of ovarian cancers are epithelial tumors, which means that they arise from the epithelial tissue, a type of tissue that lines the cavities and passageways of the body and that covers the organs—in this case, the ovary. The most common of the epithelial tumors is the serous cystadenocarcinoma, which is the cancerous form of the benign serous cystadenoma. The second most common is the mucinous cystadenocarcinoma, which is the cancerous form of a benign mucinous cystadenoma. These tumors may develop within a benign tumor or may arise initially in their cancerous form. Endometroid tumors, clear cell tumors, Brenner tumors and mixed tumors are some of the other types of epithelial tumors that may arise in the ovary and may be malignant.

Certain functioning ovarian tumors called sex cord stromal tumors may also be cancerous. There are a number of other less common types of ovarian cancer. These other tumors are also classified according to the type of tissue from which they arise. In addition, the ovary may be the site of a metastasized tumor that had its origin elsewhere in the body. Identifying the particular tissue type of the tumor is important in terms of selecting proper treatment and predicting chances of survival.

Grade

The grade (*see* p. 678) of the tumor, that is, whether the tumor cells are mature, well differentiated and low grade or immature, undifferentiated and high grade, is of particular importance in ovarian cancer, especially in the early stages of the disease. The low-grade tumors are referred to as borderline tumors or tumors of low malignant potential. They are less serious, generally result in better survival rates than the high-grade, undifferentiated ones and may require less aggressive treatment.

The concept of borderline tumors has been of great importance in the treatment of ovarian cancer. Until ovarian tumors were divided into three groups—benign, borderline and malignant—it was difficult to make sense of survival statistics and to compare the different methods of treatment used by different institutions. Survival rates for Stage I serous cystadenocarcinomas, for instance, ranged from around 60 percent to as high as 98 percent; however, once the concept of the borderline cancer was developed, the survival rates became more uniform and there was no longer such a wide variance in the statistics (see below).

Symptoms

The symptoms that may appear in ovarian cancer are the same as those that may be associated with any type of ovarian tumor (*see* p. 448). In the early stages there may be no symptoms. The most common symptom is abdominal pain. The next most frequent symptom is abdominal swelling. A change in weight, usually weight loss, may be noted and may be due to loss of appetite, intermittent nausea or occasional vomiting. As the tumor grows larger there may be symptoms of pelvic pressure, abnormal bleeding, a change in the menstrual cycle or postmenopausal bleeding, cramps, constipation or a frequent need to urinate. However, approximately one-third of women with ovarian cancer are asymptomatic at the time of diagnosis.

Diagnosis

Sometimes ovarian tumors can produce symptoms even when it is not possible for the doctor to feel a pelvic mass. Such women may have symptoms mimicking gastrointestinal tract diseases, such as gall bladder disease or spastic colon, and may be referred to an internist for treatment. If the gastrointestinal work-up is negative, the possibility of an ovarian tumor must be considered and a laparoscopic exam should be done. Sometimes women who have tumors too small to be felt but have symptoms of persistent or recurrent pelvic pain do not receive the treatment they need. If they are young, they may be treated for salpingitis, an infection of the Fallopian tube. If they are postmenopausal, they may be given a prescription for tranquilizers, in other words, the old it's-all-in-your-head-dearie diagnosis.[7] Unfortunately, some of these women actually have ovarian tumors. Women should insist on proper and complete diagnostic procedures for their symptoms.

If a woman has suspicious symptoms, the doctor should do a pelvic exam. If a suspicious mass is felt, then an operation will be necessary. However, as we have seen, women with ovarian cancer may not have symptoms until the disease is fairly advanced. Many ovarian tumors are discovered in the course of a routine physical.

Occasionally, a Pap smear will pick up a case of ovarian cancer, but in order to show up in the Pap smear the cancerous cells would have had to travel down the Fallopian tubes, through the uterus, out through the opening of the cervix and into the vagina. The Pap smear, then, is of little value in detecting ovarian cancer.

Many times the doctor will feel a suspicious mass in the pelvis but won't be able to tell, without specialized testing (see p. 453), whether the mass is actually growing on the ovary or on some other pelvic organ. If the mass is definitely an ovarian one, it is then necessary to operate, for even if the tumor is not cancerous, it must be removed, as discussed under Benign Tumors of the Ovary. Much of the information there is pertinent to diagnosis of ovarian cancer and the reader should refer to that section before continuing here.

The consistency of the tumor, whether it is bilateral or unilateral and the age of the woman may make the doctor suspicious of cancer. If there is evidence of cancer in other sites in the pelvic cavity, the doctor may suspect that the woman has advanced ovarian cancer. If cancer is suspected, some of the diagnostic steps described in the general section on cancer should be done.

Most of the time, however, there is no way to find out for sure whether an ovarian tumor is cancerous or not, short of actually operating on the woman and removing all or part of the tumor for microscopic evaluation. Whenever possible, the entire tumor will be removed. Great care must be taken with fluid-filled, cystic tumors so that the tumor capsule is not broken and the contents spilled, for if the tumor is cancerous, this could spread the disease. Sometimes, despite the surgeon's skill, the tumor will rupture and this may decrease the woman's chance of survival.

Sometimes it is not possible to remove all of the tumor, and in such cases only a portion will be removed and sent to the lab for analysis. Even though it may be quite obvious from the appearance of the tumor that the woman has cancer, this analysis is necessary to determine the tissue-type of the tumor and the grade so that appropriate treatment can be planned. The possibility that the cancer has metastasized from some other site must be ruled out as well. And even if the appearance of the tumor convinces the doctor that it is benign, this analysis should still be done, for cancer can and does arise inside of benign ovarian tumors.

The tissue removed at operation is sent to the pathology lab for analysis via frozen section. It is important that the pathologist examine all suspicious areas of the tumor and make multiple sections, for it is not uncommon for cancerous and noncancerous or borderline areas to exist in the same tumor. The pathologist makes the diagnosis on the basis of multiple frozen sections; however, permanent sections are also done.

Samples of any fluid in the area should be suctioned out and also sent to the lab for analysis. The presence of malignant cells in such fluid is an indication that the cancer has spread and will influence staging and treatment. Unfortunately, this vital step is sometimes ignored. A woman diagnosed as having Stage I should ask if samples of fluid were taken. If the answer is no, she should seek a second opinion from a cancer specialist.

If the appearance of the tumor or the abdominal cavity suggests cancer, the surgeon will proceed to explore the abdominal cavity and take other tissue samples and cell specimens while waiting for the frozen-section analysis. Even if the surgeon is not certain, s/he may still explore the abdominal cavity while waiting for the tissue analysis from the pathology lab. If the pathologist sends back a report of cancer, a thorough exploration of the abdominal cavity is mandatory.

Unless the doctor had suspected cancer prior to operation (because of the age of the woman, her symptoms, the feel and consistency of the tumor or the results of preoperative tests), the original incision for the operation may have been what is known as a Pfannenstiel incision (Illustration 52). However, if the frozen-section analysis reveals cancer, the doctor should make another muscle-cutting incision in order to do an adequate exploration of the abdominal cavity. Some doctors feel that a Pfannenstiel incision does not allow for an adequate inspection.[8] Any woman with ovarian cancer whose doctor has done only a Pfannenstiel incision should discuss this with her doctor. She may want to seek a second opinion.

If the doctor's exploration reveals other tumor areas, these must also be removed, if possible. If there is no other sign of tumor (in medical terms, "no gross tumor"), then the doctor must take cell samples and tissue biopsies from various locations. If conservative surgery (see below) is a possibility, then, in addition to these tests, the opposite ovary must be examined, using a procedure known as a wedge biopsy. This must be done even if the other ovary appears normal, for cancer could be lurking inside the ovary.[9]

It is important that the surgeon be aware of the necessity for these other procedures in addition to the biopsy of the tumor itself. These tests will help to stage the disease and to indicate the need for futher surgery. They are not always done. Any woman being operated on for an ovarian mass should discuss the possibility of ovarian cancer and the need for the above-described tests with her doctor. If possible, she should have a board-certified doctor doing her surgery. If a woman discovered to have ovarian

Illustration52   *Pfannenstiel Incision*

cancer has not had an opportunity prior to her operation to assure that adequate exploratory cell samples and biopsies were taken, she should investigate this afterward. If these tests have not been done, a "second look" operation (see below) by a cancer specialist should take place.

The skill and experience of the pathologist are of critical importance, as explained in detail in the general section on cancer (*see* p. 674). In the past, all that the pathologist was expected to do was to report whether the tumor was benign or malignant. Nowadays, the pathologist must also tell the surgeon the cell type of the tumor and the grade. The doctor must have a good working relationship with the pathologist. Good communication between them is essential to ensure that both are using the same terminology in the same way. Because the pathologist's job is so critical, a woman will want to make sure that the pathologist on her case is board-certified. If the operation is an emergency one, it may not be possible to arrange this ahead of time, but, here again, it can be done subsequently.

Staging

Accurate staging of ovarian cancer is critical in selecting treatment and predicting survival. Table 14 outlines the most widely used staging scheme for ovarian cancer.[10]

Staging of ovarian cancer is done after the surgeon has removed the tumor, inspected the abdominal cavity to assess the spread of the disease, taken samples of the fluid in the abdominal cavity and gathered tissue samples from the ovary and/or other locations, to detect possible microscopic spread. Depending on the surgeon's findings, the pathologist's report and other standard tests to determine metastasis (*see* p. 676), the proper stage is assigned.

Treatment

Treatment of ovarian cancer usually involves surgery followed by some form of radiation therapy or, more commonly, chemotherapy. There are, however, important exceptions. The stage-by-stage treatments outlined below are general ones, and of course the specific treatment recommended by a woman's doctor may differ according to the particulars of her case. In some cases there is not yet uniform agreement among experts as to what is the best treatment in a given situation. The treatment program outlined here is not prescriptive, but is intended to provide enough information to enable women to understand the issues, to ask intelligent questions, to begin to evaluate their doctor's recommendations and to recognize those instances in which they might be wise to seek a second opinion.

Table 14
Stages of Ovarian Cancer

Stage I: Growth limited to the ovaries

  Stage I A: Growth limited to one ovary; no ascites*

1. Tumor capsule unruptured and no tumor growth on the external surface of the tumor

2. Tumor capsule ruptured and/or tumor growth on external surface of the tumor

  Stage I B: Growth limited to both ovaries; no ascites*

1. Capsule unruptured and no tumor growth on the external surface of the tumor

2. Capsule ruptured and/or tumor growth on external surface of the tumor

  Stage I C: Growth limited to one or both ovaries; ascites with malignant cells

Stage II: Growth involving one or both ovaries with pelvic extension

  Stage II A: Extension and/or metastasis to uterus and tubes only

  Stage II B: Extension/metastasis to other pelvic tissues

  Stage II C: Either II A or II B, with ascites present

Stage III: Growth involving one or both ovaries, with widespread metastasis in the abdominal cavity

Stage IV: Growth involving one or both ovaries, with distant metastasis outside the abdominal cavity

*Some amount of fluid is normal; the surgeon must judge whether the fluid exceeds normal amounts.

Stage I

Most Stage I cases are treated by removal of the ovaries, tubes and uterus in operations known as bilateral salpingo-oophorectomies and hysterectomies. All or part of the omentum, a fold of fat tissue that hangs from the bowels, may be removed as well. Sometimes the appendix is also removed.

In certain Stage I cases it may be possible to do less radical surgery, removing only the affected ovary and leaving the other ovary and the uterus intact.[11] This can be done only in certain carefully selected cases and only if the woman is particularly anxious to retain her ability to bear children. Not all doctors have precisely the same criteria for selecting cases to be treated conservatively. Most doctors would restrict this conservative surgery to Stage IA (1) cancers. In this stage, the tumor is confined to one ovary, there is no tumor growth on the outside of the tumor capsule, the tumor has not ruptured and there is no ascites. Further, the ovary must be nonadherent, which means that it must not be stuck to other pelvic organs.

The cancer must be growing inside a cystic tumor. The pathologist's report must indicate that the tumor is a low-grade, borderline, well-differentiated type of tumor. Before this type of treatment is given, the surgeon must have removed the tumor, taken samples of any fluid in the cavity, taken biopsies from various key areas, such as the omentum and all samples from various areas, such as the liver. In addition, the pathologist's report on the fluid samples and biopsy specimens must be negative. A wedge biopsy of the opposite ovary must also be done. Since this important procedure is not always done, a woman who may be a candidate for conservative surgery should discuss the wedge biopsy with her doctor prior to surgery.

Some doctors might extend the criteria for conservative surgery, but performing conservative surgery in other cases is controversial. Women should discuss their doctor's criteria for conservative surgery prior to the surgery and seek a second opinion if necessary.

The other Stage I cases—Stage IA(2), IB, IC, those Stage IA(1) cases in which the tumor was not a well-differentiated, low-grade borderline tumor and those State IA(1) cases in which the woman does not have future childbearing plans—will usually be treated by the more radical form of surgery outlined above.

Stage I cases may also be treated with adjuvant therapy—preventive treatment to destroy any microscopic cancer that may remain after surgery. It is sometimes difficult to determine the desirability of using adjuvant therapy, or to decide upon the optimum type. When adjuvant therapy is given, chemotherapy may be used. In the past, external beam radiation therapy was used in these cases, but it has a higher rate of complications and involves greater expense in terms of hospital cost and medical-personnel time, so it is rarely used in Stage I cases anymore.[12] Sometimes, radioactive colloid therapy, in which a solution containing radioactive substances is circulated throughout the abdominal cavity, is used.[13] But this too has fallen out of favor. If your doctor suggests colloid therapy, make sure you understand why s/he is recommending this instead of chemotherapy. Second opinions are, of course, always a good idea.

Chemotherapy in the form of alkalyting agents has been used in adjuvant therapy in Stage I disease. There are several alkalyting agents available, but the one most widely used for these cases is melphalan (Alkeran), which is well tolerated by most women. The drug is given for 12 to 18 months after surgery in an effort to eradicate any microscopic residual cancer. However, the use of melphalan in Stage I cancers has been seriously questioned. A recent study published in a major medical journal assessed the risks of acute leukemia following treatment of ovarian cancer by alkalyting agents and found that the risk was greatly increased.[14] Although there were a number of problems with the study and it could hardly be called "conclusive," it did raise serious questions about the advisability of using chemotherapy in Stage IA(1) cases.[15] The problem is that only about 10 percent of the women with Stage IA(1) cases actually have unrecognized microscopic cancer after surgery; 90 percent do not. Only 10 percent would actually benefit from chemotherapy. According to this study, about that number could be expected to develop leukemia from the chemotherapy. Because of these findings, some doctors have discontinued chemotherapy in these cases.[16*]

Women should discuss this issue with their doctors and should request an update on the most recent developments. If your doctor recommends chemotherapy for Stage IA or IB, you may want to seek a second opinion. Doctors are more inclined to give chemotherapy in Stage IC, but even here, you may want to seek a second opinion.

Stage II

Stage II cases are treated by removing the ovaries, tubes, uterus, omentum, appendix and as much of the tumor as possible. In some Stage II cases, all of the tumor can be removed, but in others this is not possible without causing damage to vital organs.

Further therapy is needed for Stage II cases. Even if the doctor has removed all of the tumor, there is a high likelihood that microscopic cancer may remain. If some cancer remains after operation, either chemotherapy (as outlined above) or, in some instances, external beam therapy may be used.[17] In the past, external beam therapy played a major role in the treatment of ovarian cancer, but chemotherapy has taken its place in most cases; however, in certain Stage II cases, external beam therapy may still be used. A woman has a right to a full discussion of the type of therapy available for her case and the pros and cons of each. She should certainly seek second opinions from both radiologists and chemotherapists (*see* p. 226) before deciding on a course of therapy.

Stages III and IV

The aim of surgery in Stages III and IV is to remove as much of the tumor as possible without endangering the woman's life or producing excessive complications. Sometimes complete removal is possible. At the very least, the ovaries and omentum should be removed, for relief of discomfort. Surgery in these cases calls for experienced judgment and great skill on the part of the surgeon. If all areas of tumor greater than two cm in diameter can be removed, the survival chances are significantly better, but if the

---

*See note 15 in the Ovary footnotes at the end of this book for more details about chemotherapy in Stage I disease.

tumor cannot be reduced this much, radical surgery won't significantly improve the woman's chance of survival.[18] In some cases, radical surgery, such as partial or total pelvic exenteration, which involves removing all the pelvic organs, including the bladder and/or rectum, may be done. But this is done only if one of two possibilities exist: 1. this radical surgery would result in such complete removal of the tumor that no single area of tumor larger than two cm in diameter would remain following surgery; or 2. areas greater than two cm remained, but in the surgeon's opinion, subsequent chemotherapy or radiation therapy could reduce the tumor to the point where the doctor could, in a second operation, reduce all the remaining areas of tumor to less than two cm in diameter.

Obviously, having a skilled surgeon who is experienced and knowledgeable about chemotherapy and radiation therapy and the ability of these therapies to reduce tumor bulk in various circumstances is of utmost importance. A less knowledgeable surgeon may be overwhelmed by the discovery of extensive tumor on operation. The woman might then be given only minimal surgery, be closed back up and given some form of subsequent therapy, whereas another, more qualified, surgeon might have been able to reduce the tumor to the point where subsequent therapy would have a better chance of success. A woman should discuss her surgeon's qualifications prior to surgery and find out whether or not the doctor is qualified and experienced enough to do radical pelvic surgery, or if another doctor who is qualified can be called in, should the need for consultation arise. If she has not had the benefit of consultation with or surgery by a cancer specialist—either a surgical or gynecological oncologist—prior to diagnosis, *she should insist* that a second opinion be obtained before beginning chemotherapy.

Stages III and IV will always require further therapy. Chemotherapy has pretty much supplanted external beam therapy as the treatment of choice in these cases. In the past a single agent, melphalan, was given; however, studies now underway seem to indicate that various combinations of drugs may be more effective than a single agent. On the other hand, combinations may be more toxic than single drugs. Changes in chemotherapy for advanced ovarian cancer are taking place all the time, which is why it is important to have a doctor who is up-to-date on the latest developments in research and to seek second chemotherapy opinions.

Special Treatment Cases

The treatment program discussed so far holds true for the majority of ovarian cancers; however, less common types may require different treatment. Dysgerminomas often present as Stage IA(1) and can be treated conservatively; however, biopsy of the other ovary is essential, for in 15

469

percent of cases the other, seemingly normal ovary will be involved. All other stages will require further therapy, which is given by external beam radiation since these tumors are very responsive to radiation.[19]

Granulosa cell tumors can also be treated conservatively in many cases. However, if the uterus is not removed, a D&C must be done since these tumors are often associated with endometrial cancer. (If the D&C indicates cancer, the uterus must, of course, be removed.) Advanced-stage cases may be treated with radiation, as these tumors are also sensitive to radiation. It is important to note that women are frequently diagnosed as having this tumor when, in fact, their tumor is of another cell type.[20] Since granulosa cell tumors are treated differently, accurate diagnosis is important. Women who are told they have granulosa cella tumors should, therefore, confirm the diagnosis with second opinions from pathologists at cancer centers (see appendix).

Malignant embryonal tumors, endodermal sinus tumors and choriocarcinomas can never be treated conservatively because of their aggressive nature. They always require further therapy after surgery, usually consisting of combination chemotherapy rather than a single drug.[21]

Follow-up

Follow-up care is extremely important in ovarian cancer, in order to detect recurrent or persistent cancer and to monitor the success of adjuvant therapy so that the therapy can be changed if necessary or discontinued if it has been successful. In the case of chemotherapy, for instance, because of the associated leukemia risk, therapy should be discontinued as soon as it has proven successful.

Careful questioning about possible symptoms and a thorough pelvic exam are the foundation of follow-up care. Breast exam by the doctor and self-exam by the woman are also of vital importance since women with ovarian cancer are at higher risk for the development of breast cancer. The woman's weight, appetite and general well-being should be given careful attention. Nutrition is particularly important for women with ovarian cancer. Persistent ascites and abdominal swelling, signs of intestinal obstruction, nausea, vomiting and pain are important symptoms.

A "second-look" operation may be done in certain cases.[22] If the woman had only a biopsy of the tumor and did not have samples of ascites and the appropriate tissue biopsies or optimum surgery to remove the bulk of the tumor, she is a candidate for a second operation. Those women in whom it was not possible to remove all of the tumor and who are receiving subsequent therapy are also candidates for a second-look operation. The subsequent therapy may have reduced the tumor to a point where it can all be removed surgically or where the remaining tumor could at least be reduced to less than two cm in diameter by further surgery. Moreover, the presence or absence of tumor will be a guide to determining further chemotherapy.

Women who had all gross tumors removed, who have no signs or symptoms of recurrence and who received adjuvant therapy may also be candidates for a second-look operation, which might allow the doctor to discontinue the adjuvant therapy and thereby cut the risks involved in such therapy.

If a woman's tumor is known to be growing larger, however, there is no point in a second operation, for by the time a recurrence is large enough to be felt, the tumor is growing out of control and neither chemotherapy nor radiation can hope to control it. A second operation, which poses risks in and of itself, will do no good in these cases.

It is said that about one out of every eight women will be a candidate for second-look operations. There is not total agreement among doctors as to exactly which women are candidates for these operations or precisely when it should be done. Women should discuss this issue with their doctors, again seeking second opinions if necessary.

Sometimes laparoscopy rather than a second major operation may be possible. This second-look procedure will involve the same sorts of abdominal investigations, cell specimens and tissue biopsies as done in the original diagnostic procedure.

Culdocentesis, a method of extracting fluid via a needle inserted into the abdominal cavity, may be very useful in following some cases. Chest and abdominal X-rays, intravenous pyelogram, liver scans and ultrasound examinations may all be used in follow-up. Certain rather rare forms of ovarian cancer may be followed up with special blood tests that allow the doctor to detect recurrences before the recurrent tumor has grown large enough to be felt and, hence, too large to control.

Survival Rates

The overall five-year survival rate for ovarian cancer is about 30-35 percent; however, many factors will influence the survival rates.[23] Table 15 breaks survival rates down by stage and cell type. The grade of the tumor will also influence survival rates. For instance, survival rates better than 95 percent have been reported for Stage I borderline serous and mucinous tumors at some institutions.[24] In the more advanced cases, whether or not all or most of the tumor was removed during surgery will affect survival rates. A woman's doctor should be able to quote survival statistics for her particular situation.

Table 15
Five-Year Survival Rates for Various Stage and Cell-Type Ovarian Cancers

Type	Percent
Stage I	
Serous	70
Mucinous	84
Endometroid	73
Solid	58
Stage II	
Serous	39
Mucinous	68
Endometroid	79
Solid	24
Stage III	
Serous	6
Mucinous	17
Endometroid	28
Solid	2

*SOURCE: Adapted from Decker, D. G.: "The Diagnosis and Management of Ovarian Cancer," *South Me. J.,* 66:369-374, 1973.

It should be mentioned that survival rates vary, sometimes considerably, from one institution to another. This may be due to the fact that borderline tumors are sometimes included along with frankly cancerous ones. It has also been suggested that high cure rates may be due to misdiagnosis, where borderline or even benign tumors were incorrectly identified as cancerous, thus artificially raising the five-year survival rates.

The Breast

The anatomy and function of the breast are discussed in Chapter Three. In this section we are concerned with diseases of the breast, which may be either benign or malignant. These cancerous and noncancerous breast diseases can produce identical symptoms, so that it is generally impossible to distinguish between them on the basis of the symptoms alone.

Symptoms

The following symptoms, also listed in the appendix at the back of this book, may be associated with either benign or malignant breast diseases.
- □ A lump or thickening in the breast
- □ A depressed or bulging area in the skin or any change in the shape or symmetry of the breast
- □ A thickening on the skin of the breast that may feel warm to the touch
- □ Dilated veins in the breast. Some women normally have visible bluish-colored veins in their breasts; however, the appearance of such veins in a woman who has not had them previously or a change in the appearance of such veins in a woman who has previously had them calls for medical attention
- □ A change in the texture or color of the skin of the breast. The appearance of areas of skin with the texture of an orange peel, a condition known as peau d'orange, is particularly important

☐ Any change in the condition of the nipple or the areola. Changes in the size or shape, skin texture or direction in which the nipple points, retraction of the nipple, cracks in the nipple or scaling of the skin around the nipple are important
☐ Discharge from the nipple
☐ A lump in the axilla (armpit)
☐ A sore on the breast or nipple that does not heal
☐ A hot, swollen or sore breast
☐ Unusual ache or pain that persists and is not associated with cyclical changes and tenderness

A woman may have only one of these symptoms or any combination of them. If you have any of these symptoms, you should see a doctor, but many of us don't do so because we are afraid of what we might find. Our fear is that we will discover that we have cancer and that we will lose our breast or even our lives. Feeling upset and afraid is quite natural, but try to remember that the vast majority of women who discover these symptoms do not have cancer. Eight out of every ten lumps biopsied are benign.[1] Although 7 percent of women do develop cancer, the other 93 percent of them don't.[2] The odds are on your side.

Moreover, if it is cancer, you may save both your breast and your life by seeking prompt medical attention. Studies have shown that the earlier a cancer is detected, the greater the chances of survival.[3] Delaying treatment could cost you your life. There is nothing to be gained by waiting.

Having breast cancer does not necessarily mean that you will lose your breast. Today there are less radical therapies that hardly alter the appearance of the breast. While these less radical therapies are still experimental, there has been enough evidence suggesting their effectiveness to have brought about large-scale studies at the nation's top cancer centers. No responsible investigator would treat a woman with these forms of therapy unless there was good, strong evidence to suggest their effectiveness. But women are eligible for these less disfiguring therapies only if their cancer has been discovered while it is still in the early stages. Here again, there is nothing to be gained by waiting, and everything, including your life and your breast, to be lost by delaying.

Breast Self-Exam

Every woman should practice monthly breast self-exam. If she discovers anything suspicious, she should consult her doctor. Even nonsymptoms, like a bruise that doesn't fade or a vague, indefinite feeling of thickening, deserve prompt attention.

Diagnostic Work-Up

If you have found a suspicious symptom, the doctor may do one of a number of things, starting with a careful palpation (feeling) of the breast. A needle biopsy may be done. This involves applying a local anesthetic to the breast and inserting a needle into the suspicious area. X-ray studies of the breast, known as mammograms, may be done. It may be necessary to do a surgical biopsy, in which all or part of the lump is removed and examined microscopically.

The many things that you as a consumer should know about the procedures involved in diagnosing breast cancer are discussed in detail in the section on breast cancer.

There is a great deal of information in the following pages. If you are reading this section because you have a suspicious symptom and are in the process of having a diagnostic work-up, you may be feeling very apprehensive, which, of course, makes it difficult to absorb so much new information. Ask a friend or relative to help you. It may be easier for your friend to absorb the information and think clearly than it is for you right now. Both of you should take notes and make lists of questions. Remember, you have the right to take someone else along with you on your doctor visits and to ask questions and receive answers to your questions.

CYSTIC DISEASE OF THE BREAST

AKA: adenofibrosis, fibroadenomatosis, fibrocystic disease, mastodynia, mammary dysplasia, chronic cystic mastitis, blunt duct adenosis, aprocrine metaplasia, sclerosing adenosis, or ductal dysplasia

Cystic disease, often called fibrocystic disease, or mammary dysplasia, is a group of disorders that are an exaggeration of the normal changes that take place in the breast each month during a woman's reproductive years. Just as the lining of the uterus, in response to hormonal stimulation, thickens and prepares itself for the possibility of pregnancy each month, so the breast tissues respond to hormones and begin to prepare themselves for milk production each month.

In the first half of the menstrual cycle, when the hormone estrogen predominates, the cells of the milk-secreting glands, the ducts that carry the milk and the supporting fibrous tissue multiply. Once ovulation has occurred, the levels of the hormone progesterone rise and this triggers the first steps of the secreting process in the milk-gland cells. If pregnancy does not occur, the secretory process stops and the newly grown gland, duct and fibrous tissue breaks down, just as the thick, rich lining of the uterus breaks down and is shed in the form of menstrual blood. In the breast, however, there is no place for the debris to go, so it must be reabsorbed by the breast tissues. In the case of fibrocystic disease the process of growing the new cells and starting the secretory process goes too far and/or the process of breaking down and reabsorbing does not function correctly. Hence, small pockets of cellular debris and trapped secretions (cysts) are formed. These may coalesce together to form larger cysts.

Incidence

Since cystic conditions are related to hormone production, it is not surprising that they are most often found in women in their reproductive years. They can occur at any time between the first menstruation and menopause. After menopause, when the influence of hormones diminishes, the condition usually, but not always, subsides. A woman may develop cystic disease only to find that it disappears after a few menstrual cycles, or she may be bothered by it continually. Sometimes, it disappears only to reappear years later.

Cystic disease is the most common benign condition of the breast. About 50 percent of female bodies autopsied will show some degree of cystic disease.[4]

Causes

The cause of cystic disease is not known; however, there is some indication that the tendency to develop the disease is hereditary. Pregnancy, birth control pills and menopause, because of their hormonal effects, usually cause the disease to regress. The disease may also regress spontaneously.

It seems clear that cystic disease is related to hormone levels. Fibrocystic changes are apt to become more exaggerated if the menstrual cycle becomes irregular because of some other problem. According to some authorities, irregularities in menstruation in normal women happen most often in late August and September for women in the northern hemisphere, especially when they are approaching menopause.[5] Also, in the months from December to May the ovaries are at their peak production for women living in the northern hemisphere. Women who usually have some tenderness and swelling are likely to notice fibrocystic lumps more often during these months.

There is also some evidence to indicate that fibrocystic disease may be related to diet (see below).

476

Cystic Disease and Cancer

One of the biggest concerns about fibrocystic disease is its relationship to cancer. Women with fibrocystic diseases are four times more likely to develop breast cancer than women who do not have these conditions.[6] It now looks as if certain forms of cystic disease may be more significantly related to cancer than others. Some doctors feel that the age at which a woman first develops cystic disease is a particularly important factor, and that women who develop it before the age of 20 are at higher risk than those who develop it later on.[7]

A mammogram, an X-ray study of the breast, is often done as part of the diagnostic work-up for cystic disease. Mammograms can be classified into one of four categories: N_1, P_1, P_2 and DY. These are known as Wolfe's classifications. According to some experts, women whose mammograms fall into the N_1 or P_1 classification are at low risk for developing cancer, while those that fall into the P_2 and DY classifications seem to be at high risk.[8] This does not mean that all women who have P_2 or DY mammograms will develop cancer or that women with N_1 or P_1 mammograms will never develop the disease. Moreover, scientists are not in complete agreement about the significance of these mammogram patterns. Still women who fall into one of these high risk classifications may want to be followed very closely.

Research is now being done to help pinpoint the particular forms of cystic disease that are related to cancer and to refine our estimates of increased risk for women with early versus late cystic disease. Until then, any woman with cystic disease, particularly those with early onset and high-risk mammogram patterns, should consider themselves at increased risk and should carefully examine their breasts each month, as described in Chapter Three. Moreover, such women should have their breasts examined by a doctor who is well informed about breast disease every six months.

Symptoms

In the early stages of cystic disease, a woman may feel nothing more than a general thickening about the size and shape of a thick pancake or a mass with indefinite borders, the edges of which seem to blend into the surrounding breast tissue. As her period approaches, her breast may become tender, or painful or swollen. These symptoms tend to disappear with the onset of the menstrual flow.

There seem to be two distinct types of cystic disease as far as symptoms go. One type is more diffuse and is characterized by lumpiness and tenderness, usually in both breasts, which is most pronounced in the week before the onset of the period. After menstruation there is usually less lumpiness and pain. The second type tends to occur in one breast, although it may occur in both, and is manifested by one, two or even three larger, rounded lumps that are usually quite distinct and freely movable within the breast tissue. If the larger cyst is actually a collection of smaller cysts, it may not be clearly separate from the rest of the breast tissue but may tend to shade off into the surrounding tissue and not be movable. This type of cystic disease is also likely to be more tender or painful in the week preceding menstruation and may also regress once the period starts, although usually not as much as the more diffuse type does. A single cyst may be relatively soft to firm or hard, depending on how much fluid it contains and the phase of the menstrual cycle in which it is noted. When it is full of compressed fluid or if the cyst is of long-standing, it may feel quite hard.

The severity of the symptoms depends largely on how many of these cysts a woman has, their size and their location and how rapidly they enlarge. A woman with widely dispersed small cysts may not even be aware of them or may just feel small nodular lumps throughout her breasts. On the other hand, an accumulation of relatively small cysts in the upper outer quarter of the breast near the armpit may cause considerable discomfort or pain in the days preceding the onset of the menstrual cycle, when hormone levels are fluctuating. A large cyst, responding to the same hormone stimulation, may become exceedingly painful as the fluids within the cyst press against the cyst walls. It too may shrink, or regress, as the period begins, but this tends not to be as noticeable with the large cysts. The off-again-on-again nature of the symptoms is characteristic of cystic disease and distinguishes benign cystic lumps from cancerous ones.

For some women the pain associated with fibrocystic disease can last as long as three weeks and may be quite excruciating. With large cysts, removal of them will alleviate pain, but pain is often associated with the more diffuse, generalized form of cystic disease as well. Removal of these multiple, small cysts is often impractical. Some women find that wearing a good bra helps. Some studies suggest diet may be important. Avoiding excess salt, sugar, coffee, tea, alcohol and refined sugar will help relieve the symptoms.[9] Using oral contraceptives may help alleviate the pain. Some doctors prescribe Depo-Provera for relief of pain in cystic disease, but many others question the wisdom of using the drug in this way. For severe forms, some doctors have been experimenting with a new drug called bromocriptine (Parlodel),[10] but this drug has numerous side effects and its use in this manner is also questioned by many.

Diagnosis

The main aim of diagnosis is to distinguish cystic disease from cancer. The elements that help in the diagnosis are the mobility of the lumps, the absence of any suggestion of skin retraction, the feelings of tenderness and the typical waxing and waning of symptoms according to the phases of the menstrual cycle. These factors indicate that the cyst is more apt to be benign than cancerous; however, there are many forms of cystic disease, and the way in which symptoms manifest themselves may vary from woman to woman. Not all of these symptoms will be present in each case. For instance, the waxing and waning during the menstrual cycle may not be evident.

The first step in diagnosis is a needle aspiration, a simple office procedure whereby a fine needle is inserted into the suspicious area and fluid or cells are drawn out. This may cause the cyst to collapse entirely, although it may refill at a later date. The fluid or any other material extracted is then sent to the lab to make sure there are no cancerous cells. If the cyst has collapsed, the lab report comes back negative (indicating that no cancer cells are present) and the symptoms indicate cystic disease, the doctor may decide that further tests and treatment are unnecessary. A "wait-and-see" policy is adopted, and the woman's breasts are examined in a month or two and then every six months. However, even if the lab report says benign, this does not guarantee that no cancer is present—just that there were no cancer cells in the fluid extracted. If there is any reason to be suspicious, the doctor may do further tests.

If no fluid is extracted, this may indicate that the tumor is a more serious one; however, many times fluid cannot be extracted in cystic disease. In this case the doctor may try another procedure, using a wider needle to remove a sample of tissue from the breast. Not all doctors are well versed in this procedure or have access to laboratories with pathologists who are trained to interpret such tissue samples. Even if the needle aspiration or needle biopsy indicates benign disease, a mammogram, which is an X-ray examination of the breast, is usually done. Sometimes, the lump must actually be removed and examined microscopically to rule out the possibility of cancer. Breast biopsies are discussed in greater detail under the heading Breast Cancer.

MASTITIS

AKA: infections of the breast

Associated terms: breast abscesses

Infections of the breast are rather rare in women who are not nursing a child, but are not uncommon among those who are. The source of the infection is usually bacteria that enter through a crack, or fissure, in the nipple. Because the breast has a great deal of fatty tissue and a rather widely dispersed blood supply, the infection does not spread rapidly but tends to remain localized in an area of the breast.

Symptoms

The symptoms include swelling, redness, a sensation of heat in the infected area and pain or tenderness. The overlying skin may be red, and if the process continues for a long time, the infected area may become hardened. The infection may be mild, producing only an area of tenderness and a slight redness in the overlying skin, or it may be more severe, triggering a defense mechanism in the surrounding tissue. In such cases, special cells in the neighboring tissue pour out secretions that harden and wall off the infected area, thus protecting the healthy tissue. This walled-off area, full of pus and infection, is called an abscess.

Diagnosis

Diagnosis is usually a fairly simple matter, at least in the woman who is, or has recently been, breastfeeding. However, the symptoms—pain, heat, redness, nipple discharge and a feeling of hardness—may be produced by certain forms of cancer as well, so there may be some difficulty in diagnosis, especially in the nonnursing woman.

If the woman has been breastfeeding, treatment is usually given for one week. In women who fail to respond to treatment or who don't have a recent history of breastfeeding, a needle biopsy may be done. The fluid aspirated by needle biopsy is examined microscopically and will usually reveal signs of infection indicating that this is a breast abscess and not a cancerous process. A mammogram or an excisional biopsy may be necessary in doubtful cases.

Treatment

When an infection occurs, the woman must discontinue breastfeeding, at least temporarily. Bed rest and treatment with a broad-spectrum antibiotic will sometimes clear up the infection in a few days, in which case breastfeeding can continue. However, because the breast is made up of separate compartments of fatty tissue, it is sometimes difficult for antibiotics to reach the site of the infection. Thus, antibiotic therapy is often ineffective, especially when the infection has progressed to the point of abscess.

In such cases, the doctor must cut into the breast and drain the infected area. Here again the architecture of the breast, with all its little compartments of fatty tissue, can make treatment difficult. The cutting and draining must be extensive enough to include all the compartments where infection may be present. Treatment of small abscesses in the area of the areola are particularly tricky since they tend to recur. This happens because the sinus tracts in the area, which are the drainage channels for blood and lymph, tend to become overgrown with cells as a result of defensive scar-tissue response on the part of the body. Antibiotics are frequently ineffective in this situation, as are incision and drainage. Small pockets of pus may remain in the sinus tracts and give rise to repeated abscesses. If this happens, the sinus tracts may have to be removed, but this procedure is not too damaging and heals with minimal scarring.

FAT NECROSIS OF THE BREAST

The breast has a good deal of fat tissue. Any blow or injury to this fat tissue can cause fat necrosis or death of the fat tissue, either because the blow has actually destroyed the tissue by crushing it or because it has damaged the blood vessels, which restricts the flow of blood to the fat tissue, and causes it to die. The condition can occur in any age group.

Symptoms

Fat necrosis tends to form a stony hard mass, or tumor, due to a process of calcification that may take place in fat tissue. In response to the breakdown and decay of the fat tissue, the surrounding tissue exudes a fibrous substance that hardens and attempts to wall off the area of fat necrosis from the neighboring healthy tissue. This is called fibrotic response, and it tends to fix the mass of fat necrosis in place. If the fibrotic reaction is taking place just below the skin, it can cause retraction, or dimpling, of the skin.

These symptoms—a firm, fixed mass with skin retraction— may also suggest breast cancer. Furthermore, after injury an area of fat necrosis may enlarge gradually in much the same manner of certain forms of cancer. Moreover, areas of fat necrosis may break down and decay, setting up an inflammatory process and producing increased heat, tenderness and redness of the overlying skin; unfortunately, cancer may behave in this manner as well, so it is not easy to distinguish between fat necrosis and breast cancer.

Diagnosis and Treatment

If there is no bruise from the original blow, or if the bruise has subsided by the time the doctor feels the mass, s/he is apt to strongly suspect cancer. The diagnostic steps, described in the section on breast cancer, may be done, but since this condition can produce the same symptoms and even mimic cancer on a mammogram, an excisional biopsy, which is also curative, may be necessary.

FIBROADENOMAS

Types: adenofibromas
fibromas
adenomas

Fibroadenomas are benign tumors of the breast that are usually composed of fibrous (*fibro*) and gland (*adeno*) tissue. Other terms such as "adenofibromas," "fibromas" and "adenomas" may be used, depending on which type of tissue predominates.

Incidence

Fibroadenomas usually occur during a woman's menstruating years, most often in women 20-40 years of age. They are also the most common breast tumor found among adolescent girls (among whom breast tumors are uncommon).

Signs and Symptoms

Fibroadenomas are usually felt as firm, rounded tumors with a somewhat rubbery texture. They are usually sharply delineated from the surrounding breast tissue, are freely movable and are not attached to the skin. Usually they occur singly, but in about 15 percent of the cases they are multiple. They are generally found around the nipple or in the upper sides of the breasts. They tend to be small (one to five cm), not to be tender and to produce no other symptoms.

There is a less common (7 percent of the cases) so-called juvenile type of fibroadenoma that affects teenage girls. This juvenile type behaves quite differently from the so-called adult type (which, despite its name, also appears in young girls). Unlike the adult type, it tends to have dilated veins covering its surface. The skin over the tumor may be tense, but the tumor is not fixed to it. The juvenile tumor is generally larger and grows much faster, so this is the type that is most often mistaken for cancer, but it is a benign condition.

On very rare occasions a single fibroadenoma growing among a group of small tumors may take on an exaggerated growth pattern and produce what is called a massive fibroadenoma. The size varies, but they have been reported to reach 10-19 cm (see Cystosarcoma Phyllodes below).

The fibroadenoma is not significantly related to cancer or considered precancerous in any sense. In adolescents there are few other conditions it may be confused with; however, in older women it may be confused with other, possibly precancerous conditions, such as fibrocystic disease. Certain types of cancer that occur almost exclusively in older women can also mimic the appearance of a fibroadenoma.

Treatment

Since there does not seem to be any significant association between fibroadenoma and cancer, it is sometimes best to delay treatment in young girls, since surgery may interfere with the development of the breast that is taking place at this stage of life. Although growth of these tumors is usually slow in young women, they can take on an accelerated growth rate, especially during pregnancy. If this happens, it is usually wise to remove the tumor, along with a margin of normal tissue.

In older women, the doctor will want to do the usual diagnostic tests for evaluating any breast lump (see the section on breast cancer) to eliminate the possibility of cancer. Treatment of this benign condition in older women consists of the removal of the tumor, along with a wide margin of surrounding tissue, for even though the condition is benign in the overwhelming majority of cases, there have been a few cases where cancer has arisen in adjacent tissues.

CYSTOSARCOMA PHYLLODES

AKA: giant or massive fibroadenoma

To anyone familiar with medical terminology, "cystosarcoma phyllodes" has an ominous ring, since the term "sarcoma" usually implies cancer. The name is highly misleading, however, for only about 10 percent of these growths are actually cancerous.

Cystosarcoma phyllodes is a variant of the fibroadenoma, and some authorities consider it merely an overgrown or giant fibroadenoma. These tumors are most often found in the breasts of postmenopausal women, although some cases have been reported in younger women and even in teenagers.

Signs and Symptoms

They are generally rather large, 15 cm or more, although some may be only 2-3 cm in size. The small ones, however, tend to grow rapidly in size. They are usually rather firm and freely movable within the breast. In some cases, they become so large and the overlying skin so tightly stretched that it ulcerates (forms sores).

Diagnosis

The problem in diagnosis is, of course, to eliminate the possibility of cancer, particularly in postmenopausal women, so the usual diagnostic steps (described in the section on breast cancer), must be done.

Treatment

Medical opinion on the type of treatment for a benign cystosarcoma phyllodes is somewhat divided. Some doctors, perhaps because of the ominous-sounding term "sarcoma," will treat the condition with a radical masectomy. Most experts, however, consider this overtreatment. They generally recommend simple removal of the tumor, along with a wide margin of the surrounding healthy tissue. This wide margin will help prevent recurrences. Even if the tumor recurs, more radical surgery may not be necessary as long as the second tumor is similar to the first one and doesn't show any suspicious, cancer-type changes. In some cases the tumor may be too extensive for local excision, so that a simple masectomy, amputation of the breast, may be necessary.

LIPOMAS AND OTHER SOFT TUMORS OF THE BREAST

Types: adenolipomas
leiomyomas
myoblastomas
rhabdomyomas

Lipomas are noncancerous tumors of fat tissue. They are relatively uncommon, but may occur in any age group. On rare occasions they may include glandular elements (adenolipomas). Other benign tumors may occur in the smooth muscle of the erective tissue of the nipple area (leiomyomas) or may involve certain other types of muscle tissue (myoblastoma or rhabdomyoma).

Symptoms

These tumors usually occur singly and are firm, but soft rather than hard. Their size depends on how long they have been present. They are freely movable and do not produce skin retraction. They are well encapsulated, but at times their outline is not distinct because they may blend into the surrounding fatty tissue of the breast.

Diagnosis and Treatment

Once they are discovered, the doctor may do any of the diagnostic tests used to rule out cancer (see the section on breast cancer).

Once the true nature of the lump is determined, it is not always necessary to remove it; however, it is frequently removed as part of the diagnostic work-up.

INTRADUCTAL PAPILLOMAS

Types: simple papillomas
duct papillomatosis

Intraductal papillomas are overgrowths of the lining of the duct system of the breast. Simple papillomas are entirely benign. Duct papillomatosis, though, is a form of cystic disease and is considered by many experts to be a precancerous condition.

Symptoms

The chief symptom is a bloody discharge from the nipple; however, this symptom is not always present. Lumps or thickenings in the breast may also appear.

Diagnosis and Treatment

Diagnosis may involve any of the procedures used in the diagnosis of breast lumps (see the section on breast cancer). If a definite mass can be

485

felt, treatment of simple papillomas is surgical removal. In older women with duct papillomatosis and other risk factors for breast cancer, a subcutaneous mastectomy may be recommended. If no lump can be felt, the doctor may recommend careful follow-up, including bi-annual mammograms.

MAMMARY DUCT ECTASIA

AKA: plasma cell mastitis

Mammary duct ectasia is a condition in which the tissue that lines the milk duct breaks down. It usually occurs in postmenopausal women and is one of the few noncancerous conditions that can cause a firm mass in women of this age group.

Symptoms

The process starts in the collecting ducts just beneath the nipple and areola. The lining of the ducts starts to break down and the stagnant duct contents begin to irritate the walls of the ducts. There is a fibrotic response to this irritation, which means that cells in the area secrete a fibrous substance that hardens and attempts to wall off the inflamed tissue, separating it from the surrounding healthy tissue. This fibrotic response and the resultant thickening of the ducts may shorten the ducts and cause nipple retraction. There may also be a nipple discharge as a result of the infection.

The process continues slowly and may take years. Eventually, the ducts themselves "spring a leak" and the irritation spreads to the surrounding tissue. As the duct contents continue to leak, a chronic inflammation is set up, along with an accompanying attempt by the body to defend itself by the fibrotic reaction described above. A firm, hard, fixed mass of fibrous tissue is formed. As it grows larger it grows downward into the breast. There may be pain and discomfort. The tumor has a tendency to break down. Portions of it begin to die, and there may then be redness, tenderness and warmth of the overlying skin. In extreme cases, the whole breast and even the axillary lymph nodes may be involved.

Diagnosis and Treatment

The diagnostic steps used to evaluate any suspicious breast lump (see the section on breast cancer) are done. Most of the time a definite diagnosis cannot be made short of an actual biopsy, for the symptoms mimic those of cancer. Treatment consists of removal of the lump.

GALACTORRHEA

AKA: abnormal production of breast milk

Associated terms: Forbes-Albright syndrome, Chiari-Frommel syndrome, hypothyroidism, acromegaly, chromophore adenoma, idiopathic galactorrhea

Galactorrhea is defined as abnormal secretion of breast milk. Actually galactorrhea is not a disease of the breast; in fact, it is not a disease at all but a possible symptom of a number of different problems that may have nothing to do with the breast per se. However, since the symptom involves the breast and the presence of this symptom often brings a woman to the doctor, we have chosen to consider it here along with breast diseases.

Symptoms

The thin, milky-white, watery discharge may be constant or intermittent; it may be present for a short time or for years; it may flow spontaneously or may be noticeable only when the breast is expressed, or "milked." It can occur both in women who have borne children, whether they breast fed them or not, and in women who have never borne children at all.

Many times the menstrual period is also disturbed. There may be abnormal uterine bleeding, a total absence of menstrual bleeding or only occasional menstrual periods. Depending on the nature of the underlying cause, there may be additional symptoms, as described below.

It should be noted that an occasional woman with normal menstrual periods will have a slight nipple discharge at certain points in her menstrual cycle. If this is her only symptom and there are no other abnormalities, such a woman does not usually require the complete diagnostic work-up or the treatment described below. Such a woman would be wise, however, to discuss this symptom with her doctor because galactorrhea can be an indication of serious problems. Similarly, women with post-Pill amenorrhea, that is, women who fail to resume their menstrual periods after discontinuing the use of birth control pills, may also experience galactorrhea. This may not be serious, but women who have both an absence of menstrual periods *and* galactorrhea must have the diagnostic work-up described here to rule out more serious possibilities, whether they have been on the Pill or not. We have come across women who have had both these symptoms whose doctors have told them not to worry about it unless they want to become pregnant. One such woman whom we saw recently turned out to have a brain tumor. Luckily, she did not heed her doctor's "not-to-worry" advice and sought a second opinion. The combination of these two symptoms *always* demands a complete diagnostic work-up.

Causes

Galactorrhea may be caused by a number of different factors. Many times, but not always, the galactorrhea is associated with abnormal levels of the hormone prolactin. Prolactin is manufactured in the pituitary gland and causes the breast to produce milk. Overproduction of prolactin may be due to problems in the pituitary itself, to abnormal levels of certain other hormones, which alter the delicate interrelationships of hormones that stimulate or inhibit prolactin production, or to other substances that affect the chemical process through which brain messages are transmitted.

Hypothyroidism, a condition in which the thyroid gland produces insufficient amounts of thyroid, can produce galactorrhea as well as other distinctive symptoms, which are detailed elsewhere in this book. Injury to the chest or the use of certain tranquilizers can also cause galactorrhea.

Tumors in the pituitary glands sometimes, but not always, produce galactorrhea. There may be headaches and visual disturbances as well, although these may appear only after the tumor has grown rather large. A slow-growing tumor might be present for years before these sorts of symptoms appear. The term "Forbes-Albright syndrome" is used to describe a certain type of pituitary tumor known as a chromophore adenoma if the tumor is also associated with galactorrhea. Women with this rather rare syndrome tend to be somewhat overweight and don't usually have menstrual periods. If the tumor is successfully treated, the galactorrhea will disappear, and after a course of hormone therapy, the menstrual cycle will return to normal. Other pituitary tumors may cause galactorrhea as well.

A condition known as Chiari-Frommel syndrome is also associated with galactorrhea. This rare syndrome follows childbirth. The woman fails to resume her normal menstrual periods and has persistent galactorrhea whether she nursed her child or not. She may also have abdominal pain, backache and depression or other emotional upsets. The problem is thought to lie in the hypothalamus, the brain center that controls hormone production. Such women may also show signs of acromegaly, another condition associated with galactorrhea, in which the hands, feet, nose and lower jaw grow excessively large due to a disturbance in growth hormones.

Sometimes it is not possible to identify a specific cause for the galactorrhea, in which case we call it idiopathic galactorrhea. Generally, this kind of diagnosis is good news, for it means that more serious causes have been ruled out. However, the fact that a woman has a diagnosis of idiopathic galactorrhea today does not mean that the cause of her galactorrhea will always be a mystery. It may be that she has a pituitary tumor too small to be detected even by our most sophisticated X-ray techniques or a thyroid problem that has not yet advanced to the point where it could be detected by our present methods of measuring thyroid levels. Thus, the diagnosis of idiopathic galactorrhea may be changed in a year or two to a pituitary tumor or hypothyroidism. Women with idiopathic galactorrhea, then, need to be followed closely.

Diagnosis and Treatment

The first step in diagnosing galactorrhea involves expressing some of the discharge from the breast and examining it microscopically to make sure that it is actually breast milk and not discharge associated with a breast abscess or breast cancer. It is important that the doctor actually express, that is, "milk" the breast, for a simple breast palpation (feeling) that is normally done to detect tumors may not produce the discharge.

Once the doctor is sure that the discharge is actually breast milk, the next step is to get a test for hypothyroidism. If this test (a good one is the serum TSH) shows an abnormal level of thyroid, then the woman is started on thyroid therapy and followed up with regular serum TSH tests and tests to assess the level of prolactin. If the prolactin production returns to normal during thyroid therapy, the diagnosis of hypothyroidism is confirmed and treatment for hypothyroidism is continued.

If the woman's TSH level is normal, the next step is to do a blood test to measure the level of prolactin in her body. If it's high (above 200 nanograms, or ng, per milliliters), 90 percent of such women will have a pituitary tumor.[11] If moderately high, (the 100-200 ng range, about two-thirds of the women will have pituitary tumors. If close to normal (20-100 ng range), about one-third of these women will have pituitary tumors. Pituitary tumors are, however, rather rare.

If the woman's prolactin level is normal, some doctors believe she still should have X-rays to rule out the possibility of a tumor. While it is highly unlikely that such a woman would have a tumor, they feel that the X-rays should be taken just to be safe. Still other doctors will order tomograms, a special type of X-ray study, but simpler X-rays, referred to as A/P laterals and cone-down views, which involve only about one-ninth as much radiation as a tomogram and only a quarter of the cost, are all that is necessary.[12] Only rarely will tomograms be necessary.

Table 16
Diagnosing and Treating Galactorrhea

⊥ indicates that this step is controversial.
≢ See accompanying text for details.

If the X-rays are normal, then the woman has idiopathic galactorrhea, which needs to be followed. Some doctors will do prolactin tests every six months and A/P laterals and cone-down views every two years (this may change to every three to four years pending the results of studies now being done) just in case a tumor is present but is too small to be picked up by X-ray.[13] Other doctors don't feel this is necessary.

If the X-rays show some abnormality, then the woman is referred to a specialist, who may do tomograms or very sophisticated X-ray tests known as CAT scans. Treatment for a pituitary tumor is generally brain surgery to remove the tumor, although if the tumor is very small, a drug called bromocriptine, sold under the brand name Parlodel, may be used to destroy the tumor.[14]

If the prolactin levels are high, the woman will also need A/P laterals and cone-down views. Here again the tomogram is not necessary. If the X-rays show some abnormality, then the woman needs to be referred to a specialist, as described above. If the X-rays are normal, this is one case in which your doctor would be justified in ordering a tomogram. If the tomogram is abnormal, the woman should be referred to the specialist. If the tomogram is normal in these women with elevated prolactin, some doctors will treat the woman with the drug described above. However, because this drug has so many side effects, some doctors feel it should not be given to women such as these who have no demonstrable abnormalities.

Table 16 summarizes the diagnostic steps and treatment of women with galactorrhea.

BREAST CANCER

AKA: carcinoma of the breast

Breast cancer is one of the most controversial subjects in medicine today, and for this reason it is especially important that women understand the issues and become informed patients.

Breast cancer is a complex topic. It would take a book many times this size to thoroughly cover the subject. In the following pages the major issues are discussed. Vital information about symptoms, diagnosis and treatment is covered. Other important information about the emotional impact of the disease, recovering from the operation, dealing with having lost a breast, being fitted for an artificial breast and so forth is not covered in this section, for these topics have been dealt with in other books. In addition, the reader is referred to the introduction to this section, Chapter 3, which discusses the anatomy of the breast and breast self-exam, and to the general background information on cancer, all of which will help to make the information in the following pages more comprehensible.

Incidence

Of the women in this country, seven percent, or about 1 out of every 14, will develop breast cancer at some time in their lives. There are approximately 90,000 new cases each year.[15] It is the leading cause of cancer deaths in women and the leading cause of death from any cause in women ages 40-44.[16] Every 17 minutes another woman in the United States dies of this disease.[17] According to some authorities, the incidence rates are rising; others disagree with this and attribute the apparent rise to changes in the methods of collecting statistics.[18]

Risk Factors

Some women are more likely to get breast cancer than others. Risk factors have not been precisely defined, but the following conditions seem to be associated with increased risk:[19]

Previous Breast Cancer

The risk is highest for women who have previously had cancer in the other breast.

Other Forms of Cancer

Women with uterine cancer have about a two-fold increase in risk of developing breast cancer and vice versa. Similarly, having ovarian cancer increases a woman's risk for developing breast cancer and vice versa. It is not known whether this is because having the other form of cancer increases risk per se or because these diseases have some common risk factors that would predispose a woman to all of them.

Women who have had cancer of the colon seem to be at increased risk for the development of breast cancer; however, the opposite is not true. Women who have cancer in a major salivary gland are thought to have a risk about four times greater than that of the general population.

Family History

A family history (mother, sister, paternal or maternal aunts and grandmothers) of breast cancer puts a woman at a two- to three-fold increased risk. There is some indication that the age at which a woman's mother or sister developed breast cancer is significant. It seems that if the mother or sister developed breast cancer after the age of menopause, the risk is less than if she developed it earlier. If the mother or sister developed the cancer in her 30s, then the risk could be severe. At any rate, it does seem that the woman with a family history is likely to develop her cancer at a younger age than her relative did and that the cancer is apt to be more virulent.

Childbearing

Breast cancer risk increases with the age at which a woman bears her first child. Women who have their first child before the age of 18 have about one-third the breast cancer risk of those whose first delivery is delayed until 35 or older. To be protective a pregnancy must occur before the age of 30. In fact, women who have their first child after the age of 30 are at higher risk than those who have never had children. The protective effect of pregnancy is apparently limited to the first birth. Subsequent births convey little or no added protection. Only full-term pregnancy affords protection. An aborted pregnancy does not decrease risk.

Breastfeeding

The information about breastfeeding as a risk factor is rather contradictory. In the past, it was thought that it was a protective factor. Several studies done in the last decade have failed to show any correlation between breastfeeding and lower cancer rates, but most of these studies were done in countries that had generally high rates of breast cancer. One study done in Japan, a country with low rates, indicated that there was a correlation. This may be due to the fact that women in this country breastfeed for only relatively short periods of time whereas women in Japan breastfeed for considerably longer periods, thus perhaps giving any protective influence a chance to manifest itself. No one is quite certain, then, about the significance of breastfeeding, but it is thought that if breastfeeding is indeed protective, the effect is probably not a very dramatic one.

Menstrual History

Women who begin to menstruate at an earlier age are more likely to develop breast cancer. If a woman experiences menopause, either naturally or artificially at a younger age, then she is less likely to develop breast cancer. Women who go through menopause after the age of 55 are twice as likely to get breast cancer as those who experience menopause before 45.

Fibrocystic Disease

Most studies show that women with a· previous history of fibrocystic disease are four times more likely to develop breast cancer. Critics of these studies point out that many of the women studied were lost in the follow-up, and that the ones who are lost are probably the ones who never developed cancer, while the ones who do develop cancer are more likely to be the ones who stay in contract with the doctor and stay in the follow-up; hence, the results of these studies may be heavily weighted on the side of a positive association between breast cancer and fibrocystic breast disease.

There is some indication that only certain types of cystic disease are precancerous, but not enough is known yet to refine the odds about exactly which types are precancerous. One clue may be the age of onset. Cystic disease that is diagnosed before the age of 20 is considered by some experts to be particularly related to subsequent cancer.[20]

Diagnosing benign disease usually involves a special type of X-ray known as a mammogram. The pictures taken via mammograph can be divided into categories according to their common characteristics. These categories, known as Wolfe's classifications are called N_1, P_1, P_2 and DY. Classifications P_2 and DY may be associated with a higher risk of developing breast cancer (*see* p. 477).[21]

Ethnic Background, Socioeconomic Class, Geography

All of these factors play a role in increased risk, but since these things are often cross-related, it is sometimes difficult to sort them out. Affluent white women living in northern climates have the highest rates. Women living in Japan have considerably lower rates than do any women living in this country.

The incidence rates are higher in colder climates than in warmer ones, with the exception of Israel, which has high rates. These geographic variations may be due to differences in childbearing practices in various climates, but this is hard to substantiate.

Heredity suggests itself as an explanation for ethnic and racial differences; however, the fact that women from low-risk racial or ethnic backgrounds increase their risk when they move to a high-risk country indicates that environmental factors rather than inherited ones are at work.

Diet

Recently there has been a good deal of speculation that diet may be the factor that accounts for the racial, geographic and economic variables. A diet high in animal fats seems to be associated with increased risk. This could account for the fact that people in warmer climates have lower rates, for these people consume less animal fat. Moreover, women in Japan have lower rates and less animal fat in their diets. Overweight women who seem to be at higher risk often have diets higher in animal fat. The fact that low-risk women increase their risk when they move to a country where the diets are high in animal fat also supports the idea that diet and nutrition are crucial factors.

An affluent Jewish woman over the age of 40 with a history of breast cancer either in herself or in her family, a history of benign breast disease with suspicious mammogram patterns, early menstruation, no children or a child born after the age of 35, late menopause, a history of long-term use of estrogens (see below) and a diet high in animal fats and proteins would be at highest risk. A low-income Oriental woman with no family history of cancer, no prior breast disease, late menstruation, a child born before the age of 18, a surgical menopause before the age of 35 and a diet low in animal fats would be at lowest risk. Most authorities consider a personal or family history of cancer to be the most important risk factor.

Causes

The cause of breast cancer, like the cause of all cancer, is not known. For one thing, breast cancer is not one disease but perhaps fifteen or more different diseases. However, the epidemological studies that have helped to identify risk factors and studies of laboratory animals have suggested some causes.

The discovery of a virus in the milk of mice with breast cancer that seems to be associated with tumor growth in mice suggested that there might be a viral factor transmitted by breast milk in humans. The identification of a virus structurally similar to the mouse-milk virus in human milk of breast cancer patients further strengthened the theory; however, the virus was found with equal frequency in women with a family history of breast cancer and in those without. Moreover, women who were breastfed do not have a higher rate of breast cancer. Then, too, it is difficult to apply animal studies to humans, especially in cancer, which is an extremely species-specific disease, that is, it behaves quite differently in different animals. Breast cancer in mice does not usually metastasize and is generally not responsive to hormones, and the effect of pregnancy is to increase rather than decrease incidence rates. Breast cancer in rats, however, seems to mimic human breast cancer more closely. There is not persuasive evidence for a breast-milk—transmitted cancer-causing virus in rats. Thus, although the idea that cancer is caused by a virus transmitted through breast milk cannot be ruled out, the evidence is not strong.

The evidence that hormones play a role in breast cancer is suggestive but often contradictory. The fact that women who have their first menstrual period late and their menopause early are at lower risk suggests that the ovarian hormones, estrogen and progesterone, may be a factor. The fact that overweight women, who produce higher levels of estrogen, are at high risk is also suggestive. We also know that the growth rate of some human breast cancer is affected by estrogen. Estrogen has been used to induce breast cancer in rats. However, if estrogen is a causal factor, it is hard to understand why only the first pregnancy seems to offer any protective effect and why breastfeeding, which also alters estrogen levels, doesn't necessarily have a protective effect. Moreover, estrogen in birth control pills has not been shown to increase breast cancer incidence. However, as critics of the Pill point out, the Pill has not yet been in use for a long enough period of time for all the effects to have manifested themselves. Then, too, there is some evidence that women who have taken estrogen replacement therapy for menopausal symptoms are at increased risk.[22]

Just to make things more confusing, it has also been demonstrated that women with low levels of certain hormones from the adrenal glands that are related to the body's production of estrogen have higher rates of breast cancer. Since these women with low levels of adrenal hormones are thought to have low levels of estrogen as well, this would suggest that low levels of estrogen increase the risk of breast cancer—which runs contrary to the other data we have. Recently, there has been some indication that the ratio of certain types of estrogen to certain other types is the critical factor. These particular ratios have been found to occur more frequently in Asian women, who have lower incidence rates, than in American women, who have higher rates.

Other hormones have also been implicated. Prolactin, the hormone that stimulates the production of breast milk, has been related to the development of breast cancer. Here again, though, the evidence is contradictory. In some instances, low prolactin seems to bear a relationship to low rates of breast cancer. At other times, high rates of prolactin are associated with low incidence.

Progesterone, the hormone produced during the second half of the menstrual cycle, has also been studied. Women who do not ovulate regularly and hence do not produce progesterone regularly have higher rates of breast cancer, but progesterone has been used to induce breast tumors in some species of laboratory animals. Progesterone receptors, which make a tumor sensitive to the hormone, have been found in some breast tumors. Human pregnancy, which is accompanied by very high levels of progesterone, is usually associated with lower disease rates. Here again there is contradictory information.

It seems clear that hormone levels have some sort of relationshp to breast cancer, but the relationship is not a straightforward one. Many doctors are therefore concerned about the widespread use of hormones in the form of birth control pills and estrogen replacement therapy used to treat menopausal problems. There is no evidence that women on birth control pills have higher rates of breast cancer, but the Pill has been widely used for only about ten years and breast cancers may take 15-20 years to develop. Moreover, even though evidence for hormones as a causative factor is controversial, we do know that estrogen, if not a seed, is at least a fertilizer, causing some existing cancers to accelerate their growth rate. For this reason many doctors are hesitant about prescribing oral contraceptives for women who are at high risk. Certainly women with a personal or family history of breast cancer should avoid use of any hormone medications unless specifically prescribed as part of their cancer treatment (see Treatment below).

Another, more clearly understood causative factor is exposure to radiation. Women treated for tuberculosis with radiation therapy are known to be at increased risk. Female survivors of the atomic bomb exploded at Hiroshima in the Second World War also had increased incidence rates. Radiation has been used to induce breast cancer in laboratory animals. While it is clear that radiation can increase breast cancer incidence in exposed women, the doses of radiation received have been quite large, far greater than those to which most women are exposed, so most authorities feel that only a fraction of human breast cancers are related to radiation exposure. This topic has been hotly debated and is discussed in greater detail below (see Mammography).

Symptoms

Unfortunately, breast cancer may be present for quite some time before it produces any symptoms. In about 80 percent of cases, the disease will already have spread beyond the breast before the diagnosis is made.[23] Any of the symptoms listed in the introduction to this section may be associated with breast cancer; however, the presence of one of these symptoms does not necessarily mean that a woman has breast cancer. These symptoms could also be caused by benign diseases of the breast. In fact, eight out of every ten lumps biopsied will be benign; only two will be cancerous. Nevertheless, the presence of any suspicious symptoms deserves prompt medical attention.

Diagnosis

There are a number of important issues in the diagnosis of breast abnormalities that every woman should know about, including:

- ☐ The importance of monthly self-breast exam
- ☐ What constitutes a good breast exam, so that you know whether or not an exam is adequate

□ The risks and benefits of mammography, an X-ray procedure used to detect breast cancer, and how to minimize risks

□ The unnecessary expense and risk involved in certain types of breast biopsies

□ The controversy about whether certain types of breast abnormalities are malignant or benign and the importance of getting multiple pathology opinions

□ The fact that certain tests, known as hormone receptor assays, which could be of critical importance in planning treatment, are not done routinely at all hospitals and may have to be specially requested

These issues are discussed in more detail in the following pages.

Physical Exam

Most breast cancers are first discovered by the woman herself, which is why breast self-exam, described in Chapter Three, is so important. Studies have shown that tumors discovered by self-exam tend to be diagnosed in an earlier stage than tumors that are discovered by accident.[24] Every woman should examine herself once a month, and women at high risk need to be especially conscientious about breast exam. Women should enlist their doctor's help in learning breast self-exam and should also have an experienced doctor examine their breasts every six months.

Most women have their breasts examined by a gynecologist. Unfortunately many gynecologists give only the most cursory of breast exams, just a few quick pats. The exam should be quite thorough. The doctor should examine the woman while she is sitting up with her arms resting at her sides to judge the symmetry of the breasts and to note any differences in the direction in which her nipples point or any irregularities in the contours of the breasts. The arms should then be raised over the head and the breasts carefully examined for the same things. Next, the woman should lay on her back and the breasts and armpits should be palpated in the manner described in Chapter Three. It has been suggested that a woman at high risk make a point at least once in her life of having a breast exam by a specialist, even if it means traveling to a breast-cancer care facility (see the appendix), so that she will know what a really thorough exam is like.

Any woman who discovers a suspicous symptom should consult a doctor right away. There is nothing to be gained by waiting. Sometimes we may feel hesitant about consulting the doctor about a lump in our breasts, especially if we aren't quite sure whether or not the lump is actually there. We may feel particularly hesitant to bother the doctor about certain symptoms, such as a vague pain or a bruise that doesn't go away. We may also fear losing our breast. But breast cancer is a serious disease; no abnormality should be ignored. Early detection can literally save a woman's life—and, in certain instances, her breast.

Any woman whose doctor dismisses her symptoms without a thorough investigation should look for another doctor. Studies have shown that doctors are sometimes responsible for significant delays in the diagnosis of suspicious breast symptoms, delays that affect a woman's chances of survival.

Mammography

Another important part of the diagnostic work-up is the mammogram. Mammography is a special type of X-ray procedure that can detect the presence of abnormal tissue because such tissue absorbs radiation differently from normal tissue, and this shows up as a contrast on the X-ray film. There are two types of mammography: low-dose film mammography and xeromammography, or xerography that produces a paper, Xerox-type print as opposed to the film print produced by the low-dose film mammography.

There has been considerable debate about which type of mammography is best. When xerography first became available, it was considered superior by many radiologists since it took less time and produced a picture that had greater contrast and accuracy. However, since that time, film mammography techniques have been greatly improved. Studies comparing the accuracy of the two methods are now underway. Thus far, the accuracy of one method over the other seems to be related to the skill, experience and training of the person "reading" the mammogram.[25]

But even in the best of hands, mammography is plagued by a 6 percent false negative rate (in 6 percent of cases, it fails to detect a cancer that is actually there) and an 11 percent false positive rate (in 11 percent of cases, it notes a cancer that *isn't* there).[26] And that's in the best of hands; its accuracy can be considerably lower. We've heard reports of accuracy rates as low as 50 percent when used by supposedly well-trained radiologists.[27] Women should make sure that their mammograms are read by a board-certified (*see* p. 223) radiologist.

Where the mammography is done is as important as who reads the mammogram. The amount of radiation received during the mammographic exam will depend on the type of X-ray machine and equipment used, how carefully the machine is monitored, the manner in which the film is processed and the skill of the technician running the machine. The amount of radiation received is of crucial importance, for as outlined earlier, and discussed in more detail below, mammography involves exposure to radiation, which itself is known to increase the incidence of breast cancer.

The amount of radiation exposure a woman receives can vary

considerably. Not all centers have the newer types of low-dose mammography machines. One survey indicated that 10 percent of the radiologists were still using the older Egan machines, which expose women to unacceptably high levels of radiation.[28] Women should make sure that their mammograms are done on the newer, low-dose machines.

Even if the machine is one of the newer, low-dose machines, a woman may still receive an unacceptably high dose of radiation. If the machine is not maintained and adjusted properly or if proper techniques are not used to process the film, the dose may be too high. Indeed, the very same machine may give higher exposures at one center than another.[29] Sometimes higher doses are needed to get a more accurate picture of thick, glandular breasts, but some centers do not have their machines adjusted for the lowest possible dose.

The amount of radiation emitted from a machine is measured in units called roentgens, but the really critical factor is the number of rads. A rad is a unit of absorbed radiation. Skin dose refers to the number of rads absorbed on the surface of the skin. Midbreast dose refers to the number of rads absorbed in the midbreast area. The density and size of the breast will affect the number of rads received at the midbreast. It is not possible for anyone to tell exactly how many rads will be received at midbreast, but it is estimated that the breast absorbs about 25 percent of the roentgens emitted by a machine. According to the guidelines issued by the National Cancer Institute, the total number of roentgens per mammographic exam (usually two breasts, three exposures per breast) should not exceed the number that will give a woman a maximum of one rad. A woman having mammograms should ask about the estimated dose of rads she will be receiving. If the answer is more than one, she should look for another machine. The best place to find a well-calibrated, low-dose machine is at one of the major cancer-care facilities (see appendix).

Since the mammogram has a significant false negative rate, no woman should rely solely on a negative mammogram report if she has a suspicious symptom. A negative mammogram does not entirely rule out the possibility that a woman does not have cancer, for as noted above, mammography has a significant false negative rate. In certain cases, a doctor may rely on the negative mammogram and decide to follow the woman carefully. This might be done if 1. the tumor looks and feels benign to the doctor (that is, it is soft, freely movable and there is no skin retraction) and 2. the woman is young (and therefore unlikely to have cancer) and 3. the negative mammogram is not one of the high-risk types (see above). Otherwise, further tests are necessary. Similarly, a positive mammogram doesn't always mean that the woman has cancer, for there is a significant false positive rate. But, a positive mammogram definitely calls for further tests (see below).

Despite the fact that the mammography is not 100 percent accurate, it is still a valuable tool. It can detect cancers that are too small to be felt either by the doctor or the woman herself. Other, coexisting lumps may be discovered. It can indicate suspicious areas and help the doctor to decide what areas to biopsy. Moreover, the mammogram can be used as a record for the doctor to use in future comparisons.

Diagnostic mammography, as discussed above, is done on a woman who has a suspicious symptom—a lump, discharge, thickening of the skin and so forth—to help the doctor decide whether or not a lump is cancerous and where the biopsy should be done, or as part of the follow-up program for women who have been treated for breast cancer. In such cases, the benefits of mammography clearly outweigh the possible radiation risks. However, when mammography is used as a screening device, that is, when regular, periodic mammograms are done on women who have no suspicious symptoms, in hopes of detecting cancer early, the question of risks versus benefits comes up. Do the potential benefits of screening—early detection and higher survival rates—outweight the risks—radiation-induced cancer?

The complete answer to this question is not in yet. The whole mammography controversy is rather complex, but deserves attention since women have to make a decision about whether or not to have routine mammograms and if so, at what age and how often. Originally the National Cancer Institute recommended that mammography be used as a routine yearly screening device for asymptomatic women over the age of 35.[30] This recommendation was based on the initial encouraging results of a wide-scale, carefully controlled study done under the auspices of the Health Insurance Plan (HIP) of Greater New York.[31] In the HIP study, two groups of women were carefully matched. One group was merely followed, the other was given regular mammograms and physical exams (palpation) by experts. The final results of this study indicated that in women over 50 the combination of mammography and palpation proved effective in detecting cancer earlier and in achieving higher survival rates. But in women under the age of 50 no such effect was demonstrated. This was probably due to the fact that mammography is more effective in detecting lumps in the breasts of postmenopausal women than in the denser, more glandular breasts of younger women.

Before these final results were in, on the basis of initial results that had seemed quite encouraging, 27 Breast Cancer Detection Demonstration Projects (BCDDP) were set up around the country where women over the age of 35 could come for annual screening exams involving mammography, palpation and thermography, another method of visualizing the interior of the breast (see below).

Meanwhile, however, many scientists were becoming concerned about the liberal use of mammography and the risks of radiation. We actually know very little about how radiation affects the human body. Most of our information on this subject comes from women who have been exposed to large amounts of radiation, for example, survivors of the atomic bomb dropped at Hiroshima. We know that these women have a higher incidence of breast cancer than those who did not receive such radiation. We also know that the effects of radiation are cumulative—they add up. In other words, it is thought that repeated exposure to small amounts of radiation over many years may be just as bad as exposure to a lot of radiation at any one time.

The National Academy of Science attempted to estimate radiation risks on the basis of the data available.[32] According to their elaborate—and debatable—calculations, at an exposure of one rad per mammographic exam, a single exam of a woman at 35 years of age would increase her lifetime average risk of developing breast cancer from 7.58 percent to between 7.59 and 7.61 percent. Or, to put it in another way, there would be between 110-240 excess cases of cancer per one million women; if repeated annually, the test would increase the estimated risk of developing cancer during a lifetime to between 7.90 and 8.25 percent—or about 3,100-6,700 excess cases of cancer per one million women.[33]

Many assumptions have gone into this estimate. Perhaps it is not correct to assume a linear relationship between the amount of radiation exposure and cancer incidence. Maybe half the amount of radiation would still produce the same number of cancers or perhaps half that amount wouldn't produce any cancers at all. However, the Academy's estimation, although considered by some authorities to be too high and by others to be too low, is accepted by the majority of the scientific community.

In 1976, using the National Academy's official estimate of radiation risks, Dr. John C. Bailer, III, reanalyzed the results of the HIP study.[34] He pointed out that although there were a number of cancers detected in this study, they were discovered by the combined use of mammography and palpation by a skilled, experienced doctor. When Dr. Bailer tried to separate out the cases of cancer detected by mammography alone, the number of cancers detected was much lower.

Next, he tried to assess the radiation exposure given to the women involved in the study. He assumed that each woman received about two rads per exam. Two rads was actually lower than the amount of radiation received by many women in the study; however, because newer equipment developed since the time of the HIP study had reduced the radiation exposure, Dr. Bailer used the two rad figure, which was considered a good average from the best equipment available in 1976, the time of his study. Then, he calculated the number of lives saved by the use of mammography and the number of cancers that would eventually be produced as a result of the radiation exposure. After making his calculations, Dr. Bailer was forced to "regretfully conclude" that there seems to be a possibility that the routine use of mammography in screening asymptomatic women may eventually take as many lives as it saves.

He also pointed out that younger women are at a greater risk from irradiation (because they have a longer future lifetime in which to develop induced cancers) and that younger women are less likely to benefit from mammography screening, both because they have a lower incidence of breast cancer and because mammograms are less accurate in screening their breasts, which are dense.

Dr. Bailer's work led to new interim guidelines from the National Cancer Institute: Mammography was recommended for all women *over the age of 50* on a yearly basis as a screening device, but the use of mammograms as a screening device in women in the 35-49-year-old group was restricted to those at high risk for developing breast cancer. The committee continued to recommend mammography as a screening device for women over 50 because these women are at higher risk for breast cancer and lower risk for radiation-induced cancer (because their shorter lifespans mean fewer years in which to develop such cancers).

Not everyone was happy with these new guidelines. Many doctors felt that mammography was a valuable tool whose use was being too severely restricted. They pointed out that the newer mammography techniques were more accurate and involved lower doses of radiation, in some cases only a fraction of a rad. They also pointed to the results coming out of the BCDDP, which showed that there was a benefit for women under the age of 50. And the newer machines, they argued, were good enough to detect cancers in the denser, more glandular breasts of younger women.

Critics of mammography attacked this reasoning. They agreed that the BCDDP results were encouraging; however, they pointed out that the demonstration projects were operated on a self-selected basis. In other words, the woman who came to these projects were either referred by their doctors or chose voluntarily to come. Women concerned enough to go to a center might well have been women who were at high risk; and even though some of these women may have reported that they had no symptoms, they may actually have had some ill-defined symptom that prompted their concern but seemed too vague to be considered worth mentioning.

In the midst of all this controversy, the National Cancer Institute convened a panel of experts to review the data and make recommendations.[35] They recognized the fact that the BCDDP data could not be used to assess the risk/benefit ratio for asymptomatic women, but they also noted both the reduction in radiation exposure and the more accurate pictures produced by the newer machines. After reviewing the data, they recommended that mammography be used as a *routine screening device* for

1. All women 50 years of age and older

2. Women 40-49 years of age only if they have a personal history of breast cancer or a mother or sister who has had breast cancer
3. Women 35-39 only if they have a personal history of breast cancer

The panel of experts also suggested that although the results looked promising, the BCDDP data was not sufficient to evaluate the possibility that newer, more accurate low-dose machines might make screening for younger women a viable alternative, and recommended that further studies be done. The panel further suggested that investigations be carried out to determine whether a mammogram was necessary every year or whether less frequent mammograms, which would mean less exposure, would be as effective in detecting the cancer early. Recommendations for mammography may change again in the future, pending the results of these new studies.

It should be noted, however, that the NCI guidelines for safe use of the mammograph apply only to machines that deliver exposure of one rad or less. The use of such mammography in asymptomatic women over the age of 50 is considered worthwhile because by virtue of their age alone they have fewer years left in which to develop radiation-induced cancer. Higher doses, however, may not be safe for any woman, regardless of her age.

Women should realize that the NCI guidelines are just that—guidelines, not laws. Individual doctors may use mammography more or less liberally. While we generally feel comfortable about the latest NCI guidelines, we do wonder about the value of mammograms in asymptomatic women over the age of 50 who are at extremely low risk, as, for instance, the hypothetical low-risk woman described earlier. Moreover, there are some instances in which we might recommend mammograms more liberally than the guidelines suggest.

We have already discussed the fact that women with a history of benign breast disease who have certain characteristic mammogram patterns (*see* p. 477) seem to be at higher risk. The panel reviewing the BCDDPs alluded to these high-risk mammogram patterns but didn't consider them in making their guidelines since the BCDDPs did not collect data on them. Whether or not such women should have regular mammograms and if so, at what age they should have them and how frequently, is a matter of debate. All we can tell you is that one of the authors of this book has a history of benign breast disease, but of the high-risk type, and has been having yearly mammograms since the age of 35.

(Note: Since this manuscript was prepared, new guidelines have been issued. The NCI recommendations have remained essentially the same, except that one baseline mammogram, which will serve as a basis for future comparisons, is now recommended after the age of 35 for all women).

Thermography, Ultrasound, GST and Other Diagnostic Tools

Thermography is another method of visualizing the interior of the breast. It relies on differences in heat patterns between normal and abnormal tissues. Initially, researchers were enthusiastic about the potential of thermography, which unlike mammography involves no radiation exposure and little risk. Studies have shown, however, that thermography is not very accurate; it has a 30-35 percent false negative rate.[36] Indeed, it is only slightly more accurate than choosing women at random and flipping a coin to determine if they have breast cancer. Although some experimental work is still being done, most centers have abandoned thermography. A woman should never rely on thermography alone as a screening or diagnostic technique.

Ultrasound, a method of visualizing internal tissues by means of high-frequency sound, is now being used experimentally. While the technique is not yet reliable or practical enough for wide-scale use, it may play a role in the future.

GST, or graphic stress telethermometry, another experimental diagnostic tool, also involves studying heat patterns in the breast tissue. The test can detect and distinguish between benign and cancerous breast tumors. It does not involve any radiation. This diagnostic tool is currently being tested, and if it proves effective, it may become the ideal method for mass screening of asymptomatic women. New, more precise X-ray procedures that involve similar or lower-dose radiation exposure also look promising. Experiments now underway may also yield simple blood tests that could be useful in diagnosing breast cancer.

Biopsy

The only way to tell for sure whether or not a lump is cancerous is to do a biopsy. There are several types of biopsies. Needle biopsy, or needle aspiration, is one type. This simple office procedure involves injecting a local anesthetic into the breast, inserting a needle into the lump and attempting to aspirate fluid. The fluid is then sent to the laboratory for analysis. If the laboratory report is negative and the lump collapses, a more extensive biopsy may not be necessary. If the pathology report is positive, cancer treatment can be planned. If, as sometimes happens, no fluid can be extracted, a more extensive biopsy is necessary. Similarly, if the pathology report is negative but the lump has not collapsed, a more extensive biopsy must be done, for the needle aspiration is not 100 percent accurate and the remaining lump may contain cancerous cells.

The next step is another type of needle biopsy known as a tru-cut, or wide-bore biopsy. This involves inserting a hollow needle into the lump and extracting a core of tissue. If the report from the lab is negative, a more extensive surgical biopsy is still required, for this type of biopsy also is not 100 percent accurate. Although there may not have been any cancer in the tissue sample, cancer might be lurking elsewhere in the lump. But if the lab report is positive, no further biopsy need be done, for the diagnosis has been made and treatment can be planned.

The surgical biopsy may be either an incisional biopsy, in which part of the tumor is removed, or, whenever possible, an excisional biopsy, in which the entire lump is removed. The tissue is then sent to the lab for analysis.

One-Step vs. Two-Step Biopsies

In the past, most breast biopsies were done in the hospital, using a general anesthetic. The woman was admitted to the hospital as a patient, prepared for surgery, wheeled into the operating room and given an anesthetic. The surgeon then performed the excisional or incisional biopsy and sent the tissue to the pathology lab for analysis. While the surgeon waited in the operating room, the pathologist examined the tissue in a quick procedure known as frozen-section analysis. Prior to the operation the woman had signed a consent form authorizing the doctor to remove the breast, a procedure known as mastectomy (see below), should the lump prove cancerous. If the report from the pathologist came back positive, the surgeon removed the woman's breast.

This one-step biopsy/operation has come under a lot of criticism in the past few years. Many doctors are now doing a two-step procedure. The biopsy is done on an outpatient basis, using a local anesthetic. The woman comes into the office or hospital in the morning and is home again the same day.

This has several advantages. First of all, it is less expensive. Biopsies in which the woman is admitted to the hospital as a patient and in which a general anesthetic is used cost about seven times more than biopsies done on an outpatient basis using a local anesthetic.[37] Moreover, only about two out of every ten lumps biopsied will actually be cancerous. When one-step biopsies are done, eight of these ten women are paying unnecessary hospital and doctor costs. Moreover, the two-step procedure frees up badly needed hospital beds, and since there is no postoperative hospital recovery time, the woman doesn't lose time from work.

Cost is not the only advantage to the two-step procedure. There is also less risk involved. Any time a general anesthetic is used there are risks and possible complications, sometimes fatal ones. One out of every 1,600 people requiring a general anesthetic will die just from the anesthetic alone.[38] Use of a local anesthetic involves less risk. The argument is sometimes made that by using a one-step biopsy the doctor can avoid subjecting the woman to two anesthetics—one for the biopsy and one for the mastectomy—but this argument is a fallacious one. First of all, a local rather than a general can be used. Secondly, only two out of every ten women will actually need the second anesthetic, for the other eight will not have cancer. With the two-step procedure, then, only those women who actually need it will be subjected to the risks of a general anesthetic.

In addition to lowering costs and reducing risk, the two-step biopsy has other advantages. Instead of relying on the frozen section, which is done while the woman lies on the operating table, the pathologist can do a more accurate, but more time-consuming, permanent-section analysis. The frozen-section method sometimes distorts the cells, making it difficult for the pathologist to "read" the biopsy specimen. Admittedly, however, even if the one-step procedure and frozen-section analysis are done, it is unlikely that the pathologist would misread the slide and make an incorrect positive report to the surgeon, for if there is any doubt at all, the pathologist will await the permanent section. Only on extremely rare occasions will an unnecessary mastectomy be done because of a misreading of a frozen section. Still, mistakes can happen, and the permanent section is therefore preferable.

More importantly, use of a two-step biopsy means that the woman has time to seek a second pathology opinion before operation. Often this is done as a matter of routine. In small hospitals, however, this may not always be the case and, as explained in the general discussion of cancer, second pathology reports are always a good idea. Moreover, as explained below, in certain cases of breast cancer there is considerable debate even among experts about whether or not certain abnormalities are benign or malignant. Women who fall into this category will want to get second, third and perhaps even more pathology opinions from the very best experts in the field before deciding on a course of treatment. If they have a one-step biopsy, this will not be possible.

Another important advantage to the two-step procedure is the fact that it allows the doctor to do proper tests to detect metastasis prior to treatment. If a two-step procedure is done and the lump is malignant, the doctor will do chest X-rays, liver function tests and bone scans before beginning the cancer treatment. Many doctors feel that if these tests indicate metastasis, there is no point in doing a mastectomy, for it won't enhance survival rates. Simple removal of the lump will suffice.

If a one-step biopsy is done, the doctor has two choices: S/he may either do the tests after the biopsy/mastectomy, though, as explained above, this might mean that a needless mastectomy was done, or s/he could do the tests prior to biopsy, though this might mean that if the woman turns out to have a benign lump, she will have been subjected to the needless expense and radiation risks involved in these tests. Only by doing a two-step procedure can these problems be avoided.

Another extremely important advantage to the two-step procedure is that it allows time for the woman to consider the various treatments available and make an informed decision about what type of therapy she wants, for, as discussed in more detail below, different doctors favor different types of therapy, some much less mutilating than others. It also allows the woman time to shop around for the doctor she wants to perform the therapy she chooses. A general surgeon might be quite competent to perform a biopsy, but if a woman elects to have a mastectomy, she should have her surgery done by a skilled and experienced surgeon who specializes in this type of operation, not by a doctor who only performs a few mastectomies a year. Moreover, for those women who are considering breast reconstruction (see below), the two-step procedure allows for consultation with a plastic surgeon prior to the operation.

The two-step procedure has so many obvious advantages that it is hard to understand why the one-step procedure is done. In the past, the arguments were made that the cancer might be spread by disturbing the tumor during surgical removal and that the delay between biopsy and treatment would be dangerous; however, studies have shown this not to be true.[39] Delays of up to two weeks have not been shown to have any negative effect on survival rates. However, there are some very large lumps that might be technically difficult to remove without discomfort to the woman if she has only a local anesthetic. And there are tumors so small that they cannot be felt and are detectable only by mammography. These cases might require a general anesthetic. A one-step procedure might be done in these cases, but they are a minority. The vast majority of women can and should have two-step biopsies. In fact, a special committee set up by the National Cancer Institute has now endorsed the two-step procedure.[40]

Given that it is rarely necessary to do a one-step biopsy, it seems obvious that the motivation for a one-step is largely financial. The one-step procedure is more lucrative for the anesthesiologist. If two-step procedures were done routinely, then the anesthesiologist would do a major procedure only on the two women who actually had cancer—thereby losing the income from the other eight women in whom the less lucrative outpatient biopsy revealed benign disease. Hospital costs are also reduced when a two-step procedure is done.

Every woman should ask her doctor whether a one-step or two-step biopsy is planned and why. If the doctor is adamant about doing a one-step procedure, the woman should, by all means, seek a second opinion.

Biopsy Incision

Women should also ask about the type of incision the doctor plans to make in order to do the biopsy. In some cases, the location of the tumor will dictate the type of incision that is made. Many times, however, it is possible to make the incision along the outer edge of the areola, which makes for a superior cosmetic result. In most cases such incisions are practically invisible once they have healed.

Pathology

Another important issue that women having breast biopsies should consider is the skill of the pathologist. As explained in the general section on cancer, the accuracy of the pathology report is a critical factor. This is especially important in breast cancer. Today, with the use of mammography, breast abnormalities of only five mm or less are being discovered. These small abnormalities are often noninvasive, that is, the cells are cancerous but there is no sign that they have actually invaded the neighboring healthy tissues. These are sometimes referred to as carcinomas in situ, cancers that are "in place." Some pathologists feel that these growths will eventually become invasive. Other pathologists have questioned this interpretation. They point to the fact that microscopic examinations of the breasts of women over the age of 70 revealed evidence of these types of minimal cancers at a rate 19 times higher than the reported incidence of breast cancer.[41] It may well be that not all of these minimal abnormalities will actually become invasive cancer. Obviously, this has important implications for treatment: Is it necessary to remove these minimal abnormalities, let alone remove the entire breast? This issue is discussed in greater detail under Treatment below. It also has implications for pathology: How should these abnormalities be classified, as benign or malignant?

Pathology is not a hard-and-fast science. Evidence of this fact comes from a pathology review of BCDDP findings in which a board of pathologists analyzed the minimal cancers discovered in the various BCDDP centers.[42] A total of 1,810 breast cancers had been discovered in the BCDDPs at the time of the review, of which 592 had been found to meet the definition of minimal cancer, that is, an abnormality that is either noninfiltrating (in situ) or infiltrating less than one cm. Of these, 506 were reviewed by the board, all top-notch pathologists. In 83 percent of the cases they reviewed, the pathologists agreed that the abnormalities found were indeed cancerous. In 66 cases, or 13 percent of the cases they reviewed, the board found that the original diagnosis of cancer was

509

incorrect and that the abnormalities were, after all, benign. In 22 cases, or 4 percent of the cases reviewed, even the experts were unable to agree.* The review board thus found that 3.5 to 5 percent of the 1,810 cancers found in the BCDDPs were initially misdiagnosed.

How does all of this sort out and what implications does it have? Well, first of all, it underscores the need for second opinions. Women who are diagnosed as having noninfiltrating cancers—in situ cancers—or infiltrating cancers less than one cm in size should, without exception, have two, three or even more pathology opinions before accepting treatment. Moreover, these second opinions should come from top-notch pathologists, the heads of departments of pathology at major university teaching hospitals or cancer-care facilities (see appendix). It is not necessary for women to travel to these locations to get second opinions. The woman or her doctor can arrange to have her slides sent to the pathologist for review.

Although second pathology opinions are always a good idea, studies have not shown these kinds of discrepancies in diagnosis when larger, infiltrating cancers have been reviewed by teams of pathologists.[44] Every woman should ask her doctor to explain the pathology report. Terms such as "noninvasive," "in situ," "noninfiltrating," "minimal" or "early" may all be used to describe the types of cases for which we feel multiple pathology opinions are essential. Women should ask their doctors specifically, "Is my cancer an in situ cancer or an infiltrating cancer that is less than one cm?" If the answer is yes, multiple opinions from top-notch pathologists are in order.

Hormone Receptor Assays

The last but certainly not the least test that should be considered by any woman having a breast biopsy is one known as a hormone receptor assay. The results of this test, which is also called a steroid receptor assay, could be of vital importance in planning further therapy in cases where the cancer recurs and in advanced disease. Unfortunately, it is not yet done routinely at all hospitals, so you may have to request it specially.

At the time of the biopsy a small segment of the tumor is removed. The segment is then analyzed to determine how sensitive the tumor is to hormones. We have known for many years that estrogen can stimulate the growth of certain breast tumors.

After careful research and investigation, it was discovered that the presence of a certain number of estrogen "receptors," which seem to

*Women who had minimal cancers diagnosed at BCDDP centers should read the important information given in note 43 at the end of this chapter. In addition, more detailed and precise information about the number of cases misdiagnosed is also given there.

sensitize the tumor to hormones, could be used to predict which if any treatment—surgical destruction of her ovaries, radiation, hormone therapy—would reduce a woman's tumor. The test is not always 100 percent accurate in its prediction, but it is a valuable tool that can help the doctor in planning should the cancer recur.[45]

The test should be done at the time of the biopsy, or if a one-step procedure is done, at the time of mastectomy. If it is not done and cancer should recur in some inaccessible place, for instance in the bones, there is no way to then biopsy the cancer and do a hormone receptor test. Since the test is not done routinely, a woman should check with her doctor prior to biopsy. If the doctor has not made arrangements to have the test done, she should ask him or her to do so. If the hospital is not equipped to perform the test, there are a number of commercial labs across the country that can do so. But advance arrangements are necessary because the malignant tissue must be frozen for testing within 15 minutes. *All* women having biopsies should make sure that this test will be done if the biopsy shows malignancy. It should be noted, however, that the test depends on having one gram of malignant tissue, so the test may not be possible for women fortunate enough to have very small tumors.

Staging

There are a number of different staging schemes used for breast cancer. Table 17 outlines one widely used classification scheme.[46] TNM classifications like those described in Table 18 are now used more frequently.[47]

One factor that is extremely important in staging, regardless of what classification scheme is used, is the size of the tumor. Generally speaking, the larger the tumor, the greater the chance that the disease has spread

Table 17
Staging Scheme for Breast Cancer

Stage I:	Tumor less than two cm in diameter; nodes clinically negative; no distant metastasis
Stage II:	Tumor less than five cm in diameter; nodes, if palpable, not fixed; no distant metastasis
Stage III:	Tumor greater than five cm, any size tumor that is fixed in place or evidences invasion of the skin or any tumor that is accompanied by nodes other than the axillary nodes that are clinically positive; no distant metastasis
Stage IV:	Tumor of any size accompanied by distant metastasis

Table 18
TNM Classifications for Breast Cancer

T = Tumor size

T1S: Preinvasive cancer, carcinoma in situ, noninfiltrating intraductal carcinoma or Pagent's disease of the nipple with no obvious tumor

TO: No tumor can be felt

T1:* Tumor two cm or less
    T1a: Tumor not fixed to underlying pectoral muscles
    T1b: Tumor fixed to underlying pectoral muscles

T2:* Tumor more than two cm, but less than five cm
    T2a/T2b: Same as above

T3:* Tumor more than five cm
    T3a/T3b: Same as above

T4: Tumor of any size with direct extension to the skin or ribs or underlying muscles other than the pectoral muscles
    T4a: Tumor fixed
    T4b: Swelling, sores or cancerous nodules on the skin of the breast, peau d'orange
    T4c: Both of the above

N = axillary lymph nodes

NO: No palpable nodes

N1: Palpable but freely movable nodes
    N1a: Nodes not considered to contain cancer
    N1b: Nodes considered to contain cancer

N2: Nodes that are considered to contain growths and that are fixed

N3: Nodes other than axillary nodes considered to contain growths or swelling of the arm

M = distant metastasis

MO: No evidence of distant metastasis

M1: Distant metastasis (including skin involvement beyond the breast area)

---

*Dimpling of the skin, nipple retraction or other skin changes except those noted in T4b may occur in T1, T2, or T3 without changing the classification.

beyond the breast. This is not always the case, for there are some cancers that apparently grow relatively large within the breast before they spread.

The condition of the lymph nodes is also important. After careful palpation (feeling) of the nodes the doctor will decide whether the nodes are "clinically negative" (thought not to contain cancer) or "clinically positive" (thought to contain cancer). Clinical estimates of nodal status are incorrect in about a third of cases,[48] for nodes may be swollen without containing cancer or may feel normal even though cancer is present. The only way to tell for sure whether or not there is cancer in the lymph nodes is to remove them and examine them microscopically.

If the tumor is fixed in place and not freely movable, this is a serious sign. If there are open sores on the breast, swelling of the breast tissue, peau d'orange or cancerous nodules on the skin, these also indicate that the disease is more advanced.

Treatment

The treatment of breast cancer is one of the most controversial subjects in medicine today. At times the particulars of a woman's case, especially the stage of her disease, will dictate a specific form of treatment, but at other times, particularly during Stages I and II, the form of treatment recommended may depend on the doctor's philosophy and personal preference. Most doctors recommend some form of mastectomy (Illustration 53), or removal of the breast, but treatments may range from a segmental mastectomy, or simple removal of the lump and surrounding tissue, to removal of one or both breasts as well as the axillary lymph nodes and the major and minor pectorals (the muscles of the upper chest). Sometimes hormone therapy, chemotherapy and radiation therapy are used as well.

Stages I and II

Before discussing the various forms of treatment used and the pros and cons of each, it is necessary to consider the problems involved in the studies that have compared the results of the various forms of therapy. The proponents of the various therapies each point to studies that they claim "prove" the superiority of their particular form of treatment. For example, there are some very well-known doctors at major medical schools who will contend that in certain cases a segmental mastectomy, which may be followed by chemotherapy or radiation therapy, is just as effective as a modified mastectomy (removal of the breast and all the axillary lymph nodes). The segmental mastectomy is preferable, they claim, because the survival rates are on par with those obtained via other types of mastectomy while the cosmetic results are much better, since the entire breast is not removed.

In our opinion, any doctor who claims or implies that there is proof that treatments involving anything less than removal of the breast and the axillary lymph nodes are as effective as these other, more extensive

SEGMENTAL

MODIFIED RADICAL

RADICAL

Illustration 53   *Types of Mastectomies*

procedures is highly irresponsible. This is not to say that the less mutilating forms of therapy such as the segmental mastectomy might not, in the end, turn out to be equally effective but that, at the present time, on the basis of available data it is impossible to make this claim. *We simply do not know,* and therein lies the whole crux of the breast cancer controversy.

Radical Mastectomy

Perhaps a bit of the history of breast cancer treatment is in order.[49] The first major breakthrough came with the development of the radical mastectomy, also called the Halstead mastectomy, after the doctor who pioneered this form of therapy. This operation involves removal of the breast, the lymph nodes in the axillary area and the major and minor pectorals, which are the muscles of the upper chest. Proponents of this form of treatment believe that the entire breast rather than just the tumor must be removed, for breast cancer is multicentric—has many points of origin. Merely removing the tumor would, they feel, be taking too great a risk, for the microscopic residual cancer left behind could metastasize before it were detected. The lymph nodes are removed because the cancer frequently spreads to this area. Even if the lymph nodes do not appear to be enlarged, microscopic cancer could be lurking in the nodes. The only way to tell is to remove the nodes and examine them microscopically. If positive nodes are found, then chemotherapy (see below) is given.

The rationale for removing the pectorals is three-fold. First, proponents of the radical mastectomy argue that it is difficult to remove all the lymph nodes without removing the pectorals. Secondly, they argue that removing the pectorals through which the lymph passes assures that any lymph vessels embedded in the muscle tissue that might contain cancer cells will also be removed. Lastly, removal of the pectorals allows for what is known in medical circles as en bloc dissection. This means that all the tissue is removed in one piece, which supposedly lessens the chance of spilling tumor cells into adjacent tissue or into the lymph and blood systems.

This operation is, to say the least, disfiguring. Not only is the breast itself removed but also the chest muscles, which creates a hollow in the upper part of the chest. The scar is a long one and is hard to cover over with anything but high-necked dresses and tops. Sometimes skin grafts, or layers of skin transplanted from another area of the body to the wound area, must be done in order to close the wound. The destruction of the lymph network can cause a condition known as lymphedema, in which the lymph fluid that normally travels from the arm through the axillary area becomes trapped, causing the arm to swell up. Also known as milk arm, this condition can grossly distort the arm and cause grinding pain. In addition, the axillary muscles have to take over for the pectorals and for some women it is never possible to completely regain use of the arm.

515

Modified Radical Mastectomy

Because of these complications, changing notions about the spread of the disease, and the fact that women seemed to be dying, not from local recurrences in the breast/chest/axillary area, but from distant metastasis, there was increasing interest in an operation known as the modified radical mastectomy. This operation involves removal of the breast and the lymph nodes, but the pectoral muscles are left intact. Although on paper it doesn't sound much different from the radical, the modified is a much less disfiguring operation. It has a much lower complication rate and has much better cosmetic results.[50] The incision is transverse rather than horizontal and is much easier to cover over with clothing. The chances for breast reconstruction (see below) are much better. Lymphedema and muscle disability are reduced. Skin grafts are not usually necessary and recuperation is much more rapid.

Most cancer specialists now prefer the modified radical for Stages I and II. Studies have shown that it is possible to remove just as many lymph nodes with a modified radical as with a radical mastectomy.[51] The fact that most women who die of breast cancer don't die from local recurrences but from disease that has already spread through the body first suggested that removal of the pectorals—at least in Stages I and II—may not be necessary. Moreover, small-scale studies that gathered data about women who had had one or the other operation in the past indicated that in these cases there was no advantage in terms of survival, whether a modified or a radical was done.[52] Many doctors therefore felt that the modified was an acceptable alternative.

There were, however, many doctors who were hesitant to accept the superiority of the modified radical to the radical on the basis of the studies that had been done. Their hesitancy had to do with problems concerning statistical methods and the experimental design of the studies comparing the two methods of treatment. In order to understand these objections it is important to remember that breast cancer is not just one but probably fifteen or more different diseases. Different forms of the disease behave differently. Although we know that, generally speaking, the larger the tumor in the breast, the more likely it is that the tumor has spread to the lymph nodes and other parts of the body, we also know that some tumors grow quite large in the breast before they metastasize. Alternately, some very small tumors have already metastasized by the time they are discovered. Some tumors are extremely virulent and grow rapidly, while others are much less deadly and grow at a relatively slow pace.

The virulence (deadliness) of a tumor may depend not only on the particular type of tumor but also on the way in which a particular woman's body responds to the cancer. This is called host resistance. The outcome in two women with tumors of the same size and type who are treated in the same manner may be different. One may live and the other die. Apparently one woman's body is better able to combat the cancer. Thus, although the stage of a woman's disease is a rough predictor of the outcome of her case, it is not entirely accurate. As yet, we don't have a precise, clear-cut understanding of the growth pattern of all types of cancers. Nor do we understand or find it possible to predict or measure host resistance.

Any study that attempts to compare the results of various treatments must take into account the fact that there are many different types of cancer and variations in host response. If, for instance, 100 women are given radical mastectomies and another 100 are given modified radical mastectomies, the fact that there is no difference in survival rates doesn't prove equal effectiveness. Even though the women who had the modified radical had Stage I disease, they may have had a less virulent form of cancer, while those who had the radical may have had a more deadly type of cancer. Or perhaps the women who had modified radicals just happened to be those who had superior host resistance. Even just a small proportion of the less favorable type of cancer or less adequate host resistance in one of the groups studied could bias the results. In order to provide reliable information, then, studies must include large numbers of women. The laws of statistics tell us that with small numbers we are likely to get biased results, but as the numbers increase, the chances of biased results decrease. Only by including large numbers of women is it possible to insure the proper "mix" of unknown factors.

It is especially important for a researcher to have large numbers and a proper mix of unknown factors anytime s/he wants to distinguish small differences between groups and treatments being studied. If big differences exist, large numbers are not so important. If, for instance, a researcher compares two methods of treatment and finds an 80 percent cure rate with one and a 10 percent cure rate with another, then that researcher can feel fairly confident that the treatment with the 80 percent cure rate is superior and not just a statistical fluke arising from the presence of more women with poor host resistance in one group, for example, or more virulent tumors in the other. But although the studies that compare modified radicals and radicals indicated that if there were differences in survival rates, they were going to be small ones, these studies nonetheless involved only small groups of women.

Another problem with many of these studies was that they were retrospective studies, that is, they "looked backward" and collected results from groups of women who had in the past been treated by one method or another. Then they compared these results. However, it is impossible to compare such results with any assurance, for even when the women all had the same stage of disease, different definitions of stage were sometimes used at that time by different surgeons. The skill of the surgeon was also a factor. One surgeon may simply have been more adept than another. Definitions of surgery are different as well. What one doctor called a modified radical was sometimes more or sometimes less extensive a procedure than what another doctor meant by that term. In short, there are simply too many variables for any researcher to compare historical data and have complete confidence in the results. These sorts of studies are valuable as guidelines, but they can't yield definitive results.

NSABP Studies

It became obvious that in order to make a clear-cut comparison of various methods, it would be necessary to do new studies. Thus, in 1971, after almost a decade of planning, the National Surgical Adjuvant Breast Project (NSABP) studies of treatment options for Stages I and II breast cancer, under the direction of Dr. Bernard Fisher of the University of Pittsburgh, were begun.[53] These studies, which were called protocols, were carefully designed to include large numbers of women. The definitions of eligibility for the study were carefully delineated so that they were uniform and so that the women being compared were as well-matched as possible. The types of surgery were also precisely defined so that the women were receiving comparable operations.

The first widescale NSABP study was called Protocol B—04. Women who were eligible for the study were broken down into two main groups: those who had clinically positive nodes (nodes that were suspected of being cancer on the basis of the doctor's palpation) and those who had clinically negative nodes. These women were then randomly assigned by a computer to receive one form of treatment or another. The form of treatment was called the arm of the protocol. By having a computer randomly assign the woman to one arm of the protocol, any bias on the part of the doctor that could affect the outcome of the study was eliminated.

By August 1974 a large enough number of women had been entered into the study. This study is now in its seventh year, and when the first official results were reported, the women had been in the study for an average of three years. In these results, all forms of treatment were shown to be equivalent: No form of therapy studied proved superior to another in terms of survival rates. Updates at four and five years have not changed the picture. Although five-year survival rates for breast cancer do not hold the same significance as they do for other cancers (see Survival Rates below), enough time has elapsed so that trends are firmly established.

The NSABP Protocol B—04 has provided valuable information about the treatment of breast cancer.*

*See note 54 for details.

The study was designed in such a way that it answered the question about whether removing the pectoral muscles would really enhance survival rates, which was, of course, the key point that advocates of the radical mastectomy were making.[55] Since the removal of the pectorals was not shown to increase survival rates, the NSABP study showed, indirectly, that the modified could produce survival rates equivalent to the radical.

Secondly, the NSABP studies showed that total mastectomy followed by radiation therapy did not produce results superior to those of the modified radical. The total mastectomy, also called a simple mastectomy, involves removal of only the breast itself. The chest muscles and lymph nodes are not removed. Surgery can then be followed by radiation to the axillary area that destroys the cancer in the lymph nodes and axillary area. Proponents of this method of therapy had argued that radiation might be more effective than surgery in treating the axillary area. They felt that even though the radical mastectomy employed en bloc dissection, tumor cells could still be spread by surgical intervention. Moreover, radiating the armpit avoided the necessity for removing the chest muscles, so the total mastectomy plus radiation was a less disfiguring procedure. Because of the NSABP studies we know now that this method could not produce superior results to the radical.

The modified radical mastectomy, like the total mastectomy with radiation, also allows for preservation of the chest muscles. Moreover, the modified allows the doctor to actually remove the lymph nodes and examine them microscopically for signs of cancer, which the total plus radiation does not. This has become increasingly important in recent years, for we now have chemotherapy that can provide better survival rates in cases where the disease has spread beyond the breast. However, as explained below, chemotherapy involves certain risks and should be given only to women who actually need it. The only way to tell whether the woman needs it is to remove the lymph nodes and examine them microscopically for signs of cancer. (Remember, although palpation of the nodes yields a finding of "clinically" positive or negative, it is not totally accurate; only the microscopic examination can tell for certain whether cancer is present in the nodes.) Thus, we can now conclude that for Stages I and II, the modified radical is equivalent to both the radical mastectomy and the total mastectomy plus radiation therapy; since the modified offers better cosmetic results than the radical and unlike the total plus radiation allows for microscopic examination of the lymph nodes, it is generally considered the best treatment for Stages I and II. There are still some doctors who do radical mastectomies in these cases, but given the results of the NSABP studies, this more disfiguring and disabling operation can hardly be justified. There are still some doctors who will do a total mastectomy plus radiation therapy, but with the development of chemotherapy, it is essential that the lymph nodes be removed in order to determine whether chemotherapy is indicated.* Although there are a few cases (deep tumor near chest wall and pectorals) in which a radical of some sort may be necessary, we suggest that women with Stage I and II disease whose doctors suggest a radical mastectomy or a total mastectomy plus radiation therapy seek second opinions.

Segmental Mastectomy

Women with Stages I and II disease may also be eligible for another less extensive form of therapy than the modified radical; however, this other form of therapy, known as segmental mastectomy, is still considered experimental, and while it may yet prove to be as effective as the modified, we still can't be sure. Another term for segmental mastectomy is "partial mastectomy."* Basically this form of therapy involves removal of the lump itself, along with a generous portion of breast tissue, with or without radiation or chemotherapy. The lymph nodes in the armpit should also be removed. There are some doctors who will perform segmental mastectomy without axillary dissection, a procedure in which the lymph nodes in the armpit are removed. We strongly urge women to insist on an axillary dissection, for without actually removing the lymph nodes and examining them microscopically, there is no way of knowing whether or not cancer is present in them. Clinical estimates of whether or not the nodes are involved are too often inaccurate. If cancer-bearing lymph nodes are left behind, the disease could spread to other parts of the body. Moreover, accurate decisions about the use of chemotherapy cannot be made unless the lymph nodes are examined microscopically. There are also some doctors who will perform a segmental mastectomy without a complete axillary dissection: They may remove only the lower lymph nodes. We feel this is unwise. Removal of all the lymph nodes doesn't distract significantly from the cosmetic effects. Moreover, we know that cancer can "skip" lymph nodes; if the lower nodes are negative, this does not necessarily mean that the higher ones are not positive. Women should insist on an axillary dissection, and the axillary dissection should be a complete one.

In the past, the notion of doing a segmental mastectomy was considered too risky because it has long been known that cancer is a multicentric

---

*Using radiation therapy also has another disadvantage—exposure to radiation. Concern has been expressed over the relatively small number of rads involved in mammography. Women are exposed to thousands of rads when radiation is used to treat breast cancer.
*The terms "tylectomy" and "lumpectomy" are not actually synonymous with segmental mastectomy although some doctors use them in that way.

disease.[56] Multiple microscopic cancerous areas have been found in breasts removed via mastectomy. Doctors were afraid that if these small cancerous areas were left behind, they would continue to develop and might metastasize before they became large enough to be discovered. However, new developments in the field of breast cancer have led to a rethinking of this issue. Autopsies of women who have died have shown the presence of microscopic breast cancers even though the women never had breast cancer during their lifetimes. Autopsies of the breasts of women over the age of 70 who have died from other causes have revealed the presence of microscopic cancerous areas at a rate 19 times higher than the actual rate of breast cancer in this age group.[57] This suggests that some cancers will never actually become truly invasive cancers, but will remain localized within the breast. The question then arises: Do we really need to remove the entire breast in all cases?

We also now know that a large portion of women with breast cancer will have cancer in their lymph nodes at the time of diagnosis. Once the cancer has reached the lymph nodes, the chances are greater that it has spread to other parts of the body. Since chemotherapy is needed to treat metastasized disease, is the removal of the entire breast really worthwhile? Will it prolong life or increase survival rates? Or will a segmental mastectomy suffice? The answers to these and other questions are not known. However, studies of women who have refused mastectomy or who were for health reasons unable to have this surgery, along with the development of effective chemotherapy, have stimulated interest in the possibility that for certain women segmental mastectomy could be an acceptable alternative to the modified radical mastectomy.[58]

A number of doctors have been using the segmental mastectomy, either alone or in combination with chemotherapy or radiation therapy in the past decade. The results, at least in Stage I and sometimes in Stage II, seem to be on par with the modified radical mastectomy; however, their studies have the same sorts of problems we discussed earlier, so there is as yet no real proof that segmental mastectomy is as good as a modified radical.

The indications are strong enough, however, to justify experiments. Thus, a new protocol has been developed by the NSABP, again under the direction of Dr. Bernard Fisher and again with the same careful study design.[59] In order to be eligible, women must have tumors smaller than four cm in size. The nodes may be clinically positive or negative, but they cannot be fixed to the chest wall. There cannot be any ulceration (open sores) or any peau d'orange (skin textured like an orange peel). There can be no signs of distant metastasis. Basically, this means Stages I and II. Also, the cancer cannot be located near the nipple, for tumors in this location are more likely to have metastasized and may have done so even though the chest X-rays and liver and bone scans give negative reports.

521

Just as in the earlier NSABP studies, women who are eligible are randomly assigned to different treatment programs by computer to prevent bias on the part of the doctor giving the treatment. There are three treatment arms: 1. total mastectomy and axillary dissection (in other words, modified radical mastectomy); 2. segmental mastectomy plus axillary dissection; and 3. segmental mastectomy plus axillary dissection plus radiation to the breast. In categories 2. and 3. any women who subsequently develop tumors in the remaining breast tissue will receive a total mastectomy. All women who are found to have positive nodes will receive chemotherapy. The treatment protocol is outlined in Table 19.

Currently, women are still being accepted into this study, so it will be some time before results are available. In the meantime, what are women with Stages I and II breast cancer to do? Well, the women who want to play it safest should have a modified radical mastectomy. We know how that will work. These less extensive therapies will at best give equivalent survival rates. The only point of having one of these less extensive therapies is to preserve the breast, that is, to obtain better cosmetic results. Having a modified eliminates the problem of what will happen to the multicentric areas of breast cancer, for the entire breast is removed.

Table 19
NSABP Protocol B-6

*If microscopic examination of the nodes indicates the presence of cancer, the woman is treated with chemotherapy.

We would encourage all women—those desiring modifieds, those who are undecided and those who are interested in these less extensive therapies—to seek treatment consultation from a doctor participating in a NSABP study. A list of participating doctors and hospitals is included in the appendix. Only by participating in these studies will we ever be able to answer the questions that now exist about breast cancer. While the results may not help those of us who have breast cancer at this time, they will help our sisters and our daughters who may develop it in the future.

Women making the decision between a segmental mastectomy with axillary node dissection and a segmental and node dissection with radiation to the breast should know, if they have positive nodes and will therefore require chemotherapy, that some doctors feel that the radiation therapy will limit the effectiveness of chemotherapy. Others feel that radiation therapy will suffice anyway. Still others feel that radiation therapy will actually cause the development of breast cancers in the future.* Here again, these issues cannot be resolved at the present time.

Radiation Implants

No discussion of Stages I and II cancer would be complete without a discussion of yet another method of treatment known as radiation implants. In this form of therapy, hollow needles are inserted into the tumor area (Illustration 54)[60]. A radioactive substance is loaded into the needles and left in place for a specified amount of time, until the proper dosage of radiation is achieved. This may or may not be done in combination with axillary dissection (although we feel it should).

Proponents of radiation implants claim superior cosmetic results, but radiation therapy can also damage the breast. Whether superior cosmetic results are obtained with radiation or with a segmental mastectomy is highly debatable. Women who are interested in this form of therapy should know that the type of biopsy they receive may preclude it. Women who opt for radiation implants should also be aware of the fact that this type of treatment is only what is called "phase two." In studying and evaluating the efficiency and desirability of any form of treatment, there are three phases. Phase one involves trying the treatment out on people who for medical or personal reasons cannot have the standard form of therapy—in the case of breast cancer, mastectomy. If the results seem promising, a phase-two study is done. In phase two, a number of subjects are given the treatment and the results are compared with the results achieved in the past by giving the standard form of therapy to a comparable group. Phase-

---

*The issue of radiation-induced breast cancer has been discussed earlier under the heading Mammography (p. 499). Radiation therapy involves much, much more exposure to radiation than mammography, but the magnitude of the risk is not known.

Illustration 54 *Radiation Implants: Hollow needles are inserted into the breast in the tumor area. Radioactive material is inserted into the tubes and left in place for a specified amount of time.*

two studies are retrospective studies, which have the limitations described earlier. If these results seem promising, phase-three studies are done. The NSABP studies are examples of phase-three studies—large-scale, randomized, prospective, carefully controlled studies. Perhaps in the future radiation implants will prove to be as valuable as the modified radical or the other types of treatment for Stages I and II now being studied; however, at the present time such treatment must be considered experimental. Many doctors point out that this form of therapy, which does not always offer superior cosmetic results to those obtained with segmental mastectomy, also involves exposure to high amounts of radiation, which can cause cancer as well as cure it.

Carcinoma in Situ

Before discussing the treatment of more advanced cancer, a word or two should be said about the treatment of carcinoma in situ of the breast. Carcinoma in situ, if you will recall, means cancer that has not invaded the surrounding tissue. We have discussed the problems in the pathology diagnosis of this form of cancer elsewhere. Carcinoma in situ is highly controversial: in terms of defining the condition, determining whether or not it even exists and predicting whether it will develop into cancer. It is also not clear how to decide upon the best treatment. With the improvement of mammography, cancer is being detected at earlier and earlier stages and more minimal cancers are being found. It is only in recent years that we have been able to detect cancers in this stage, for they are generally too small to be felt. It has not yet been determined which is the best form of treatment for this type of cancer. As a result, the type of treatment recommended varies widely, from radical mastectomy to modified radical to segmental mastectomy. Many doctors recommend an operation known as a subcutaneous mastectomy, an operation whereby most of the internal breast tissue (about 85 percent) is scooped out but enough skin and tissue is left to accommodate a silicone implant, which may be inserted at the time the subcutaneous mastectomy is done or during a second operation later on.[61]

A woman with in situ cancer of the breast has a difficult choice to make. First of all, as outlined above, she should have multiple pathology opinions before accepting any form of treatment. Like the woman with Stage I and II disease, she could opt to be on the safe side and have a modified radical. Having this operation assures the woman that even if her pathology diagnosis were incorrect, and even if the multicentric areas that are quite possibly present in other areas of her breast were to become full-blown cancers, she would not have a problem, for the breast has been removed.

On the other hand, the fact that lesser surgeries are being done for Stages I and II (NSABP studies outlined in Table 19, for example) certainly suggests that lesser therapies may be appropriate for carcinoma in situ. Both a subcutaneous and a segmental mastectomy are viable alternatives. The subcutaneous removes 85 percent of the breast and if multicentricity turns out to be a problem, this form of treatment has the advantage of having removed more tissue than the segmental. However, there are some doctors who argue that the silicone implants will make it harder to feel recurrences in the small amount of breast tissue that remains, or may create confusing shadows on mammography.

The NSABP trials discussed above will shed some light on the behavior of the multicentric areas of cancer in the breast that may have implications for the treatment of carcinoma in situ as well. Until that time, there is not much information on which to base treatment decisions.

Prophylactic Subcutaneous Mastectomy

It should also be noted that a prophylactic (preventive) subcutaneous mastectomy may be recommended for women who don't actually have breast cancer but who are at high risk for developing it. When we first heard about this practice, we were, quite frankly, horrified at the idea of removing perfectly normal tissue just to prevent the possible development of breast cancer. While we're all for preventive medicine, this seemed, to say the least, a bit radical. Since that time, we have changed our thinking somewhat. We realized that the average woman has about a one in 14 chance of developing breast cancer. As explained under the heading Risk Factors, for a woman who has a mother or sister with the disease, the chances are increased two- to three-fold, and perhaps even more if her mother developed breast cancer before menopause. Moreover, women with certain types of benign breast disease are at greater risk as well. Reports of a four-fold and even higher increase in risk have been noted. Unfortunately, we have not yet been able to define risk factors precisely enough to say exactly how much having a combination of factors will affect a woman's chances of developing the disease, but women with a family history of breast cancer and a history of benign breast disease may have a better than 50-50 chance of getting the disease. Certainly, a high-risk woman who has undergone the trauma of repeated breast biopsies for suspicious lumps might want to consider the possibility of having a subcutaneous mastectomy. At this time, however, the value of this procedure is highly debatable. Although 85-90 percent of the breast tissue is removed, the 10-15 percent of tissue that remains is still at high risk. Some doctors also feel that the implants make it difficult to detect cancer in the remaining tissue. Women interested in this procedure should have multiple opinions from experts at cancer-care centers.

Stages III and IV

Anyone who has read this far will not be surprised to discover that the treatment of advanced breast cancer is also controversial. Radical and modified radical mastectomies, radiation and even less extensive therapies may be used. In certain Stage IV cancers, many doctors feel that the mastectomy is useless and that simply removing the lump and using some form of adjuvant therapy will suffice.[62] In Stage III, there are some cases in which the particulars of a woman's case will dictate the form of treatment. Radiation therapy is sometimes used. Chemotherapy is always used in these advanced cases. Hormone therapy and immunotherapy may also be used (see below). Because there is so much controversy and so many unanswered questions about the proper method of treatment in these cases and because opinions are needed from surgeons, radiologists, chemotherapists and experts in immunology, we feel that it is especially important for women with advanced disease to have the benefit of consultation by a team of experts, which is best obtained at a cancer-care facility or approved cancer hospital (see appendix).

Chemotherapy

Chemotherapy, the treatment of cancer by the use of drugs, has been one of the most promising developments in recent years. In the past chemotherapy was only given to women whose pretreatment diagnostic tests to detect metastasis showed that the cancer had already spread beyond the breast or who suffered a recurrence following the original treatment. While the drugs were effective in relieving pain and shrinking tumors, they could not totally eradicate the cancer.

As a result of studies on laboratory animals, it became evident that the smaller the tumor, the better the chances that the chemotherapy will be able to eliminate it. If, then, women could be given the chemotherapy before the metastatic cancer was large enough to be detected, it was thought that the chances of the chemotherapy's being effective were much greater.

We know that in about 80 percent of the women diagnosed as having breast cancer, the disease has already spread beyond the breast; however, in 20 percent the disease has not spread. These 20 percent will not need chemotherapy. If it weren't for the fact that chemotherapy can have serious side effects, including the development of other forms of cancer in future years, it might make sense to give all women with breast cancer chemotherapy. As yet, however, there is no "safe" form of chemotherapy. We can't always tell for sure which women have disease confined to the breast and which have systemic disease.

Most women whose lymph nodes are examined microscopically and found to contain cancer will have a recurrence of the disease within ten years,[63] so chemotherapy is considered appropriate for these women. If microscopic examination of the lymph nodes is negative, chemotherapy is not usually given, for the risks are thought to outweigh the benefits. Chemotherapists have a general rule of thumb: Unless the woman has less than a 50 percent chance of survival, chemotherapy risks are thought to outweigh the benefits, so it is not given. Women with the minimal or early cancers discussed above have a 90 percent survival rate, so most chemotherapists feel that chemotherapy should not be given to these women.[64] Women with Stages I and II disease and nodes judged negative on the basis of microscopic examination have about a 65 percent survival rate,[65] so chemotherapy is generally not given to these women. This may, however, change in the future. Some doctors are advocating using a single drug in the treatment of women with Stages I and II even if they have negative nodes. Although single-drug therapy has been shown to be less

527

effective than combinations of drugs in the treatment of more advanced disease, it is also less dangerous. So, in the future, studies to evaluate the effectiveness of single-drug chemotherapy in Stages I and II disease may be done.

If a woman has advanced disease, recurrent cancer or positive nodes, chemotherapy is given. In the past, a single agent was used, but NSABP studies have shown that combinations of two drugs can give superior results.[66] NSABP studies are now being done comparing two-drug combinations with three-drug combinations.[67] Women in this protocol are given either a combination of L-Phenylalanine (L-Pam) and 5-Fluorouracil (5-FU) or L-Pam, 5-FU, and methotrexate (MTX). Enthusiasm for a three-drug combination was originally generated by results from a study sponsored by the National Cancer Institute and conducted by Dr. G. Bonnadonna in Milan, Italy, in which a three-drug combination known as CMF was used.[68] The initial results were positive not only for premenopausal women but also for postmenopausal women, who have, in the past, not done as well on chemotherapy. The NSABP studies comparing two-drug and three-drug therapy have not shown any benefit from the addition of the third drug, but it is too early to clearly evaluate these studies.

Chemotherapy in combination with hormone therapy and immunotherapy is also being studied by the NSABP. These experiments are described below.[69] Again, we urge women who need chemotherapy to consult with one of the doctors participating in these NSABP studies. The only way we will ever answer these important questions is if women participate in carefully designed studies like those being done by the NSABP. Women who have had radicals and modified radicals and positive nodes are eligible, regardless of whether their original surgery was done by an NSABP doctor. Being part of an NSABP protocol also assures the woman that she is getting treatment from a doctor who is knowledgeable and up-to-date on the most recent developments in the field of chemotherapy.

Radiation Therapy

We have already discussed the ongoing NSABP protocol in which segmental mastectomy is followed by irradiation designed to destroy any residual cancer in the remaining breast tissue. We have also discussed the experimental use of radium implants and the use of radiation to the axillary area following a simple, or total, mastectomy. As explained above, this last form of therapy has fallen out of favor as a result of NSABP trials and the advent of chemotherapy.

Another use of radiation in the treatment of breast cancer that has fallen out of favor is the so-called prophylactic, or preventive radiation to the armpit following radical or modified radical mastectomy for Stages I and II disease. At one time radiation was given in these cases to "dry up" any remaining cancer cells. However, carefully controlled studies have failed to show any benefit.[70] In fact, prophylactic radiation may even be harmful, in that the remaining healthy tissue can be damaged by radiation. Then, too, there is the danger of the development of radiation-induced cancer in ten or twenty years.* Moreover, radiation therapy may hinder the effectiveness of chemotherapy. Today most, if not all, experts are opposed to radiation to the axillary area following modified or radical mastectomy or any form of therapy that involves removal of the lymph nodes. Unfortunately, the word has not yet percolated down through the ranks, and there are still some doctors who use radiation in Stages I and II disease following axillary dissection. Women who are Stage I or II whose doctors recommend axillary radiation should seek a second opinion (*see* p. 226).

Some Stage III cases may require radiation. In Stage IV cases where the cancer has spread to the bone, some doctors use radiation therapy to treat these areas of bony metastasis; however, many doctors feel that by the time the disease has gotten to the point where metastasis can be detected in the bone, there is no point in radiation, for the disease has already spread throughout the system.[71] Radiation, like surgery, is only a local form of therapy. Only chemotherapy can hope to control the disease once it has involved the whole system.

Since radiation may inhibit the effectiveness of chemotherapy, these doctors prefer to go right to chemotherapy without wasting time on radiation. Many of these doctors will, however, use radiation if the cancer is in a weight-bearing bone like the leg since the cancer could weaken the bone and cause it to break. At the present time this question as to whether small areas of bony metastasis should be treated by chemotherapy or radiation has not been answered.

A similar question comes up with regard to cancers that occur near the middle of the chest.[72] This area is drained by a group of lymph nodes known as the internal mammary chain, which runs along the breast bones under the ribs. Some doctors favor radiation to destroy these nodes, but there is no way of telling whether or not they are involved, so the use of radiation in these cases is controversial. Others favor chemotherapy because they feel that by the time the internal mammary chain nodes are involved, the disease, in all likelihood, has spread throughout the body and chemotherapy should be done.

Radiation is also used in advanced disease for palliation, or relief of symptoms. If, for instance, the cancer has metastasized to the brain or the bones, radiation may be given to shrink the tumor and provide relief.

*Radiation risks are discussed under the heading Mammography.

Hormone Therapy

It has long been known that some breast cancer tumors are sensitive to hormones. At one time, it was standard practice to remove the ovaries of all women who had breast cancer; however, the results of this type of therapy were rather unpredictable.[73] Some women seemed to benefit; others did not. Today we have the hormone assay receptor tests described above to help us predict whether or not a woman will respond to hormone therapy.

Hormone therapy has not provided cures, but it has offered temporary relief of symptoms and slowed the growth of some cancers for a time. It is generally only used to treat recurrent cancer and advanced disease; however, experiments are now being done that combine hormone therapy with chemotherapy.

In addition to hormone therapy in the form of drugs to suppress hormone production, there are also surgical hormone therapies. The ovaries of a woman with recurrent cancer may be removed, a procedure known as oophorectomy, or the ovaries may be destroyed by radiation. This is generally only done for premenopausal women.

Two other forms of surgery designed to curtail hormone production are sometimes done. The adrenal glands, two small glands located near the kidneys that produce essential hormones, including cortisone (which helps the body metabolize sugar), and are apparently able to produce some estrogen as well, may be removed. This operation, known as an adrenalectomy, may be done following oophorectomy in premenopausal women with recurrent cancer. It may also be done in postmenopausal women whose tumors are thought to be estrogen-sensitive, in an effort to remove a potential source of estrogen. The operation is a difficult one, however. Today, cortisone and other drugs can be used to suppress the action of the adrenal glands. Although adrenalectomies are still done in some cases, drug therapy has pretty much replaced adrenalectomy.

Another surgical procedure used in the treatment of recurrent breast cancer is hypophysectomy, which involves removal of the anterior pituitary gland in the brain. The pituitary produces hormones that in turn stimulate the ovaries and the adrenal glands. By removing the anterior pituitary, the functioning of the ovaries and adrenals falls to a low level, almost as low as if the woman had had an oophorectomy and adrenalectomy. In addition, destruction of the pituitary effectively stops the production of growth hormone and of prolactin (the hormone responsible for milk production), both of which have been implicated in the stimulation of breast tumors. However, this operation requires major brain surgery and some risk. Even though the pituitary can now be destroyed by radiation instead of surgery, the procedure is not often done, for it is now known that estrogen can be produced in fatty tissues of the body, so even this extensive a procedure may not succeed in removing all the estrogen from a woman's body.

In the treatment of recurrent cancer, in addition to surgery, radiation or drugs used to destroy or suppress the body's production of hormones, sometimes large doses of hormones are given. For example, some women respond well to massive doses of estrogen. It seems that a change in the hormone climate of the woman's body—oophorectomy if she is premenopausal or, in certain cases, large doses of hormones if she is postmenopausal—will sometimes be helpful in relieving symptoms or slowing the growth of the tumor. Eventually, though, the tumor will return. Recently, experiments combining hormone and chemotherapy have begun and it is hoped that this combination will prove useful to postmenopausal women who have not responded as well to chemotherapy as premenopausal women.

Immunotherapy

Immunotherapy, which makes use of drugs that bolster the body's immune system, is also being used experimentally in the treatment of breast cancer. NSABP studies are evaluating the effectiveness of immunological agents in combination with chemotherapy. However, it may be some time bfore the results of these trials are available.

Breast Reconstruction[74]

Breast reconstruction is a procedure made possible by some of the same techniques plastic surgeons first devised for cosmetic reshaping of the breast. In the past, less than 1 percent of all women who had mastectomies had breast reconstruction. The techniques have improved greatly, however, and since many insurance companies now provide partial or total coverage for the procedure, more and more women are choosing to have it done.

The procedure and the outcome vary considerably. Sometimes the reconstruction can be done at the time of surgery. Most of the time, however, a waiting period of at least three months is necessary. Reconstruction may also be done many years after surgery. In fact, successful reconstructions have been done as long as 20 years after mastectomy.

The reconstruction may require more than one operation, especially if the woman had a radical mastectomy, which leaves a hollow in the chest wall. Tissue from other parts of the body may be transplanted to fill in the hollow. More than one operation is sometimes needed if the nipple is also reconstructed. A new nipple can sometimes be constructed using tissue from the vulvar lips or other areas of the body. Depending on the size of the other breast and the amount of muscle and skin remaining after mastectomy, it may be necessary to reduce the size of the other breast to restore symmetry. Sometimes this procedure, known as reductive mammoplasty, can be done at the same time as the reconstruction; at other times, a separate operation must be done.

Basically, reconstruction involves inserting a plastic bag of silicone gel under the skin or muscle. The silicone gel implant, unlike silicone injections, which are now banned in most states, is not thought to be harmful to the body in any way. Some doctors do worry that the presence of the silicone implant might make it difficult to feel recurrent cancer on the chest wall under the implant or might create confusing shadows on a mammogram.

The results of reconstruction vary considerably. In some cases a very satisfactory result is obtained, but in others the results are disappointing. Women should not expect the breast to look the same as it did prior to mastectomy. The reconstructed breast is intended to look good under a bra, but in the nude, its appearance may be marred by scarring and other imperfections. The woman's doctor should be able to give her an idea of how the reconstructed breast will look. Most good doctors will have "before and after" photos of other women. Women may wish to ask the surgeon if it's possible to talk with some of his or her previous patients, if any have given the doctor permission to offer their names to prospective patients. There is also an organization, AFTER (Ask a Friend to Explain Reconstruction), 99 Park Avenue, New York, New York 10016, that puts women in touch with other women who've had reconstructive surgery. The organization also publishes a pamphlet on the subject.

Reconstruction is a fairly new technique, so it is important to find a doctor who is skilled and experienced in this procedure. Ideally, the doctor should be a board-certified plastic surgeon who is experienced in performing the operation. A woman should shop around before making a decision, asking how many operations the doctor has done, talking with former patients and viewing before and after shots. The surgeon who is doing the mastectomy may be able to provide referrals. Cancer hot lines or medical-school—related hospitals may also provide names. Women can also contact the American Society of Plastic and Reconstructive Surgeons, 29 East Madison Street, Suite 807, Chicago, Illinois 60602, for a list of surgeons in their area. The Society also publishes an informative pamphlet on the subject. If possible, the plastic surgeon should consult with the doctor performing the cancer surgery prior to operation. Although the cancer operation should never be compromised for the sake of better reconstruction, sometimes it is possible to perform the cancer operation in such a way that the plastic surgeon's job will be easier.

Not all women can have breast reconstruction. Sometimes the skin is too tight to allow for a successful reconstruction. If radiation therapy has been used, the remaining tissue may be too badly damaged to allow for reconstruction. Many doctors discourage reconstruction in cases where the cancer has recurred or metastasized. Women on chemotherapy may have to wait until the chemotherapy is discontinued, for the drugs may suppress the white blood cell count, making surgery inadvisable.

Breast reconstruction can be very costly, especially if more than one operation is required. While a number of insurance companies now cover these costs, some do not, so it is important to discuss finances prior to surgery.

Breast reconstruction, like any form of surgery, carries risks. There may be bleeding, infection and extensive scar formation. Occasionally, the blood supply of the skin may be inadequate and there may be partial skin loss. The implant may be rejected by the body. There may be distortion in shape or hardening of the areas around the implant, or the implant may fall. In these instances further surgery may be needed. However, many women have been very pleased with reconstruction results, and the possibility of reconstruction should be considered.

Breast Prosthesis

Women who have had mastectomies are usually fitted for artificial breasts, called prostheses. This is done both for appearance and for medical reasons. The prosthesis will counterbalance the weight of the remaining breast, eliminating back strain, which can be caused by uneven weight distribution. The American Cancer Society sponsors a program, Reach to Recovery, run by volunteers who have had mastectomies themselves. These women can provide important information on fitting prostheses and can also offer invaluable assistance to women who've had mastectomies. Your doctor can put you in touch with this group.

Survival Rates

Survival rates for most forms of cancer are given in terms of five years because most of those who are alive at five years will be disease-free at ten years. With breast cancer, five-year survival rates do not mean as much, for a significant number of women will have recurrences ten or even twenty years later. Table 20 lists survival rates according to both stage and nodal involvement.

Table 20
Survival Rates for Breast Cancer by Stage

Stage	Five-Year Survival Rate (%) by Stage
I	82−94
II	47−74
III	7−8
IV	−

Survival Rates for Breast Cancer by Nodal Status

Condition of Nodes	Five-Year Survival Rates (%)	Ten-Year Survival Rates (%)
Negative axillary lymph nodes	78.1	64.9
Positive axillary lymph nodes	46.5	24.9
1−3 positive nodes	62.2	37.5
More than 4 positive nodes	32.0	13.4

SOURCE: Adapted from Craig Henderson, M.D., and George P. Canellos, M.D., "Cancer of the Breast: The Past Decade," *New England Journal of Medicine*, 302:1 (Jan. 3, 1980), pp. 17−30.

Follow-Up

Women with breast cancer will need careful follow-up for the rest of their lives. Follow-up has three objectives:

1. The detection of metastasis
2. The detection of a possible second cancer in the opposite breast or in the remaining breast tissue if a segmental mastectomy has been done
3. The detection of other forms of cancer.

Metastasis usually occurs first in the lungs and soft tissues such as the liver. Metastasis frequently occurs in the bones. Women who have had breast cancer are at higher risk for other forms of cancer, especially endometrial and ovarian cancer. Follow-up will then pay special attention to the remaining breast, the soft tissues, the skeletal system and the uterus and ovaries.

Many women we have spoken with in the course of writing this book have received less than adequate follow-up. Table 21 outlines a widely recommended follow-up program. The tests listed in this table are those

Table 21
Follow-Up Program for Breast Cancer Patients

I   Monthly breast self-exam

II   First Year:
- Complete physical exam at three-month intervals, with special attention to inspection and palpation of mastectomy area, remaining breast and lymph nodes and abdomen, liver, chest, pelvic and rectal areas, oral cavity, skin, chest and bones
- CBC blood exam at six-month intervals
- SMA12 blood chemistry at six-month intervals
- X-ray of chest at six-month intervals
- Mammogram once a year
- Liver, bone and brain scans as indicated

III   Second Year:
- All tests and examinations listed above should be performed twice a year, except for mammography, which should be done once a year

IV   Third and Subsequent Years:
- All tests and examinations listed above should be performed on an annual basis

recommended routinely in the absence of symptoms or signs. If symptoms appear, further tests will be needed. Significant symptoms include: bone or chest pain, persistent cough, appetite or weight loss, weakness, headaches, falls, seizures and changes in behavior or psychological changes.

Sexually Transmitted Diseases

Imagine what would happen if we were having an epidemic of a group of diseases that were transmitted by shaking hands, diseases that could, if not treated in time, lead to serious complications, including birth defects, infertility, arthritis, blindness, heart failure, mental retardation, insanity and even death. To complicate matters further, suppose that some people didn't have symptoms in the early stages of these diseases and therefore didn't have any way of knowing they had been infected unless the person who had infected them passed the word on. Not only that, but what if the diseases were so widespread that only colds were more common. Indeed, what if every 15 seconds another person came down with one of them. Suppose that just caring for the psychiatric and blinded victims cost taxpayers 50 million dollars each year.

Well, for starters, a lot of people would wear gloves. Health officials would be passing out free pairs at clinics across the country. A massive education program would be launched to educate people about these diseases. The signs and symptoms of the diseases and how to recognize and prevent them would be the most important items in the curriculum of public school health classes. Conscientious doctors would report each case to the state health department, and social workers would diligently track down the infected person's contacts, warning them of the dangers and helping to stop the spread of the diseases. The government would pour vast sums of money into medical research projects in an effort to develop a vaccine. In a few short years, immunizations would be available, and the "shaking hands" disease would join the ranks of smallpox, polio, diphtheria, whooping cough and other conquered diseases.

You can stop imagining now, for as it turns out, we do have an epidemic of a group of diseases that can have the serious complications outlined above. But there aren't any massive education programs. The topic is ignored in most public schools. Doctors, despite legal requirements, aren't reporting the cases they treat to state health officials. Infectors aren't passing the word along to infectees. Methods of prevention are a well-kept secret. A mere pittance is spent on research; there is no vaccine.

Why not? Because you don't get these diseases by shaking hands, you get them by having sex with an infected person. They're called venereal disease (VD), or, if you prefer (as we do) the more direct term, sexually transmitted diseases (STD).

Because these diseases are transmitted sexually, the whole issue has been clouded by fear, guilt, moralizing and sexual hypocrisy. Since early childhood most of us have been taught to think of our genital organs as something unclean and of sex as something to be ashamed of, something "nice girls" don't do—don't even like to do. Getting VD, like getting pregnant, is an obvious indication that you've been "doin' it." Since most of us have at least some difficulty in talking about sex and in confronting our sexuality, dealing with veneral disease, with all its sleazy connotations, is especially difficult. On both a personal and social level, we've tended to ignore the VD problem, shoving it back into some dark, guilty corner, hoping it will go away.

But, it won't go away. Indeed, VD is on the rise. In 1978, there were an estimated 468.3 cases of gonorrhea per 100,000 people, a rise from 466.8 per 100,000 in 1977.[1] Incidence rates for syphilis have risen too, and it's anybody's guess how many cases of herpes there are, since it is not a disease that must be reported, but clinics and private doctors are now seeing it more frequently than gonorrhea.

Apparently, "nice girls" *do* like to do it; either that or else there are an awful lot of "not-nice" girls around. A popular bit of folklore holds that nice people, meaning of course upper- and middle-class people, don't get VD, that it's a disease of the poor and of prostitutes. Not true. The disease occurs in the suburbs as well as the ghettos. The organisms that cause these diseases don't make moral judgments, aren't social snobs and make no distinctions as to race, color or creed. They'll attack anybody. Unfortunately, many in the medical profession don't seem to know this, so a lot of people who need testing don't get it because their doctors have decided that they are "nice, middle-class people" who don't get such diseases. Conversely, many poor people can't get any kind of medical treatment without first being tested for VD.

Although most of these diseases are readily cured in their early stages, they can have serious, even fatal, complications. Although the symptoms may disappear, sometimes for years, most of these diseases don't go away by themselves. It is often possible to infect someone else even when you don't have symptoms.

Prevention

There are ways of protecting yourself—and your partners—against STDs, although these methods aren't receiving the public attention they deserve. Perhaps this stems from the old sex-is-bad-and-VD-is-a-punishment-for-your-sins school of thought. Moreover, these methods are not 100 percent effective, so many public information services, including some VD hotlines, don't tell people about them. They fear that people will think that these methods offer absolute protection and will therefore go ahead and have sex, even though they know they (or their partner) have one of these diseases. We don't think people are that dumb, however, and believe that it's important for people to know about any possible forms of protection. Even if these protective measures were only 25 percent effective, they'd make a big dent in the current epidemic.

At any rate, we'll say it again: There are ways of protecting yourself and your partners, but these methods don't offer 100 percent protection. If you know for sure that you—or someone else—has the disease, you'd be a fool to rely on one of these protective devices and go ahead and have sex.

One of the best ways to protect yourself is to have your partners use condoms. Condoms, also called rubbers, have been shown to cut down on your chances of getting most sexually transmitted diseases.[2] Widespread promotion and use of condoms in Sweden has cut the rate of sexually transmitted diseases dramatically.[3] Condoms may not be as effective in preventing viral diseases like herpes, however, because viruses are smaller than bacteria and can more easily penetrate the rubber. The condoms also don't protect your outer genitals. Still, they do afford some protection against herpes.

Certain foaming spermicides and various creams and jellies used with diaphragms, such as Delfen Foam, Emko Foam, Ortho-Cream, Perceptin Gel, Ortho-Gynol Jelly and Koromex A-II Vaginal Jelly, have been shown in laboratory studies to be effective against some of the organisms that cause sexually transmitted diseases.[4] Whether or not they will be as effective in actual use has not yet been determined.*

*We do not recommend these jellies and creams for birth control unless they are used with a diaphragm. Using a condom along with one of the foams will offer both better protection against STDs *and* better birth control.

You should also know that if you use the birth control pill, you are much more susceptible to certain STDs. This is because the Pill alters the acid/alkaline balance, or pH level, of your vagina, making it more conducive to the growth of some of the organisms that cause STDs. For instance, if you have sex with someone who has gonorrhea, you normally have about 40-50 percent chance of catching it, but if you're on the Pill, you have nearly a 100 percent chance.[5]

Urinating and washing the genitals with soap and water before and after sex will help, for the urine will help flush out germs and soap and water will kill some of them; however, although these sorts of precautions are of value, they are not highly reliable.

Another way of protecting yourself is to inspect your partner's sex organs for signs and symptoms of disease before having sex, which may require a bit of finesse. Look for sores, reddened areas and/or warts on the penis, scrotum (balls), anus and buttocks. If the man is not circumcised, pull back the foreskin, the flap of skin that covers the tip of the penis, and check there. Obviously, if your sex partner has any sores or symptoms, you should not have sex with him or her, and since some people can have the disease without obvious symptoms, you should use a condom and spermicide in heterosexual sex unless you have good reason to believe your partner is not infected.

Now, all of this doesn't sound terribly romantic. If you don't feel comfortable saying, "Hey, I want to check you for VD before we have sex," you can be a bit more subtle about it. Incorporate a quick check into your foreplay (men like foreplay too, you know). This is very important for those of us who have sex with a number of different partners, especially if the partners are not people we know well whom we could count on to contact us if they were to discover later that they had one of these diseases.

In the case of herpes, you'd be wise to ask your partners specifically if they have a history of herpes. You can figure out a way to bring it up in conversation if you don't want to ask point-blank. Many people don't realize that they can pass herpes on to others even though they don't have active symptoms.[6] This disease can be particularly devastating, for there is no cure, and having herpes may increase your chances of getting cervical cancer. Those planning to have children in the future should know that it has been implicated in birth defects, miscarriages and premature labor.[7]

Getting Treatment

It's important to learn the signs and symptoms of these diseases and not to ignore them if they do develop. In some of these diseases, the early signs and symptoms may go away but the disease is still in your body. It is important, too, that you familiarize yourself with the tests available since some tests are not reliable for women or won't detect the disease until it has been in your body for a certain amount of time. If you are sexually active and have more than one sex partner (or if your sex partner does), you should have regular tests every three to six months. For lesbians who have sex only with other lesbians (not bisexuals), this precaution may not apply, as they rarely get syphilis or gonorrhea. If you are married or fall into the class that some doctors vaguely define as "nice" people, you may have to insist that your doctor do the test. The doctor may pooh-pooh the idea, saying something like, "Oh, you couldn't possibly...," but you should insist upon the test or seek treatment elsewhere. If you have oral or anal sex, you may specifically have to ask your doctor to take cultures from these areas.

If you think you have an STD or have had sexual contact with someone who has, you should get medical help right away. Do not take any medications or douche before being tested, as this could lead to false negative test results. "Waiting to see" if you develop symptoms is dangerous. Eighty percent of the women who get gonorrhea and 90 percent who get syphilis have no early symptoms. The diseases are readily cured in their early stages, but waiting could lead to serious complications.

Getting treatment for STDs is not always easy. First of all, a disease—any disease—is not a pleasant thing. If we feel uncomfortable with our sexuality and with talking about sexuality, asking for tests and treatment for STDs may not be easy. To make matters worse, many doctors have a very moralistic or judgmental attitude about sexuality and about STDs. Finding a doctor or clinic that can provide, at a price you can afford, good medical care, accurate information and nonjudgmental support isn't always easy, but it can be done.

One place to try might be a community "free clinic." These may be listed in the telephone book, or the information operator may be able to help you find the number. Local hotlines, help hotlines, rape hotlines, gay counseling centers, crisis intervention hotlines and so forth may be able to refer you to a free clinic or to a VD hotline, which in turn can refer you for testing and treatment. There is a national VD hotline that can answer questions and help you find treatment. You don't have to give your name to get information, and the numbers are toll-free. In California, call 800-982-5883; in the rest of the country, call 800-227-8922. Most state or county public health departments have a VD control or infectious disease section. They may be able to provide answers to the questions you have. They can usually refer you to a clinic, where you can at least get adequate testing and treatment at little or no cost. In some areas, Planned Parenthood clinics which provide birth control counseling, also provide testing and/or treatment for sexually transmitted diseases or can refer you if they do not. They usually have sensitive, supportive, nonjudgmental staffs. If you prefer to be tested and treated by a private doctor, see Finding a Doctor in Chapter Six.

Minors

In most states, minors can be treated confidentially. In California, for instance, the law says that doctors can treat anyone over the age of 12 for venereal disease without a parent's consent. Puerto Rico and Wisconsin don't yet have such laws, but hopefully they will in the future. However, the specific age used to define a minor may vary from state to state, and the laws simply say the doctor doesn't have to notify the parents, not that they *can't* notify the parents. So if you are a minor and don't want your parents to know, you can do one of two things. First, once you have a list of community free clinics or county health department clinics, call and ask what their policy regarding minors is. Second, remember that you don't have to give your parents' address or telephone number in order to get treatment.

Reporting

The law requires that a doctor treating you for syphilis or gonorrhea report your name to the state health department. This is done so that a special public health investigator can contact you and ask for your help in contacting the people you may have gotten the disease from or who may have given it to you. You are not required by law to provide any names. However, reporting the disease is important. Consider, for instance, a group of 10 people, each of whom has gonorrhea. If they each give it to one other person, that's a total of 20 people, and if each of the 10 newly infected people in turn pass it on to one other person, then that's a total of 30 people, then 40, then 50 and so on. If that first group of 10 people were all reported and their 10 contacts tracked down, then the next 10, 20, 30, 40 people wouldn't have gotten the disease.

Despite the law, not all doctors report the names of the people they treat for gonorrhea and syphilis. The failure of physicians to report these diseases has contributed to our inability to control VD. If you are being treated by a doctor who does not report your name, s/he is, in a sense, responsible for your having the disease, for if physicians were conscientious about this, others who have the disease would thus also get treatment and we wouldn't have an epidemic. You might want to point this out to your doctor.

The reporting of the diseases to the state health department may cause special problems for some people. If you have had sexual contact with a person who is a minor living with parents or with someone who is married or living with another sexual partner, this can be a bit sticky. You might then want to assume the burden of informing your sex partner yourself, in the most discreet way possible. You can't count on the public health investigator's discretion, which varies considerably from state to state and even from case to case. In the very best of circumstances, investigators will try to visit the person. They are usually quite discreet about this. The information you give them will help them to be discreet, and they aren't beyond telling white lies. In the case of a minor, for instance, the contact might be made through the school nurse, or a female investigator might call the home, saying that the school nurse needs to do "a routine eye test" or "bring the immunization records" up to date. Not all investigators are so discreet, and in the wake of cut-back state budgets, there simply aren't funds available for this sort of fancy footwork. As a result, in some cases a postcard (which, of course, anyone can read) telling the person to contact the public health service may be sent to the home of your sexual contact. You have a right to know exactly what kind of notification will be made and to meet the person making the contact before you provide names. But remember that we are dealing with diseases that can, for you, your contacts or someone else down the line, have serious and even fatal complications.

Herpes is not a disease that must be reported, although there are efforts being made to change this. It is especially important that anyone with herpes inform everyone they sleep with, for there is no cure for herpes. Once you have it, you always have it, and some authorities consider it the most serious of all the venereal diseases.

In the following pages, the most common STDs—gonorrhea, herpes, crabs, syphilis and venereal warts are discussed along with the less common chancroid, granuloma inguinale, and lymphogranuloma venereum. A special heading, Other Sexually Transmitted Diseases, includes information on diseases that may be transmitted sexually but are frequently transmitted in other ways, and on a certain group of little-understood diseases that are suspected of being sexually transmitted. Other diseases such as trich, yeast infections, hemophilus and nonspecific vaginitis that can be transmitted sexually are discussed in detail under the section of the vagina. In addition, there is a growing body of evidence suggesting that invasive cervical cancer and the early forms of cervical cancer, such as carcinoma in situ and dysplasia, may also be caused by a sexually transmitted agent. This topic is discussed in more detail under the heading Cervical Cancer.

GONORRHEA

AKA: dose, clap

Gonorrhea is an extremely widespread disease, which, if untreated, may have serious consequences. Information on how to prevent this disease and where to seek treatment, which may be of particular interest to minors, is discussed in the general introduction to this section (above).

Incidence

Gonorrhea has the dubious distinction of having the highest incidence rate of any venereal disease in this country.[8] It is epidemic, and, if not treated properly, can be a serious disease.

Cause and Transmission

The disease is caused by a very delicate, very discriminating germ, the *Neisseria gonorrhoeae,* or gonococcus, which can live only in the mucous membranes of the human body where there is both warmth and moisture—places such as the inside of the cheek, the throat, the genital organs, the rectum, the urethra and, occasionally, the eye. Air, sunlight, soap, water and a variation of only 3° in temperature supposedly destroy the gonococcus. Thus, it is virtually impossible to get it other than through vaginal, oral-genital or anal sex with an infected person, the only exceptions being babies, who may get it from their mothers and young girls, who may receive it via the hands of an adult and then unknowingly, transfer it to their vulvar tissues. Gonorrheal eye infections can also be spread as a result of hands touching an infected area and then rubbing the eyes.

Gonorrhea is usually transmitted by sexual contact when the mucous membranes of two people are in contact. A man need not ejaculate in order to infect a partner. Not every contact with an infected sex partner results in the other person's contracting the disease. Women, who are more likely to get it, have about a 50 percent chance of contracting it from one infected contact, unless they use birth control pills, in which case they have nearly a 100 percent likelihood of getting it. Men run about a 20-40 percent chance.

Symptoms and Complications

Part of the problem with gonorrhea is that somewhere between 70 and 80 percent of the women who have the disease are asymptomatic. Some

543

women don't have any noticeable symptoms or signs until weeks or even months after first contracting the disease. Men generally have obvious enough symptoms so that the majority seek treatment within one to two weeks. Only about 10 percent of the males with gonorrhea are thought to be asymptomatic.

In women the disease most commonly affects the cervix, the urinary opening, the Skene's duct, the Bartholin's gland and the anus. The gonococci enter through minute cracks in the skin in these areas. Since the openings to the vagina, urinary tracts, ducts and rectum are so close together, menstrual blood, vaginal discharges, sanitary napkins and/or careless wiping may spread the infection to one or more of these openings. Anal or oral-genital sex may spread the infection to the rectum or throat.

In women, the first signs, if there are any, appear within three to eleven (usually three to five) days after infection. The chief early symptoms, which may be so slight as to be unnoticeable, are pain or burning on urination, urinary frequency and an increase in vaginal discharge.

On speculum exam, the cervix may appear red and swollen. The vagina is not usually the seat of gonorrheal infection, although in young children, pregnant women and older women the vagina itself is sometimes infected. The tissues of the normal adult vagina seem to provide protection against the penetrating power of the gonococci. In the young, the old and in pregnant women, however, this normal tissue either has not yet developed or has changed with age or with shifting hormone levels and does not afford the same protection. If the vaginal canal does appear to be red and swollen, this most often is because the cervix is infected and the vagina is subsequently irritated. In those cases where the vagina itself is actually infected, there may be a good deal of pain, and pus may cover literally every crevice of the vaginal walls.

The vulva, which is subject to discharges from all these openings, may become red and swollen. The lips may become so swollen that they fuse together and voiding may become painful. Occasionally, the vulva is so irritated that genital warts caused by a symbiotic virus appear. If the rectum is involved, there may be painful and bloody stools and a mucus discharge from the anus. If the Skene's and Bartholin's glands are infected, it may be possible to milk pus from the opening of the glands and they may become quite swollen (see Skeneitis and Bartholinitis).

Although any of the symptoms described here may appear in women in the early stages of the disease, most of the time they are not present or are so slight that they go unnoticed.

Unlike women, most men have obvious early symptoms that are usually recognized and treated early, so that the more serious complications and the chronic form of the disease do not affect them as often.

If the gonorrhea is not recognized and treated in its early stages, it can spread upward beyond the cervix and infect the uterus and tubes. This is known as pelvic inflammatory disease (PID). Gonorrhea is more likely to progress to PID in women who use birth control pills.

The gonoccocci may even spill out through the tubes into the pelvic cavity. Symptoms like pain on one or both sides of the lower abdomen, vomiting, fever and irregularities in the menstrual period may occur. The time interval from the initial contact until the appearance of symptoms of pelvic infection is quite variable and unpredictable. It may take months or years. Most of the time, however, the upward spread of the gonococci takes place during the first menstrual period after infection, because the cervix opens up at this time and because the menstrual debris is a rich environment on which gonococci feed and thrive. When the disease does spread above the cervix, serious complications may result. If the Fallopian tubes are infected, they may become permanently blocked. In some cases a hysterectomy may be necessary, and the disease may even be fatal. Even if the disease can be treated with drugs, the damage done may be permanent, and infertility and chronic pelvic pain are not uncommon. The symptoms and complications of gonorrhea that has spread beyond the cervix are discussed in more detail under the heading Pelvic Inflammatory Disease.

In addition to PID, gonorrhea may have other serious complications. The organisms may get into the bloodstream and septicemia, or blood poisoning, may develop. The gonococci circulating in the blood can attack any organ in the body. Gonorrheal arthritis can occur if the circulating gonococci settle in the joints—the wrist, knees, knuckles or other joints—causing them to fill with pus. The surrounding tissue becomes inflamed and swollen. The elastic cartilage tissue of the joints may be destroyed, causing the adjacent bones to atrophy. The joints may stiffen permanently. The symptoms vary; sometimes there is excruciating pain and marked swelling of the joints, and at other times, there are intermittent attacks that recur over time. Carditis, an inflammation of the lining of the heart, and meningitis, an inflammation that causes destruction of the membrane covering the brain and spinal cord, may also be associated with gonorrhea. With the use of modern antibiotics, these complications are rare; however, they do exist and may be fatal.

Nonsexual Transmission

Adults with germs on their hands can pass gonorrhea on to female children, which is one of the few instances of the nonsexual spread of the disease. The immature tissue of the child's vulva makes the child more susceptible to what is called gonorrheal vulvitis, or vulvovaginitis. Fortunately, this infection is usually confined to the vulva and lower two-thirds of the vagina and does not progress beyond the cervix. There may be a vaginal discharge, but quite extensive infection may be present with little discharge or pain.

A pregnant woman who contracts gonorrhea is usually protected from the spread of the disease through her Fallopian tubes and out into the pelvic cavity by the fact that the tubes normally close up shortly after pregnancy. Though there is a short-term protection for the mother, this is not so for the child. The gonorrhea doesn't affect the baby until delivery, when its eyes come in contact with the infected membranes of the mother. The gonococci eat away at the delicate lining of the eyes. Before antibiotics, this was a major cause of blindness, but now the law requires that all newborns be treated with silver nitrate drops or penicillin. Gonorrheal eye infections also occur in older children and adults as a result of rubbing the eyes after touching an infected area. When this disease does occur, the damage ranges from a slight scarring of the cornea to such serious infection of one or both eyeballs that surgical removal is required.

Diagnosis

There are two methods of diagnosing gonorrhea: the smear and the culture. The smear involves using a swab to obtain discharges from various areas that are then wiped on a glass slide, stained with a special dye and examined under a microscope for the presence of the coffee-bean—shaped gonococci. The culture involves obtaining discharges with a swab and placing them in a special container with a culture medium that stimulates the growth of the gonococci. Since the gonococci are so easily destroyed by air and heat, it was not until the mid-1960s that a suitable culture medium was developed that would keep the gonococci alive and yet would not be conducive to the growth of other organisms that might mask the gonococci. Now that such a medium is available, the gonococci can be put in the culture dishes, mailed to a laboratory, incubated for 16 to 24 hours and then examined to determine whether or not gonococci are present.

The smear is 99 percent accurate in diagnosing symptomatic men but is practically worthless in both asymptomatic men and in all women unless pus can be squeezed from the woman's urinary opening or gland ducts or is dripping from the cervix. The culture is 88 to 93 percent accurate in these women if a swab is taken from the cervix alone. If swabs are taken from both the cervix and anus, the culture is 92 to 94 percent accurate. Most doctors do not take a swab from the anus if they are doing just a routine culture, for extra cultures cost more money. However, people who practice anal intercourse should have a swab taken from the anus even in a routine smear. They will probably have to ask for it specifically since many doctors are too embarrassed to ask their patients if they practice anal intercourse. Similarly, people who practice oral-genital sex should have throat cultures taken. People who have symptoms or who have reason to think they've been exposed should *always* have both cervical and anal discharges cultured.

There are a number of reasons why the culture test is not 100 percent accurate: The woman may have douched before the doctor's visit (don't!) or may have tried to treat herself by taking a few antibiotic pills (again, don't!). The culture may have already spread above the cervix, leaving only a few organisms at the original infection site. The disease may have retreated deep into the glands of the cervix or vulva. The discharge on the swab may have contained only dead gonococci, so that there were none that could grow in the culture. The culture might not have been processed properly.

Given that undiagnosed gonorrhea can cause such serious problems, that the tests are unreliable and that women, especially those on the Pill, are highly susceptible, any woman who knows or even suspects that she has been exposed should be satisfied until she has had negative test findings from *two consecutive sets of cultures* taken during her menstrual flow.

Treatment

The best time to treat gonorrhea is early, before it spreads. The most effective treatment is penicillin given by injection into the buttocks, usually in a single treatment. About an hour before the penicillin injection, a drug called probenecid (Benemid) is given orally that inhibits excretion (so that the penicillin is not eliminated from the body) and increases sensitivity to penicillin.

If a person is allergic to probenecid or penicillin, another antibiotic, tetracycline, is given orally. Since tetracycline can cause problems in certain people and should not be taken by pregnant women, ampicillin with probenecid is sometimes used. One gram of probenecid is followed by oral ampicillin. Tetracycline or ampicillin is given orally by some doctors at six-hour intervals in cases of anorectal (anus and rectum) gonorrhea because the bacteria tend to get caught up in the feces, and once the level of penicillin given in the shot drops, the bacteria may cause a new infection. A spectacularly effective new drug called spectinomycin hydrochloride, sold under brand names like Trobicin, has been developed that is effective against strains of gonococci that may have become resistant to tetracycline and penicillin. It seems to have little in the way of side effects; however, it is more expensive and for some unexplained reason is not effective against gonorrhea in the throat. Treatment of gonorrhea may change in the future, for although the drugs available can cure the disease, it is taking increasing amounts of them to be effective against some of the particularly virulent strains.

Follow-up is essential, since cures are not always effective. The dosage may not have been high enough to combat a resistant strain, or the person's particular body chemistry may have affected the absorption and retention of the medicine. If single-dose oral therapy is given, it has a lower cure rate. An incorrect choice of antibiotic and the problems that arise when the gonococci are present in more than one location both contribute to treatment failures. Since one out of every ten people will require further treatment, it is essential to return one week after medication to have another culture taken. Then, in one more week, another should be taken.

There is no immunity to gonorrhea. A person could be treated and get reinfected immediately. *No one should have intercourse until they have had two consecutive negative cultures.* Even if you have no symptoms and your partner is also undergoing treatment, you face a very real risk of reinfection if you have intercourse before you both have had two negative cultures.

HERPES

AKA: herpes simplex, herpes virus hominis, herpes genitalis, herpes vaginitis

Types: herpes type I, or HSV-1
herpes type II, or HSV-2

Herpes is a widespread and little understood disease for which there is no cure. Once a person contracts it, he or she has it for life. Since the disease may have serious consequences, including birth defects and possibly cancer, prevention, which is discussed in the general introduction to this section, is of prime importance.

Incidence

Despite the fact that herpes is a widespread disease with serious implications for its sufferers' health and sexuality, it is not a disease that must be reported, so there are no really accurate figures as to how prevalent it is. Based on samplings from clinics, some researchers have estimated that there are 500,000 new cases of herpes in the United States each year and that somewhere between 5 to 14 million people have the disease.[9]

Cause and Transmission

Herpes of the genitals is caused by a virus known as herpes type II (HSV-II). It is closely related to herpes type I (HSV-I), which causes the common cold sore or fever blister. HSV-I usually affects the lips, mouth and face; while HSV-2 usually affects the genital area.

Herpes is usually transmitted through sexual intercourse. Oral-genital sex may account for the appearance of type I in what are normally type II locations and vice versa. Other methods of transfer may exist. It's been suggested, for instance, that HSV-2 may survive on warm, moist surfaces, so an infected washcloth, for instance, could transfer the disease. Although herpes type I can cause the same symptoms as type II and be equally uncomfortable, it is not implicated in the serious complications associated with type II and is therefore not considered to be as serious a disease.

Both men and women may be carriers of the disease. This means that although they have no history of the disease and have never shown a single symptom, they nonetheless carry the active virus in their bodies and can transmit it to others. No one knows how widespread this is.

When herpes first became a topic of news stories and magazine articles, it was generally supposed that the disease could be transmitted only by someone with active symptoms. Some writers suggested that a very tiny sore, not particularly painful, might go unrecognized and that this undetected symptom could lead to inadvertent infection of another. We now know that some people are carriers and also that a woman can have a recurrence whose only active symptom might be a sore on the inside of her vagina or on her cervix.[10] Unless she had her own speculum, she probably wouldn't be aware of a sore in such a location, yet would still be contagious. Moreover, it has recently been determined that a person can continue to infect others even though the symptoms of an attack have subsided. In fact, one doctor noted a woman who had active virus 132 days after the last of her symptoms had faded.[11] Also, active virus may be present for a period of time before the sores erupt. It is, then, quite possible to transmit herpes even when you don't have active symptoms.

Sexual intercourse should be avoided while active sores are present, although if both people have the disease, this may not be necessary. However, many people are in too much pain to attempt intercourse.

Although a person is less likely to transmit the disease during the dormant period between acute attacks, it is, as we have seen, still possible even in this latent stage to transmit it, so people with a history of herpes should always use condoms. Since condoms do not provide total protection, it is only fair that all sexual partners be warned of the potential risk in advance.

Symptoms

As mentioned earlier, herpes may be asymptomatic. In some cases, the initial attack may be very mild and go unnoticed, although usually the first attack is the most severe. No one knows why some people have only mild attacks and others have severe ones. It has been suggested that if a person has previously had a type I infection, they are apt to have a less severe attack.

The first symptoms usually appear within three to seven days of exposure to the virus; however, cases have been reported in which symptoms appeared in as few as two days or took as many as twenty days to manifest themselves.

The first attack, referred to as primary herpes, is generally the most painful and is usually more severe for women than for men. It usually begins with a slight tingling or burning sensation, or perhaps an itching or rash, in the genital area. The whole genital area may be swollen and inflamed. This may be followed by the appearance of small, raised, fluid-filled blisters on the genitals. In women, these may also be seen on the cervix and vaginal walls. In both men and women, they sometimes appear on the urethra, or on the buttocks and thighs, but this is less common.

In women, the sores may appear on the cervix or the vaginal walls without involvement of the external genitals, but in the majority of cases, internal sores are accompanied by external sores. There may be a burning sensation and an increase in the amount of vaginal discharge. This watery discharge may be mild or it may be more profuse and irritating. Typically, the cervix and walls of the vagina will be covered with this discharge. In men, irritation to the urethra may produce a watery discharge from the tip of the penis.

The skin around these blisterlike sores may be inflamed, swollen and hardened. The sores themselves are not hardened or raised, which distinguishes them from other sores that may appear on the vulva. They are usually grayish in the center and red around the edges. They are tender, but do not usually bleed. They may rupture and ooze discharge that is often yellowish in color. Scabs may form over the ruptured sore. The sores are more likely to rupture if they are located on the moist inner lips of the vulva. For the most part, the sores are small, although they may coalesce and appear as a single larger sore, and there may then be a swelling in the lymph glands on both sides of the groin.

The sores may persist for three to six weeks and are usually accompanied by pain, which can range from moderate tenderness to an intense, sharp burning pain. In fact, in extreme cases, the person cannot even be examined without hospitalization and a general anesthetic.

Urination can be particularly painful, as a result of the urine passing over the open sores. If there are sores inside the urethra, this, of course, increases the pain. The pain with urination can be so severe that it becomes impossible to urinate. In extreme cases, the person must be hospitalized and sedated so that a tube can be inserted into the bladder to drain the urine.

Sexual intercourse is painful. Indeed, it may be so painful as to become impossible. The primary, or first, attack may be accompanied by flulike symptoms of fever, headache and a general feeling of malaise.

Although some people have only the one primary attack, most people have recurrent attacks within a few days or a few months. Over 50 percent of those infected will have a second attack within six months.[12] These recurrent attacks are generally progressively less severe and heal much more quickly. There is no way to predict when recurrences will happen, and no one knows what causes them. Physical and emotional stress seem to be factors. The hormonal changes associated with pregnancy and menstruation can trigger attacks. Some people report that sexual stimulation, even if there is only manual stimulation and no genital-to-genital contact, will trigger an attack.

In about 35 percent of herpes cases, there is also another venereal disease present at the same time, so symptoms of these diseases may appear as well.[13]

Complications

In the past decade, there has been growing evidence linking herpes infection to cervical cancer.[14] Women with a history of herpes infection are eight times more likely to develop cervical cancer than women who have not had herpes. Herpes-type viral material has been found in malignant cervical tumors. The evidence suggesting that herpes is a causative factor (or one factor in a string of causes that eventually leads to cervical cancer in some women) is not conclusive, but any woman with a history of herpes should have Pap smears at least twice a year. The association between herpes and cervical cancer is discussed in more detail under the heading Cervical Cancer.

The other serious complications that herpes may cause involve pregnancy and childbirth. Women with herpes have a rate of miscarriages that may be three times higher than normal.[15] Herpes infection increases the risk for a premature delivery. Herpes simplex virus can also cause severe disease in infected infants. It is not common for babies to be infected, but when it does occur, it is apt to be serious. The closer to term, the more dangerous the infection is for the infant, for the fetus has not yet had time to develop its own protective antibodies. The risk of infection is greater if the infant is exposed to an active infection in the mother's birth canal during delivery. In such a case, the baby has a 40 to 50 percent chance of being infected.[16] The mortality rate from herpes in infected babies may be as high as 50 percent.[17] Even if the infection is not fatal, there may be birth defects, including blindness and diseases of the central nervous system. Because of the risk of infection during normal delivery, many doctors and women feel that Caesarean delivery, that is, cutting open the abdomen to deliver rather than allowing the baby to move through the birth canal, should be done. Others feel that this may not be necessary in some cases.[18] Some doctors will isolate the newborn and keep the baby in the hospital for a week or two after delivery to avoid transmission of the disease and in case the baby might be sick. Other doctors have found that transmission can be controlled by careful handwashing and other precautions. A pregnant woman with a history of herpes should try to find a doctor who is experienced with herpes deliveries; however, this may not be easy. Another alternative is for the woman or her doctor to contact a large university teaching hospital, where up-to-date information may be available.

Standford University Medical Center in Palo Alto, California, Division of Pediatric Infectious Diseases, has a Perinatal Herpes Simplex Program, headed by Dr. Anne S. Yeager, where new procedures for testing HSV are being investigated. By assessing risk to the infant late in pregnancy on the basis of antibody levels, indications of virus shedding and the timing of active lesions, they have been able to avoid Caesarean deliveries in certain cases. They have also developed a protocol (treatment procedure) that minimizes the risk of infection during birth and avoids separating the mother and infant. Another way to get up-to-date information about herpes and pregnancy is through a program known as HELP (for more information, see Treatment below).

Diagnosis

The symptoms of herpes, the sores, pain, etc., are often enough to indicate to the doctor that herpes is present. In pregnant women, the doctor will want to be absolutely sure of the diagnosis. Since other venereal diseases often occur at the same time, the doctor may test for these as well as for herpes.

A Pap smear will show characteristic changes in your cells that indicate the presence of herpes. It is 90 percent accurate if sores are present at the time of testing.[19] Viral cultures grown from a sample taken from the sores can also be used, but they have less accuracy (65-75 percent).[20] They should be done when the sores first appear, for that is when the concentration of HSV-2 in the sores is highest. A certain blood test, known as an antibody titer, can be used to detect herpes. A sample of blood is taken when the sore first appears and a second one is taken two to four weeks later. In most people, the body naturally produces its own infection fighters in the form of antibodies, in an attempt to fight the herpes. They take a couple of weeks to build up enough strength to show up in blood tests. The first sample, then, will not show antibodies, or only a very low level. If there is an infection, the second test will show a jump in the level, or titer, of herpes antibodies, an indirect yet unmistakable sign indicating that herpes has attacked. However, in a small percentage of people, for some unknown reason, no antibodies are produced.

Treatment

There is at present no cure for herpes, since it is caused by a virus and we have very little in the way of antiviral medications. Nor are there any proven measures for preventing recurrences. However, there are ways to relieve the symptoms, and there are some things that may possibly speed up the healing process.

The problem in finding a cure for herpes is that after the sores heal, the inactive virus retreats into the nerve cells, where it may remain dormant or periodically flare up again. It is thought that this retreat to the nerve cells prevents the body's immune system from dealing effectively with the virus. Although there are some drugs that can work against the active virus in the sores, these drugs work on the viruses only when they are in the process of reproducing, or replicating, themselves and thus are powerless against the dormant virus.

A number of different treatments have been suggested for herpes in the past few years, among them smallpox vaccine, Flagyl, flu vaccine and a process called photodynamic activation, which involves painting the open sores with a special dye. The virus absorbs the dye and is then inactivated by exposure to a light source; however, this treatment is no longer used, for it has not been proven effective and may cause cancerous changes in normal cells.[21] Many times the initial reports of these sorts of cures have been quite good; however, subsequent, more careful studies have always yielded disappointing results. There are a number of proposed cures now in the experimental stage at various centers across the country, but until one or more are proven effective and become available in the marketplace, treatment must generally consist of alleviating the symptoms and speeding up the healing process. A person with herpes may find that pouring water over the genital area while urinating or even voiding in a tub full of water will make the pain more bearable. In general, it's best to avoid creams and jellies but, if necessary, K-Y Lubricating Jelly can be applied to the sores to ease the irritation on urination. It should be washed off afterward, however, as any ointment will prolong the symptoms. Sitting in a hot (not warm) tub may help relieve the pain. Wet dressings applied with a soft cloth for 15 to 30 minutes three or four times a day will also help relieve the pain. The wet dressings can be soaked in solutions of potassium permanganate, benzalkonium chloride, saturated boric acid solutions, Borrow's solution diluted 1:20 in water or 0.25 percent aluminum subacetate diluted 1:16 in tap water. Some doctors prescribe Stoxil cream applied every three to four hours. Pain relievers may be prescribed; sometimes a topical anesthetic such as xylocaine is helpful. If ulcers have formed and a secondary infection ensues, the doctor may prescribe antibiotics, probably in cream form, to fight the secondary infection, although antibiotics, of course, have no effect on the herpes virus.

Although the reason for its effectiveness is not at all clear, there have been some reports advocating the use of aspirin—one to two tablets every four hours, five days before the menstrual period—to prevent recurrences that are known to flare up at this time. Proper nutrition and avoidance of stress and direct sunlight are also thought to be factors in preventing recurrences. Taking a zinc pill three to four times a day is helpful for some people.

It is hoped that in the not-too-distant future there will be a cure for herpes. One way to keep abreast of the latest developments in herpes research is through an organization called HELP, which puts out an informative newsletter every 12 weeks for its members. Subscriptions cost $8 a year. (Pregnant women should get their special report "Herpes and Pregnancy," Vol. 1, No. 2). For information, write to HELP, Box 100, Palo Alto, California 94302. PLEASE, PLEASE send a stamped, self-addressed NO. 10 (business-size) envelope along with your request.

SYPHILIS

AKA: Ives, bad blood

Many people think syphilis is a thing of the past, but this is not true. Although the disease is readily cured in the early stages, it may not be detected, especially in women, until later, when it may be harder to cure. Information about prevention and how minors can get treatment without their parents being notified is discussed in the introduction to this section.

Incidence

Syphilis, like almost all venereal diseases, is on the rise. In 1977, 66,625 cases were reported, and it is estimated that another 500,000 cases either went undetected or unreported.[22]

Cause and Transmission

The disease is usually transmitted through sexual contact. It is caused by a strain of bacteria called *Treponema pallidum*, which dies rapidly without warmth and moisture, so that it is virtually impossible to get syphilis from toilet seats or infected clothing or towels. However, it is possible to get the disease by kissing someone with an open sore or by touching the infected sore. Anal-genital, oral-genital or genital-genital sexual contact can spread the disease. Although the disease is quite prevalent in the male homosexual population, lesbians (with no bisexual involvement) rarely get it. It may also be spread during pregnancy or during delivery to an infant by an infected mother. Although it is uncommon, a man who is in the tertiary stage (see below) of the disease can transmit it to a woman, but *only* if his sperm impregnates her ovum. Then the blood of both the mother and her infant become contaminated. This type of infection initially produces only a mild form of the disease, which may, therefore, go untreated for years.

Symptoms

The first symptoms of syphilis may appear anywhere from 10 to 90 days following the initial contact, the average being around 21 days. The disease is divided into stages. The first stage, called early, or primary, syphilis, is usually marked by the appearance of a small, reddish brown spot that may range from the size of a pinprick to the size of a dime and may look like a pimple, sore or blister. This sore, or chancre, as it is called, is located at the exact spot where the germs entered the body and is a by-product of the attempt of the body's white cells to fight the infection. It may grow to about the size of a marble and ulcerate, producing a round or oval-shaped sore with hard, raised edges and a depression in the center. It is generally painless, does not itch and usually lasts for anywhere from six to ten weeks, although it may disappear more quickly. It may leave a scar or disappear leaving no trace at all. In most cases it eventually goes away by itself, even if not treated. While the sore is present, as well as for some time preceding and following it, the person is contagious and can pass the disease along to others. The sore usually appears on the vulva or penis but can appear inside the vagina or on the cervix, anus, lips, mouth, fingers or breast. There may be an associated swelling of the lymph glands in the area around the groin.

Since the sore is painless, often very small and disappears quickly, it may not be noticed, particularly in women. A woman who practices self-exam on a regular basis has a much better chance of detecting it early, but about 90 percent of the women with syphilis don't remember ever having seen the primary symptoms. Men are more apt (40–60 percent) to notice the primary symptoms. People who do notice primary symptoms should seek treatment immediately, for even though the symptoms go away, the disease is still there. All sexual contacts in the previous six weeks should be notified.

The second, or secondary, stage of syphilis may occur anywhere from one week to six months after the initial contact. The symptoms vary from person to person, but generally they begin as slightly raised blotches—a skin rash about the color of raw ham that may change to a copper-red color. The rash may resemble measles, chicken pox, scarlet fever or other infectious diseases. It is generally not painful, nor does it itch. It may appear on dry areas, like the palms of the hands or the soles of the feet, or may even cover the entire body. In moist areas, especially on black people, it may appear as slightly raised, round or oval sores with flat, grayish surfaces that ooze a clear liquid. This liquid is full of germs, and the sores are highly contagious. The lymph glands in the groin, armpit, neck or elsewhere in the body may swell and feel tender. There may be a mild fever, headache, sore throat, hoarseness, lack of appetite, a dull ache in the joints and bones and a general feeling of illness. In some people the rash may cover the head and scalp and cause patches of hair to fall out. The untreated symptoms may last for three to six months and can even come and go for a period of years. Most people, however, notice the symptoms and seek treatment at this point.

Next, during the latent phase, there is an apparent remission of the disease. The rash is gone and the infected person may look and feel fine. There is no limit as to how long this phase may last. It may even last a lifetime. During the first year or so after the symptoms disappear, a person may still pass the disease along to someone else; but after that time, with the exception of during pregnancy (when the fetus can be infected) they are generally no longer able to infect others.

No one knows what causes the disease to become active and flare up again during the third stage, which is also referred to as tertiary, or late, syphilis. About 25 percent of those with untreated syphilis will go on to the third stage.

When the disease does flare up, it can attack with an incredible virulence. It may attack the skin, muscles, eyes, lungs, digestive system, liver, endocrine glands or the walls of the blood vessels. An internal, chancrelike sore called a gumma attacks the organs and eats away at them. The progress of the disease may be halted at this stage, but the damage already done is permanent.

The effects of syphilis in this stage can be devastating. Cardiovascular syphilis will affect the heart and blood vessels and may be fatal. Neurosyphilis destroys the fragile sensory nerves, so that the person is unable to sense what his or her legs are doing without looking at them. Walking becomes difficult, and the person may develop a peculiar gait. If untreated, neurosyphilis can cause lightning pain, feelings of pins and needles being stuck into the skin all over the body and severe pains and spasms in the throat. Syphilis can also cause a condition known as general paresis, which involves the cranial nerves and affects the facial muscles. Paresis can cause total personality changes, insanity or death. People with paresis may pass through a series of very pleasant and/or extremely unpleasant hallucinations until they are finally cut off totally from outside sensory impressions and are the sole occupants of a disease-induced fantasy world. Luckily, there are now treatments that can prevent the disease from progressing this far, provided that it is diagnosed and treated early enough.

Syphilis and Pregnancy

It is important to know that a pregnant woman with syphilis, regardless of which stage of the disease she is in, may pass the disease on to her unborn infant (in which case it is called congenital syphilis). Both the primary chancre and the secondary rash are generally quite mild in pregnant women and may pass by unnoticed. Syphilis in pregnant women may, therefore, go untreated for a longer period of time. The mother may pass the syphilis through the placenta to the fetus, or the infant may contract the disease if a secondary rash is present on the vagina or vulva during delivery. If the mother is treated before the fourth month, the child usually won't develop any symptoms. The fetus is cured as the mother is cured. However, if untreated, the placenta may be damaged, resulting in miscarriage or stillbirth or in the child's being born with the disease. Since the baby has received the syphilis bacteria directly into the bloodstream, there may be no primary or early secondary stages. The child may be born with latent syphilis that remains latent for anywhere from two years until the time of puberty. In some children there are birth defects and symptoms or problems that develop soon after birth, including distorted bones, misformed teeth, inflamed and clouded eyes, deafness, blindness and mental retardation. Every pregnant woman should be tested for syphilis at least twice during her pregnancy, once at the initial visit and again just before delivery.

Diagnosis

All people who develop a sore on the genitals should be tested for syphilis. The diagnosis of syphilis is made in a couple of ways. The doctor can examine scrapings of the chancre, or sore, under a special dark-field microscope that makes the spirochetes show up brightly. If you practice anal or oral-genital sex and have sores in these areas, make sure the doctor tests them as well. Since the *T. pallidum* may be confused with other organisms, it is important that this test be done by a highly skilled person. If such a microscope is available in the doctor's office or clinic, test results may be ready in a few minutes; otherwise, the sample can be sealed and sent to a laboratory for testing. The testing is done free of charge by the Public Health Service. It is important not to put any cream or lotion on the sore before seeing the doctor, as this may kill germs on the surface and upset test results.

All men and women believed to have syphilis are given a blood test, no matter what the results of a dark-field examination. All blood tests for syphilis rely on detecting the antibodies that the person's body has produced in reaction to the invading syphilis germs. The most widely used test is one called the VDRL, but it cannot detect syphilis until it has been in the body long enough to form antibodies, or for about four to six weeks. Even then, it is only about 76 percent accurate in detecting primary syphilis. It can give both false positive and false negative results. The FTA-ABS is a more accurate test that requires more expensive equipment and is more difficult to perform. It can detect syphilis earlier than the VDRL and is about 86 percent accurate in detecting primary syphilis. If you have been exposed to syphilis less than four weeks previously, request that an FTA-ABS be done rather than a VDRL. If you have had intercourse with an infected person, or with someone you suspect may be infected, and yet your test results indicate that you do not have syphilis, you should have the tests repeated in six weeks and again in 90 days. There is a third test, the TPI, that is used in special, confusing cases and is expensive and difficult to perform. In latent syphilis, this test may be necessary to make sure that the disease is not continuing quietly in the central nervous system. In the TPI, a needle is inserted between the bones of the spine and a sample of the spinal fluid that surrounds the spine is withdrawn for testing.

Treatment

The usual treatment for syphilis is penicillin, injected into the buttocks. Two injections, one in each buttock each time, must be given on at least two separate occasions, usually three days apart. Patients who are allergic to penicillin are treated with oral tetracycline. For pregnant women and others who cannot use tetracycline, another drug, erythromycin stearate (Erythromycin), is given by mouth for a couple of weeks, but since Erythromycin does not cross the placenta very easily, two new drugs that show promise, cephaloridine and, less often, doxycycline, may be used instead.

The introduction of the antibiotic will kill large numbers of the germs suddenly, and in dying the organisms break open and release their contents into the bloodstream. This can cause a fever of 101°-102°, and if a chancre is present, it may become swollen and enlarged, but the reaction usually lasts only a few hours.

Everyone treated for syphilis needs several follow-up exams to make sure the disease is completely cleared up. If it is a case of primary or secondary syphilis, a follow-up blood test should be done one month later and then once every three months for one year. People with latent or late syphilis must be seen more often.

CRABS

AKA: pubic lice, cooties, pediculosis pubis, phthiriasis pubis

Pubic lice are tiny, wingless insects that attach themselves to pubic hairs by means of their crablike claws. They insert their sucking-type mouths into the hair follicle and feed on the tiny blood vessels in the area. These perfectly loathsome creatures, which look like props from a grade-B monster film, are about the size of a pinhead and are a nondescript white/yellow/gray sort of color that makes them very difficult to see on light-skinned people. They appear to be a small scab or flake of skin until you look very closely and see movement of the legs. They may be a bit easier to see after they have just finished a "meal," when they are gorged with blood and are consequently rather rust-colored. Although they prefer pubic hair, it is also possible for them to exist in any hairy part of the body, including eyelashes, underarms, eyebrows and hairy parts of the chest.

The lice cannot survive for more than 24 hours unless they are attached to a human body. They have a lifespan of about 30 days and apparently have no knowledge of birth control—they put rabbits to shame, mating frequently and laying three eggs a day. The eggs, called nits, are oval in shape, whitish, hard and glistening. The female cements the eggs to the side of a pubic hair, usually near the junction of the hair and skin. The eggs hatch in seven to nine days. By the time they are 17 days old, the newly hatched lice can reproduce.

Transmission

Pubic lice are usually transmitted during sexual contact; however, a mere hug while nude will suffice. It is even possible to pick up crabs from articles of clothing, bed linen, mattresses, toilet seats—or anything that has been infested with the lice or their eggs.

Symptoms

The telltale symptom is an intolerable itching, often worse in the middle of the night. It is believed that the itching is caused by an allergic reaction to the saliva that the crabs secrete while feeding. Not all people develop this allergic reaction, so it is possible to have crabs without any symptoms. The itching causes scratching, which gives no relief and only intensifies the sensation. In some people, the bites cause a mild rash of small bluish dots, which are the result of hemorrhage (bleeding) in the tiny blood vessels just below the surface of the skin.

Diagnosis

No special tests are required to diagnose crabs, for they are large enough to be seen with the naked eye; however, since the initial infestation involves only six to eight of these tiny creatures, they may be difficult to locate at first. Sometimes it is easier to see the glistening tiny eggs (nits) glued to the pubic hairs.

Treatment

Treatment involves killing the lice and their eggs on the body and sterilizing any clothing, bed linen, towels, mattresses, washcloths, toilet seats and such that may harbor the lice or their eggs. It's best to see your doctor, who can prescribe a product called Kwell that kills both the lice and their eggs. It comes in a shampoo or a cream lotion. There are also certain over-the-counter preparations that can be purchased in drugstores or pharmacies without a doctor's prescription, but they are usually not as effective as Kwell. Home remedies, such as kerosene and shaving the pubic hair, are rather extreme and can cause irritation of the genital skin. They also may not be as effective as Kwell.

Kwell lotion is used by applying a thin coating to the hair and skin of the pubic area, thighs, trunk and underarms. It is rubbed into the hair and skin, left in place for 12 hours and followed by a thorough washing. The Kwell shampoo is a bit easier to use. First apply enough shampoo to wet the hair and skin of the hairy areas of the body. Once thoroughly wetted, add water a bit at a time to work up a good lather. Then shampoo for four minutes. Rinse well and towel-dry briskly. A second treatment is sometimes necessary. Check yourself again in seven days and repeat treatment if necessary. The dead nits can sometimes be removed with a fine-tooth comb. If not, you may have to resort to the ancient art of nit picking.

Avoid getting Kwell on mucous membranes, the area between the lips of the vulva, the penis and the eyes, as it may irritate them. Kwell should be used with caution on children and by pregnant women because the active ingredient can penetrate the skin and could potentially poison the central nervous system. Crabs in the eyelashes may be treated with mercuric oxide ointment, available in pharmacies without a prescription.

Since the crabs can live briefly on clothing, bed linen mattresses and can also lay their eggs in such places, it will be necessary to treat these things as well. This can be quite a hassle. Drycleaning or washing the items in boiling water will kill the lice and their eggs; however, if you can't afford to dryclean your underwear and haven't got a kettle big enough to boil all the clothing, sheets and towels you've used in the last couple of weeks (not to mention your mattress), you can simply leave everything undisturbed and away from human contact for two weeks. The hatched crabs will die within 24 hours. The eggs take a week to ten days to hatch and without a human host won't survive more than 24 hours once they've hatched. If you treat yourself and any sexual partners or other contacts who might have crabs, scrub your toilet seat and stay away from everything for two weeks, your life will once again be crab-free.

GENITAL WARTS

AKA: condyloma acuminatum; verruca acuminata; verrucous lesions; pointed condyloma; papilloma acuminatum; papilloma venereum; fig, moist, wet, pointed or venereal warts

Despite the string of rather complicated medical terms by which it is known, the condyloma acuminatum is just a simple wart that grows in the genital area. It is thought to be caused by a virus closely related to the virus that causes warts on other parts of the body. It is sometimes confused with the condyloma latum associated with secondary syphilis.

Transmission

Genital warts are usually transmitted through vaginal, anal or oral sex, but it is possible to pick them up through others types of contact. The warts are more contagious in their early stages than when they have been present for a long time. About 70 percent of the people who have intercourse with an infected partner will develop warts.

Incidence

Like all venereal diseases, it is especially prevalent among the sexually active, and the incidence is on the rise. It occurs more frequently in women who have other sexually transmitted diseases or one of the common vaginal infections, use birth control pills or are pregnant, and in uncircumcized men. In all these instances, a damp, moist environment is provided that is ideal for genital warts.

Symptoms

The warts may appear anywhere from one to four months following the initial contact with an infected person. They may grow near the vaginal opening or on the labia, the anus, or elsewhere in the genital area. On men, they usually grow on the tip or shaft of the penis or on the scrotum. If the warts grow on dry skin, like that on the outer vulva or the shaft of the penis, they look very similar to the warts that grow on other parts of the body. If they grow on the moist areas, they may appear as small, dark pink bumps about the size of a grain of rice. They may grow singly or there may be several. In the moist areas they tend to grow together, forming clumps that look like small cauliflowers. There may be a foul-smelling discharge and intolerable itching; however, the warts, though annoying, are generally not serious. Their growth, however, is stimulated by pregnancy, and in extreme cases they may block the vaginal opening, bleed during delivery or even necessitate a Caesearean delivery.

The warts can produce an abnormal Pap smear. But venereal warts are not related to cancer, and the Pap smear will return to normal once they have been successfully treated.

Diagnosis and Treatment

The doctor can usually diagnose the warts simply by their appearance. Although in some cases the warts will disappear spontaneously, they

562

should be treated promptly, since they tend to rapidly increase in size and number. Treating vaginal warts can be a bit tricky in women who have another vaginal infection that is causing a lot of moisture and discharge. The first step will be to dry up the area by treating any related infections. In some cases it may be necessary for a woman to temporarily stop using the birth control pill in order to get rid of the warts.

The specific treatment will depend on the size, number and location of the warts. Most people can be treated successfully with a solution of a substance called podophyllin. The solution is painted on the warts, left on for six hours and then washed off. In a few days, the warts fall off; however, the treatment may have to be applied a few times in order to get rid of all the warts. If you don't get all the warts, the whole mess usually recurs.

Generally, the podophyllin is applied by a doctor or nurse since the solution is quite irritating to the skin and care must be taken to apply it only to the wart itself. Six hours after treatment, the area is washed thoroughly with soap and water. If a burning sensation develops, the area must be washed off right away. If there is pain, aspirin and/or hot sitz baths are suggested. If these measures don't relieve the pain, the doctor can prescribe a cream to soothe the area.

Podophyllin cannot be used by pregnant women since it has been known to cause miscarriage and premature labor. It cannot be used to treat extensive cases, for if the warts are too large, then only the outer layers of tissue will be killed, the wart will not disappear completely and the dying tissue will be particularly susceptible to infection.

In the past, extensive or stubborn warts were treated with chemical or electric burning (cautery); however, it is now possible to destroy them by freezing, a procedure known as cryosurgery, which is more effective and more comfortable for the woman. In extreme cases, an operation known as a "skinning" vulvectomy, which removes the outer layers of vulvar skin, may be done.

GRANULOMA INGUINALE

AKA: granuloma pudendi, ulcerating granuloma of the pudenda

Granuloma inguinale is usually lumped in with venereal diseases because the disease is thought to be transmitted sexually; however, this has not been conclusively proven. Perhaps the only nice thing about this disease is that you are not likely to get it unless you live in a tropical climate. Only a few hundred cases are reported in this country each year, mostly in the southern states.[23]

Symptoms

The symptoms may be quite delayed, appearing anywhere from four days to twelve weeks after infection. The first symptoms are small bumps or blisters, which may appear in the area of the vulva, anus or, occasionally, on the cervix. In the man they may be found on the tip of the penis, under the foreskin and in the area of the anus as well. The blisters rapidly turn into raw, oozing sores that are reddish and may bleed or exude pus. Secondary infection is common, with painful, tender sores or bumps that emit a pungent odor. The spreading sores may affect the urinary and rectal openings, making elimination difficult. Contraction of the vaginal opening and tenderness in the area limit sexual activity. Indeed, even sitting or walking may be uncomfortable.

Diagnosis and Treatment

The diagnosis is made on the basis of the symptoms and microscopic examination that reveals the presence of the organism, *Donovania granulomatis*, which causes the disease.

Treatment usually consists of tetracycline taken by mouth every six hours for two to three weeks. For pregnant women and others who cannot take tetracycline, another antibiotic, ampicillin, is given orally over a period of three to twelve weeks. Patients should be followed up every three to four months after they start treatment.

CHANCROID

AKA: soft chancre, ulcus molle

On a worldwide basis, chancroid is more common than syphilis; however, it is usually found only in tropical climates. Less than 1,000 cases are resported in the United States each year, and most of these occur in the southeastern states.[24]

Causes and Symptoms

The disease is caused by a tiny rod-shaped bacterum, the *Haemophilus ducreyi*, which usually enters the body through some preexisting cut, scrape or crack in the skin of the genital organs. In the United States, the disease is usually transmitted through vaginal, anal or oral-genital sex. In other parts of the world where it is more widespread, it is probably transmitted through other forms of contact as well.

It is possible to have the disease without having any symptoms. When symptoms do appear, it is usually within one to five days after intercourse with the infected person; however, it can be as long as ten days. The first symptom is the appearance of one or more small raised bumps with a narrow red border that may be located on the vulva, vagina, cervix, anal opening or urethra. In men, they may appear on the shaft of the penis, the foreskin or the anal opening. They may look like small pimples or blisters that soon rupture to form small, red, saucer-shaped sores. The sores may produce a great deal of foul-smelling pus. They are usually soft and painful or tender and may bleed easily when touched. They may spread to adjacent areas, like the groin, thighs, abdomen and stomach.

The lymph glands in the groin may also swell and, if untreated, the enlarged glands will gather into a large, red painful swelling called a bubo. The bubo usually ruptures and pus may drain out, in which case a person is highly susceptible to secondary infection. There may be such acute pain that the person has difficulty in even walking.

Diagnosis and Treatment

The disease is difficult to diagnose. It is easily confused with syphilis and lymphogranuloma venereum. No one test is completely accurate, so the doctor will have to make several.

Different doctors will choose different methods of treating the disease, for there is no clear indication of which treatment is most effective. Most of the time, sulfa drugs or tetracycline are used.

Since there is no immunity to chancroid, reinfections are common. It is important to be examined every two to three months for one year after treatment.

LYMPHOGRANULOMA VENEREUM

AKA: LGV, lymphopathia, lymphopathia venereum

LGV is widespread through the world, especially in tropical areas, but until recently was fairly rare in the United States. There are only a few thousand cases reported each year; however, the incidence is increasing, possibly because servicemen brought the disease back from Southeast Asia.[25]

Cause and Transmission

The organism that causes LGV displays characteristics of both a virus and a bacteria and is not yet fully understood. The disease is usually spread by vaginal, anal or oral-genital sex, although in tropical climates it is probably spread by other forms of contact as well. It is not as contagious as syphilis or gonorrhea and is more common in men.

Symptoms

Symptoms may appear anywhere from one to twelve weeks after the infected contact but usually appear within seven to twelve days. A small painless sore or blister appears on the sex organs. In women it may appear on the cervix, vulva or interior walls of the vagina. In men it usually appears on the tip of the penis or in the urethra. Since the sore is painless, may be hidden from view and disappears rapidly, it often goes unnoticed. Within a few days, the infection spreads to the lymph glands. If the sore appears on the external genitals, the lymph glands in the groin may become swollen and inflamed. If the initial sore is in the vagina, or in the rectum as the result of anal intercourse, the deeper pelvic lymph nodes may be affected.

The tender, enlarged glands may fuse together to form a hard, painful swelling called a bubo. The skin over the bubo may be bluish-red in color. The lymph nodes may be destroyed. The buboes may break through the skin and drain pus. This bubo formation usually occurs anywhere from 10 to 30 days after the appearance of the first sore. If it involves the deep pelvic lymph nodes, it may go unnoticed. In both men and women there may be fever, chills, pain, an aching in the joints and a loss of appetite.

The untreated disease can cause a number of complications that may appear in the first several months or as late as 20 years afterward. The swollen lymph vessels in the penis or vagina may block the normal flow of lymph. The fluids back up and cause an enormous swelling called genital elephantiasis. This occurs more often in women and can cause unbearable pain. It may require plastic surgery to restore the vulva to its normal size.

Complications involving the anus occur more frequently in women and homosexual men. Pain and bloody discharge are common symptoms. If the disease isn't treated, scar tissue may form, partially blocking the rectum and causing painful bowel movements. This may require surgery to correct.

Diagnosis and Treatment

The diagnosis of the disease cannot be based on symptoms alone, for they are easily confused with other STDs and other nonvenereal diseases as well. In the presence of swollen lymph glands, the doctor may want to test for all these possibilities. There are also special skin and blood tests for LGV.

LGV responds slowly to treatment. The treatment of first choice is tetracycline, given orally for a few weeks. Sulfa drugs may also be used.

LGV is a difficult disease to get out of the system and needs to be checked frequently. An LGV blood test should be taken every three months for the first year and then once a year for at least two years.

OTHER SEXUALLY TRANSMITTED DISEASES

Types: chlamydial infections
  mycoplasmas
  cytomegalovivus, or CMV
  hepatitis B
  scabies
  molluscum contagiosum

In addition to the common and not so common sexually transmitted diseases described in the preceding pages, there are a number of other diseases that may be associated with sexual intercourse. First there are the common vaginal infections, such as trich, hemophilus, nonspecific vaginitis and yeast infections, although the latter are more frequently caused by nonsexual means. There is also a growing body of evidence that dysplasia, carcinoma in situ and invasive cancer of the cervix may be caused by some sexually transmitted agent. In addition, there are certain diseases that are suspected of being transmitted sexually or are known to be sexually transmitted although they are more frequently passed in other ways. These diseases are discussed below.

Chlamydial Infections

These infections are caused by chlamydiae, unusual bacteria that have many of the characteristics of viruses. Chlamydiae cause nongonococcal urethritis (NGU). NGU, which is an inflammation of the tube that conducts urine from the bladder to the outside of the body, is characterized by discharge and pain on urination, the same symptoms that gonococcal urethritis can produce. Urethritis may also be caused by other organisms beside chlamydiae and gonococci. Indeed, men may catch urethritis just as easily as they catch the common cold.

There is no doubt that chlamydiae cause urethritis in men. NGU sometimes coexists with gonorrhea. If a man's gonorrheal-type symptoms persist after penicillin treatment, this may be due to the chlamydiae, for unlike gonococci, chlamydiae are not killed by penicillin. Such men maybe misdiagnosed as having drug-resistant gonorrhea. Persistent gonorrhea symptoms in women may have the same origins. However, in women the

567

disease is not so clearly understood. It is thought that some women's urethritis or cervical infections may be caused by chlamydiae, but it is also known that the organism may be present without causing any problems. Doctors are not sure what the complications of untreated chlamydial infections in women are. There is evidence that many untreated cases clear up by themselves in four to six weeks. On the other hand, there is evidence that chlamydiae can cause PID. Although it is suspected that the organism can be transmitted sexually, this has not been confirmed.

Because chlamydiae cause some 2.5 million cases of urethritis in men each year,[26] some doctors prescribe medication for the female sexual partners of these men even though the doctor has not actually examined the woman or done any diagnostic tests. Since it is unwise to take any medication unless it is necessary, and since the antibiotics used to treat chlamydiae often cause yeast infections in women, a woman would be wise to insist on proper diagnostic tests—to make sure she does indeed have the organism in her body—before taking such medication.

Mycoplasmas

Mycoplasmas are unique organisms that, like chlamydiae, are now considered bacteria, although they also have characteristics of viruses. It is known that they can be passed through sexual intercourse, but their exact role in genital infections is unclear. Although they can be cultured from sex organs, it is not known whether they actually cause diseases.

Cytomegalovirus (CMV)

CMV belongs to the same group of viruses as the herpes simplex virus and, like herpes, may infect infants. In fact, CMV is one of the most common causes of such birth defects as mental retardation, blindness and deafness. There is increasing evidence that the disease may be sexually transmitted among adults; however, it causes few, if any symptoms in adults. It is thought that the mother may in turn pass it on to the infant. At present, there is no treatment. Further research is needed to determine how the disease is transmitted and to develop ways to treat and prevent these infections.

Hepatitis B

Hepatitis B, or serum hepatitis, is a form of viral hepatitis, an infection of the liver. It was once thought that this disease could be transmitted only through contaminated blood transfusions or through injections using a contaminated needle. It is now recognized that the disease can be transmitted in other ways, including sexual contact. Symptoms include fever, loss of appetite, weakness, nausea, hives and a yellowing of the skin. There is no specific medical treatment available. Although most cases clear up by themselves, some do not, and the disease may have serious, even fatal, complications. There is no way to prevent the disease except to avoid exposure to people known to have it.

Scabies

Scabies, which are caused by small parasitic mites (bugs), cannot technically be called a sexually transmitted disease, for the bugs are often passed through nonsexual contact. Scabies often occur in children and tend to affect warm, moist areas of skin around the wrists, between the fingers and on the elbows. However, recently scabies have become quite common on the external genitals. The symptoms include severe itching and the appearance of small red bumps or lines caused by the female mite burrowing under the skin to lay her eggs. Diagnosis involves extracting the mite from the burrows and examining it microscopically. Treatment is the same as that used for crabs.

Molluscum Contagiosum

Molluscum contagiosum is a condition in which small, smooth, white, raised growths with a depression in their center appear on the male or female genital organs. There may be as few as one or as many as 20 of these growths. They may fuse together to form larger growths. In the past the disease occurred mainly in children on other areas of the body, but in recent years it has been found with increasing frequency on the genital organs in adults, which has led many doctors to believe that it is sexually transmitted. However, the evidence is far from conclusive, for the sexual partners of people with molluscum contagiosum are frequently not affected. The disease is often confused with vulvar folliculitis, and definite diagnosis can be made only by microscopic examination. For some unknown reason the disease seems to disappear spontaneously, but in extreme cases this may take as long as two to four years. It is generally not worthwhile to treat the growths unless they become infected, in which case treatment consists of removing them and painting the area with a special solution to prevent scarring.

Problems Related to the Menstrual Cycle

The conditions discussed in this section are not really diseases; rather they are symptoms of some underlying problem whose cause may or may not be understood. For instance, the first heading in this section, Premenstrual Syndrome, describes the changes that many women experience in the days preceding the menstrual flow. Although there are some theories to explain these changes, no one knows for sure what causes them. The same is true for menstrual cramps. In the case of the third condition in this section, amenorrhea, a term which refers to an absence of menstrual periods, it is sometimes possible to pinpoint a cause, but not always. Similarly, abnormal uterine bleeding, which includes any variation from the usual menstrual pattern as well as any other abnormal bleeding from the vagina, can sometimes but not always be traced to a specific cause.

The last three conditions in this section, precocious puberty, menopausal problems, and premature menopause, are related to the larger cycles of a woman's life stages rather than to the monthly cycle of menstruation. Here again, these conditions are symptoms rather than diseases, and the cause of these symptoms cannot always be identified.

Women seeking medical treatment for the conditions described in this section may not be taken seriously by their doctors. In part the doctor's response will depend on exactly which of these conditions a woman has. If a girl is experiencing precocious puberty, her problem is not likely to be dismissed by her doctor. Likewise, a woman who has a premature menopause will probably receive serious consideration from her doctor, for there is usually a history of surgical or radiation damage to the ovaries to explain her condition. Even when there isn't, there are tests the doctor can do to confirm the fact that her ovaries really have stopped functioning. Abnormal uterine bleeding is also likely to be viewed by doctors as a "real" problem since there is an observable symptom—blood loss—and since medical science can often pinpoint the cause of the abnormal bleeding. Moreover, even if the doctors can't explain why a woman is bleeding, they can always "cure" her problem by removing her uterus.

If you have amenorrhea, you can also expect to have your condition considered in an objective, rational manner, at least initially. Again, you have an observable symptom—lack of menstrual flow—and the doctor has lots of tests s/he can perform to find out why. If, however, the doctor's tests fail to explain your condition, you, along with those women seeking treatment for premenstrual syndrome, menstrual cramps and menopausal problems, are apt to find yourself up against the old it's-all-in-your-head-dearie diagnosis or the I-can't-figure-out-what's-wrong-with-you-so-you - must-be-crazy syndrome.

Consider, for example, what the most recent edition of one of the most widely used gynecological textbooks in this country has to say about the diagnosis of puzzling cases of amenorrhea.[1] After pointing out that even the most exhaustive tests administered by the most conscientious doctors will sometimes fail to pinpoint a cause for amenorrhea, the authors conclude, "It is undoubtedly incorrect to classify all such cases as of psychogenic origin, but such a practice is not uncommon and, until additional evidence is available, no more satisfactory solution can be suggested."

"Psychogenic" means "of emotional or mental origin"—in other words, it's-all-in-your-head. The authors of this widely read textbook, who apparently feel that it's perfectly all right to diagnose a woman as neurotic just because they have failed to find out what's wrong with her, are obviously suffering from the I-can't-figure-out-what's-wrong-with-you-so-you-must-be-crazy syndrome. These women aren't even given the benefit of the traditional judicial principle, innocent till proven guilty; instead, they are to be judged as crazy (or to put it in more polite, medical terminology, as having problems of psychogenic origin) until "additional evidence" proves otherwise. The doctors who authored this text can't suggest a "more satisfactory solution" to their inability to diagnose the cause of a woman's amenorrhea, but we can. How about a simple, honest "I don't know"?

If this sort of thing happened only after doctors had performed exhaustive tests and given women the benefit of what medical science had to offer, it wouldn't be such a problem. Women could perhaps learn to recognize this as one of the peculiar foibles to which doctors are prone and take such a diagnosis with an appropriate grain of salt. But all too often these attitudes prevent doctors from giving their women patients proper medical care.

Menstrual cramps, which have traditionally received the psychogenic "diagnosis" are an excellent example of how this works. One woman we know had cramps and vomited each time she had her period. Her gynecologist (who had no psychiatric training) decided she was neurotic and referred her to a psychiatrist. After extensive and expensive therapy, in which her male therapist helped her explore "her rejection of her femininity" as symbolized by her menstrual problems, she finally consulted another gynecologist. This doctor did not assume her problems were psychogenic and performed a thorough diagnostic work-up, including a laparoscopic exam. It was then discovered that this woman had a condition known as endometriosis that was affecting her bowels. We don't know whether she ever got around to accepting whatever it was she'd been rejecting, but once the endometriosis was treated she did stop vomiting and having pain each month. This is just one example of the ways in which doctors' prejudices and assumptions can negatively affect the health care a woman receives.

Women who suffer from cramps and other unpleasant symptoms prior to the onset of menstruation may have trouble in finding relief. The idea that these symptoms, which cannot be observed, measured or otherwise verified by the doctor, are imaginary, made-up or psychosomatic has been so firmly ingrained in doctors' thinking that the medical profession has paid little attention to them. However, some recent research, including some fascinating studies about the levels of little understood substances called prostaglandins, which are found in higher concentrations among women who suffer menstrual pain, is leading toward a tangible, physiological explanation for menstrual cramps. Perhaps now that doctors are beginning to understand the reasons for menstrual cramps, they will finally admit that they actually do exist and are not imaginary problems made up by hysterical women.

Women seeking treatment for these sorts of medical problems should insist on a complete and thorough investigation of their symptoms. The appropriate diagnostic steps are outlined in the following pages. (Reviewing the discussion of the menstrual cycle in Chapter Four, making notes on the terminology and referring to these notes may be helpful as you read through the information in this section.)

If, after a thorough diagnostic work-up, your doctor is unable to identify the source of your problem, don't allow yourself to be made to feel that you have psychological problems. In all likelihood, the problem is that medical science just hasn't advanced far enough yet to understand your condition.

PREMENSTRUAL SYNDROME

AKA: PMS, premenstrual tension or congestive dysmenorrhea

In contrast to men, whose hormone levels rise dramatically at puberty and then level off and remain constant until about middle age, women's hormone levels fluctuate constantly throughout the month from the time of puberty until menopause, when they level off. Almost every woman who charts her menstrual cycles will notice some sort of changes in her body as these powerful hormones, which affect virtually every type of tissue in her body, wax and wane. "Premenstrual syndrome" (PMS) is the term used to describe the changes many women notice during the premenstruum, the time that precedes the onset of the menstrual flow.

PMS is described in largely negative terms in the medical literature, but as discussed in the chapter on menstruation, probably as many women find positive changes as negative ones. The women who experience positive changes don't, of course, consult doctors, so the medical point of view about menstrual changes is rather unbalanced.

Symptoms

A wide variety of symptoms may appear at this time. These symptoms may be so mild as to be hardly noticeable, or they may be so dramatic that they are undeniably obvious. The way in which any given woman experiences these symptoms will depend largely on her personal body chemistry. The thing that these premenstrual symptoms have in common is that they begin in the days immediately prior to the onset of the menstrual flow in contrast, for instance, to menstrual cramps, which start with the actual flow.

There may be swelling of the abdomen, breasts, genitals, ankles, feet and hands, which may or may not be uncomfortable. Some women experience nausea, vomiting, diarrhea, constipation, headaches, depression, lethargy, fatigue, anger, anxiety, a dull ache in the lower abdomen, skin problems, respiratory problems related to asthma and allergies and urinary infections. About 30 percent of women will experience a weight gain of three or more pounds. Some women have a runny nose or sores in their mouths, others experience insomnia or a change in normal sleep patterns. Increased appetite, thirst and a craving for sweets are not uncommon. Alternatively, some women experience an elevation in mood, a rosy glow in their cheeks, extra energy, a dramatic increase in sexual desire and a general feeling of well-being. Any combination of the symptoms described here can occur. These symptoms may vary from month to month or year to year.

PMS is most often noticed by women in their 30s. Women on birth control pills generally don't experience symptoms of PMS, although some complain of depression that is particularly bad during the premenstruum.

Cause

Research into the cause of PMS has been rather limited and has often emphasized psychological and cultural rather than physical, chemical or hormonal aspects of the problem. Women with PMS are apt to be told that their problem is psychological.

The limited research into possible physiological causes of PMS indicates that the hormone progesterone may play a role in PMS symptoms, but the evidence is contradictory. The fact that women who use birth control pills or who don't ovulate and therefore do not produce progesterone are less likely to have PMS symptoms has led some researchers to conclude that progesterone, the hormone produced during the second half of the menstrual cycle, is responsible for PMS. Yet others have claimed to get good results by treating PMS symptoms *with* progesterone. Making the issue even more confusing is the fact that the results of this type of treatment have been mixed. In some cases there is relief of symptoms, but in others no effect has been demonstrated. Perhaps one explanation for this apparent discrepancy lies in the fact that different types of progestational drugs have been used. Dr. Katherine Dalton, the pioneer of progestational therapy, suggests that using progestins, the synthetic progesterone in birth control pills, won't relieve PMS symptoms.[2] But if pure progesterone is used, the symptoms will be relieved, because of the differences in the way in which the body metabolizes these substances.

Nutrition may also be a factor. It is known that some women on birth control pills experience depression due to a deficiency of vitamin B_6 caused by the Pill. If the B_6 is replaced, the depression usually disappears.[3] Supplementary vitamin B complex, foods rich in potassium (bananas), balanced calcium and magnesium supplements and extra vitamin C have proven effective for some women whether they are Pill users or not. Prunes, a natural laxative, bran and a high-bulk diet (whole-grain foods, raw vegetables and fruits), as well as a diet high in protein and vegetables but low in refined sugar and carbohydrates, have served to relieve PMS symptoms in some women.

Many of the symptoms of PMS may be related to fluid and salt retention. All women tend to retain fluid and salt in their bodies during the latter half of the menstrual cycle. These are released during the period. In addition to the obvious effects of swelling, this fluid retention may also be responsible for the emotional changes—the mood swings, both positive and negative—that women experience at this time in their menstrual cycles. It may be that the brain tissues also retain fluid; hence, the mood swings.

Treatment

If these changes are unpleasant for a woman, she may find that cutting down on her salt and fluid intake beginning 14 days prior to the expected onset of her menstrual cycle will provide relief of symptoms. A mild diuretic, a drug which helps the body eliminate fluids, may also be helpful.

We have only rarely encountered women who have had such severe PMS symptoms that medical treatment has been needed. In the rare instance where a woman does have severe symptoms, we have used a mild tranquilizer and a diuretic taken a week before the onset of menstruation. Progesterone therapy has seemed too drastic for most of the cases we have encountered. However, if the symptoms are severe and none of the less drastic forms of therapy are successful, progesterone therapy, although it involves certain risks (*see* p. 103), may be worth a try.

MENSTRUAL CRAMPS

AKA: dysmenorrhea

Types: primary, or essential, dysmenorrhea
secondary dysmenorrhea
congestive dysmenorrhea, or premenstrual tension
spasmodic dysmenorrhea

"Dysmenorrhea" is a fancy medical term for "menstrual cramps." Dysmenorrhea may be either secondary or primary. Secondary dysmenorrhea is menstrual pain that is caused by some associated disease—pain that is secondary to some other illness. Primary dysmenorrhea is menstrual pain that is not associated with some other disease—in other words, menstrual cramps whose cause is unknown.

Incidence

Menstrual cramps are extremely common. Indeed, it is rare to find a woman who has never experienced some degree of menstrual pain. Secondary dysmenorrhea typically appears for the first time in women who are in their 20s and 30s. Primary dysmenorrhea usually makes its appearance in the early teens and is usually less severe after about the age of 25 or after childbirth. Primary dysmenorrhea doesn't occur as frequently in women who are not ovulating, which explains why young girls during the first year or two after menarche don't have cramps, for they usually are not yet actually ovulating. It also explains why most women who use birth control pills, which suppresses ovulation, don't experience menstrual cramps. However, dysmenorrhea can occur in women of any age and may persist until menopause.

Symptoms

The pain may vary in severity from mild to severe and may also vary from month to month or from year to year. Some doctors recognize two different types of menstrual pain, spasmodic and congestive. Congestive dysmenorrhea is really a form of premenstrual syndrome and occurs just before the menstrual period begins. There may be a dull, achey feeling in the lower abdomen, painful swelling of the abdomen, breast, genitals, hands and/or feet, headache, backache, depression, fatigue, diarrhea or constipation, to mention just some of the symptoms. This type of pain may continue throughout life, and it doesn't usually abate with pregnancy and in fact may get worse. There may be a hereditary factor involved.

Spasmodic dysmenorrhea, as the name implies, involves spasms of dull or acute pain in the lower abdomen. It is usually a localized pain involving only the lower abdomen and genitals but may include the entire pelvic area, the inside of the thighs and the lower back. The pain usually begins on the first day of the menstrual cycle and is usually relieved by the third or fourth day but may affect some women for the entire period. Some women are plagued by this type of dysmenorrhea for their entire lives, but many gain relief after they have had a child. The severity may vary from a vague sense of pelvic heaviness (which one friend quite aptly calls "lead vagina") to severe, incapacitating pain.

If the dysmenorrhea is secondary, the symptoms may have certain characteristics that are related to the underlying cause. For instance, if the dysmenorrhea is due to a uterine fibroid tumor, there may be a gushing, flooding type of menstrual bleeding that is followed by cramping. If endometriosis is the cause, there may be premenstrual staining as well as pain on intercourse, and the pain tends to get progressively worse with each period. If pelvic inflammatory disease is the causative factor, the pain tends to be bilateral. If the pain is associated with adenomyosis, it may not abate after the first few days but may continue through the entire menstrual period.

Cause

Secondary dysmenorrhea may be caused by endometriosis, pelvic inflammatory disease, fibroid tumors, cervical polyps, adenomyosis, cervical stenosis or endometrial polyps.

The cause of primary dysmenorrhea is not well understood. There are a number of theories, each of which may partially explain primary dysmenorrhea. An old but popular theory holds that women with narrow cervical canals have cramps because the menstrual flow is obstructed. On one hand, the fact that bearing children or having a D&C, a surgical procedure in which the lining of the uterus is removed, both of which stretch the cervical opening, often relieves menstrual cramps seems to support this theory. On the other hand, the fact that X-ray studies of women who experience menstrual pain have failed to correlate cramps with narrow cervical canals, as well as the fact that many women with cervical stenosis don't experience menstrual pain, tend to discredit this theory.

Another theory holds that cramps occur because the uterus is excessively sensitive to progesterone. The uterus may have an allergic reaction to progesterone that causes it to contract sharply, leading to pain. This theory could account for the fact that primary dysmenorrhea often starts when ovulation first occurs, a year or two after the first menstrual period. This is when progesterone is first introduced into the body, and sensitivity would therefore be greatest at that time. It could also account for the fact that primary dysmenorrhea tends to become less severe as the woman gets older, for according to this theory, the uterus is desensitized to the progesterone over time and the allergic reaction is therefore less severe. Moreover, it could also account for the relief of pain that occurs in women who have borne children, for during pregnancy the body is flooded with progesterone, thus desensitizing the uterus and quelling the allergic reaction. This theory would, however, fail to account for the fact that cramps are experienced by some women who have borne children and by some women who use birth control pills and therefore don't ovulate or produce large amounts of progesterone. Another problem with this theory is that progesterone is thought to have a relaxing effect on the uterus.

Hormonal imbalances have long been blamed for menstrual cramps. Some researchers feel that spasmodic dysmenorrhea occurs when there is too much progesterone in relation to estrogen. By giving the woman extra estrogen they claim to relieve such cases. But not all doctors have had equally good results with this type of treatment. These same researchers also argue that congestive dysmenorrhea, or premenstrual tension, results from too much estrogen in relation to progesterone (in which case birth control pills would make the cramps worse). They therefore use progesterone to treat this type of menstrual pain. Again, not all doctors report equally good results, casting doubts on the ability of this theory to explain all cases of menstrual pain.

A theory that has received a lot of publicity lately is that menstrual cramps are the result of overproduction of substances called prostaglandins. There are many different types of prostaglandins in the body, and one type is apparently responsible for causing uterine contractions. Some studies have shown that women with menstrual cramps have higher levels of prostaglandins in their body, and antiprostaglandin medication has been effective in relieving pain in some, but not all, women with menstrual cramps.[4]

Despite the fact that so many women experience at least some amount of menstrual pain at some point in their lives, comparatively little research has been done in this area. Not surprisingly the old its-all-in-your-head-dearie diagnosis has been widely used to explain menstrual cramps. Some doctors point out that women whose mothers have a history of menstrual discomfort are more likely to suffer themselves, suggesting that such women may "learn" to have menstrual cramps because their mothers "made such a fuss." This interpretation of facts ignores the possibility that there is indeed some physical cause for menstrual cramps that may be an inherited problem.

While it is undoubtedly true that there are some women who consciously or unconsciously create their own menstrual pain, it is hardly logical to explain a phenomena as widespread as cramps as being psychological in origin. On some level it may be true that all disease has a psychological component; however, it is only in the field of gynecology, which deals with women's ailments, that medical science so readily accepts the notion that disease is psychosomatic and is so willing to ignore physical causes.

Diagnosis and Treatment

The first step in diagnosis is to obtain a thorough medical and menstrual history, including the type, severity and time of onset of pain and a description of any associated symptoms as well.

Next, the doctor should do a careful pelvic examination. If there are signs of endometriosis, fibroids, polyps, pelvic inflammatory disease or any of the other conditions that can cause secondary dysmenorrhea, the diagnostic procedures appropriate to those conditions should be done.

If these steps fail to turn up anything and the woman is over 25, making her a less likely candidate for primary dysmenorrhea, a more thorough investigation, including perhaps a D&C and/or laparoscopic examination, a method of examining the pelvic cavity by means of a lighted viewing instrument, may be in order to rule out the possibility that the cramps are due to some disease or abnormality known to cause secondary dysmenorrhea. Too many times such women are merely dismissed as neurotic and are not given a thorough diagnostic work-up. Women have a right to and should insist upon a complete work-up.

The treatment of secondary dysmenorrhea depends on the nature of the underlying cause. The various treatments are described under the appropriate headings elsewhere in this book.

The treatment of primary dysmenorrhea depends on the severity of the symptoms. A number of different natural or home remedies have proven successful. Sometimes having an orgasm, either by masturbation or by having sex with another person, can help relieve menstrual pain, for it relaxes the uterus and draws blood to the cramped muscles. Heat methods, such as hot baths, applying heat to the area and massaging the area, will, like orgasm, promote blood flow to the muscles and relax spasms. Yoga, pelvic exercises, deep breathing, acupuncture, acupressure and herbal remedies have all been used successfully. It should be noted, however, that herbal remedies are often powerful medicines and should be used only by people knowledgeable about herbs. For instance, pennyroyal, an herb used for menstrual cramps, can cause serious, even fatal, poisoning.

Another approach to treating cramps is the use of analgesics. The most popular analgesic, aspirin, will relieve the pain for some women. Interestingly, aspirin as well as being a pain reliever is an antiprostaglandin agent. Nonaspirin pain relievers such as Tylenol are also effective for some women. A number of other over-the-counter drugs, such as Midol, Pamprin, Trendar, Femicin, and Humphrey's No. 11, work for some women. They usually contain aspirin, caffeine, an antispasmodic and, sometimes, a diuretic. Alcohol is sometimes helpful. Prescription painkillers such as codeine compounds work for some women. Darvon and other prescription painkillers are often prescribed, although double-blind randomized studies have proven that Darvon is only slightly more effective than a sugar pill in relieving pain of any sort. In the past a drug called Edrisal, which contained aspirin and amphetamine, was available, but the FDA removed it from the market in an effort to control the prescription of amphetamines. Although amphetamines are dangerous drugs, their careful use may be justified in women who suffer from severe cramps and for whom other remedies are unsuccessful. A doctor can, of course, still write a prescription for the same amounts of amphetamine and other drugs that were contained in Edrisal, as long as the prescriptions are filed separately.

Birth control pills have been used to treat dysmenorrhea. They prevent ovulation and hence the production of progesterone, which may account for their effectiveness. Progesterone alone has been successful in treating women with spasmodic dysmenorrhea, while estrogen has been useful in treating congestive dysmenorrhea, or premenstrual tension. However, estrogen therapy may actually make the pain worse if prescribed for spasmodic dysmenorrhea, whereas progesterone may make congestive dysmenorrhea worse, so careful attention must be given to the type of symptoms before treatment is prescribed. Moreover, the safety of hormone therapy has been seriously questioned (*see* p. 103). Sometimes the hormones need only be prescribed for a few months, after which the woman's system may adjust itself. Short-term use of hormones may not involve as serious risks as prolonged use for purposes of birth control.

Recently, antiprostaglandin agents such as indomethacin (Indocin) have been studied and seem to be effective.[5] However, this drug may have unpleasant side effects in some women. Other antiprostaglandin medications such as naproxen (Naprosyn)[6] and mefenamic acid (Ponstel)[7] have been studied. These drugs seem to be effective in relieving pain but may not have any effect on the vomiting and diarrhea that some women experience. Doctors convinced of the efficacy of prostaglandin inhibitors also emphasize their safety and practicality relative to oral contraceptives. The prostaglandin inhibitors are needed only for one to three days, and in very low doses compared to oral contraceptives or hormones, which must be given for 21 days.

Another new treatment for menstrual cramps now being investigated involves dilating the cervix with a slender, dry rod of sterile seaweed called a lamanaria. The rod, which gradually expands as it absorbs water and dilates the cervix painlessly, is inserted in the doctor's office without an anesthetic and is left in place for about six hours.

A D&C, which may be done as part of the diagnostic work-up for menstrual pain, may also provide relief for some women. Another surgical procedure, known as a presacral neurectomy, in which the nerve passageways that transmit pain messages from the lower abdomen to the brain are severed, has been effective in preventing menstrual pain in 60-70 percent of the cases in which it has been tried; however, the operation involves risk and complications.[8] As with any operation requiring a general anesthetic, the possibility of fatal complications exists. Moreover, the surgery may result in damage to the sensory fibers of the bladder; a number of women gradually lose control of their bladder after the operation and experience problems in retaining urine that may last anywhere from a few weeks to a lifetime. It should also be noted that women who have this procedure done may not feel any contractions in the early stages of labor. This operation should be done only by a surgeon experienced in this type of therapy and only after less drastic forms of treatment have failed. Recently a new form of surgery called uterosacral ligament resection has been used.[9] This is thought by some doctors to have the same effect but without any interference, even temporarily, with bladder function. It has been effective in 75-80 percent of cases in which it has been tried and in women who have borne children can be done vaginally, without making an abdominal incision.

Sometimes it is hard for a woman to get adequate treatment for her menstrual cramps. In mild to moderate cases she may get nothing more than advice to "grin and bear it." If her pain is severe enough for her to persist in seeking treatment, she may wind up with a referral to a psychiatrist. All women, and particularly those over the age of 25, deserve a thorough gynecological investigation of their menstrual pain, for it may be the symptom of an underlying disease that needs treatment. Any woman whose doctor suggests psychiatric referral without first giving her an exhaustive diagnostic work-up as outlined above should find herself another doctor.

AMENORRHEA

AKA: absence of menstrual periods

Types: primary amenorrhea, delayed menarche, or delayed puberty
secondary amenorrhea
physiologic amenorrhea

Associated terms: cryptomenorrhea, galactorrhea, hirsutism

Amenorrhea means without (*a*) menstruation (*menorrhea*), or the absence of menstrual periods. Amenorrhea may be either primary or secondary. Primary amenorrhea, which is also called delayed puberty or delayed menarche, is defined as the failure to have a menstrual period by the age of 14, 16 or 18, depending on who's doing the defining. The majority of women will have had their first menstrual period by the age of 14. Some women, although they are completely normal, simply won't have theirs until the age of 16, and a small minority won't menstruate until age 18. There have been cases of completely normal women who didn't start menstruating until they were in their 20s, but, generally, failure to menstruate by the age of 18 is an indication that something is wrong. Certainly it would be wise to at least consult a doctor if menstruation fails to occur by the age of 14.

Secondary amenorrhea is the absence of menstrual periods in a woman who has previously menstruated. It is not uncommon for a woman to miss an occasional menstrual period, or even two or more in a row. For this reason most doctors define secondary amenorrhea as the absence of menstruation for a period of six months or longer. In our opinion, any woman who goes to the trouble and expense of consulting a doctor because

581

she is concerned about her failure to menstruate can legitimately consider herself as having amenorrhea. She deserves a complete physical exam and medical history and certainly, if pregnancy is even a remote possibility, a pregnancy test. If the physical exam or medical history leads the doctor to suspect one of the specific causes outlined below, appropriate tests should be done. If, however, as is often the case, no specific abnormalities suggest themselves and the woman is not particularly anxious to get pregnant, we recommend that she wait until she has missed her period for at least three to six months before subjecting herself to the progesterone withdrawal test (described below), a standard part of the diagnostic work-up. In most cases, this will prevent unnecessary doctor's visits and unnecessary use of progesterone, which carries certain risks (*see* p. 103), since most women will resume their periods normally within six months.

Another type of amenorrhea is known as physiologic amenorrhea. One obvious example of this would be pregnancy, for pregnant women do not menstruate.* Menopausal women also experience physiologic amenorrhea as they go through the change of life. After childbirth the majority of women do not menstruate for anywhere from six weeks to three months. If a woman is breastfeeding, this period of physiologic amenorrhea may be even longer. Some women don't menstruate again until they stop breastfeeding.

Symptoms

Amenorrhea is not, in and of itself, a disease, but it may be a symptom of some underlying hormonal problem, often an imbalance, which may either be serious or just a minor, temporary imbalance. Sometimes, depending on the underlying cause, other symptoms will occur along with the amenorrhea. For instance, some women with amenorrhea also have galactorrhea, a milky-white, watery discharge that can be expressed or may flow spontaneously from the nipples. Hirsutism—male hair-growth patterns—may appear in certain women with amenorrhea. The various other symptoms that may accompany amenorrhea are considered in more detail in the following discussion of causes.

Causes

As indicated by Table 22, amenorrhea can be caused by a multitude of factors. Some of these underlying causes fall within the realm of

*There is an occasional woman who has menstrual-type bleeding during the first month or two of pregnancy.

Table 22
Causes of Amenorrhea

Physiologic Causes:
    Pregnancy
    Childbirth
    Breastfeeding
    Menopause

End Organ Problems:
    Imperforate hymen
    Septate vagina
    Transverse vaginal septum
    Double vagina
    Congenital abnormalities of the
      uterus
    Cervical stenosis
    Vaginal stenosis
    Asherman's syndrome
    Congenital absence of the uterus

Ovarian Problems:
    Congenital developmental defects
    Congenital abnormalities of the
      ovary
    Premature menopause
    Benign ovarian tumors
    Malignant ovarian tumors
    Tubo-ovarian abscesses
    Functioning ovarian tumors
    Polycystic ovarian disease

Hypothalamic Problems:
    Emotional stress or shock
    Organic brain disease
    Idiopathic hypothalamic
     insufficiency
    Chiari-Frommel syndrome
    Birth control pills
    Drugs
    Anorexia nervosa
    Psychiatric problems

Pituitarian Problems:
    Simmonds' disease
    Sheehan's syndrome
    Pituitary tumors
    Hypogonadotropic eunuchoidism

Chronic Diseases:
    Tuberculosis
    Hepatitis
    Cirrhosis of the liver
    Other chronic systemic diseases

Pancreatic Problems:
    Diabetes (insufficiency in the
      pancreas)

Thyroid Problems:
    Hyperthyroidism
    Hypothyroidism

Adrenal Problems:
    Addison's disease
    Congenital adrenal hyperplasia
    Cushing's disease or syndrome

Other Causes:
    Malnutrition
    Excessive weight gain
    Excessive weight loss
    Rigorous athletic training

gynecology, and since they are discussed elsewhere in the book, they are mentioned only briefly here. Amenorrhea can also be caused by diseases or conditions that are not strictly gynecological, and these are discussed in more detail. It may be helpful to review Chapter Four before reading the following pages.

End Organ Problems

A woman's amenorrhea may be due to what is called an end organ problem, that is, one involving the uterus, cervix or vagina, and it may be either an acquired problem or a congenital one (one that has been present since birth). A woman may have an imperforate hymen, a condition in which a thin sheet of tissue completely covers the vaginal opening, so that no blood can escape. Or she may have a septate vagina, a transverse vaginal septum, a double vagina or a complete absence of the vagina, any of which could result in amenorrhea. Likewise she may have certain congenital abnormalities of the uterus or stenosis (blockage) of the cervix or of the vagina, which could also block the menstrual flow. In all of the conditions mentioned thus far, the woman may actually be menstruating and may notice cyclical signs of menstruation, such as weight gain, breast tenderness and mood swings, but no blood flow, due to the blockage. This is called cryptomenorrhea. The diagnosis can usually be made by physical examination, although certain types of uterine abnormalities may require more extensive diagnostic procedures.

Another type of end organ problem that can cause amenorrhea is a condition known as Asherman's syndrome, in which the endometrial lining has been damaged so badly that it can no longer respond to hormonal stimulation. A history of certain types of surgery coupled with a careful physical examination will lead to a diagnosis of Asherman's syndrome.

A woman may also miss her menstrual periods because she does not have a uterus. She may simply have been born without one or she may have a condition known as testicular feminization syndrome. A careful physical examination will reveal the fact that the woman doesn't have a uterus but won't tell the doctor which of these two conditions she has. Diagnosis of such women is discussed in more detail below.

Ovarian Problems

Amenorrhea may also be caused by problems involving the ovaries. If the ovaries are not working properly and thus are not producing the proper amounts of estrogen and progesterone, the woman may have amenorrhea. Women with congenital developmental defects such as Turner's syndrome, hermaphroditism or the testicular feminization syndrome mentioned above will have primary amenorrhea. Other congenital abnormalities of the ovary can also produce amenorrhea. In addition, a woman might have a premature menopause, the result of irradiation, surgery or other factors. The ovaries might be destroyed or impaired by benign or malignant ovarian tumors or a tubo-ovarian abcess. Certain ovarian tumors, called functioning ovarian tumors, can produce hormones and thus cause amenorrhea.

Hypothalamic Problems

Sometimes when the ovary is not producing its hormones it's because the ovary is not receiving proper stimulation from the pituitary gland. In some cases, the pituitary itself is the source of the problem. In other cases, the pituitary per se may be normal but may function improperly because *it* is not receiving sufficient stimulation from the hypothalamus. For instance, polycystic ovarian disease, a condition associated with amenorrhea in which the follicles in the ovary never release their eggs, may be due to either a problem in the ovary itself or to a problem in the hypothalamus.

There are a number of reasons why the hypothalamus could fail to function properly, for it is a finely tuned organ that is sensitive to all sorts of outside events. Indeed, the hypothalamus is so sensitive that even the sound of a baby crying in the next room is sometimes enough to trigger substances within it that could, in turn, cause milk to flow from a nursing mother's breasts. In a similar fashion stress, perhaps from the death of someone close or from problems at work or with love relationships, can cause a woman to miss one or more periods. This may be due to some sort of protective mechanism cleverly designed by mother nature to prevent us from adding the demands of pregnancy to our bodies when we are stressed and therefore have lowered resistance to disease or other abnormalities. Less dramatic types of emotional stress may also cause amenorrhea, presumably because of the effect on the hypothalamus. Even after the initial stress has passed, the amenorrhea may persist, for the hypothalamus may not get back into synch all by itself.

Hypothalamic amenorrhea is also associated with anorexia nervosa, a condition that most often occurs in adolescents and women in their early 20s. The woman develops a distaste or aversion for food and consequently eats nothing or next to nothing, losing a great deal of weight. Unlike the woman with Simmonds' disease (discussed below), a woman with anorexia nervosa is not usually lethargic and may have a considerable amount of energy. The loss of weight and extreme malnutrition may be the cause of the amenorrhea, but in most cases the amenorrhea precedes the dramatic loss in weight. In 10-20 percent of cases, anorexia nervosa results in irreversible, fatal malnutrition. If the woman can regain her normal weight, which sometimes requires hospitalization and intravenous feeding, menstruation may be restored.

Although anorexia nervosa is commonly held to be the result of a psychological disturbance, one wonders about the accuracy of this diagnosis. It is true that the hypothalamus is profoundly influenced by emotional states, and as we have seen, psychological stress or problems can and undoubtedly do disrupt its normal functioning. However, it may be that some supposedly psychologically caused conditions are the result of an as yet mysterious organic disruption of normal glandular process. Certainly, in this case, the fact that the amenorrhea precedes the weight loss and that patients who are receiving certain forms of cancer treatment often experience anorexia nervosa, presumably because of drug or radiation upset to their systems, should alert us to the possibility that there may be a physical cause for this disease.

In general, women diagnosed as having psychogenic amenorrhea who do not have a history of psychological stress should view this diagnosis with a good deal of skepticism. In the future, medical science may find, just as we have found with menstrual cramps, that so-called psychological problems have a physiological basis. Even removing the stigma of "psychological problem" from the diagnosis could provide a certain relief. In the case of anorexia nervosa, for instance, it might help relieve parental guilt and thus temper the parents' incessant and unsuccessful efforts to nag the patient into eating.

Hypothalamic amenorrhea can also be caused by prolonged use of certain drugs. Some women who have used birth control pills for long periods of time stop menstruating once the Pill is discontinued. There is some disagreement as to whether this post-Pill amenorrhea is actually caused by the birth control pill, since many of the women who experience it had irregular menstrual patterns before going on the Pill. At any rate, most of the women with post-Pill amenorrhea eventually resume menstruation. Some, however, do not, and such women may also experience premature menopause.

Certain drugs used to treat psychiatric problems, some tranquilizers and some of the drugs used to treat hypertension, a condition characterized by high blood pressure, may, if used for long periods of time, cause amenorrhea. Heroin addicts and women on methadone may also have amenorrhea. Most cases of drug or medicine-related amenorrhea will revert to normal once the drug is discontinued.

There are a number of other factors that can cause the hypothalamus to malfunction. Organic brain disease, which can be caused by encephalitis, a viral infection of the brain, other related infections, head injuries, scars, tumors and exposure to poisonous substances all can interfere with hypothalamic function and hence produce amenorrhea. A history of such disease, along with symptoms such as unconsciousness, dizziness, headache, bleeding from the mouth, nose or ears, vomiting, drowsiness, confusion and/or fever, will help the doctor make the diagnosis. If the underlying problem can be treated, the menstrual cycle will usually return to normal. If, however, portions of the brain have been permanently damaged, it may be necessary to give the woman some form of oral medication to take the place of the substances her body is unable to produce (see below).

Some women are apparently born with a hypothalamus that just doesn't secrete the usual amounts of hormone-releasing factors or that is particularly sensitive to the "turn-off" messages that are sent to it by means of ovarian hormones at certain points in the menstrual cycle. In medical jargon, this is known as idiopathic hypothalamic insufficiency. Such women will have amenorrhea punctuated by an occasional menstrual period. There is often a family history of menstrual irregularities. Once the diagnosis has been clearly established (see below), there is usually no need to treat these women.

Another type of amenorrhea thought to be related to a problem in the hypothalamus is the Chiari-Frommel syndrome. It occurs in women after childbirth. Galactorrhea, in which there is a milky-white discharge from the nipples, accompanies the amenorrhea in these women. Such women are usually somewhat overweight and may have some excessive hair growth. The uterus and ovaries are small. It is thought that the factor in the hypothalamus that normally supresses the pituitary hormone prolactin (which causes the breast to produce milk) is absent. Without this inhibiting factor from the hypothalamus the pituitary overproduces prolactin. This throws the rest of the hormone balance out of whack, causing amenorrhea. Diagnosis is made by the symptoms, the history of childbirth and X-rays to rule out a pituitary tumor. The Chiari-Frommel syndrome is often resistant to treatment.

Pituitary Problems

The pituitary gland itself can also be the source of the problem, even if the hypothalamus is functioning normally. There may be an insufficiency of pituitary hormones as a result of either Simmonds' disease or Sheehan's syndrome. Simmonds' disease, which usually occurs after traumatic or infected childbirth but which may occasionally be caused in other ways, involves destruction of the pituitary gland. The woman with Simmonds' disease may have amenorrhea, a smaller uterus, postmenopausal vaginitis, a decline in breast size and other symptoms of menopause, due to ovarian failure. Such failure is the result of insufficent stimulation of the ovary by the pituitary hormones. The thyroid gland also is insufficiently stimulated, and any of the symptoms of hypothyroidism (described below) may also appear. There may be a deterioration of connective and muscle tissue. Typically, the hair begins to fall out, first from the armpits and later from the scalp and pubic area. The woman may give the appearance of having aged prematurely and may be severely emaciated.

Sheehan's syndrome, which is also associated with blood loss and shock due to childbirth or severe infection after childbirth, likewise results in damage to the pituitary gland, though usually not as extensive as in Simmonds' disease. However, the woman with Sheehan's syndrome is apt to maintain her body weight or to become overweight. It may take years for the symptoms of Sheehan's disease to become obvious. The classic symptoms include amenorrhea, inability to produce breast milk, menopausal-type changes in the vagina and uterus, loss of armpit and pubic hair, gradual thinning of the eyebrows, dry, pale skin that is sensitive to cold and does not perspire, loss of appetite, vomiting, a tendency to spells of weakness and fainting and lethargy.

Diagnosis of both of these conditions is suggested by the symptoms and a history of bleeding and infection associated with childbirth, it may be confirmed by laboratory tests. Treatment will depend on the extent of the damage to the pituitary gland. Cortisone-type drugs to replace the missing pituitary hormones may be given. Estrogen replacement therapy may be given to make up for the lack of ovarian hormone. Progesterone-type drugs may be given as well. Thyroid may be given to make up for the lack of natural thyroid. Women with minimal Sheehan's syndrome may only need temporary replacement therapy, for after a rest, the unimpaired portions of the pituitary gland may resume function and the woman may return to normal. For some women, however, cortisone, estrogen and thyroid therapy may have to be continued. Sometimes, although the estrogen, thyroid and cortisone therapy may relieve the symptoms, including the amenorrhea, a cure may not be possible, and in some cases death can occur.

Pituitary tumors can cause amenorrhea. Such women may have headaches and visual disturbances as well, although these may appear only in the late stages. A slow-growing tumor might be present for years before these two symptoms appeared. One type of pituitary tumor, called a chromophobe adenoma, produces amenorrhea because it destroys so much of the pituitary gland. Sometimes these tumors produce the hormone prolactin and the woman may have a milky discharge from her breasts, in which case the term "Forbes-Albright syndrome" is used to describe the condition.

Another type of pituitary tumor, the acidophilic adenoma, is associated with amenorrhea. Women with this condition may also have a condition known as acromegaly, in which the hands, feet, nose and lower jaw grow excessively large due to a disturbance of growth hormones. The tumors are radiosensitive and are often treated by radiation therapy. Menstrual periods generally resume after successful treatment, but if the pituitary has been destroyed, the amenorrhea will persist.

In addition to these pituitary diseases and tumors, there are apparently some women who are born with a pituitary that is not capable of producing the proper amounts of hormones. This is referred to as hypogonadotrophic eunuchoidism. Diagnosis involves a complete hormone work-up by a specialist (see below).

Pancreatic Problems

Disturbances in the pancreas, the gland that produces substances to help the body convert the food we eat into a usable form, can also cause amenorrhea. Women who have diabetes mellitus, a disease in which the pancreas fails to produce the hormone insulin, so that the body is unable to metabolize nutriments—in particular, to utilize sugar properly—may have amenorrhea, although excessive menstrual bleeding is a more common symptom for such women. Other symptoms may include excessive thirst, urination or hunger; weight loss; generalized weakness; skin disorders; yeast infections of the vagina; blurred vision; numbness; dry mouth; and cramps in the legs. Diagnosis is made by blood tests. Proper diet and exercise may control mild forms of the disease. Medication, usually insulin by mouth or injection, may be required. Amenorrhea should disappear with successful treatment of the diabetes.

Thyroid Problems

Excessive or inadequate amounts of thyroid, conditions known as hyperthyroidism and hypothyroidism respectively, may both be associated with menstrual abnormalities, including amenorrhea.

Hypothyroidism may be caused by a birth defect, and such children may have impaired mental and physical development. The disease may also be acquired later in life as a result of destruction of the thyroid gland through radiation or surgery, too much or too little iodine in the diet or certain drugs and foods; however, the cause is not always clear. Symptoms may include apathy; sluggishness; increased sensitivity to cold; brittle hair; low, husky voice; dry, cool rough skin; puffy hands, face and eyelids; discolored fingernails; weak muscles; slow pulse rate; weight gain; slow reflexes; constipation; and anemia. The symptoms may be mild or severe. Diagnosis is made by specific tests used to measure thyroid levels. Treatment consists of iodine supplements, which may succeed in some cases, but daily thyroid tablets are usually necessary.

Hyperthyroidism, whose exact cause is unknown, may cause an enlarged thyroid gland; nervousness; emotional outbursts; excessive sweating; intolerance to heat; hyperactivity; weight loss; weakness; tiredness; thin hair; diarrhea; warm, moist smooth skin; rapid pulse; bulging eyes; and vision disturbances. Diagnosis is made on the basis of the amenorrhea and other symptoms and confirmed by special tests designed to measure thyroid levels. Treatment may include surgical removal of part of the thyroid gland or radiation treatment.

Adrenal Problems

Over- or underproduction of the adrenal glands may also cause amenorrhea. In the past, tuberculosis infections were responsible for most cases of Addison's disease, in which there is underactivity of the adrenal glands. Today, with TB under control, wasting of the glands from unknown causes, a tumor, infection or insufficient pituitary hormones are the main causes of Addison's disease. Symptoms include weakness, lethargy, nausea, vomiting, abdominal pain, drop in blood pressure, depression, anemia and irritability. The disease may develop slowly, and severe attacks may be brought on by stress, injury or infection. Diagnosis is made by the symptoms, which indicate to the doctor that tests measuring adrenal hormone levels in the blood and in urine should be done. Once the tests have confirmed the diagnosis, treatment involves daily doses of the adrenal hormones. Although women may have amenorrhea in the later stages of Addison's disease, it is not clear whether this is actually due to the lack of adrenal hormones or to associated malnutrition.

Overproduction of the adrenal glands can also cause amenorrhea. One cause of such overproduction is a condition known as congenital adrenal hyperplasia. Such women usually have deformities of the external genitals. For instance, the clitoris may be enlarged and may resemble the tip of a penis. The condition may be diagnosed at birth, or at puberty when male hair-patterns develop and menstruation fails to occur. Milder forms may not be recognized until later in life, when whiskers, chest hair and other male-type hair patterns appear in the woman. The breasts may get smaller, the clitoris may enlarge, baldness and acne may occur, the voice can deepen and a male-type body structure may develop. The menstrual cycle is altered until, finally, menstruation stops altogether. Treatment may include the removal of the tumor or one or both adrenal glands; in rare cases, radiation of the pituitary may be recommended.

Conditions known as Cushing's disease, or Cushing's syndrome, are also associated with amenorrhea. These conditions may be caused by tumors in the pituitary or in the adrenal glands or by other problems in the pituitary or adrenals. Women with these conditions may bruise easily and have male hair-growth patterns, acne, a deepening of the voice, muscle weakness and smaller breasts, uterus and ovaries. These women are typically overweight. They tend to have large abdomens but thin arms and legs and a round "moon" face. They may have pads of fat over their shoulders, a condition that has been described as "buffalo hump." They may have purplish lines or stretch marks, called striae, in certain areas of their bodies. Diagnosis is made by the physical appearance and confirmed by laboratory tests.

Treatment depends on the exact site of the problem and may include surgical removal of the tumor, removal of one or more of the adrenal glands or, in rare cases, irradiation of the pituitary gland. Symptoms usually regress after treatment.

Chronic Disease

Chronic diseases may exert their influence on proper hormone interaction between the pituitary, hypothalamus and ovaries and thus be associated with amenorrhea. Tuberculosis, for instance, can cause amenorrhea, either through a specific attack on the ovary or uterus or through its effects on the whole system.

Since hormones are eliminated from the body through the urine, a chronic kidney disease called nephritis, which interferes with this normal elimination process, can alter the proper hormone balance and result in amenorrhea. In addition to amenorrhea, symptoms may include puffiness of the face, eyelids and ankles, a swollen abdomen, high blood pressure, headache, insomnia, poor vision, excessive urination at night, anemia and shortness of breath. Diagnosis is confirmed by urine tests, which may show blood and certain proteins in the urine. Treatment includes bed rest; a high-vitamin, low-salt diet; sedatives and medication to control high blood pressure; iron compounds for anemia; and, in extreme cases, blood transfusions. If the kidney is severely damaged, hemodialysis, in which blood is circulated through an artificial kidney machine that washes the blood clean of wastes and poisons, may be necessary. If the disease itself can be treated, the amenorrhea will usually disappear.

Similarly, the liver plays a role in metabolizing estrogen. Disturbances in liver function, such as cirrhosis of the liver, a condition that is usually associated with alcholism but is occasionally caused by B-virus hepatitis, can result in excessive menstrual bleeding, followed by periods of amenorrhea. Other symptoms include nausea, vomiting, gas, weight loss, liver enlargement, bad breath, puffiness of the feet and legs, reddened palms, enlarged blood vessels in the chest and shoulders, swollen abdomen, nose bleeds, hemorrhoids, vomiting of blood and blood in the feces. The treatment includes abstinence from alcohol, a diet rich in proteins and low in salt, and medications to help the body eliminate fluids. A woman who has such severe cirrhosis that she misses her menstrual periods may not resume menstruation.

Other Causes

Excessive and rapid weight gain or weight loss or poor eating habits and malnutrition may cause amenorrhea. Women athletes involved in unusually strenuous conditioning programs sometimes experience amenorrhea. This is because they have altered the ratio of body fat and muscle in their bodies and a certain proportion of fat is apparently necessary for ovulation.

Diagnosis and Treatment

As we have seen, amenorrhea can be caused by a number of different factors. Diagnosis, then, is pretty much a process of elimination and involves trying to identify the cause or at least to rule out the more grave possibilities. Once the cause has been identified, proper treatment, if indeed treatment is actually needed, can be given.

A careful medical history, physical exam and bimanual pelvic exam are the first steps in diagnosis. A pregnancy test should also be done, to rule out that possibility. A careful medical history is quite important, but some doctors don't spend a sufficient amount of time on it. This is another instance in which nurse practitioners can be of great value, for they can afford to take the time to get a really thorough history. For instance, past psychological stress may have thrown the hypothalamus out of whack, and although the stress may have passed, the hypothalamus may simply never have gotten back in synch. Careful questioning in the course of a thorough medical history might reveal such a situation. Similarly, a history of diabetes in the family, an abortion, a D&C, difficulties in childbirth, rapid weight gain or loss, poor eating habits and other suggestive information that could point to a diagnosis may be discovered in the course of a thorough medical history. The age of the woman, a recent history of childbirth or breast-feeding may point to physiologic causes. A bimanual pelvic exam may rule out end organ problems or detect ovarian tumors or abcesses.

If a woman has been taking birth control pills, she may have post-Pill amenorrhea, so the doctor should ask the woman if she has had any nipple discharge and carefully examine the woman's breasts trying to express any discharge. If there is or has been a discharge, then the woman requires further testing, which is described in the section on galactorrhea. If the woman has no nipple discharge problem, then the doctor will want to know how long ago she stopped taking the Pill. If she has been off the Pill for less than six months, the doctor will not usually do anything, for the vast majority of women who have troubles with amenorrhea after they stop the Pill will resume menstruation by the time six months have passed. If, however, she fails to resume menstruation after six months, she should return to the doctor at that time for further diagnostic work-up, as described below.

Sometimes the physical exam will reveal the classic signs of pituitary, adrenal or thyroid problems, in which case the doctor will prescribe certain tests that can lead to a diagnosis. If the woman has the signs of Cushing's disease, for instance, the doctor should do a simple test known as a dexamethasone suppression test.[10] At 11 PM the woman takes one mg of a drug called dexamethasone by mouth. She may also be given a tranquilizer. Between 8 AM and 9 AM the next morning, she reports to the doctor and has a blood sample taken and then analyzed. If the level of the substances measured in this test are low, then she does not have Cushing's disease. If they are high, she may or may not have Cushing's and must be referred to a specialist known as a medical endocrinologist for a more complex and more expensive series of tests. Some doctors neglect to do this simple dexamethasone screening test and either refer the woman directly to a specialist or immediately order the more elaborate, expensive series of tests. Any woman with amenorrhea and symptoms suggestive of Cushing's syndrome whose doctor orders the extensive tests or refers her to a specialist without first doing the simpler test should discuss this with her doctor and should consider getting a second medical opinion (*see* p. 226) before undergoing more elaborate testing.

If the dexamethasone suppression test results show high levels, the woman, along with anyone who shows signs of specific pituitary or adrenal problems, will need a complete endocrinology work-up, with elaborate urine and blood tests. Hospitalization, in order to draw blood from certain veins deep inside the body, may be necessary, but this is rare. Although in the past many women were subjected to these tests, most of them were unnecessary. Today a simple test, known as a progesterone-withdrawal, or progesterone-challenge test, which is described below, is done instead.

If the physical exam, medical history or accompanying symptoms fail to indicate the cause of the amenorrhea, then the woman will fall into one of three groups. The characteristics of each of these groups, along with the appropriate diagnostic steps, are outlined in Table 23 on pages 594-96 and are explained in detail in the following text.

Here again, jotting down notes on the terminology and abbreviations used to describe the menstrual cycle and keeping the notes handy will help you to sort through the somewhat complex process of diagnosing amenorrhea.

Group One

In the first group are those women with primary amenorrhea (that is, they've never had a period) who have a normal uterus and cervix but do not have the secondary sex characteristics, like breast development and pubic hair, that normally appear during puberty in response to rising levels of estrogen. The first step is to do a hormone test, known as a serum FSH,

Table 23
Diagnosing Amenorrhea

Physical Signs and Symptoms

Group One

Woman with:
- primary amenorrhea
- normal uterus
- no breast development or other secondary sex characteristics
- no nipple discharge

Do a serum FSH test

Low levels of FSH → High levels of FSH

Low levels of FSH → Hypothalamic or pituitary problem—Do GRFR stimulation test

High levels of FSH → Ovarian problem—Do karyotype to detect abnormal chromosomes

No response | Normal response | Abnormal karyotype | Normal karyotype

Pituitary problem: refer to specialist for complete work-up to rule out tumors or other pituitary disease.

Hypothalamic problem: refer to specialist to rule out brain tumors or other brain abnormalities.

Congenital chromosomal abnormality of the ovary: possibly Turner's syndrome. Treat as necessary.

Diagnosis: primary ovarian failure. See Premature menopause.

that measures levels of FSH, the follicle-stimulating hormone from the pituitary that stimulates the follicles inside the ovary to produce estrogen. Women who don't have secondary sex characteristics are lacking in estrogen. The doctor wants to know whether this lack of estrogen is the result of a problem in the ovary or in the brain, either in the pituitary or in the hypothalamus.

If the FSH test comes back indicating high levels of FSH, the doctor knows that the pituitary and hypothalamus are both doing their part, for if they weren't, the FSH levels would be low. So it must be that it is the ovary that is for some reason failing to produce estrogen. Unfortunately, not all

Table 23
Diagnosing Amenorrhea

Physical Signs and Symptoms

Group Two

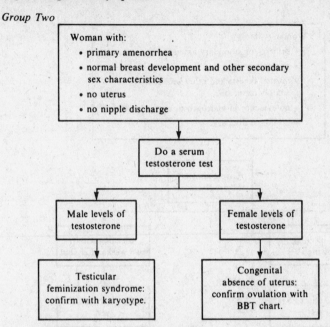

```
Woman with:
  • primary amenorrhea
  • normal breast development and other secondary
    sex characteristics
  • no uterus
  • no nipple discharge
```

```
Do a serum
testosterone test
```

```
Male levels of        Female levels of
testosterone          testosterone
```

```
Testicular            Congenital
feminization syndrome:  absence of uterus:
confirm with karyotype.  confirm ovulation with
                      BBT chart.
```

doctors have a clear understanding of how hormones work in the female body. Some doctors will mistakenly refer women with high FSH levels to a medical center for an elaborate series of tests looking for tumors or other brain abnormalities when the problem is actually in the ovary.* Women (or parents of these females, for they are often young girls) who have primary amenorrhea, normal uteri, no secondary sex characteristics and high FSH levels should seek a second opinion if the doctor recommends X-ray studies.

If the FSH is high, the next step is to do a karyotype, which is a study of the chromosomes. If the karyotype is abnormal, then the doctor knows (depending on the exact nature of the test results) that the woman has Turner's syndrome or one of the other congenital developmental abnormalities of the ovary. If the karyotype is normal, the doctor will suspect primary ovarian failure. Treatment of these conditions is discussed in detail elsewhere, and may include some form of estrogen replacement therapy to stimulate secondary sex characteristics.

If the FSH is low, this indicates that the pituitary isn't making enough

*There is no such thing as an FSH-producing brain tumor.

Table 23
Diagnosing Amenorrhea

Physical Signs and Symptoms

Group Three

FSH to stimulate the ovaries to make estrogen; hence, there are no secondary sex characteristics. This may be due to a malfunctioning pituitary that isn't producing enough hormone to stimulate the ovary. Or, it may be due to a malfunctioning hypothalamus that isn't producing enough of its FSH-releasing factor. Without the FSH-releasing factor from the hypothalamus, the pituitary can't produce FSH, which in turn means no estrogen from the ovaries and, again, no menstrual periods or secondary sex characteristics.

It should also be noted that some women may get back FSH test results that indicate FSH levels in the normal range. These are not actually normal, but what doctors call pseudonormal, for they are actually low for the particular woman's body.[11]

A further test may be done to tell whether the problem is in the hypothalamus or the pituitary. This test is done by injecting some of the releasing factor substances normally made by the hypothalamus into the woman's body and then doing blood tests to measure the levels of pituitary hormones in her body. It is called a gonadotropin-releasing-factor response (GRFR) test. If there is no response to the test, the doctor will know that it is the pituitary gland that is not doing its job and will refer the woman to a specialist who will do X-rays and other tests to rule out the possibility of a brain tumor or other pituitary abnormalities. If the GRFR test results are normal, then the doctor will know that the pituitary is quite capable of responding to these releasing factors. There must, then, be an insufficiency of releasing factors from the hypothalamus. Again, a specialist is needed to perform certain tests to rule out brain tumors. Depending on the results of the test, the woman may be given replacement therapy, that is, drugs to replace the substances her body is unable to produce.

Group Two

In the next group of women are those who have primary amenorrhea (that is, they have never had a period), and who do have normal breast development and other secondary sex characteristics, but who on physical examination turn out to be missing a uterus. These women fall into one of two categories: those who were simply born without a uterus, a condition known as congenital absence of the uterus, and those with testicular feminization syndrome, a condition associated with chromosomal abnormalities in which a woman normal in other ways has male-type testicular tissue instead of ovaries. Women with the syndrome need to have this testicular-type tissue removed because it is subject to cancerous tumors, so it is important to distinguish between the two conditions. This is done by giving a blood test known as a serum testosterone test.

If the test shows that the woman has female levels of the hormone testosterone in her body, then the doctor can be fairly sure that the woman has congenital absence of the uterus. Such women usually ovulate and don't require estrogen replacement therapy. A careful questioning may reveal that the woman has cyclical swelling of the breasts, weight gain, mood changes or other symptoms related to the menstrual cycle, which would indicate that the ovaries and other hormone-producing organs are functioning properly and that it is just the absence of the uterus that is causing the problem. A basal body temperature chart will confirm the diagnosis.

If the testosterone serum levels are at male levels, then the diagnosis of testicular feminization can be confirmed by a karyotype test, which will reveal the chromosomal abnormalities characteristic of women with this condition. The testicular-type tissue must be removed because of the potential of developing cancer. Again, the woman may be put on estrogen replacement therapy; however, estrogen involves certain risks, so it must be used with caution.

Group Three

In the third group are women with either primary or secondary amenorrhea, a normal uterus, normal breasts and other secondary sex characteristics, no signs of adrenal problems (excessive hair growth, etc.) and no nipple discharge. This is by far the largest of the three groups. These women should have, as the first step in diagnosis, a simple progesterone-withdrawal test. They should not allow themselves to be subjected to the expense, inconvenience and risk of a complete work-up (which may include blood and urine tests and X-rays) unless this simple test has first been done. On the other hand, women with secondary amenorrhea (women who have menstruated previously) but no other symptoms should probably not have a progesterone-withdrawal test done until they have missed at least three, or possibly six, periods, for the use of progesterone carries certain risks (*see* p. 103) and the shot can be quite painful. Because of the possibility of birth defects caused by progesterone, no one should have this test unless pregnancy has been ruled out by the most sensitive tests (*see* p. 756).

The first thing the doctor wants to know is whether or not the woman is making estrogen. That is why she is given the shot of progesterone. The progesterone will gradually be excreted by the body over a two-week period. As the levels of progesterone fall, the endometrial lining, which you will recall from Chapter Four is built up by estrogen in the first place, will break down and be shed, causing bleeding from the uterus.

Bleeding Following Progesterone Shot

If the woman does start bleeding (usually within two weeks), this will tell the doctor that the ovary is indeed producing estrogen, for if it weren't, there wouldn't be any endometrial lining to be shed and hence there wouldn't be any bleeding. If bleeding does occur, the doctor also knows that the pituitary gland is functioning normally, for without the proper follicle-stimulating hormone from the pituitary, the follicles in the ovary wouldn't be stimulated to produce their estrogen and, again, there would be no endometrial lining and thus no bleeding after the progesterone shot.

Since the woman who bleeds following the progesterone-withdrawal test isn't lacking estrogen, the doctor knows that her problem must be a lack of the other hormone that regulates the menstrual cycle, progesterone. The next step is to figure out *why* she is lacking progesterone. There are two possibilities. The first is that the woman has polycystic ovarian disease, a condition in which the egg follicles that produce estrogen never make it to the surface of the ovary to release their eggs at ovulation. Since the follicle never bursts open, the corpus luteum, which is formed from the remnants of the burst follicle after ovulation, never develops. The absence of the corpus luteum, whose job it is to produce progesterone in the second half of the cycle, accounts for the lack of this hormone in women with this condition. Although these women do produce enough estrogen to stimulate the growth of the endometrium and to trigger the surge of luteinizing hormone (LH) that would normally trigger ovulation, some other factor, perhaps something in the follicle itself, prevents the LH from causing ovulation, so that there is no progesterone.

The second possible explanation for a woman's inability to produce progesterone is that the ovary is simply not getting enough luteinizing hormone, so that there is not enough stimulation to cause the follicle to burst open and release its egg. Again, without ovulation there is no corpus luteum and therefore no progesterone. Theoretically, the lack of luteinizing hormone could be due to a problem in the pituitary or hypothalamus. However, since the woman has bled following the shot of progesterone, the doctor already knows the pituitary is functioning normally or, as outlined above, she would not have estrogen and would not have bled. Thus, her problem must be in the hypothalamus.

In order to tell whether the problem is in the hypothalamus or in the ovary, the next step is to do a blood test to measure levels of luteinizing hormone. This test is called a serum LH. If the test indicates high levels of LH, then the doctor knows the woman has polycystic ovarian disease. The explanation for the diagnosis is as follows: In polycystic ovarian disease, the pituitary is constantly sending out FSH, which keeps stimulating more follicles to develop and thus creates high levels of estrogen (which is made in the follicle). The high levels of estrogen keep stimulating the pituitary to produce luteinizing hormone, so the woman has high levels of this hormone as well. Since there is no progesterone to tell the pituitary to "stop producing FSH," the pituitary continues to churn out both FSH and LH. This series of events is confirmed by the serum LH test. Once the diagnosis of polycystic ovarian disease is indicated by the high LH levels, treatment, which is described under the heading Polycystic Ovarian Disease, may be given.

The serum LH test may also indicate low levels of luteinizing hormone. It should be noted that some women may get back test results that indicate the LH is in the normal range, but the LH is not really normal.[12] Here again, it is what doctors call pseudonormal and is really low for that particular woman. Low or pseudonormal LH levels indicate a problem in the hypothalamus. There is some LH because there is estrogen that is stimulating the pituitary to put out a certain amount of LH. But there is not enough LH to trigger ovulation because the hypothalamus is not producing its luteinizing-hormone—releasing factor (LHRF), without which the pituitary is unable to produce the surge of LH that causes ovulation.

This woman does not, however, need a work-up to detect brain tumors or other such abnormalities, for the fact that the hypothalamus is producing follicle-stimulating—releasing factors (as evidenced by the fact that the pituitary is indeed releasing FSH, which in turn is causing the ovary to produce estrogen, as demonstrated by the fact that the woman bled following the shot of progesterone) shows that a serious abnormality is not present. These are the cases in which the women have psychological stress problems, weight gains or losses or other problems that are not well understood. These women will often resume menstruation on their own accord. Generally, treatment involves inducing a menstrual period every two to three months by giving oral progesterone. This will prevent the uterine lining from growing too thick, a condition known as endometrial hyperplasia that is sometimes a precursor to cancer, and will also serve as a follow-up, a way of checking to see that the woman is indeed still producing estrogen.

It should be noted that some women will have long periods of amenorrhea punctuated by an occasional menstrual period. This can be the result of any one of the problems outlined earlier or it may simply be normal for that woman's body. Her hypothalamus may simply work differently. If serious problems have been ruled out, and pregnancy is not a concern, then these women don't need treatment.

Before discussing the woman who fails to bleed from the shot of progesterone, a word or two about the progesterone shot itself is in order.

As noted earlier, in the past women were given a battery of fancy tests instead of the shot of progesterone. There are still some doctors who prescribe these tests, but in the vast majority of women with amenorrhea they are unnecessary; 50 cents' worth of progesterone will do the trick.

A particular type of progesterone, called IM progesterone, is used for this purpose. Depo-Provera, Delalutin and other, similar progesterones cannot be used for this purpose because when they are given by injection, they often cause long periods of amenorrhea.

600

The IM progesterone can be given mixed either with oil or with water; however, progesterone mixed with water has caused abscesses in some women, so oil is preferred.[13] Usually 100 mg of IM progesterone is injected into the buttocks. This should cause the woman to bleed within two weeks.

If the woman fails to bleed from a 100 mg injection, the doctor will give a second injection of 200 mg. Some doctors will give the 200 mg right away, but most women who are going to bleed will do so on 100 mg, and since the 200 mg shot can be rather painful, the doctor will usually try 100 mg first, unless the woman lives far away. Rubbing down the area where the shot is given for the first couple of hours afterward can help eliminate much of the subsequent discomfort.

Women who are given progesterone shots may bleed quite noticeably, or there may be only a slight brownish staining. This slight brownish staining is also blood. It is brown because it is old blood, but it is still a sign that estrogen is being produced, so women should examine their underclothes carefully to make sure they don't miss this vital sign.

After being given the shot of progesterone, the woman is then asked to return to the doctor's office in three weeks. One of two things will have happened: either the woman will have had bleeding, as we have discussed, or she will not have had any bleeding.

Failure to Bleed Following Progesterone Shot

The woman who fails to bleed following the shot of progesterone has a somewhat more serious problem. The next test the doctor should do is a serum FSH. If the FSH is high, this indicates (in the woman who has failed to bleed from a shot of progesterone) that the ovaries have failed, for there is plenty of FSH to stimulate the follicles and produce estrogen. The problem is in the ovary, and this woman has premature menopause.

If the woman fails to bleed following the shot of progesterone but the FSH levels are low or pseudonormal, then this woman has a problem in either the pituitary, which is the source of FSH, or the hypothalamus, which is indirectly responsible for FSH production. She must be referred to a specialist for X-rays and other studies to rule out a tumor or other abnormality.

Once a woman with amenorrhea has received a complete diagnostic work-up, as described above, treatment may be given. In those cases where brain tumors or disease have been ruled out but the woman remains amenorrheic, menstruation may be induced every few months as follow-up and to prevent hyperplasia. If, however, these women want to get pregnant and are not ovulating because of a hormone imbalance, it is sometimes possible to use fertility drugs to achieve pregnancy.

ABNORMAL UTERINE BLEEDING

Types: anatomical uterine bleeding
dysfunctional uterine bleeding

Associated Terms: hypomenorrhea, hypermenorrhea, oligomenorrhea, polymenorrhea, menorrhagia, intermenstrual bleeding, contact bleeding, metorrhagia, postmenopausal bleeding, breakthrough bleeding, withdrawal bleeding

Abnormal uterine bleeding is not really a disease but a symptom. It may be caused by a wide variety of factors, and sometimes its exact cause is not understood. The bleeding may vary from mild to severe and may take on a number of different patterns. It may be indicative of a serious problem or may be only a temporary, minor problem. Any persistent abnormalities in the usual monthly bleeding pattern or unexpected vaginal bleeding should be brought to a doctor's attention.

Incidence

Abnormal bleeding is common in young women who have just begun to menstruate, for their cycles have not yet stabilized. It is also common during menopause, when the menstrual cycle is tapering off.

Types and Causes

Abnormal uterine bleeding may take many different forms. The menstrual period may be disturbed. The flow may be scanty (hypomenorrhea) or it may be excessive, requiring more than six to eight napkins or tampons a day to control the flow (hypermenorrhea). The interval between periods (which may range from 20 to 36 or 40 days and still be considered normal) may be excessively long (oligomenorrhea), or too short (polymenorrhea). If the bleeding is profuse and the period is prolonged as well, the term "menorrhagia" is used.

The menstrual period may be late and the bleeding very heavy. This can happen with an ectopic pregnancy or a miscarriage. Women who don't ovulate for one reason or another may also have this sort of bleeding pattern.

The bleeding may occur at regular intervals, but it might be prolonged or heavy. Pelvic inflammatory disease, endometrial polyps, fibroid tumors, and adenomyosis are all examples of diseases or conditions that could cause this type of abnormal uterine bleeding. The use of an IUD may be a factor. Women who have certain blood disorders, such as severe anemia or leukemia, or whose blood doesn't clot properly because of medications they are taking or because they have a particular disease may also have long, heavy periods.

The bleeding may take the form of spotting in between periods or light bleeding that occurs at the time of ovulation. About 10 percent of women experience bleeding at ovulation, probably because of the drop in estrogen levels that occurs at that time. If a woman has this type of bleeding, which is harmless, her period should start almost exactly 14 days later.

Sometimes the bleeding will be irregular and unpredictable. In such cases, the term "metrorrhagia" may be used. The bleeding may be continuous or the woman may bleed for several days, then stop for a few days, then start again. The bleeding may be slight or it may be profuse. This type of bleeding may be caused by pelvic inflammatory disease, endometrial polyps, birth control pills, an IUD, thyroid deficiency, ectopic pregnancy, uterine cancer, cervical cancer, endometrial hyperplasia, or any disturbance in hormone balance.

Abnormal bleeding that occurs in postmenopausal women may be a result of estrogen replacement therapy, postmenopausal vaginitis or endometrial hyperplasia, but it may also be caused by cervical or uterine cancer.

Since women in this age group are more likely to have cancer than are younger women, postmenopausal abnormal bleeding requires prompt attention.

Hormonal imbalances may be responsible for a variety of abnormal uterine bleeding patterns. Problems in the hypothalamus, the master gland that orchestrates the menstrual cycle, the pituitary glands or the ovaries can be responsible for abnormal bleeding. Sometimes the hormones are disturbed in such a way that ovulation fails to occur. This is called anovulatory bleeding. Sometimes the corpus luteum, the remnants of the follicle containing the ripe egg that bursts open at ovulation and that produces progesterone, functions improperly, producing too little or too much progesterone. If the thyroid gland isn't producing enough thyroid, this too may upset the delicate hormone balance. Since the kidney is responsible for eliminating estrogen from the body, chronic kidney infections can interfere with the body's elimination, causing too high a level of estrogen in the body. In a similar fashion, chronic liver problems can lead to hormone imbalances.

Table 24 lists the many causes of abnormal uterine bleeding.

Diagnosis

The diagnosis of the cause of abnormal uterine bleeding is basically a process of elimination. A careful medical history, bimanual pelvic and speculum exams, pregnancy tests and a Pap smear may lead to the

Table 24
Causes of Abnormal Uterine Bleeding

Pelvic inflammatory disease	Cervical polyps
Endometrial polyps	Uterine cancer
Endometrial hyperplasia	Estrogen replacement therapy
Uterine fibroids	Chronic kidney or liver problems
Adenomyosis	Benign ovarian tumors
Endometriosis	Physiologic cysts of the ovaries
Intrauterine devices	Functioning ovarian tumors
Severe anemia	Ovarian cancer
Blood disorders	Cancer of the Fallopian tubes
Birth control pills	Tumors of the Fallopian tubes
Ectopic pregnancy	Miscarriage
Thyroid deficiency	Hormone imbalances
Cervical cancer	Trophoblastic disease
Cervical erosion	Ovulation

discovery of the cause of the abnormal bleeding. Blood tests may also pinpoint the cause of the disease. Thyroid tests may also be useful. X-ray studies of the uterus called hysterosalpingograms may be done. In some cases, laparoscopic or culdoscopic examination may be necessary.

A dilation and curettage (D&C), a process by which the cervix is dilated, the endometrial lining removed and the inside of the cervix carefully explored for abnormalities, may also be called for. In teenage girls, the doctor will try to avoid the D&C. Abnormal uterine bleeding often occurs in this age group when the menstrual cycle is just starting up and the system is not yet perfectly synchronized, and the cycle often stabilizes itself with the passage of time. In older women, particularly in postmenopausal women, a D&C must be done to rule out cancer and other causes.

One important diagnostic question is whether or not the woman is ovulating. Vaginal smears, endometrial biopsies, basal body temperature charts or urinary tests to detect progesterone may help the doctor decide whether or not the woman is ovulating. If a D&C is done, examination of the tissue removed will indicate whether or not the woman has been ovulating. If the woman is ovulating, the search for an organic or anatomical cause must be very thorough, for dysfunctional bleeding occurs with ovulating cycles in only about 10 percent of cases. When such cases do occur, it's usually because the corpus luteum, the source of progesterone, has failed to regress completely.

If the woman's cycles are anovulatory and no specific disease that could cause failure of ovulation is found, a complete hormone work-up done by a specialist may be necessary.

Treatment

Treatment of abnormal uterine bleeding will depend on the severity of the bleeding, the suspected cause of the bleeding and the age of the patient.

If a D&C has been done as part of the diagnostic work-up, further treatment may not be required, because for reasons that are not clear, the cleaning out of the uterus puts an end to the abnormal bleeding problems in 40 to 60 percent of such cases. Sometimes, even if the first D&C has no effect, a repeat D&C may be successful. If, however, the problem is a polyp, a submucous fibroid tumor, or a hormone imbalance, the D&C cannot cure the problem.

Hormone therapy may be used to treat abnormal uterine bleeding. This type of therapy may be used in young girls in whom the doctor is trying to avoid a D&C, in women whose diagnostic tests have suggested a hormonal cause for the bleeding and in women whose first D&C proved unsuccessful.

The aim of hormonal therapy is usually two-fold: to stop severe bleeding and, once that is accomplished, to restore normal menstrual cycles. Estrogen, progesterone and combinations of the two have all been used, and all of these will stop the bleeding. However, most authorities today feel that it is best to use a drug that is predominately progesterone but that also has mild estrogen and androgen (male-type hormone) effects, such as norethindrone (Norlutin). This type of drug gives the promptest relief of bleeding, is well tolerated by most women, isn't associated with the severe side effects caused by the other drugs, and doesn't cause breakthrough bleeding. Provera may also be used. The drug is given continuously for various amounts of time, depending on how heavy the bleeding is. If it's severe, the woman may be kept on the drug for several weeks to allow her blood levels to return to normal. (It should be noted that hormone therapy should not be started until pregnancy has been ruled out since hormones have been associated with birth defects.)

Once the bleeding has been stopped for the appropriate amount of time, the medication is discontinued. This will usually cause the bleeding to begin again in a few days.

The bleeding occurs as a result of a process similar to that which takes place in a normal menstrual cycle: The constant progesterone stimulation of the medication causes the endometrial lining to thicken, just as it does in response to the progesterone normally produced by the body during the second half of the menstrual cycle. In the normal menstrual cycle, if pregnancy does not occur, the levels of progesterone gradually diminish, causing the endometrial lining to break down and shed. Discontinuing the medication has the same effect. The levels of progesterone in the body fall, the lining breaks down and is shed; hence bleeding resumes. In effect, the medication has the same effect as a D&C, removing the endometrial lining by a sort of "medical curettage."

After the bleeding has continued for four days, the medication is given again from day five to day 25 of the menstrual cycle. This is continued for a few months. The medication is then discontinued altogether, to allow the woman's body to resume normal menstrual function all by itself. Many times this sort of hormonal therapy will have the effect of "priming the pump"; the boost of the hormone treatment will be enough to return the woman's cycles to normal.

Unfortunately, some doctors don't have a clear understanding of the underlying hormonal problems that can cause abnormal uterine bleeding or the effects of the various types of hormone medications available. According to authorities in the field, the four most common mistakes made in medical treatment are as follows:[14]

1. The doctor may choose a drug that has an estrogen/progesterone balance unfavorable to the prompt relief of bleeding
2. The doctor may not prescribe an adequate dose of the hormone, prescribing an amount sufficient for contraception but not sufficient for treatment of abnormal bleeding
3. The doctor may interpret the initial stoppage of the bleeding as success of the treatment and discontinue the drug
4. The doctor may misinterpret the initial withdrawal bleeding after the drug is discontinued as failure of treatment and reoccurrence of the abnormal bleeding problem

These kinds of mistakes could lead to unnecessary D&C or even to unnecessary hysterectomies.

The type of hormone therapy described here is just one of many possibilities. It has particular applications for abnormal uterine bleeding associated with anovulatory cycles. Other instances may require different therapies. For instance, Clomid, a drug that stimulates ovulation, may be effective in treating cases where the problem is related to persistent activity of the corpus luteum. In such cases, although the bleeding is not anovulatory, Clomid has proven to be effective. It is also effective in women who have anovulatory cycles who wish to become pregnant. Women who have anovulatory cycles but who have recurrent bleeding after a D&C or hormone therapy, may be successfully treated with Clomid as well. Many doctors, however, don't like to use Clomid unless a woman is particularly desirous of pregnancy since use of the drug carries certain risks.

It is impossible to describe all the varieties of hormone therapy, but since, as outlined above, mistakes are made by doctors, a woman whose doctor suggests another type of hormone therapy would do well to take this book with her and ask the doctor why s/he is suggesting this particular form of therapy. That way, the woman will be sure that her doctor is acting from a legitimate medical basis rather than from ignorance.

A hysterectomy, a surgical removal of the uterus, is sometimes necessary. If the bleeding is associated with fibroid tumors, endometriosis or pelvic inflammatory disease and if less drastic forms of treatment for these conditions are not successful—or if the cause of the bleeding cannot be identified and repeated D&Cs and hormone therapy have not been successful—then in all of these cases a hysterectomy may be in order, depending on the severity of the bleeding.

PRECOCIOUS PUBERTY

Types: true, or constitutional, precocious puberty
  pseudoprecocious puberty

Definitions differ somewhat, but generally, if breast development, pubic hair and other signs of puberty appear before the age of eight, the girl is said to have precocious puberty.

Types and Causes

Basically, there are two types of precocious puberty, true, or constitutional, precocious puberty and pseudoprecocious puberty. In true precocious puberty, the whole maturation process has for some reason been stepped up. Girls with this type of precocious puberty go through the normal sequence of developmental stages and actually ovulate and function as completely normal women; however, they do so abnormally early in life. Pseudoprecocious puberty, on the other hand, is not an acceleration of the normal maturation process. Instead, some disease or abnormality has caused the body to produce estrogen. These girls are not really biologically mature, for they do not actually ovulate (produce a ripe egg from the ovary each month). They do, however, show signs of sexual development, due to the abnormal amounts of estrogen in their bodies.

Pseudoprecocious puberty may be caused by an ovarian tumor, hypothyroidism, a tumor of the adrenal glands, a brain tumor or some other form of brain disease.

Symptoms

The symptoms of both types of precocious puberty are pretty much the same and are the changes normally associated with puberty: development of breast buds, darkening of the skin around the nipple and the lips of the vulva, the growth of pubic and underarm hair and bleeding from the uterus. In true precocious puberty this bleeding is true menstrual bleeding: The estrogen stimulates the lining to grow thicker and thicker; a ripe egg bursts out of its follicular sac in the ovary; the remnants of this burst follicular sac then produce progesterone. If pregnancy does not occur, progesterone levels fall and the lining of the uterus, which has grown thick and rich in response to the progesterone and estrogen, breaks down and is shed, just as it does in normal females.

In pseudoprecocious puberty, the girl may also bleed from the uterus on a fairly regular basis, but this is not true menstrual bleeding, and she doesn't ovulate or produce progesterone. However, the estrogen in her body stimulates the uterine lining to grow rich and thick and finally it gets so thick that pieces of it break away and are shed, mimicking menstrual bleeding.

Girls with precocious puberty differ from normal girls in several noteworthy respects: Although they are tall for their age when they first begin to develop symptoms, this growth spurt is not sustained, and such girls often end up being shorter than average by the time they reach their 20s. Moreover, their heads tend to be larger than normal and they tend to have a long trunk and short legs.

Diagnosis and Treatment

It is important to distinguish between true and pseudoprecocious puberty. In the former case the girl can get pregnant, and in the second case there is an underlying disease that needs treatment. Electroencephalograms, tests that measure brain waves, hormone tests and X-rays may be needed. Girls with true precocious puberty generally do not need treatment. Girls with pseudoprecocious puberty need to have surgery or other appropriate forms of treatment. Sometimes treatment is not possible and such children may die. The cause of such deaths is not well understood, but luckily they are rare.

MENOPAUSAL PROBLEMS

AKA: menopausal syndrome, problems related to the change of life, problems related to the climacteric

The transition from the reproductive phase of life to the postreproductive phase is called the climacteric. Menopause, the cessation of menstrual periods, is the most obvious change, but there are other changes as well. Even though they don't mean the same thing, the terms "climacteric" and "menopause" are often used interchangeably.

In the past, the average age at menopause for American women was 48, but in recent years, this average has risen. Nowadays it is not uncommon to find women in their mid 50s who are still menstruating.

It used to be that doctors thought of menopause as a deficiency disease, for during this time the ovaries stop producing estrogen. Many of the changes women go through at this period in their lives were thought to be the result of estrogen deficiency. We now know that only a few of these changes are actually related to lower levels of estrogen.

Signs and Symptoms

Although some women experience severe problems with menopause, the vast majority do not. Many women find this time of their lives the most pleasurable of all.

There are a number of physical and emotional changes that women may experience during the climacteric. Some of these are related to menopause and changes in hormone levels, but many are not, although in the past they all used to be attributed to these hormonal changes.

The most obvious signs are a cessation of menstrual periods. Some women menstruate normally until they come to an abrupt stop; others experience a gradual decrease in the amount of the flow and longer times between periods, alternating perhaps with regular periods or with missed periods, until finally the periods cease altogether. These types of bleeding patterns are all quite normal. If, however, there is a heavy or gushing flow, periods that last longer than usual, periods that occur more frequently than every 21 days or bleeding that starts again a year or more after the last period, there may be something wrong and such women should consult their doctors.

Hot flashes, or flushes, are the most common complaint of climacteric women. A hot flush is a discomfitting sensation of being heated-up from within. It usually begins as a feeling of heat in the chest that spreads to the neck and head; at times the entire body is affected. The skin may become bright red. Some women perspire quite profusely and are chilled afterward. The flash may last from a few seconds to several minutes, and may occur several times a day or only once or twice a week. About 65 percent of menopausal women experience hot flashes, but only about 20 percent have serious problems with them. Some women have them so frequently during the night that they are unable to sleep and suffer from insomnia.

609

The flashes may persist for quite some time, although rarely longer than a year, or they may be short-lived.

During a hot flash the blood vessels dilate and blood rushes to the surface of the skin. This causes the feeling of heat. No one knows exactly why this happens. Just as mysteriously, the blood vessels return to their normal state and the symptoms subside. Some researchers feel that hot flashes are caused by estrogen deficiency; others feel that the high levels of the pituitary hormones FSH and LH in menopausal women are responsible.

As levels of estrogen decline, the vaginal, vulvar and urinary tissues become thinner. The thinning of the vulvar tissues, a condition known as postmenopausal vulvitis, can cause dryness and itching. The thinning of the tissues of the urinary tract can make a woman more susceptible to urinary tract infections. The thinning of the vaginal tissues can cause a vaginal discharge, a condition known as postmenopausal vaginitis. The vaginal lubrications diminish in some women and this may make intercourse painful. In some women, the thinning of the urinary and vaginal tissues is associated with a prolapse (falling down) of the urinary organs, conditions known as cystoceles and urethroceles. The acid/alkaline balance of the vagina is also altered by the decline in estrogen, making postmenopausal women more susceptible to vaginal infections.

Another condition that may be associated with menopause and decreased estrogen production is osteoporosis, a condition in which bone density is decreased. Osteoporosis is not always a serious condition. Some people have extensive osteoporosis (as revealed by X-rays taken for other reasons) without ever having problems. Other people suffer pain and multiple fractures of the bones. Hip fractures are not uncommon, and these are serious injuries in older women, for they are sometimes accompanied by fatal complications.

It is not entirely clear whether osteoporosis is actually related to menopause and decreased estrogen or not. The fact that the incidence rate is higher in postmenopausal women and that women who have premature menopause sometimes develop the condition in their 40s, an age at which osteoporosis is rarely seen otherwise, suggests that the condition is related to estrogen. Moreover, the fact that there is some evidence that estrogen-replacement therapy (ERT) improves and can prevent the condition also suggests that it is related to estrogen deficiency.[15] However, there is also evidence that other factors, such as lack of exercise and an inadequate supply of certain vitamins and minerals, particularly, calcium, are implicated in the disease. It may be that lower levels of estrogen indirectly affect the way in which a woman's body metabolizes these nutrients, making a woman more susceptible to osteoporosis.

The evidence that osteoporosis is truly a menopausal symptom related to estrogen deprivation is contradictory, and as we shall see, this causes some controversy as to the proper treatment of menopausal women.

Some women in this age group put on extra weight, but weight gain has nothing to do with estrogen deficiency or menopause; rather, women in this age group tend to get less exercise and yet may not reduce their calorie intake. Weight gain is not an estrogen-associated phenomenon.

Depression, irritability, nervousness and psychological instability have long been associated with menopause. Actually, menopausal women have only about a 7 percent incidence of depression and emotional problems serious enough to require psychiatric care, as compared to a 6 percent incidence for other age groups.[16] According to some studies, climacteric women report a slightly higher incidence of nervousness, irritability, headaches and "feeling blue" than other age groups.[17] Other studies fail to confirm these feelings. Not surprisingly, women who experience severe hot flashes that disturb their sleep are more likely to experience psychological tension than women who don't experience insomnia. This is not to discount the psychological upset some women experience during these years. In our culture, with its sexist stereotypes and limited roles for women, the menopausal woman who has been a homemaker may find that her children have left home and she feels as if she is suddenly unemployed. Like any person forced into retirement, she may feel useless and inadequate, but these feelings and the psychological problems they create have nothing to do with menopause per se.

It has long been a popular myth that menopausal women lose interest in sex. While it is true that middle-aged men experience a change in sexual responsiveness—a longer time period between erection and subsequent ejaculation, due to decreased hormone levels—sexual responsiveness in females is not related to menopause per se. Estrogen is not thought to have much of an impact on sexuality. Androgen, another hormone apparently does, but it is still produced during and after menopause. Women's psychological problems with sex during this time may be caused by men who are bewildered by the changes in their sexual performance and somehow shift the blame to their partners.

Given our society's preoccupation with youth, our rather restricted, Madison Avenue notions of beauty and our cultural notions that a woman's femininity is tied up with her ability to bear children, it is not surprising that some women feel less sexually desirable during menopause. But many women experience an increase in sexual responsiveness after menopause, when pregnancy and birth control are no longer a problem. Changes in sexual responsiveness, if they occur, are not related to menopause itself.

611

Treatment

Many times estrogen replacement therapy (ERT) is prescribed for menopausal women whether they have symptoms or not. Sometimes it is prescribed for symptoms that are not actually related to estrogen deficiency and cannot be relieved by giving ERT (see the section on ERT for details). The use of ERT carries certain risks, including the risk of cancer, so it should be avoided if at all possible. The only menopausal problems for which ERT is effective are hot flashes, conditions related to the drying and thinning of vaginal, vulvar and urinary tissues and, possibly, osteoporosis. There are alternative forms of therapy for these conditions, and we suggest women try these first and not use ERT unless absolutely necessary. Alternative cures for vaginal, vulvar and urinary problems are discussed under the headings Postmenopausal Vulvitis, Postmenopausal Vaginitis and Cystoceles and Urethroceles. Alternatives to ERT are discussed in the section on estrogen replacement therapy.

PREMATURE MENOPAUSE

AKA: early menopause

Types: artificial, or induced, menopause
       primary ovarian failure

Premature menopause is a condition in which a woman experiences menopause, the cessation of menstrual periods, before the usual age. An artificial, or induced, menopause occurs when both of the ovaries are destroyed by surgery, radiation therapy, disease or, in rare cases, by the use of certain medications. Sometimes, even though a woman hasn't had an induced menopause, her ovaries cease to function normally. This is called primary ovarian failure.

Any induced menopause is a premature menopause. If a woman has primary ovarian failure and experiences menopause before the age of 40, most doctors would call this a premature menopause; others use the age of 35 and still others the age of 45 to define premature menopause.

Causes

As noted, artificial or induced menopause can be caused by radiation therapy, disease, the use of large doses of fertility drugs and in very rare instances by tubal ligation done for sterilization purposes.

Sometimes the ovaries are destroyed by ovarian tumors, pelvic inflammatory disease or cancer and are then removed in an operation known as bilateral oophorectomy. Sometimes, however, the ovaries will be removed even though they are perfectly healthy. Some doctors will remove the ovaries as well as the uterus in all women over the age of 35 who are having hysterectomies. Others will remove the ovaries in their hysterectomy patients over 40; still others will use the age of 45 as a cut-off point. The pros and cons of combining the removal of healthy ovaries in women having hysterectomies are discussed in greater detail under the heading Hysterectomy. Whether the ovaries removed are diseased or healthy, this type of surgery generally resuls in premature menopause.

Although the causes of primary ovarian failure are not well understood, it is thought that some women are born with ovaries that have a fewer number of eggs and hence "run out" of eggs at an earlier age; or it may be that the ovaries have received too much stimulation from the pituitary gland, causing the ovary to exhaust its supply of eggs and thus bringing on a premature menopause.

Symptoms

The symptoms of premature menopause are the same as those of a natural menopause, only they are usually more severe. In the case of artificial menopause, instead of a gradual decline in hormone production, there is an abrupt cessation. Since the body doesn't adjust gradually, the abrupt transition may be that much more difficult and the menopausal symptoms intensified.

In women who have primary ovarian failure the most obvious symptom will be the absence of menstruation. The diagnosis of women with primary ovarian failure is covered in more detail under the heading Amenorrhea.

Women who have a premature menopause may be at higher risk for the development of heart disease, hypertension, a condition characterized by high blood pressure, and osteoporosis, a condition in which there is a loss of bone density, making the woman more susceptible to bone fractures. However, women who have a premature menopause may be at decreased risk for the development of breast cancer.

Treatment

Premature menopause may not require any treatment at all. If, however, a woman has severe symptoms, these may be dealt with in the same manner as severe menopausal symptoms.

There is disagreement among doctors as to whether or not women who

613

experience menopause at a particularly early age, yet do not have symptoms, should be given estrogen replacement therapy. This is discussed more fully under the heading ERT.

TOXIC SHOCK SYNDROME

AKA: TSS

Toxic shock syndrome (TSS) is not, strictly speaking, a menstrual problem. In actuality it is an overwhelming systemic infection that can begin in the vagina, but since the majority of women who get TSS get it during their menstrual periods and since it seems to be related to the use of tampons, we have chosen to include it here in the section on menstrual problems.

TSS is a newly defined disease about which there are still many unanswered questions. Some doctors believe that the disease has been around, although not defined as such, for over 60 years. Others believe that TSS, at least the form of the disease that affects menstruating women, is a fairly recent phenomenon.

Incidence

TSS is supposedly a relatively rare disease. The official incidence rate is only three cases per 100,000 menstruating women. Some researchers believe the actual incidence rate may be much higher.[18] They point out that milder cases may go unrecognized or unreported. Moreover, the Center for Disease Control has only recently begun to publicize the syndrome and to collect statistics, so this estimated incidence rate may be revised in the future.

TSS usually affects menstruating women under the age of 30, but men and children, as well as non-menstruating and older women, have been affected by what may be the same disease.

Cause

The disease is caused by Staphylococcus aureus, a bacterium that is often found in the nose and mouth. Approximately 5-15 percent of women have this organism in their vaginas. The organisms produce a toxin. If a sufficient number of organisms are present and enough toxin is released into the bloodstream, the women may develop an overwhelming infection that may have fatal consequences.

Tampons apparently play a role in the disease. The majority of women with the disease have been tampon users. One brand in particular, Rely tampons, has been associated with the disease, but other brands and the natural sponges some women use to collect the menstrual flow have been associated with TSS. The syndrome was first identified about the time that Rely came on the market. Rely contained new super absorbent fibers and quickly captured 20 percent of the market. The competitors followed suit and reconstituted their tampons, so that most of the tampons now on the market contain some sort of super absorbent fiber.

No one is certain exactly how tampon usage contributes to the disease. The most widely held theory is that tampons trap the blood and staph organisms, thereby providing a breeding ground for the staph. Because the super absorbent tampons tend to be left in for longer periods of time, they may be giving the organisms more of a chance to produce their toxins. However, it should be noted that the disease has also occurred in women who have changed their tampons frequently. Another theory holds that the tampons absorb the normal vaginal secretions as well as the menstrual blood, thereby altering the acid/alkaline environment of the vagina and making it more conducive to the growth of the staph organisms (*see* p. 273).

Another possibility is that the staph can get into the bloodstream more easily because of microscopic lacerations or abrasions that these super absorbent fibers can create on the vaginal wall. Still another possibility is that there is something about the makeup of the fibers themselves that aids the growth of the staph organism.

Symptoms

The disease is characterized by the sudden onset of fever, vomiting and diarrhea. Sometimes there is accompanying headache, sore throat and aching muscles. Within about 48 hours there may be a dramatic drop in blood pressure. The woman may go into shock, become disoriented, and her kidneys may fail. At the same time a red rash that peels like sunburn may develop. The disease tends to recur in about 30 percent of the cases and may be fatal. In milder cases only some of these symptoms may be evident.

If you experience a sudden high fever (usually over 102°) accompanied by vomiting and/or diarrhea, contact your doctor immediately. If you are wearing a tampon, remove it.

Treatment

Medication to stabilize the blood pressure and fluids may be given. Large doses of antibiotics are given to combat the infection. Antibiotics are important even in milder cases as they have been shown to cut down on recurrences.

Prevention

The best prevention is to stop using tampons, at least until more is known. If you continue to wear them, don't use the Rely brand (they've been withdrawn by manufacturers); change your tampons at least four times a day; alternate between tampons and pads (this has been shown to reduce your chances of getting TSS).

Some women are using natural sponges instead of tampons, but at least one case of TSS has been associated with natural sponge usage. Some researchers have found sand and other impurities in these sponges, so if their use becomes more widespread, we may see more cases of sponge-related TSS.

If you do develop TSS, do not use tampons even after the disease has cleared up because of the possibility of recurrence.

Complications

TSS may produce aneurysms—dilations of the blood vessels—that can lead to heart and vascular problems. Some researchers advise women who've had TSS to keep to a low cholesterol diet and to have frequent check-ups for cardiovascular irregularities.[19]

Problems Related to Pregnancy and Fertility

The conditions described in this section are related to pregnancy and fertility. A complete survey of the medical considerations of pregnancy is beyond the scope of this book; however, we have chosen to include certain of these conditions because they occur in the early stages of pregnancy, in some cases before a woman is even aware that she is pregnant, and can produce symptoms such as vaginal bleeding and lower abdominal pain that may be associated with any number of gynecological problems in the nonpregnant woman.

All of the conditions described here involve either the inability to get pregnant—infertility—or the involuntary termination of a pregnancy, either because of a miscarriage, an ectopic pregnancy, trophoblastic disease or repeated miscarriages. Women who don't have menstrual periods, a condition known as amenorrhea, will also have an infertility problem, but this is discussed in the section on menstrual problems.

Myths About Infertility

There are a number of myths surrounding infertility, some of which can make the emotionally difficult task of dealing with this problem even harder. One myth is that infertility is largely a psychological problem, that, deep down, infertile couples, or more specifically, infertile women, really don't want to become pregnant. This is simply not true; in 70-90 percent of cases, a specific medical explanation for the infertility can be found.

617

Moreover, this does not necessarily mean, in the remaining cases, for which no medical explanation can be discovered, that "psychological factors" are responsible; it merely means that medical science has not advanced enough to identify the problem.

Another myth is that infertile couples often conceive after having adopted a child. Again, this is simply not true. About 5 percent of infertile couples will indeed conceive after adopting, but 5 percent of all infertile couples will experience a spontaneous cure of their problem whether they have adopted a child or not.[1]

Yet another myth is that female factors are most often the cause of fertility problems—also not true. In about 35-40 percent of the cases in which a specific cause for the problem can be found, female factors are responsible; in another 35-40 percent it's male factors. In the 20-30 percent that remain, it is either a shared problem or there is a cause that cannot be identified.

Emotional Stress and Infertility

A couple with an infertility problem is likely to encounter a lot of social pressure. Relatives are apt to come up with questions such as "When are you going to give us the grandchild we're waiting for?" People who hardly know us are apt to question us about our childless state or our future childbearing plans. Because of all the myths and misinformation about infertility, people often interpret the anxiety, frustration and depression an infertile couple is likely to experience as the *cause* rather than the *result* of the problem. "Just relax, and you'll get pregnant" is a typical piece of advice. Such advice not only shows an ignorance of the medical realities of the situation but is also a huge put-down, implying that it is the couple's fault—their own uptightness—that is keeping them from conceiving.

Cultural expectations and assumptions about sexuality, femininity, masculinity and fertility add to the problem. Most of us, either consciously or unconsciously, feel that a man's ability to father children is somehow tied up with his virility, with his worth as a man, and that a woman's ability to become pregnant is somehow a sign of her womanliness, an indication of her femininity. These old roles and notions are changing, but they still exert a strong influence on our emotional selves. Men and women with infertility problems are likely to have questions about their sexual selves. There may be terrible doubts about their adequacy and their worth as human beings.

The process of being diagnosed for an infertility problem can also put a strain on the infertile couple. Having to subject the details of their sex life to a doctor's scrutiny, scheduling lovemaking for optimum chances of conception and having to keep records and charts of sexual activity can have a bad effect on a couple's sex life. The importance that each act of lovemaking takes on—for after all, *this* could be *the* time—can be exciting, but also stressful. It is not unusual for such couples to experience impotence, a decrease in sex drive and inability to reach orgasm during this time. Not only their sex life but all aspects of their relationship may suffer, especially if one partner wants the pregnancy more than the other, or if, as is often the case, it is seen as the woman's problem and responsibility—*her* charts, *her* sexual schedules, *her* doctor's appointments. Agreeing to take a vacation from sex for a time, sharing the responsibility for keeping charts and so on, as well as talking ahead of time about the kinds of feelings you are likely to experience, can be helpful.

Finding a doctor with whom you feel comfortable and who can not only answer your questions but also offer emotional support is vitally important. Finding a support group composed of other couples who are going through the same crisis can also be helpful, and your doctor or a staff member at an infertility clinic at a large medical center should be able to put you in touch with such groups.

If the fertility work-up fails to disclose a specific cause for the fertility problem or if treatment is not possible or is unsuccessful and the couple remains childless, there are apt to be feelings of intense disappointment and grief, mourning for all the children that will never be born. Anger and resentment are natural reactions as well. If the cause has been isolated and one partner or the other is the source of the infertility problem, the infertile partner is apt to feel that the fertile partner wants to leave the relationship and is concealing terrible, negative feelings about the infertile partner. It may be quite true that the fertile partner has feelings of disappointment and anger. It is better to talk these feelings out honestly rather than to bottle them up, for they will eventually come out in other, less direct, less healthy ways. Finding a therapist to help you work through this emotional crisis can help. For many couples, this difficult experience can actually bring them closer together, creating a new and special kind of caring and feeling for each other out of their shared disappointment.

Anywhere from 30 to 50 percent of the couples being treated for infertility will become pregnant within the first two years of treatment. After that, there is still hope. Five percent of all such couples experience a spontaneous cure, sometimes after many, many years of childlessness. Then, too, new techniques are being developed all the time. But, this glimmer of hope is only that—a glimmer—and for some couples, this tiny chance may be more difficult to deal with than the absolute knowledge that they can never conceive.

Miscarriage

Miscarriages are also likely to result in emotional complications. Grief and sorrow, especially if the pregnancy was eagerly awaited, are of course the overwhelming reactions. There may also be feelings of guilt. Many couples feel their sex life was too vigorous, causing the miscarriage (not true). A woman is apt to feel that something she did or didn't do was responsible for the spontaneous abortion or that there is something wrong with her. Fear that it will happen again is also a natural response. However, 80 percent of the women who have a single miscarriage will have no problems with subsequent pregnancies.

All of these emotions may be further compounded by the frustrations a couple feels when they try to seek answers to their basic questions, "Why did this happen? Is there something wrong with me or with us? Will it happen again?"

Repeated Miscarriages

A couple or a woman who experiences a series of miscarriages, a condition known as habitual abortion, is of course likely to experience even more severe emotional trauma. One miscarriage is bad enough, but two, three, four or more can be totally wrenching. To make matters worse, the couple, in particular the woman, is likely to encounter a good deal of prejudice about her condition and a lot of sexist attitudes from the medical profession. Many, if not most, doctors have been trained to think of women who are habitual aborters as neurotic personality types and to attribute a habitual abortion problem for which they are unable to identify a specific medical cause to emotional factors, even though there is no scientific evidence to support this viewpoint. This myth is perhaps the cruelest of all, for it is believed by many doctors, the very people to whom the woman suffering from this problem must turn for help.

A look at how the topic of habitual abortion and psychological factors is treated in the most recent edition of one of the most widely used gynecological textbooks in the country, reveals the incredible prejudice that clouds doctors' thinking on this subject.[2]

"There is mounting evidence that emotional factors play a role in etiology [cause] of repeated pregnancy loss," claim the authors. The "mounting evidence" subsequently cited in this text includes the opinion of two doctors who "have *always felt* [emphasis ours] that stress and emotional problems were responsible for many cases of habitual abortion." These two doctors claim an 80 percent success rate in treating habitual abortion through psychotherapy; but as the authors themselves point out, an 80 percent cure rate is about what one would expect from the treatment of infertility cases.

The authors further inform their medical-student readers that another team of two doctors has "noted two distinct types of personality among women who abort repeatedly: (a) basically immature women who are not ready to assume the full responsibility of being either a woman or a mother, or (b) they are frustrated women who have adjusted to a man's world and whose main aspirations are beyond what they believe to be their feminine limits." Moreover, the reader is told that "a few of these women have the instinct to destroy not only themselves but others." No mention is made of the type of psychological tests employed to determine who is "immature" or "frustrated," because obviously there are no valid psychological tests to measure such sexist perceptions. The evidence that women who are habitual aborters are neurotic personality types is merely the opinion of these male doctors.

The medical student reading these texts is then told that therapy is a good idea for such women and should "proceed along common sense lines ... " The therapy, which apparently is administered not by a trained psychotherapist but by the gynecologist, is "time consuming" and requires "repetitive visits." No mention is made of how expensive these visits are for the "irresponsible" and "immature" habitual aborter who has to pay for them, nor of how profitable they are for the doctor who is going to charge her for them even though, by the authors' own admission, her chances of improving her habitual abortion problem will not be significantly improved.

The authors close with the following totally unscientific statement endorsing their common sense therapy: "This type of therapy is far more effective than the older methods of pampering the mother by putting her to bed, applying heat, giving vitamins and hormones and telling her to avoid intercourse." We do not recommend the old therapy, especially in light of new evidence that estrogen or progesterone hormone therapy is not only ineffective but may cause birth defects. Indeed, such estrogen therapy has clearly been shown to cause abnormalities, including a rare form of vaginal cancer in the teenage daughters of women who were given the hormone DES to prevent miscarriage.[3] However, the new therapy of "common sense" psychotherapy, administered by gynecologists steeped in sexist prejudices of the kind reflected in this text and untrained in psychotherapy, hardly seems much of an improvement.

If you are seeking help for an habitual abortion problem, you should remember that chances are your doctor used this very text (or, heaven forbid, an earlier edition) in medical school. While the good doc may do a bang-up job of assaying your hormone levels, any nonmedical conclusions are likely to be just so much nonsense. If the source of your problem lies beyond the limits of present medical knowledge, and the doctor can't identify the cause or find a cure, it is quite possible that instead of frankly admitting ignorance the doctor will pull the old switcheroo: "I-can't-figure-out-what's-wrong-with-you-so-you-must-be-crazy."

A woman who has gone through the trauma of three or more miscarriages and suffered the loss of new and eagerly awaited life growing in her body, may quite naturally feel shaky emotionally. She may be having terrible feelings of inadequacy and is apt to be very vulnerable. The last thing she needs is a doctor who tells her, directly or indirectly, that she is neurotic and that her emotional problems are the cause of her habitual abortion problem. Indeed, for doctors to inflict this sexist assumption, for which there is absolutely no scientific evidence, on such women is cruel and irresponsible.

If your doctor seems to be working from a "it's-all-in-your-head-dearie" diagnosis, don't buy it. Such prejudiced assumptions about your condition could stand in the way of your receiving the optimum medical care for your condition. Find another doctor.

INFERTILITY AND STERILITY

AKA: inability to get pregnant

Sterility is defined as the absolute inability to conceive. Infertility is defined as the inability to get pregnant after one year or more of regular sexual activity (without the use of contraception, of course) or the inability to carry a pregnancy to a live birth. The problems of miscarriage and habitual abortion are discussed elsewhere. Here we are concerned only with the inability to conceive. Some doctors define infertility in terms of one year; others use two years as the cut-off point. The particular length of time used in the definition is based on studies that have shown that about 56 percent of fertile couples trying for pregnancy will do so within one month and about 77 percent within the first six months. An additional 5 to 10 percent will become pregnant within the following year. However, anyone has the right to seek medical help whenever they themselves feel that infertility is a problem. Women in their thirties who are having trouble getting pregnant may want to seek help after only four or five months, for their fertility is dropping and the chances of getting pregnant are declining with the passage of time. Moreover, after 35, the incidence of birth defects is much higher. Women who are not menstruating regularly may also want to seek treatment without waiting since irregular menstrual cycles may mean that they are not ovulating. Such women are not likely to conceive without treatment. A woman who has a history of pelvic infections or a man who has a history of mumps might also forego the waiting period.

Most people seeking help for an infertility problem are couples; however, in some cases, either the male partner refuses to seek medical help or the woman is single. If the husband refuses to participate in the diagnostic tests, obviously this will limit the scope of the diagnostic investigation.

Some doctors will refuse to treat a single woman. Indeed, some may even refuse to treat an unmarried couple. A single woman seeking help for an infertility problem should read this section carefully so that she is familiar with the tests available; otherwise, she may be given only the most cursory of exams and told there is nothing wrong with her. A more extensive diagnostic work-up might have uncovered the source of the problem.

Infertility is a fairly common problem; about 10-18 percent of the population, or about one out of every six couples, is infertile at any given time. Fertility in women declines markedly with age. A woman is at the height of her fertility in her midtwenties, and this slowly tapers off to about the age of 30 and then begins to decline. A man's fertility decreases slowly until about the age of 40, and then there is a more rapid decline. The incidence of infertility is rising.

Causes and Treatment of Female Infertility

There are many possible explanations for infertility. Many people believe that infertility is usually the woman's problem, but this is not true; the problem may be traced to the female or the male, or the infertility may be a result of a factor involving both of them. Most of these causes and treatments of infertility are discussed in depth elsewhere in this book. Only a brief summary is included here.

Pelvic Scar Tissue

One of the leading causes of female infertility is scar tissue in the uterus and Fallopian tubes and around the ovary. The scar tissue may be formed as the result of infections such as gonorrhea and pelvic inflammatory disease. Indeed, any major infection in the pelvic cavity, for instance, an inflammation set up by a ruptured appendix, can cause scar tissue. The treatment for these problems may be a dilation and curettage (D&C), which may remove the scar tissue. Endometrial polyps, which may also be the result of infection, can be cured by dilation and curettage as well. If extensive scarring is present, laparoscopy or even major pelvic surgery, laparotomy, may be required to cut the scar tissue. The ligaments that hold the uterus may be tightened, lifting the entire uterus. This closes the space behind the uterus and reduces the area where scar tissue, which could bind

623

the tube, can occur. However, many doctors question the wisdom of this operation, both because its effectiveness is questionable and because the ureters, the tubes that conduct urine from the kidney to the bladder, are so close that they could easily be damaged.

Endometriosis, a condition in which the tissue that lines the inside of the uterus is found growing in abnormal locations in the pelvic cavity—for instance, on the ovaries or tubes—can also cause scar tissue and adhesions. This abnormally placed tissue tends to behave just like the normal tissue in the uterus, bleeding in response to the monthly ebb and flow of hormones. The lining of the pelvis is very sensitive to blood, and so bleeding sets up a defensive reaction in the neighboring tissue that may result in extensive adhesions and cysts on the ovaries. Treatment may be by either surgery or drugs. There is some controversy as to which is the most effective method for treating infertility associated with endometriosis. This is discussed in more detail under the heading Endometriosis.

Cervical Problems

The cervix may be the seat of a woman's infertility problem. Mucus secreted by the cervical gland changes in character and consistency over the course of a woman's menstrual cycle. At the time of ovulation, it is clear and thin. On a microscopic level, the molecules of the mucus form tunnels that facilitate the sperm on its journey into the uterus. At other times of the month it is thick and impassable. If a woman's cervical mucus is always thick and impassable, this can sometimes be corrected with low doses of the hormone estrogen; however, this may involve certain risks.* Chronic cervical infections can also cause a discharge that either slows the sperm down or makes it difficult for the sperm to pass through the cervix and up into the uterus. This condition, cervicitis, may be treated with antibiotics, and if this treatment is not successful, as is often the case, the infected tissue can be destroyed by heat or freezing. This is usually a simple office procedure. Sometimes a woman's cervical secretions are too acid, and this may create an environment that is hostile to the sperm. These overly acid secretions can sometimes be neutralized by using certain douches just prior to intercourse. If these methods of dealing with a cervical mucus problem are not successful, it is sometimes possible to mechanically inject some of the husband's sperm up into the uterus, a technique known as husband insemination. This too may involve certain risks. The fertilized egg may implant too low in the uterus or may implant poorly, causing death of the fetus and miscarriage.

Then, too, mechanical obstructions such as cervical polyps or cervical

---

*See the section on fertility drugs for details.

fibroid tumors may block the passage of the sperm. Removing polyps is usually a simple piece of surgery that can be done in the office. Removing a cervical fibroid tumor may be somewhat more difficult and less successful and is an operation that requires hospitalization.

Hormone Imbalances

In some women, the second half of the menstrual cycle, from ovulation to menstruation, is abnormally short. This is known as corpus luteum insufficiency, or luteal phase defect. The corpus luteum, the source of the hormone progesterone in the second half of the menstrual cycle, begins to degenerate after only four or five days rather than after the normal eight or ten days. Without the hormone progesterone, the lining of the uterus is not adequately prepared for implantation of the fertilized egg; hence the woman is unable to sustain a pregnancy or has continual miscarriages. Progesterone treatments have been used, but synthetic progesterone has been implicated in birth defects. Low doses of certain fertility drugs, such as HCG and Clomid, have been used as well.

If a woman frequently has menstrual cycles in which she does not ovulate (called anovulatory cycles), she can't possibly get pregnant since no ripened egg is being produced. She is likely to have menstrual irregularities as well. Failure to ovulate may be caused by a malfunction of any of the glands involved in regulating the menstrual cycle. Tests to check the function of these glands can be done, and sometimes treating the underlying imbalance will solve the infertility problem. This is discussed more fully under the heading Amenorrhea. Certain powerful fertility drugs, like Clomid and Pergonal, may be used to stimulate ovulation, but these involve certain risks.

Ovarian Problems

A condition such as Stein-Leventhal disease in which the ovary may be surrounded by a thick, fibrous capsule and in which the woman only rarely, if ever, ovulates is also associated with infertility. This disease may be treated with drugs such as Clomid or by surgery. In some rare cases a woman is simply born without ovaries, a condition called Turner's syndrome, and such women are usually completely sterile and can't achieve pregnancy. Women with Turner's syndrome usually have other symptoms that are generally evident long before the infertility. However, in some cases, these women may have rudimentary, or streak, gonads and the symptoms of ovarian absence may not be as obvious. Occasionally, one of these women will have a small number of eggs in the streak gonad and will ovulate, and on rare occasions such women have become pregnant.

The ovaries may also fail to produce eggs because there has been extensive ovarian surgery, exposure to radiation or excessive stimulation from fertility drugs or because the blood supply to the ovaries has been cut off. This is known as primary ovarian failure, or premature menopause.

Uterine Problems

Structural problems in the uterus such as fibroid tumors and congenital abnormalities of the female organs can affect a woman's ability to carry a pregnancy to term or her ability to conceive. Some of these abnormalities may be the result of certain hormones, such as DES, taken by the mothers of those women during pregnancy. Congenital abnormalities can many times be corrected surgically. Many women have what is called a tipped uterus. Such women may have to use special techniques (see below), but they usually don't need surgery in order to become pregnant. Fibroids can sometimes be removed through surgery, a procedure known as myomectomy. This is not always possible, however, for if the tumors are extensive, requiring that a lot of tissue be removed, this might weaken the walls of the uterus so much that the entire uterus would have to be removed.

The Fallopian tubes may be blocked, causing infertility. Plastic surgery known as tuboplasty may be used to repair damage. This is a rather elaborate procedure in which microsurgery is performed. The success of any tubal surgery depends on exactly where in the tube the blockage is and whether one or both tubes is affected. After surgery, there is an increased risk (5–10 percent) of ectopic pregnancy. If one tube is hopelessly blocked, some doctors will recommend that the ovary on that side be removed. Ovulation normally alternates, so that an egg is produced from the right ovary one month and from the left ovary the next. Removing the ovary on the side of the blocked tube forces the woman to ovulate from the remaining ovary, thus increasing her chances of fertility. But most doctors question this procedure and won't remove a healthy ovary in case something should ever happen to the remaining ovary.

Other

Any infection of the uterus can cause infertility, for if the uterine wall is too irritated, the egg cannot implant. Any chronic disease, thyroid conditions, alcoholism or drug abuse can affect the sensitive hypothalamus, the control center in the brain that regulates the menstrual cycle, thereby causing infertility. Exposure to radiation and environmental pollutants has been implicated in fertility problems in women as well as men (see below).

Causes and Treatment of Male Infertility

So far, we've been talking about female infertility, but male fertility may also be impaired. Basically, there are four ways in which a man's fertility can be affected: inadequate sperm production or sperm maturation, insufficient sperm motility (the sperm's ability to swim or move), a blockage or other problem somewhere in the sperm delivery system or inability to place the sperm properly in the vagina.

Sperm Count

The absence of sperm or a low sperm count can be due to any infection associated with high fever that occurs after puberty. Mumps infections have long been associated with male infertility. If a male past the age of puberty gets the mumps, he may be rendered permanently sterile. In many cases, though, only one testicle is affected. If both are affected, the situation is less hopeful; however, even in such cases a man may gradually recover his fertility, usually within a year. A number of other infections, notably the sexually transmitted diseases, can temporarily depress sperm count, and, if untreated, may render a man permanently sterile. Recovery of normal sperm production after a high-fever illness takes at least three months, for it takes the testicles that long to produce mature sperm.

If the testicles do not descend into the scrotal sack before puberty (undescended testicles) this will also affect sperm production. Fertility is affected because the testicles function at a slightly lower temperature than the rest of the body organs. They need to be within the scrotal sack to have their optimum temperature. A surgical cure for undescended testicles is possible, but best results are achieved if the surgery is done before the age of six. In some cases, there may be abnormalities within the testicle itself that affect sperm production and these cannot be corrected surgically.

Other congenital factors, for instance, Klinefelter's syndrome (which is similar to Turner's syndrome in females), can also affect sperm production. A man with Klinefelter's syndrome tends to have small testicles and an absence of sperm in his ejaculation.

The undescended testicle is not the only condition that can cause too high a temperature in the scrotal sack and hence lower sperm count. A variocele, which is a varicose or twisted vein of the testicle, can also cause this problem. This condition can be corrected surgically, and in 80 percent of cases the sperm count improves. Higher than usual heat from frequent use of athletic supporters, hot tubs, sauna baths, long, hot showers, etc., can also temporarily slow down sperm maturation. Here again, the effect is usually reversible within three months.

627

Any abnormalities in the testicles can affect sperm count; however, even if a man has only one testicle, he can still be fertile. Injury to any of the reproductive organs from a serious accident may cut off the blood supply to the tissue, resulting in the death of that tissue. In rare cases, this has also occurred as a result of a hernia operation or other type of surgery.

Radiation can render both men and women permanently sterile, although in some cases the effect on male fertility may be only temporary, for he is constantly producing new sperm, whereas a woman at birth already has all the eggs she will ever have. Once these eggs have been damaged, new, healthy ones cannot be produced.

If a man suffers from chronic illness, including alcoholism or drug addiction, fertility may also be impaired. Heavy and prolonged use of marijuana has been associated with lowered sperm counts. Stress, both physical and emotional, can likewise affect fertility. Hormone imbalances, the result of diseases of the pituitary or hypothalamus such as tumors, can also cause infertility. If these are successfully treated, fertility may be restored.

Toxic pesticides and herbicides and environmental pollutants also affect fertility.[4] Agent Orange, an herbicide used extensively in Vietnam to defoliate the jungles, has been implicated in sterility as well as miscarriage, birth defects, skin cancers and other problems. This same herbicide, 2-4-5-T, is used extensively by lumbering firms in this country. In one area in Oregon where this chemical has been used, the rate of birth defects is as high as 40 percent. Other toxic substances have also been implicated in infertility, miscarriage, birth defects and cancer. PCB, a chemical used in electric transformers, fluorescent bulbs, TV sets and even carbon paper has been found in almost all sperm tested for its presence. These and other contaminants may be responsible for the fact that the average sperm count in American men has fallen by as much as 30 percent in the last 30 years.

Sperm Motility

Many of the factors mentioned above will also cause inadequate sperm motility. Prostatitis, an infection of the prostate gland, which produces the milky fluid released with the sperm during ejaculation, or surgical removal of the gland will also affect sperm motility. Chronic illness or hormonal problems will likewise have an affect on the sperm's ability to swim. Curing the illness or infection, when possible, will usually improve fertility. Sometimes the female hormone estrogen may be given to improve a man's sperm production, but long-term use of estrogen may have feminizing effects. Some doctors use testosterone, a male hormone, to achieve a "rebound" effect from the feminization effects, but most doctors feel that this can cause the permanent suppression of sperm production. Drugs

628

called corticosteroids are also used, but only rarely, for they have also been implicated as a cause of reduced sperm production. HGC, another hormone, stimulates the production of testosterone, which improves sperm motility in some men. Clomid has also been used to stimulate sperm production and improve motility. In cases in which the man has a borderline sperm count and problems with motility, a technique known as split ejaculate in which the man catches the first half of his ejaculate (the part that has the greatest number of live sperm) in a glass jar, may be used. The sperm is then used to artificially inseminate the wife. Artificial, or donor, insemination, in which an anonymous donor's sperm is injected into the uterus, is another possibility.

Sperm Delivery

Untreated sexually transmitted diseases or other illnesses can cause a blockage in the sperm delivery system. Injury from surgery or an accident, a variocele or a vasectomy can all cause such blockage as well. Sometimes surgical repair can correct these problems, but this is not always possible, especially in the case of a vasectomy. Another problem that can affect the sperm delivery system is a condition known as retrograde ejaculation, in which the sperm are deposited in the man's bladder instead of continuing out through the urethra. This condition may be permanent or temporary and may be caused by certain drugs, injury during surgery or damage to the nerve. Men with retrograde ejaculation have no visible sperm and their urine tends to be milky-colored after sex. The condition can sometimes be treated by drugs. For a couple seriously intent on pregnancy, it may be possible to recover sperm from the bladder and impregnate the woman using the technique of husband insemination described earlier.

Impotence (the inability to get and maintain an erection), premature ejaculation ("coming" before the penis can be inserted in the vagina), and the inability to ejaculate can all cause infertility. Sometimes these forms of sexual dysfunction will have an organic, physical cause, but the problem may also be psychological. Sex therapy a la Masters and Johnson has been very effective in treating these problems.

Sperm Antibodies

In some cases, antibodies to sperm may be the source of the infertility problem. In a man, immunity to his own sperm may result from an injury or infection that allows the sperm to enter the surrounding tissue, where they may trigger his immune system and cause an antibody reaction. If the injury or infection can be treated, sometimes this will stop the production of antibodies. A woman may also have antibodies that attack the sperm.

Such women are, in essence, allergic to sperm, and each time they have intercourse, more antibodies are produced. Sometimes this problem can be successfully treated by having the man use a condom (a rubber) during intercourse for a period of three to six months. During this time, the level of a woman's antibodies are measured and when they drop, the couple can begin to have sex without a condom, but only at the time of optimum fertility, around ovulation.

Sexual Practices That May Affect Fertility

Sometimes the couple's sexual practice may affect fertility. The use of lubricants like vaseline must be discontinued, since these are known to weaken or in some cases even kill sperm. The position the couple use during intercourse may also be affecting their ability to conceive. For most couples, the best position is the missionary style, with the man on top and the woman's hips raised on a pillow. The man should penetrate as deeply as possible. If the woman draws her knees up to her chest this will facilitate deep penetration. The man should stop thrusting and hold his penis still when he experiences orgasm. The woman should hold her knees in this position for half an hour after intercourse. The exception to this rule is the woman who has a tipped uterus, for whom entry from behind may be best. The frequency of a couple's sexual activity is an important factor. The longer a man goes without ejaculating, the less sperm he generates. Having sex two or three times a week is considered optimum for conception. The timing of sexual activity is also important and charting a woman's fertile period (see the section on natural family planning) will help the couple determine the optimum time for conception. Generally, a woman will ovulate 14 days, give or take 24 hours each way, before the beginning of her next period, so her best chances of conceiving are on the 13th, 14th and 15th day before the day on which her next period is expected to begin. During these three days, the couple should have intercourse no more than once every 30 to 36 hours. This will avoid exhausting the man's sperm supply and will assure that active sperm are in the reproductive tract during the woman's fertile time. For best results, the couple should have intercourse on each of the two days before this three-day period so that the male's sperm production will be stimulated.

Diagnosis

Because there are so many different factors that can affect fertility and because more than one factor may be responsible, diagnosing the causes of infertility can be a difficult and time-consuming task. A couple should look for a doctor who specializes in fertility. The American Board of Obstetrics and Gynecology now certifies specialists in fertility, but there are few of them. Most are associated with medical schools. The American Fertility Society, 1608 13th Avenue S, Suite 101, Birmingham, Alabama 35205, has a listing of fertility centers and specialists across the country. A specialist may not be necessary for the preliminary steps, but if a test such as a laparoscopy or a procedure such as tubal surgery is needed, do seek referral to a specialist.

It should also be mentioned that nurse-practitioners are assuming an important role in fertility work-ups. The doctor still supervises the tests and diagnostic work-up, but much of the patient contact is done by the nurse-practitioner. This can have advantages for everyone. The nurse-practitioner is generally less pressed for time and is therefore able to spend the time needed to take a very thorough medical history and to answer questions and explain procedures. Many times the nurse-practitioner is actually better at explaining things in lay terms than the doctor is. Couples being treated for infertility who spend much of their time with the nurse-practitioner should not feel that they are being slighted or receiving less than adequate care. Although the nurse-practitioner works closely with the doctor, the fee for his or her time is less than for the doctor's time, which can be a particularly important factor, since fertility work-ups can be expensive and many times insurance policies don't cover these costs. People with an infertility problem should discuss the financial aspects with the doctor and with their insurance companies.

The doctor should be able to do a complete fertility work-up in two to three months and give the couple some idea of what chances they have of achieving pregnancy or what further treatment is necessary. The one-test-at-a-time approach can drag on for a year or more and can be a severe emotional drain on the couple. Step one is an initial interview that should, if at all possible, include both the man and the woman. The doctor will ask both of them about their medical history and sexual practices. A complete physical examination for both is in order. Most of the time, the couple will be asked to keep a basal body temperature chart to find out whether a woman is ovulating and, if so, to time the couple's sexual activity around these dates.

A semen analysis of the man's sperm is also part of the diagnostic work-up. This is simple procedure and should be done before the woman is asked to undergo an endometrial biopsy, X-ray exams or other more elaborate and expensive tests. The man will be asked to masturbate into a jar and to deliver the sample to the lab within one hour. Catching all of the ejaculate is particularly important since most of the sperm are in the first half of the ejaculate. The sperm must be kept at room temperature. A man should not abstain from normal sexual activity prior to the test, for this may diminish the number of healthy, fresh sperm in his ejaculate. If for religious or other reasons a man cannot masturbate, a special type of condom may be used during intercourse to collect the sperm sample. If there is a religious objection to birth control, a small pinhole can be made at the top of the condom. Coitus interruptus, or withdrawal, as a method of collecting the semen is not as satisfactory because some of the early ejaculate may be lost. If the sperm count is abnormal, a testicular biopsy, a simple office procedure done under a local anesthetic, may be done.

If the male factors are normal, study of the woman continues. There may be a postcoital, or Huhner, test, which requires that a woman arrive at the doctor's within a few hours after intercourse without having washed or douched. A sample of her cervical mucus is studied to see if the sperm have been able to penetrate the mucus and survive in this environment.

An endometrial biopsy, another method of determining ovulation, may also be done. The test can be done in the doctor's office, and since it may involve some pain, a local anesthetic will be used. Tests to determine thyroid gland function are also done. X-rays of the uterus, taken after a special contrast dye has been injected, may be done to find out whether the woman has abnormalities in her uterus. A special type of X-ray, a uterotubogram, also called a hysterosalpingogram, in which a dye that will show up on X-ray film is injected into the uterus through the cervix, may be done. Normally, the dye will fill the uterus and spill out through the Fallopian tubes into the pelvis, where it will be absorbed. If the tubes are blocked, this test will reveal such tubal blockage. In some cases, it may even be curative, because the fluid may flush out any slight blockage and the small (not harmful) amount of radiation in the special dye may stimulate the ovaries. The test may also reveal any uterine abnormalities.

A tubal insufflation, or Rubin's test, may be done, in which a small amount of gas is blown into the uterus and, if the tubes are open, out into the pelvic cavity, where it is eventually absorbed. This test is a simple, harmless procedure that can be done in a doctor's office, but it doesn't tell whether one or both tubes are open or whether the gas escaped in some other manner. Most specialists, therefore, no longer use it, relying on X-ray studies instead. Although tubal insufflation may be useful in some cases, a woman whose doctor suggests this test should question him/her carefully as to what exactly s/he hopes to accomplish, for such a doctor may be a bit behind the times.

If these tests fail to pinpoint the cause of the infertility problem, other tests should be done, including blood tests for diabetes and thyroid problems. If hormone problems are suspected, specific urine and blood tests to check hormone levels may be done. X-rays of the pituitary gland may be necessary for either the man or the woman.

If all these diagnostic tests are inconclusive, the doctor may want to do a culdoscopic or laparoscopic exam, which must be done in the hospital. A viewing instrument is inserted through a small incision in either the vagina or the abdomen, allowing the doctor to inspect the tubes, ovaries, uterus and pelvic cavity directly. If laparoscopy is done because of suspected tubal adhesions, a specialist should perhaps be consulted, because if it turns out that microsurgery is needed to correct the problem, only specially trained doctors can perform this operation. If the doctor who does the exploratory laparoscopy is unable to perform the microsurgery, then a second laparoscopy procedure will have to be done by the specialist. Expert consultation may, then, prevent a repetition of the laparoscopy.

Treatment

If a specific cause can be identified, the doctor may attempt the various treatments outlined above. Recently, some doctors have been successful in treating unexplained infertility with a new drug, danazol (*see* p. 380).[5] If treatment of infertility is not possible or is unsuccessful, techniques such as husband insemination, in which some of the male partner's sperm is injected directly into the woman's uterus, may be possible. If the male partner's sperm is not satisfactory or, in the case of a single woman desiring artificial insemination, there is no male partner, artificial donor insemination is a possibility, although there may be a higher than usual rate of miscarriage associated with this procedure. Sperm donors, usually medical students who are paid a fee for their services, are screened and, in the case of couples, matched as closely as possible to the ethnic background, height and complexion of the male partner. Frozen sperm can be used, but the use of fresh sperm is more effective. The process is strictly confidential. To insure total anonymity some doctors select two donors and use both sperm samples. Anonymity has become an issue because of questions that have been raised about the legal aspects of artificial insemination. Although it is hard to imagine a case in which a donor would sue for information about his artificially inseminated offspring, anything can happen. A doctor who had used two or more donors would not be able to testify as to whose sperm resulted in the pregnancy. Some doctors send their artificially inseminated couples to obstetricians who are unaware of the couple's history so that the man and woman will automatically be listed as mother and father on the birth certificate. Questions regarding inheritance, custody and child support in the event of divorce are other possible legal complications, and a couple may wish to discuss the legal aspects with a lawyer first.

Artificial insemination, especially when it involves a single woman, is a highly controversial topic. In recent years, some gay women have chosen to be artificially inseminated. This, needless to say, is even more controversial, and such women may have a very difficult time finding a doctor. They would probably do best to seek help from doctors who are gay and/or sympathetic to gays (see Chapter Six).

In any case, artificial insemination has legal, philosophical and emotional aspects that deserve careful consideration by anyone considering the procedure.

Equally controversial is the so-called test-tube baby, which is more properly referred to as in vitro fertilization. In this procedure, the sperm from the male and an egg taken from the female are brought together in the laboratory. The fertilized egg is then put into the mother's body and allowed to develop as in a normal pregnancy. Recently, a great deal of media attention has been focused on the first publicly acknowledged "test-tube baby," Louise Brown, born in England. The procedure is being done in this country on a very limited basis. The first publicly announced program, which has a long waiting list, is being run at the University of Virginia Medical School.

MISCARRIAGE

AKA: spontaneous abortion

Types: threatened abortion
      inevitable, or incipient, abortion
      incomplete abortion
      missed abortion
      habitual abortion

Associated terms: septic, or infected, abortion

Miscarriages, or spontaneous abortions, occur, as the name implies, spontaneously, in contrast to therapeutic, or induced, abortions, which are performed deliberately to terminate an unwanted pregnancy. There are several different types or stages of spontaneous abortion (Illustration 55). The term "threatened abortion" is used to describe a condition characterized by bleeding and, sometimes, cramplike pain, which may or may not be followed by the expulsion of the fetus. Inevitable, or incipient, abortion refers to a threatened abortion that has progressed so far that there is no longer any question as to whether the pregnancy will continue. When an abortion does occur, it may be complete, meaning that the uterus has expelled all of the fetal and placental tissue, or it may be incomplete, meaning that some of the tissue is still inside the uterus. In some cases, even though the fetus has died it is not immediately expelled. The dead tissue remains trapped inside the uterus, and this is known as a missed abortion.

THREATENED ABORTION

INEVITABLE ABORTION

INCOMPLETE ABORTION

MISSED ABORTION

Illustration 55   *Types of Spontaneous Abortions (Miscarriages)*

635

Incidence

Miscarriages are said to occur in 10-15 percent of all pregnancies. The actual figure may be much higher than this, for some abortions undoubtedly occur without a woman's having realized she was pregnant. In such a case, all that the woman might notice would be a slightly delayed, heavier-than-normal period with, perhaps, some unusually large blood clots.

Any given woman's chances of having a miscarriage depend on a couple of factors. For instance, the chances are about one in 400 if the woman is under 25, got pregnant within three months of trying and has no previous history of miscarriage. The chances are considerably higher—40 in 100—if the woman is over 35, took six months or more to get pregnant and/or has had previous miscarriages.[6]

Cause

It is not always possible to pinpoint the cause of a miscarriage. In the majority of cases there is some abnormality in either the sperm or the ovum that results in the failure of the fertilized egg to undergo its first important cell divisions properly; thus, the embryo is incapable of growing or surviving beyond 10 or 12 weeks. The abnormal tissue dies and by the second or third month of pregnancy is expelled from the body.

The fact that a fetus is abnormal and is spontaneously aborted does not necessarily mean that there is something basically wrong with the mother's ova or the father's sperm. In the majority of cases, it is thought that the deformity was just a chance event. Just because a woman has one miscarriage, it does not follow that she will have trouble with her other pregnancies. In fact, normal delivery of a healthy infant occurs in about 80 percent of the women who have had a previous miscarriage and in 60 percent of cases where there have been two previous miscarriages. If, however, a woman has three or more spontaneous abortions, a condition known as habitual abortion, the chances of her having a normal subsequent pregnancy drop considerably.

While in the past most of these single instances of miscarriage were attributed to chance, new information is accumulating to suggest possible causes. Cigarette smoking has been linked to a higher rate of miscarriage, as has poor nutrition.[7] Environmental pollutants have been linked to higher rates of miscarriage as well as birth defects, infertility, cancer and other abnormalities.[8] For instance, an herbicide known as 2-4-5-T used widely in the Northwest by lumbering firms to retard the growth of underbrush in forests has been implicated in higher rates of spontaneous abortion and birth defects. Women living in the area of Alsea, Oregon, where there has been intensive spraying of 2-4-5-T, have a 40 percent increase in the rate of birth defects or miscarriages. In one neighborhood in the Niagara Falls area near Buffalo, the birth defect rate climbed to 56 percent and the miscarriage rate to 25 percent above normal when noxious chemicals started leaking from a dump site running right through a residential area.

In addition to these sorts of problems, miscarriage may be caused by many other factors. These are described under the heading Repeated Miscarriage.

Symptoms

Most miscarriages—about 75 percent of them—occur in the first three months of pregnancy. In very early abortions, a woman might not even be aware of the fact she was pregnant.

The first indication that a miscarriage might occur is vaginal bleeding. The bleeding may appear for only one day and be quite heavy or it may continue for weeks as scanty spotting. Sometimes the blood is bright; at other times, it is dark brown, indicating that the bleeding has been going on for some time. The longer the bleeding continues and the heavier it is, the more likely it is that an abortion will occur. The later in the pregnancy that the signs and symptoms appear, the greater the chances that the pregnancy will continue.

Pain may also be a sign that an abortion is in the offing, although in some threatened abortions there is little or no pain. If there is pain, it is usually preceded by bleeding in a woman who is going to have an early abortion. Occasionally, pain and bleeding occur together. In late abortions, the pain usually precedes the bleeding. It should be noted that pain may occur in normal pregnancy, due to pressure from the growing fetus; however, women should not hesitate to consult their doctors if pain occurs.

After the initial symptoms of pain and/or bleeding indicating a threatened abortion, the situation may develop in a number of ways. The symptoms may get worse, and on speculum exam it may be possible to see parts of the fetal tissue protruding through the cervix. Once this has happened, abortion is inevitable.

The symptoms progress until a complete abortion takes place and all the fetal and placental tissue are expelled from the womb. An early miscarriage may not feel any more uncomfortable than a heavy period. There may be one or more large clots in the blood. In a late first-trimester miscarriage— one that occurs in the third month of pregnancy—there may be cramping and bleeding on and off for days, until the uterus is completely emptied. If the miscarriage occurs after the third month of pregnancy, there are usually strong, regular uterine contractions as the cervix dilates, and for many women this may be associated with a good deal of pain. Once the fetus is expelled, the bleeding should stop within a few days.

A woman who has a miscarriage and is aware of passing the fetus and placenta should try and collect the tissue in a clean container. This may be a very difficult task emotionally, but by looking at the tissue the doctor may be able to tell whether the miscarriage was a chance event or was due to some other problem that can be treated before the next pregnancy.

Another possible turn of events is an incomplete abortion, in which portions of the fetal or placental tissue remain in the uterus. In this case the cramping and bleeding do not stop and may get a good deal worse. Sometimes there is a gushing, flooding type of bleeding. This can be quite scary. While this unusual amount of bleeding needs *immediate* medical attention, it is sometimes surprising how much blood a pregnant woman can pass without the loss being threatening to her life. Here again, fragments of recognizable fetal or placental tissue may be passed, and, if possible, these should be saved.

Sometimes, even in the presence of severe symptoms, the threatened abortion never takes place. The symptoms subside. The pregnancy continues to term, and in most cases a normal baby is delivered, although there is a slight increase in the number of birth defects in such cases.

At other times, even though symptoms have subsided, the outcome is not as happy. The fetus has died, but the uterus has not expelled the dead tissue, a situation known as a missed abortion. The cervix closes up and the bleeding stops, although in some cases there may be light bleeding if the cervix does not close tightly. As the trapped tissue decays, such bleeding is apt to be brownish in color and to smell bad. In women known to be pregnant, the failure of the uterus to grow larger after the bleeding episode is another sign of a missed abortion. In women who were not yet aware of the fact that they were pregnant, missed menstrual periods may be a sign of missed abortion.

Diagnosis

It is not always immediately possible to distinguish between a threatened abortion and an inevitable abortion. The amount of blood lost is often a clue. Keeping a count of how many sanitary napkins are used will help the doctor to estimate blood loss. Once portions of the fetal tissue are seen protruding through the cervix, the diagnosis is clear.

If the fetal tissue has been passed and the bleeding doesn't stop within a few days, this is an indication that there is something wrong. The woman may have had an incomplete rather than a complete abortion. If, however, a woman is not aware of having passed the fetus, the continued bleeding may sometimes be misinterpreted as a sign of a threatened abortion. A pregnancy test is not much help, for the test may remain positive for a while. Moreover, large blood clots in the uterus may be mistakenly interpreted to mean that the fetus is still inside the uterus. Bleeding tends to be rather profuse in an incomplete abortion, but initially this may not be so. The opening to the cervix tends to be dilated, but again this may be less obvious if most of the tissue has been expelled. Thus, a clear diagnosis cannot always be made right away.

Diagnosing these conditions may be particularly difficult in very early threatened abortions, when the characteristic signs of pregnancy—the enlarged uterus and softened cervix—may not yet be obvious. If a woman has irregular periods, doesn't have a clear idea of when her last period was or, as sometimes happens, has menstruated even though she is actually pregnant, her situation may be even more confusing. Her intermittent spotting or even heavier bleeding may be caused by a number of factors. A Pap smear, pregnancy test, endometrial biopsy, or perhaps a D&C may be necessary. Even if a woman is aware of having missed a menstrual period and pregnancy is suspected—or has been confirmed—the diagnosis of the scant bleeding and cramps that accompany threatened abortion can be very difficult. One of the most common errors in diagnosis is to mistake what is really a tubal pregnancy, that is, a pregnancy that has implanted in the Fallopian tube rather than in the uterus, for an early threatened abortion.

Consider Table 5. This neat list represents the clues a doctor uses in making this diagnosis. Unfortunately, real-life situations are rarely so clear-cut. For instance, pelvic pain is often reflected and generalized, so that it may be hard to tell exactly where the source of the pain is. A woman may not know exactly when she last menstruated, so clue No. 4, which is not a hard-and-fast rule anyway, is not always an aid in diagnosis. Sometimes anemia is not present in either case, and if it is present, may be due to another condition altogether. If the threatened abortion is very early, uterine enlargement and cervical softening may not yet be obvious. Likewise, the symptoms of fever, vomiting and fainting are not always present in tubal pregnancy. Moreover, should the threatened abortion become infected, some of these same symptoms might occur.

Since tubal pregnancy is a potentially life-threatening situation that requires immediate surgery once the diagnosis has been made, the doctor may have to use some specialized diagnostic tools to rule out the possibility if the symptoms are ambiguous. These diagnostic tools might include a Culdoscope or a laparoscope, which are specialized viewing instruments that are inserted into the pelvic cavity, or culdocentesis, a procedure in

Table 25
Symptoms of Tubal Pregnancy and Early Threatened Abortion

Tubal Pregnancy	Early Threatened Abortion
1. Scanty vaginal bleeding.	1. Scanty vaginal bleeding.
2. Enlargement on one side of the uterus, due to embryo in the tube.	2. Possible enlargement on one side of the uterus, due to corpus luteum cyst of pregnancy.
3. Sharp, cramplike pain on the affected side.	3. Pain, if present, less severe; located in the middle rather than to the side.
4. The time between the last menstrual period and the onset of bleeding is apt to be shorter, usually six to eight weeks.	4. The time between the last menstrual period and the onset of bleeding is apt to be longer, usually eight to ten weeks.
5. Anemia, if present, out of proportion to observable blood loss from internal bleeding.	5. Anemia not usually present, except if there is profuse bleeding, and then it is in line with observable blood loss.
6. Uterus not enlarged, cervix not softened.	6. Uterus enlarged, cervix softened.
7. Nausea, vomiting, faintness.	7. No nausea, vomiting, faintness.

which a needle is inserted through the vagina into the pelvic cavity in order to withdraw fluid from the pelvic cavity. The reasons for using these tools are discussed under the heading Ectopic Pregnancy.

Diagnosis may be a bit easier in a woman with a previously established pregnancy who has a missed abortion. The stopping of the initial bleeding and the failure of the uterus to grow larger are telling clues. In later stages of pregnancy, absence of fetal heartbeat and movement are, of course, strong indications. If the formerly positive pregnancy test becomes negative, this pretty much cinches the diagnosis, but the possibility, although rare, does exist that the missed abortion is actually a form of trophoblastic disease, an abnormality of the developing embryo. Although a sonogram, a method of taking internal pictures by sound waves, may be helpful in differentiating between a missed abortion and trophoblastic disease, it is rarely possible to tell until the fetus has been expelled or removed.

Treatment

Once the process has begun, there is not really much that can be done to prevent a threatened abortion from taking place. Generally, a wait-and-see approach is adopted. The woman is confined to her bed and intercourse is prohibited. If the bleeding stops of its own accord, she is usually confined to bed for another couple of days. She will be given a pregnancy test to make sure that her apparent recovery was not, in fact, a missed abortion.

In the past, hormone treatment was given to help prevent miscarriages. The now infamous DES, a synthetic estrogen, was given to millions of women in the years between 1947 and 1969 to help prevent miscarriages. When some of the teenage daughters of these women developed a rare form of cancer and other abnormalities, the dangers of this treatment became apparent (see the section on DES for details). Moreover, it is now known that DES was not even effective in preventing miscarriage.

Progesterone hormone therapy is sometimes given. There is some indication that this hormone too may cause abnormalities in the fetus.[9] It should certainly not be used without tests that demonstrate an actual deficiency, and even then, its lack of success and its possible dangers make it a highly questionable treatment.

Many threatened abortions eventually do abort. Usually, the fetus will be expelled within a short period of its death, but sometimes this doesn't happen for a few days. If there is no fever and the blood loss is minimal or sporadic, there is usually no medical need to go to the hospital to have the fetus removed, so the woman will be spared this expense. The tissue will be expelled by contractions of the uterus and the bleeding should stop within a few days. If the bleeding gets too heavy, the woman must be hospitalized, blood transfusions prepared and the uterus emptied by suction curettage, a vacuumlike method of emptying the uterus. The suction curettage is often followed by gentle scraping of the uterus with a blunt instrument called a curette. This has several advantages. First, it rules out the possibility of a congenital abnormality of the uterus, a fibroid tumor or a polyp, any of which might have distorted the shape of the uterus and thereby caused the miscarriage. Certain tissue samples can be taken to help rule out the possibility that trophoblastic disease is present. Moreover, it assures that the uterus has indeed been completely emptied.

Although the tendency in treatment is to let nature take its course and to allow the uterus to expel the fetal tissue on its own, provided of course that the bleeding is not too severe, there are two factors that might suggest a more aggressive course of action. First of all, while a missed abortion will eventually be expelled, this can take some time, perhaps a month or more. Carrying the dead fetus, and not knowing when it will be expelled, may be more of an emotional strain than a woman cares to deal with and so a suction curettage may be performed.

The second factor is infection. In an incomplete abortion, the cervical os is dilated, leaving the uterus open for bacterial invasion. The dying or dead fetal tissue is fertile ground for breeding bacteria. At the first sign of infection, the uterus must be emptied. If infection does occur, it may be mild, moderate or quite severe, depending on whether or not the infection has spread beyond the uterus. Such an infection, which is called an infected, or septic, abortion, can cause high fever and chills. If the infection spreads, there may be serious complications, which are discussed under the heading Pelvic Inflammatory Disease. Given the possibility of infection, some doctors and women will decide, even when there is no heavy bleeding, to do a suction curettage as a preventive measure. Although this can be done with a local anesthetic in the doctor's office, this procedure is sometimes more painful than normal abortion procedures, so the woman may decide to have it done in the hospital with a general anesthetic, which, while more expensive and riskier, is also more comfortable.

Prevention

Since the cause of a single spontaneous abortion is not well understood and since 80 percent of the women who experience it do not have subsequent medical problems, prevention has not been emphasized. With new information about cigarette smoking, environmental pollutants, over-the-counter drugs and nutrition, many clinics are now emphasizing nutritional and genetic counseling in preparation for subsequent pregnancies, even for women who have had only one miscarriage.

REPEATED MISCARRIAGES

AKA: recurrent miscarriage, repeated spontaneous abortion, habitual abortion

In medicalese, repeated miscarriage is called habitual abortion. The term "habitual abortion" is generally used when a woman has three or more successive pregnancies that end in miscarriage. However, some authorities apply the term to women who have had only two successive miscarriages. Still others use the term to apply to any woman who has a tendency to abort, regardless of whether the abortions occur sequentially or are interspersed with live births.

Causes and Treatment

It is thought that most miscarriages are the result of a "blighted ovum," that is, a fertilized egg or embryo that is too defective to survive. Such

642

"blighted ova" are thought to be chance events, although recent research and discoveries have implicated various drugs, cigarette smoking, poor nutrition and environmental pollutants as factors in higher rates of miscarriage. While it may be true that most spontaneous abortions can be attributed to such chance abnormalities, it is statistically unlikely that successive abortions could be traced to this cause. The odds of a random mutation happening twice, let alone three times, in the same woman, are probably less than one in a million. If, on the other hand, rather than successive abortions, there were miscarriages interspersed with normal live births, a genetic factor might be suspected. Under these conditions, an analysis of the mother's and father's chromosomes, a testing process known as karyotyping, might reveal the source of the problem; however, at this time, there is no known treatment for such a genetic defect. Genetic counseling as to the possible risks involved in future pregnancies and odds for recurrence may be offered to such couples.

In some cases, abnormalities in the father's sperm may be a factor in habitual abortion. Sperm analysis may therefore help to pinpoint the cause of a woman's habitual abortion. In some instances, though certainly not in all, these sperm abnormalities can be corrected. For details, see the discussion of male factors under the heading Infertility and Sterility.

Abnormalities that distort the shape of the uterus can be a factor in habitual abortion. These abnormalities may be congenital (present since birth). For instance, a woman may have a uterus that is divided in half by a wall of tissue. Such abnormalities and their treatment are discussed in detail under the heading Congenital Abnormalities of the Uterus. Recently, congenital abnormalities of the uterus and cervix that may affect fertility have been found in the daughters of women who took the synthetic hormone DES during their pregnancies.

Such distortions may also be acquired (the result of new disease or injury that has happened since birth). For instance, a woman may have fibroid tumors of the uterus or uterine growths known as endometrial polyps. Any of these conditions may distort the uterine cavity and make it impossible for the fertilized egg to implant or the developing embryo to grow properly. These conditions may be diagnosed by the symptoms they produce, careful physical exam, a gentle scraping of the uterine lining by a process known as dilation and curettage or, in some cases, by hysterogram, an X-ray picture of the uterus taken after the injection of a contrast fluid that makes the uterus and tubes visible on the X-ray film. Treatment of these abnormalities is generally surgical and is not always successful.

An incompetent cervix, a condition in which the cervix opens up spontaneously, can cause repeated miscarriage. Incompetent cervix may be the result of injury or a congenital defect. DES daughters may have this problem. Typically, abortions linked to cervical incompetence occur in the

18th to 32nd week of pregnancy without any prior bleeding or symptoms of impending abortion, and the duration of each succeeding pregnancy is shorter. Diagnosis is made on the basis of a history of such abortions, evidence of prior injury to the cervix and, if necessary, by ultrasound, a method of visualizing the inside of the body using high-frequency sound waves. Treatment involves tying off the cervix to prevent premature dilation.

Hormone imbalances of the type discussed under the heading Infertility and Sterility may also cause habitual abortion, though there is disagreement among the experts about whether such imbalances are a frequent or rare cause. In any case, progesterone therapy, the treatment for these abnormalities, should not be given unless the various tests used to measure hormone deficiencies indicate a definite lack. Some doctors, perhaps overcome by the logic of progesterone deficiency as an explanation for habitual abortion (and it does seem to fit right in), prescribe progesterone without the preliminary assays. This practice is questioned by many. A word of caution should be injected at this point. In the past, realizing that estrogen was important in maintaining pregnancy and that a specific type of estrogen was low in patients who aborted, doctors prescribed a treatment program using estrogen substitution in the form of the now infamous synthetic estrogen DES to a large number of pregnant women to prevent miscarriage. An alarming number of abnormalities have begun to be found in the teenage daughters born to women who took DES during their pregnancies (see the section on DES for details). Recently, there have been reports suggesting that synthetic progesterone therapy may be responsible for malformations among the offspring of women who took it,[10] which may make the use of progesterone equally questionable.

There is some evidence that certain incompatibilities in the mother's and father's blood may be a factor in miscarriage, but exactly why or how is not known. Couples with a history that runs along these lines—one normal pregnancy, then perhaps a pregnancy resulting in a jaundiced baby, then recurrent abortions at earlier and earlier stages in the pregnancy—are thought by some authorities to be suffering from certain blood incompatibilities. At the present time, there is no known treatment for this condition. Women who have an Rh-negative blood type may have problems with miscarriage.

Certain bacterial and viral infections, such as herpes, have been implicated in recurrent miscarriages. Anemia, acute and chronic diseases, including alcoholism, and constitutional illness may play a role. Certainly, treatment of such problems should be attempted when possible. Nutritional factors may play a role. Cigarette smoking is also associated with a higher rate of miscarriage.[11]

644

In many cases, no specific medical cause can be identified. Many doctors attribute cases of habitual abortion for which they are unable to find a cure to "psychological factors." It may be true that psychological factors play a role in all disease processes, but it has long been the habit of the medical establishment to blame women's diseases they have not been able to understand on womens' supposed psychological problems. (Menstrual pain is an excellent case in point.) Any woman who is told that her problem is "all in her head," or is treated as if it were, should read the introduction to this section carefully and consider seeking another medical opinion.

Diagnosis and Treatment

Finding a doctor who is sensitive and skilled in treating these problems is very important. For specific information on finding a fertility specialist, see the section on Infertility and Sterility. For general information on choosing a doctor see Chapter Six.

Diagnosing a woman with an habitual abortion problem should be done with the help of laboratory tests on the aborted tissue whenever possible. Physical exams and certain tests similar to those described under the heading Infertility and Sterility may be done on both the mother and the father. Treatment for the particular problem, based on the outcome of these diagnostic tests, may then be undertaken. These treatments are discussed in detail under the specific diseases and conditions mentioned above.

ECTOPIC PREGNANCY

AKA: extrauterine pregnancy

Types: tubal, isthmic, ampullar, or infundibular, pregnancy
      cornual, or interstitial, pregnancy
      abdominal pregnancy
      cervical pregnancy
      ovarian pregnancy

Associated terms: tubal abortion; tubal rupture; hematoma, or blood tumor; hematocele, or blood cyst

In normal pregnancies, the egg is fertilized by the sperm inside the Fallopian tube. It then travels through the tube to the uterus, where it attaches itself to the lush uterine wall and begins to grow. In ectopic pregnancies, the fertilized egg doesn't attach to the uterine wall but to

645

some other inappropriate tissue. In most ectopic pregnancies the egg implants in the Fallopian tube, but as indicated in Illustration 56, other locations are also possible.

Because only the uterus, with its rich lining and its ability to expand as the fetus grows, is really equipped to nourish a fetus and to expand to accommodate a developing pregnancy, most ectopic pregnancies abort or rupture within 6 to 14 weeks. There have been cases of certain types of ectopic pregnancy in which the pregnancy was carried to term and a normal infant delivered by Caesarean section, but the incidence of birth defects in such infants is considerably higher.

Incidence

The actual incidence of ectopic pregnancy is hard to determine since many times the symptoms are vague and minimal and the embryo is reabsorbed by the body and without the woman's being aware there was an ectopic pregnancy. Also, an ectopic pregnancy may be confused with a miscarriage or other gynecologic conditions.

The reported statistics in this country range from one in 300 to one in 40 pregnancies. The incidence is related to socioeconomic status, with much

Illustration 56   *Sites of Ectopic Pregnancies*

higher rates being reported among poor, minority women, who are less likely to have the benefit of good medical care. Twice as many black women as white die from ectopic pregnancies, which are estimated to be responsible for about 6.5 percent of all maternal deaths. There is good evidence that ectopic pregnancies are on the increase. Some doctors attribute this rise to the increase in the use of the IUD as a method of birth control, while others discount the role of the IUD. The increase in the incidence of pelvic inflammatory disease, called PID for short, especially PID caused by gonorrhea, may also explain the rise in the number of ectopic pregnancies.

Cause

There are a number of theories to explain ectopic pregnancies, some of them rather far-fetched; however, in most cases, the function of the Fallopian tube is impaired in some way, which prevents the fertilized egg from making its usual journey through the tube and into the uterus. There may be an obstruction or a distortion in the shape of the tube that might have been caused by PID, endometriosis, scar tissue from previous tubal or pelvic surgery, congenital deformities of the uterus and tubes, tumors of the tube or by ovarian or fibroid tumors pressing on the tubes. In addition to actually obstructing the tube, these conditions may also cause problems with the normal muscle contractions and the action of the tiny hairlike cilia that help move the fertile egg through the tube and into the uterus. It has also been suggested that bits of the normal uterine lining tissue may be found growing in the tubes. If this is the case, it is not surprising that the egg might incorrectly implant in such tissue.

Symptoms of Tubal Pregnancy

The fertilized egg implants in the wall of the tube, which develops an increased blood supply in response to the needs of the growing pregnancy and stretches to accommodate the enlarging embryo. But since the tube was not designed to support a pregnancy, sooner or later something has to happen. As the embryo burrows into and sometimes beyond the wall of the tube in its search for sustenance and the tube stretches, there is bound to be some bleeding. One of several things may then happen (Illustration 57).

If a woman is fortunate and the embryo has implanted near the end of the tube, the bleeding may totally separate the embryo from the wall of the tube and force it backward through the tube and out into the pelvic cavity. This is called a tubal abortion. If this happens early on, the embryo may be

TUBAL RUPTURE

TUBAL ABORTION

Illustration 57 *Possible Outcomes of Ectopic Pregnancy*

completely reabsorbed by the body. As long as no major blood vessels have been injured, the bleeding stops. There may be only minimal symptoms, like a slight delay in the menstrual period and perhaps a dull aching pain for a few days, but nothing serious enough to require medical attention. This sort of ectopic pregnancy may go unrecognized or only be discovered years later when, in the course of another operation, the remnants of the tubal pregnancy are found.

If the embryo is still partially attached to the wall of the tube, the expulsion is more likely to take place gradually, over a period of two to four weeks. The bleeding is intermittent, only a portion of the embryo being detached each time. A hematoma (blood tumor) may form around the *end* of the tube, and it may get larger with each bleeding episode, eventually causing the tube to rupture, usually between the 8th and 12th weeks. Tubal rupture may also occur if blood collects *in* the tube, a condition known as a hematosalpinx.

The tubal rupture may happen suddenly, as the tube literally bursts, or it may develop more slowly, a leaking process that takes place over a period of weeks. The bleeding may be slight or profuse; sometimes it is so excessive as to be fatal. The tubal rupture may be set off by intercourse or even by straining at the bowels.

Tubal ruptures and tubal abortions can cause external as well as internal bleeding. The first sign or symptom is apt to be a 7 to 14 day delay in menstruation, followed by slight bleeding, a red or brownish vaginal discharge that persists. Usually, there is only a scant show of blood each day. Although this spotting type of bleeding is characteristic, the bleeding may be more profuse. In some cases the bleeding will occur even before the expected time of menstruation, and in other cases the external bleeding may not occur until after two or more menstrual periods have been missed.

Pain is also an early symptom, although in some cases it is mild. At first, there may be a vague soreness on the affected side or a sort of "stitch in the side" that precedes or accompanies the spotty bleeding. Later there may also be intermittent sharp, colicky pains. In either the complete tubal abortion or the tubal rupture, the pain may be very severe, and there may be faintness, nausea and vomiting. These symptoms are a result of the irritation of the lining of the pelvic cavity, which is particularly sensitive to blood. If the bleeding into the pelvic cavity is severe, there may be symptoms of shock: rapid, irregular pulse; pallor; cold, clammy skin; subnormal temperature; and difficulty in breathing. Such a case, if not treated promptly, can be fatal. In cases of excessive internal bleeding, there may be referred pain in the top of shoulder if blood has collected beneath the diaphragm. More often, though, the bleeding is slight and of an on-again/off-again nature. Then the pain may subside quickly, leaving only soreness in between more acute attacks.

Since the developing pregnancy, even if it implants ectopically, produces hormones, the hormone-induced changes that occur in a normal pregnancy may also occur in the uterus of an ectopic pregnancy. One of these changes is the formation of a decidual lining, which becomes part of the blood-rich placenta that helps nourish a fetus during pregnancy. Once the ectopic embryo dies, the hormone production stops and this decidual lining may be shed in fragments or even in one piece. Thus, there may also be vaginal bleeding of this nature. If the lining is cast off in one piece, the woman and her doctor may mistakenly assume that the woman has had a spontaneous abortion. It is important for a woman to save any such tissue so the doctor can examine it. If there are no signs of embryonic tissue, then this may suggest an ectopic pregnancy.

The usual symptoms of pregnancy—morning sickness, swelling of the breasts, etc.—are not often seen because the embryo usually dies so early; but in cases where it does survive, such symptoms may develop.

If the embryo develops to a large enough size or if the tube is sufficiently swollen with blood, the doctor may be able to feel a tender swelling on one side or the other. The whole abdomen may be swollen, possibly so swollen that it's stretched as tight as a drum, as a result of the bleeding into the abdomen. The cervix may be softened and opened up, and the uterus may be enlarged even in early tubal pregnancy, although in most early cases this may not be noticeable. If the swelling of the tube is large enough, the doctor may be able to feel a uterus that has been pushed to one side.

There is generally little or no fever unless a hematocele (blood cyst) has formed in the pelvis and has become secondarily infected.

Diagnosis

The diagnosis of ectopic pregnancy may be quite difficult, for there are a number of other conditions that may be confused with ectopic pregnancy. A threatened or incomplete abortion, for instance, is often confused with ectopic pregnancy. Both can cause a delay in the onset of menstruation, although the length of time of the delay is longer with threatened or incomplete abortion. Moreover, the uterus is likely to be softer and larger, the pain less severe and located in the middle rather than the side and the bleeding more profuse in the case of incomplete abortion. In tubal pregnancy, where there is a great deal of internal bleeding, the anemia that results is all out of proportion to the external blood loss, whereas in miscarriage, any anemia is more or less in line with the observable blood loss.

Pelvic inflammatory disease can also behave like a tubal pregnancy and vice versa, the major difference being the fact that in PID the infection of the tubes and their swelling is usually bilateral while in ectopic pregnancy it is usually one-sided. It does happen, though, that the swelling in PID may be larger on one side than the other and thus appear to be unilateral. Although ectopic pregnancy usually produces scant, spotty bleeding, it may occasionally produce bursts of bleeding, like PID. Acute PID that affects the tubes usually produces high fever and a high white blood cell count that is not seen in ectopic pregnancy, but chronic PID may not produce these signs.

The sudden onset of pain with nausea and vomiting that may accompany tubal rupture or tubal abortion may also occur with an ovarian cyst that has become twisted on its stem, but usually there is no menstrual irregularity with the latter. It really isn't too important to make the correct diagnosis in this particular situation, for both conditions constitute an emergency and surgery is done in either case.

Luteum and follicle cysts on the ovary may also cause a delay in menstruation, followed by persistent slight bleeding, just as a tubal pregnancy does. Moreover, the enlargement of the ovary produced by these cysts may be hard to distinguish from a tubal swelling in ectopic pregnancy, especially when it is near the end of the tube. In the rare case where the tubal pregnancy implants on the ovary, this may be especially difficult.

Sometimes the corpus luteum, which produces hormones in the early stages of a normal pregnancy, will bleed into the pelvic cavity. The bleeding may be so scant that it doesn't require surgery, but it may be the cause of the pain some women feel in the first three months of pregnancy. On occasion, though, this bleeding may be extensive and may be difficult to distinguish from the shock symptoms produced by certain ectopic pregnancies, even though such symptoms as external bleeding and a tender pelvic mass are absent.

Diagnosis of an ectopic pregnancy, then, can be very difficult, and often it is not made until the tube has ruptured and the woman has had to be rushed to the hospital. Because ectopic pregnancy is a potentially life-threatening situation, it used to be that all women with suspected ectopics were operated on. Now there are specific tools that can help in the diagnosis. Culdocentesis, a procedure in which a needle is inserted into the pelvic cavity through the rear wall of the vagina, may be done. If unclotted blood is aspirated, this usually indicates an ectopic pregnancy. Culdoscopy, another procedure that can be done under a local anesthetic, allows the doctor to insert a viewing instrument into the pelvis and visually inspect the uterus, tubes and ovary. Laparoscopy, although it involves more risks and possible complications, may allow a better view and a more accurate diagnosis.

Treatment

Once a tubal pregnancy has been diagnosed, surgery must be performed. Even if a woman has little in the way of symptoms, surgery must not be delayed for too long because of the risk of fatal bleeding from a tubal abortion or rupture. In those cases where the internal bleeding has been profuse, immediate surgery is necessary and blood transfusions before or during surgery may be given.

In most cases involving younger women who have future childbearing plans, only the affected tube will be removed. There are, however, some important exceptions to this general rule in which either more or less extensive surgery may be done.

On the more extensive side, there is the older woman who has long since completed her family. In her case the uterus, tubes and, if she is close to menopause, the ovaries as well may be removed. Pros and cons on the removal of the uterus and ovaries and the age at which this should or should not be done are discussed under the heading Hysterectomy. Sometimes, upon operation, the doctor will discover that the other tube is also diseased. The same sort of scar tissue or disease that affected the first tube and caused the ectopic pregnancy may have affected the second tube. If the tube is hopelessly damaged, the doctor will remove it as well. Unless the ovaries are so diseased as to be nonfunctional or are so hopelessly matted together with the tube as to require removal, the doctor will try to leave the ovaries to prevent a premature menopause. If both tubes are taken, the majority of doctors feel that the uterus should be removed as well.

On the less extensive side, there are some cases in which it may be possible to avoid removing the affected tube. If the tube has not burst and the pregnancy is located near the open end of the tube, it may be possible to "milk" it out. Even if the pregnancy is not located at the end, as long as the tube has not yet burst, it may be possible to make an incision in the tube, remove the embryo and repair the tube. This is not always possible, and some surgeons are hesitant to try, even when one of these options seems feasible. Such doctors believe that the tube was probably defective in the first place—hence, the ectopic pregnancy—or that the ectopic pregnancy has probably done irrevocable damage to it. They feel that leaving the tube in would not increase the woman's chances of having a subsequent, successful pregnancy and might even increase her chances of having another ectopic pregnancy.

Other doctors point out that there have been many cases of women whose other tube had previously been removed who have had successful pregnancies following operations such as these. A woman, especially one who has only one tube, who very much wants to have a child, may decide to assume the risks. It is important that such a woman discuss her attitudes with the doctor prior to surgery and that she feel sure that s/he is both willing to follow her wishes if possible and sufficiently competent and experienced in this special type of surgery to do it if the situation demands it.

A similar sort of dilemma may confront the woman even if her tube has already ruptured or is so damaged that there is no choice but to remove it. Often the other tube has been affected by the same underlying disease. In cases where it is feasible, the surgeon may choose to repair the other tube at the same time. In emergency ectopics, where the woman has lost a good deal of blood, such a procedure cannot be considered, for prolonging the operation even by half an hour could risk the woman's life. In less severe situations, though, this procedure may be possible. However, many women who have such operations are unable to get pregnant again, and for those who do, the rate of second ectopics is high. Only about 50 percent of such women will subsequently have successful pregnancies. Some women may decide that they are willing to assume the risks involved. Here again, women need to discuss their feelings on this matter with the surgeon before the operation. Women who want the chance to get pregnant again should know that most gynecologists are not skilled in the special type of tubal repair surgery, known as microtuboplasty, that in some cases may be necessary to save the tube. In order to avoid the risks and complications of another operation at a later date, as well as more loss of fertility time while the body readjusts after surgery (a factor that could be critical in women in their 30s), such women might decide to seek out a surgeon skilled in microtuboplasty before having an operation for what is deemed to be an ectopic pregnancy. This, of course, will not be possible in cases demanding emergency surgery.

Other Types of Ectopic Pregnancies

Thus far, this discussion of ectopic pregnancy has centered around the more common tubal pregnancies. However, as noted in the illustration at the beginning of this section, there are other possible locations. The interstitial, or cornual, pregnancy is located where the Fallopian tube joins the uterus. It is often mistaken for a soft uterine fibroid or an early miscarriage. The symptoms are similar to those of a tubal pregnancy, although the pain may not be as severe and the delay of menstruation may be a bit longer since this location is more favorable and the embryo may survive longer. Should it rupture, the bleeding into the pelvic cavity may be very heavy, producing the same sorts of symptoms and necessitating the same treatment as a heavily bleeding tubal abortion or rupture.

Most medical authorities feel that ovarian pregnancy is extremely rare, probably due to the fact that the egg given off by the ovary is not fully mature, a process that is usually completed during the egg's journey through the Fallopian tube. Thus, the immature egg cannot be fertilized and implant anywhere. Some doctors believe that the IUD may be a factor in ovarian pregnancies. Ovarian pregnancy may also be more common than is generally thought, many cases of what are assumed to be ruptured corpus luteum cysts being in reality early ectopic ovarian pregnancies.

It is also possible for an egg to be fertilized and travel into the pelvic cavity (instead of through the tube to the uterus). This is called abdominal pregnancy and can also result from tubal abortion or rupture in which the embryo and its partially detached placenta grow out from the tube and latch on to the lining of the abdominal cavity. In removing one of these, the surgeon will leave the placenta in place since detaching it may cause massive bleeding. Some doctors use a drug called methotrexate, which is sometimes used to treat cancer, to aid in the absorption of the placenta; others feel that this very toxic drug should not be used in this manner. Women should seek second opinions (*see* p. 226) before consenting to this type of therapy.

Although extremely rare, the possibility of a cervical pregnancy does exist. This bizarre type of pregnancy produces profuse bleeding that may be fatal and usually necessitates hysterectomy. There have also been cases of tubal pregnancy accompanied by normal pregnancy, simultaneous pregnancy in both tubes and twin and even triplet pregnancy in one tube. Recently there was even a case where a woman had intercourse the night before her hysterectomy, subsequently carried an abdominal pregnancy and delivered a normal baby.

Subsequent Pregnancies

Once a woman has had an ectopic pregnancy, she is at higher risk for having another one, so subsequent pregnancies should be monitored carefully. Providing that too much blood has not been lost and the woman is not anemic, pregnancy can be attempted following resumption of the first normal menstrual period.

TROPHOBLASTIC DISEASE*

AKA: gestational trophoblastic disease, TRD

Types: hydatidiform, or benign, mole
        nonmetastatic TRD, chorioadenoma destruens, or invasive mole
        metastatic TRD, choriocarcinoma, or chorioepithelioma

Trophoblastic disease (TRD) is a condition involving the trophoblast, the layer of specialized cells on the outside of the sac in which the fertilized egg develops. In normal pregnancies, the embryo attaches itself to the uterus by means of this trophoblastic tissue. The trophoblast then invades the uterine wall and develops projections called chorionic villi through which the embryo receives nourishment from the mother's bloodstream.

TRD is usually a benign (noncancerous) disease, but in some cases it may degenerate into cancer. The benign form of TRD is known as hydatidiform mole (the term "mole" here means a swelling, not the kind of mole seen on the skin). Hydatidiform mole occurs when the fetus is stunted, has died or has never developed at all. If the fetus has died, it may be expelled in a spontaneous or induced abortion, or it may remain within the uterus, as in a missed abortion. In any case, even though the fetus is dead or absent altogether, the trophoblast continues to live and, temporarily, to grow. Since the fetus is dead and its circulatory system is no longer functioning, the fluid from the chorionic villi that would normally

---

*Readers seeking information on cancerous forms of TRD should also read the general section on cancer.

be absorbed by the fetus is not utilized. Thus, the chorionic villi become swollen with fluid. The resultant mass of swollen villi has the appearance of a cluster of pale grapes. It should be mentioned that in some rare cases, a few villi will develop in the same manner in the course of a normal pregnancy and a normal baby can be delivered in those cases. Also, parts of the placenta, the tissue through which the mother's blood reaches the infant, may be retained after childbirth and may develop a few of these similarly swollen villi.

Although TRD is most often a benign disease, it does on occasion become cancerous. The cancerous forms of TRD are metastatic and nonmetastatic TRD. They may occur after a hydatidiform mole or, in some cases, after a normal delivery, an abortion or, even more rarely, after an ectopic pregnancy, but when they do occur it is always following a pregnancy, even though the pregnancy may have been of such a short duration that the woman was not even aware of the fact that she had been pregnant. Both metastatic and nonmetastatic TRD involve abnormalities of the process by which the trophoblast invades the rich uterine lining.

The exact nature of these abnormalities is not clear. Even in normal pregnancies, the process by which the trophoblast implants is not well understood. The fetus and the trophoblast are actually foreign bodies to the mother's uterus, and why they are not rejected remains a mystery. It is thought that the mother's immune system, which normally attacks foreign bodies, is somehow switched off, thereby allowing the trophoblastic tissue to make its invasion without resistance. The trophoblast is allowed to go only just so far and is stopped before it can grow into the lower levels of the uterine wall. It is thought that the mother's immune system somehow sets limits on this invasive process.

In all other instances in which one type of tissue invades another, we are talking about a malignant, or cancerous, growth pattern, the exception being the curious case of the trophoblast in a normal pregnancy. The trophoblast also has another similarity to cancer. Just as cells from a cancerous tumor may travel to other parts of the body and set up new colonies of cancerous tissue—a process known as metastasis—so cells from the trophoblast may travel via the bloodstream from the mother's uterus to her lung. In a normal pregnancy, this metastasized trophoblastic tissue in the lung causes no harm. Here again, there is probably some mechanism in the mother's immune system that prevents trophoblastic metastasis from becoming a problem.

Sometimes this little-understood process of trophoblastic invasion, which as we have seen may also include metastasis, goes awry. The trophoblast may not stop growing, continuing to grow beyond the uterine wall and even through it into the pelvis or vagina, a process that produces an alarming and sometimes even fatal amount of bleeding. If this growth pattern, which is now considered a cancerous one, is accompanied by metastatic colonies of trophoblastic tissue invading the lung, the terms "metastatic trophoblastic disease," "choriocarcinoma" or "chorioepithelioma" are used. If there is no metastasis to the lung or other points in the body but there is growth into the uterine wall or beyond, it is considered nonmetastatic trophoblastic disease, which is also known as chorioadenoma destruens or, more simply, invasive mole.

Incidence

Fortunately, trophoblastic disease is rather rare in this country, occurring in only about one in every 1,500 or 2,000 pregnancies.[12] It occurs more frequently at the extremes of reproductive life, that is, in women over 40 or under 20 years of age. Cancerous types of TRD are fortunately much less common than the benign hydatidiform mole. Two percent of the women who have a hydatidiform mole pregnancy will have moles in subsequent pregnancies, which, although it is a low incidence, is 40 times the normal rate for women who have not had previous moles.

Symptoms

The chief symptom of hydatidiform mole is painless vaginal bleeding. The bleeding occurs after at least one or two menstrual periods have been missed. There is little to distinguish this bleeding from that of an early miscarriage, except that the hydatidiform mole generally occurs later, usually beyond the tenth week of pregnancy. However, in the case of a mole the bleeding usually does not stop once it has started. It continues until the uterus has been emptied of all abnormal tissue.

About half of the women with hydatidiform mole will have enlarged uteri.[13] If a woman is known to be pregnant, the doctor may become suspicious when s/he feels a uterus that is larger than it should be for the stage of her pregnancy. An enlarged uterus in a pregnant woman with vaginal bleeding is going to make the doctor suspicious of several possibilities. However, not all women show this symptom, and some may even have uteri that are smaller than expected through the duration of the pregnancy.

Women with hydatidiform mole may show signs of toxemia, a condition that is characterized by swelling, headaches, vision disturbances (from swelling in the brain), high blood pressure, nausea and protein in the urine. About one-half of the women will have vomiting.[14] These symptoms are probably caused by the hormone HCG, human chorionic gonadotropin.

During pregnancy, this hormone is secreted by the placenta, the organ through which nutrients are filtered from mother to fetus and which develops in part from the trophoblast. In TRD, the hormone is secreted in abnormally excessive amounts. There may be an excess of other hormones as well. In about 10 percent of cases of hydatidiform mole, there will be evidence of an overactive thyroid gland.

A woman may pass pale, grapelike clusters of villi, or sometimes these may be seen on speculum exam as pale grapes protruding through the cervical os. There may be bleeding if the woman spontaneously aborts the mole. Although the vaginal bleeding discussed above is painless, the bleeding that accompanies the expulsion of the mole is usually associated with uterine cramps.

The ovaries may also be affected in TRD. Apparently, the excessive amount of the hormone HCG triggers the first steps in the process of ovulation. The stimulated eggs do not burst out of their capsules, but remain on the surface of the ovary as cysts. These cysts may be small or large; in about a third of cases of TRD they are large enough to be felt by the doctor in the course of a bimanual pelvic exam.[15] However, these same sorts of cysts may be large enough to be felt in a normal pregnancy as well.

For some unknown reason, these cysts seem to grow rapidly after the mole has been expelled from the uterus. Another curious fact is that they sometimes disappear spontaneously as the disease progresses. It has been suggested by some experts that these cysts may provide protection against the subsequent development of choriocarcinoma. The large amount of estrogen produced by these cysts seems to act as a brake against excessive trophoblastic growth; thus a woman without ovarian enlargement may be more likely to have her hydatidiform mole undergo malignant transformation.

Diagnosis of the Hydatidiform Mole

Diagnosis of a hydatidiform mole is not always a simple process. The painless vaginal bleeding is likely to be interpreted as a sign of impending miscarriage, a much more common occurrence than hydatidiform mole. A woman with such bleeding and a uterus that is overenlarged for the duration of her pregnancy should cause a doctor to be suspicious enough to run tests. Likewise, the onset of symptoms of toxemia before the 20th week of pregnancy in a woman without underlying disease to which the toxemia could be attributed should make the doctor suspicious. If the doctor can't hear fetal heart tones by the 12th week of pregnancy, or if there is no evidence of fetal movement by the 18th to 20th week, TRD should be suspected.

If all or some of these symptoms—bleeding, enlarged uterus, toxemia and absence of fetal heart tone and movement—are present, the doctor should be suspicious enough to run extensive laboratory tests. Laboratory evidence from the series of tests indicating higher than normal levels of HCG are extremely useful, though not conclusive, for HCG levels may vary in individuals. Moreover, a twin pregnancy could also yield high levels of HCG. When the high levels of the HCG are accompanied by low levels of certain other hormones normally associated with pregnancy but not with TRD, the doctor will have an almost certain diagnosis.

The next step will probably be ultrasound examination, a method of visualizing the soft tissue inside the body by the use of high-frequency sound waves. If the ultrasound examination shows fetal parts, the diagnosis of hydatidiform mole is pretty much ruled out since a developed fetus and a mole only rarely coexist. One rare example might be a twin pregnancy in which one of the pregnancies is molar and the other one normal.

X-ray examination can also be used to determine whether or not a fetal skeleton is present, but because of the possible risks involved in radiating the fetus, the X-ray examination is not used until the doctor is fairly certain that a viable fetus is not present.

Many times the diagnosis of hydatidiform mole is not made until the woman actually starts to pass the characteristic clusters of swollen, grapelike villi. Any woman who passes something unusual should save the tissue if at all possible so that her doctor can examine it.

Treatment of the Hydatidiform Mole

Treatment of a hydatidiform mole is threefold. The first step is to determine the best method of removing the mole and then to do so. The next step is to rule out the possibility that the mole has undergone cancerous transformation. The third step is to plan and execute a careful follow-up program.

If the diagnosis of hydatidiform mole is not made until the woman is spontaneously aborting the mole, then the woman is hospitalized and given a drug that aids the uterine contractions and helps in the expulsion of the mole.

In the absence of labor, a decision must be made as to how to evacuate the mole. If the woman is over 35 and has finished her family, a hysterectomy may be the treatment of choice since there is a much higher incidence of malignant TRD in women over 35. If there is cancer and it is only a localized, nonmetastatic form of TRD, then the hysterectomy will be curative. But the hysterectomy is more treatment than is really needed for 85 percent of the women with TRD since only 15 percent of TRD patients will have cancerous complications. Although in the past hysterectomy was the only alternative, today, thanks to two developments—the sensitivity of tests to detect HCG and the development of drugs that can offer close to a 100 percent cure rate—not all women with a molar pregnancy need to have their uteri removed.

In most cases, the uterus can be emptied by a D&C or a suction curettage, a vacuumlike procedure used to suck out the contents of the uterus. Once the evacuation has been accomplished by whatever method, the tissue is carefully studied for signs of cancer. Unfortunately, such studies are not conclusive; therefore, a careful follow-up program, which involves measuring levels of HCG, must be instituted to rule out the possibility of cancer.

In two to four weeks, most women's HCG levels will return to normal.[16] Even after the HCG levels drop, a woman must be tested once a month for six months, and then once every other month for six more months, since the trophoblastic tissue may still be present, either in the pelvic area or in some other location as a result of metastasis, and it might take this long for the remaining tissue to grow large enough to produce a quantity of HCG that could be measured even by the most sensitive of tests now available. A woman should not become pregnant during this time because pregnancy would create higher levels of HCG, which would confuse the picture.

Since metastasis, if it occurs, frequently affects the lungs, chest X-rays are done every two weeks until HCG levels return to normal, and then every three months for a year. Bimanual pelvic exams to check that the uterus is returning to normal size and to allow the doctor to examine the vulva and vagina for masses of TRD are also done every two weeks until the HCG level returns to normal, and then, every three months for a year.

Metastatic and Nonmetastatic Trophoblastic Disease

Invasive mole is the nonmetastatic form of TRD that occurs when the trophoblast of a hydatidiform mole takes on a cancerous growth pattern. There is apt to be bleeding beyond the normal six to eight weeks after the mole has been expelled or removed from the uterus. If the uterus has been perforated by the invasive mole, there may be a great deal of bleeding, sometimes enough to be fatal. Also, if perforation has occurred, there may be infection, chills and fever. If the mole has spread beyond the uterus, it may be possible to feel masses in the pelvis or vagina. Choriocarcinoma is a metastatic form of TRD and can produce symptoms like those of invasive moles.

If vaginal bleeding continues for too long a time after a mole has been evacuated, this may indicate that the trophoblastic tissue is still present. If the HCG levels remain elevated for more than 60 days or if the HCG rises at any time during the follow-up, this is also taken as a sign that the trophoblastic tissue is still present and that it has taken on a cancerous growth pattern. Actually, only about 40 percent of those women whose HCG levels remain elevated after 60 days actually have metastatic or nonmetastatic TRD, but it is impossible at this point to tell whether any given woman is among the 60 percent who will progress to cancer or among the 40 percent who will not.[17] Chemotherapy, treatment of cancer by drugs, must be given to all such women, for the risks of withholding treatment are simply too great.

Chemotherapy is usually given orally or by injections for five days, followed by a resting stage of one week while new tests of HCG levels are obtained. If HCG continues to decrease, subsequent chemotherapy is continued until the tests are negative. The tests are then repeated until they remain negative for one year. If during the therapy there is a rise in HCG or evidence of drug toxicity, another type of chemotherapy is used. Although a few experts recommend giving preventive drug therapy to all women with hydatidiform mole, this practice is questioned by most experts since 85 percent of these women will not develop TRD and these drugs are extremely toxic.[18] Any woman whose doctor suggests prophylactic, or preventive, chemotherapy just because she had a mole should seek a second opinion (*see* p. 226).

Cancer that starts out as a seemingly normal pregnancy and turns out to be a life-threatening, horrible disease is not a pleasant prospect for any woman. However, the progress that has been made in treating what was formerly a highly lethal disease is encouraging. Cure rates of 80-100 percent for nonmetastatic TRD and 36-95 percent for metastatic TRD have been reported.[19] Because the disease is hardly a common one, many doctors are not equipped, trained or experienced enough to properly treat it. A woman with TRD should consider contacting one of the trophoblastic-disease study centers around the country. Her doctor should be able to find out where the nearest center is located. If not, the nearest medical school should be able to answer this question.

These study centers generally have some form of counseling available. Any woman, especially one who is childless, may need counseling in these circumstances. She is apt to feel that there is something monstrous about her. Both she and her partner or family may benefit from such counseling. Normal pregnancies can and do follow drug therapy. If the woman wants to get pregnant again, she must wait until follow-up therapy has been completed. She may also find special counseling and support during pregnancy valuable.

Cancer

Madison Avenue and public health agencies, in an effort to make us aware of the cancer problem and to encourage us to seek early treatment for suspicious symptoms, have in some ways oversold cancer to the American public. Most of us are terrified of the disease, although great strides have been made in treating it and some forms are now virtually 100 percent curable. Yet, even those of us with curable forms of the disease are apt to find being diagnosed as having cancer or even going through a diagnostic work-up for a possible cancer, a frightening experience, for confronting cancer brings us face to face with the possibility of our own death.

Too many times, our fear makes us act hastily, choosing a doctor or accepting a form of treatment before we really understand our options; but these decisions are important ones, sometimes even matters of life and death and they deserve our careful consideration. The treatment of cancer is one of the most controversial subjects in medicine. The type of treatment you receive will depend on many factors, including your age, menstrual status and the type and extent of your cancer. The quality of treatment as well as the kind of treatment you receive may also depend on the particular doctor you choose. The same woman may be treated differently by different doctors.

It's especially important to be an informed consumer if you have or may possibly have cancer. But it isn't always easy to be a wise consumer when you're anxious and apprehensive, as anyone confronting cancer is apt to be. For this reason, we suggest that you enlist the help of a friend or

661

relative. The following pages provide general information about cancer and advice on how to assure yourself of getting optimum care. In addition, specific types of female cancers are discussed in greater detail in other sections of this book. Read these pages carefully, taking notes as necessary, and ask your friend or relative to do the same thing. Working together, make a list of the important issues and questions to be discussed with the doctor.

When you visit the doctor, take that person along with you. When we are upset, we may not be thinking rationally and often misunderstand what is being said. Having someone else with you can therefore be invaluable. A good doctor will not object to your bringing someone else along. If your doctor refuses to allow you to include someone else in your consultations, find another doctor.

Do not allow yourself to be rushed into a decision about treatment. By the time a cancer is discovered, it has already been in your body for quite some time. Taking a few days or, with certain types of cancer, even a week or two to fully inform yourself and to seek consultations and second opinions won't hurt and may be a lifesaving step.

In the following pages we provide basic information about cancer and how it behaves. We also define basic terms and concepts used in connection with cancer. More specific information on the various types of cancer is discussed in the section on the particular organ involved—breast cancer, for instance, is covered in the section on the breast. The information on each of the specific types of cancer is broken down into various subheadings, such as Incidence, Risk Factors, Symptoms, Diagnosis, Stage, Treatment, Follow-Up and so forth. Basic information on these topics is also included here, and you will probably find it useful to review this more general information before you turn to the discussion of the specific type of cancer with which you are concerned.

What Is Cancer?

In order to be an informed consumer of the medical services available to cancer patients, it helps to have an understanding of what cancer is. Actually, cancer is not a single disease but many different diseases that may present a variety of symptoms, may have different causes and may require different forms of treatment. The exact nature of cancer is not understood, but the one thing that all cancers have in common is irregular growth of abnormal cells.

Our bodies are a collection of organs and tissues that are made up of trillions of cells, which are microscopic bits of Jell-O-like material. Each cell has a center, called a nucleus, and is surrounded by a special membrane that acts like a filter, permitting certain substances to enter or leave the cell. Throughout the cell there are tiny "factories" that process the nutrients that have filtered through the cell membrane from the bloodstream. Each type of cell has its particular job to do. By interacting physically and chemically with each other, the cells produce energy to support the function of the particular organ in which they are located. Cancerous cells can interfere with the function of the organ in which they are located because they don't do their job properly.

There are many different types of cells, and each type has its own individual characteristics. Some are long and slender, others are rather round. The size of the nucleus also varies. Each type of cell also has its own particular architecture. Glandular cells, for instance, form circular patterns. Skin cells form flat sheets. Whatever the pattern, these cells build up, layer by layer, in a neat, orderly fashion.

Cells grow up and mature in the same sense that a person does. Young cells look different from fully mature cells. The normal cells at the same stage of growth in any given class of cells look pretty much the same. Cancerous cells sometimes look rather like the normal cells, but sometimes they look wildly different. They do not organize themselves into the same orderly architecture, although there is a tendency to mimic the normal growth patterns. Cancerous gland cells, for instance, often organize into circlelike patterns. Their circular architecture is not, however, as orderly as that of normal gland cells.

As normal cells mature and develop, so that they are able to perform their particular job, they are said to be differentiating. A fully mature cell, then, is one that is well differentiated. This term, "differentiated," is an important one in cancer, especially in certain types of cancer. If the cells of a cancerous tumor are undifferentiated, this means they are immature and look quite different from the normal, mature, differentiated cells, which generally means that the cancer is a more serious one. The term "grade" is used to refer to the degree of differentiation. Grade is discussed in more detail below.

Normal cells constantly wear out and die and are replaced by new ones. Most cells in our body reproduce by a process known as cell division, or mitosis. Inside the nucleus of each cell are strands called chromosomes, which are the bearers of substances called genes. Genes are made of the protein molecule DNA. These chromosomal strips, with their genes and DNA, are the cell's mastermind, a sort of computer headquarters that directs its behavior. When a cell is ready to reproduce itself, it grows a duplicate set of chromosomes, a process known as twinning. Once there is a complete duplicate set, the two sets begin to move apart, migrating to opposite sides of the cell. Meanwhile, the outer membrane of the cell begins to indent and then quickly starts to cleave, pinching in until it divides into two separate cells, as shown in Illustration 58.

After resting for a while, the cells begin the process of twinning and dividing all over again. Different types of cells have different resting times. Specific directions are "printed" in the DNA of the chromosome strip that let the cell know how long to rest and stay dormant until the tissue of which it is a part needs new cells to replace those that have died.

If everything goes well, the new twin strip of chromosomes is identical to the original strip and the new cell will then behave exactly like the original one in every detail, right down to the specific amount of resting time in between reproductive cycles. Sometimes, however, errors, or mutations, occur. The twinning process goes awry and the new cell is not an exact replica. If the mutation is severe, the cell may die. If it is a minor one, it may merely affect one particular behavior of that cell. If, for instance, one of the cell's jobs is to absorb iron from the bloodstream and the new cell has an error in twinning that involves the gene that regulates iron absorption, then that cell and its descendants will not absorb iron in

Illustration 58 *Twinning: The Reproductive Process of a Cell*

the usual fashion. In most cases, an error like this is not likely to affect the overall functioning of the organ. If, however, the error or mutation in the twinning process involves the gene that controls the length of time the cell spends resting in between reproduction, the result could be cancer.

Once the mutation has occurred, it is repeated each time the cell reproduces. So the one mutated cell becomes two. The two become four; the four become eight, the eight sixteen; the sixteen thirty-two; and so on, until after about 20 cell generations there are about one million cells, weighing about 1/1000 of a gram. By 30 generations, there will be about one billion cells weighing about one gram. A tumor of this size, depending on where it is located, may be large enough to be felt. The tumor grows 1,000 times larger in just half the time that it took to grow to the 1/1000 gram weight. By the 31st generation, it will increase to two grams, and by the 32nd, it will weigh four grams.

This explains a phenomenon that people often find puzzling—the fact that although cancer is said to take years to develop, once a cancer is discovered it often seems to grow at a rapid-fire pace. Actually, the rate of growth is constant. This rate, the average time required for all the cells in the tumor to reproduce, is called the doubling time. The doubling time varies according to the type of tissue. If the normal cells in an organ grow slowly, generally the cancer in that tissue will have a relatively slow rate of growth. Liver cells, for instance, are slow-growing and so are cancerous liver cells. Some cancers grow more quickly. Breast cancer has a doubling time of anywhere from 6 to 540 days, depending on the particular kind of cells involved.

A tumor that had a 100-day doubling time would take nine years to grow from a single cell to a one-gram tumor that could be felt, but in only 15 more months it would weight 16 grams—about half an ounce—and in 15 more months it would weigh almost a pound! Thus, although the doubling rate is steady—100 days—the fact that every cell in the entire tumor doubles every 100 days—a geometric progression—explains the rapid acceleration in its size.

Meanwhile, the other cells of the organ are plodding away, reproducing at the preprogrammed rate designed to assure that the proper numbers of the right kinds of cells will be in the proper ratio to each other so that the organ will function as it should. But, as we have seen, the cancer cells are not resting; they are reproducing at too fast a rate. Although the cancer cells, like normal cells, wear out and die, their birth rate far outstrips their death rate.

The invaded organ has no use for this overabundance of cells. Thus, the cancerous cells may throw the organ out of whack by their sheer bulk; because they have not matured properly, are undifferentiated and unable to do their job; or by gobbling up the food that should nourish the other cells. Not only do they endanger the proper functioning of the organ by their overabundance within a particular area, but they tend to invade other tissues as their exuberant growth continues. If one of these mutant cells gets into the blood or lymph system, it may be carried to another part of the body and start a new colony of aberrant tissue, a phenomenon known as metastasis.

Spread

Different types of cancer can spread from the tissues in which they originate in a number of different ways. The cancerous tumor may simply keep growing in the same place (in which case it is said to be localized), getting bigger and bigger, until it invades and destroys the neighboring tissue. When this happens the terms "direct extension" or "invasion" are used. As noted above, sometimes the cancer spreads because the abnormal cells get into the bloodstream or the lymph system, which is an intricate network of interconnected passageways through which a fluid known as lymph is circulated. The lymph system is part of the body's defense system. The abnormal cells may then be carried to other parts of the body, where they start growing. The tumor is then said to have metastasized. Metastatic tumors, then, are colonies of new tumors composed of cells that have been transplanted. Once either direct invasion or metastasis (plural: metastases) has taken place, the malignant disease is said to be disseminated.

Particular types of cancer have a tendency to spread to particular organs. Breast cancer, for instance, generally metastasizes from the primary site in the breast to the liver, bones, lung or brain. Even though a breast cancer has metastasized from the breast to the bones, it is still called breast cancer, for the cancer, although now located in the bones, is made of breast cancer cells, not bone cancer cells.

Sometimes it is easy to identify whether a cancer is primary, i.e., had its origin in the tissue in which it is found, or secondary, i.e., is the result of metastasis or direct invasion from some other site. But sometimes it isn't so easy. If, for instance, there is a widespread cancer involving the vulva, vagina and cervix, it may be impossible to say just where the cancer started or, indeed, if there were just one primary cancer. In the case of metastatic cancer in a distant organ, if the cancer cells are quite abnormal, it may be impossible to clearly identify the original source.

Some cancers metastasize early in the course of their development;

others tend to grow relatively large or to invade directly before they metastasize. Thus it is sometimes possible for the secondary cancer to be discovered before the primary one.

Identifying a cancer as either primary or secondary is very important for two reasons. First of all, if it's a secondary cancer, the primary one needs to be found and treated. Secondly, not all types of cancer are responsive to the same forms of treatment. A bone cancer that has metastasized from the breast will be most successfully treated by therapies effective against breast cancer cells, not treatments designed to cure bone cancer.

Causes

Why these cell abnormalities and errors in twinning occur is not known—in other words, nobody knows what causes cancer. But with all the twinning that is constantly going on inside our bodies, it's not surprising that once in a while something will go wrong.

Chemicals or even natural substances that get into our tissues in one way or another are thought to play a role. Hormones, both natural and synthetic, are also thought to be factors. Vaginal clear cell adenocarcinoma is related to the use of the synthetic hormone DES[1]. Uterine cancer is linked to both naturally produced hormones[2] and the estrogens used to treat menopausal sympoms[3]. Viruses that can penetrate the cell membrane and alter the DNA have been implicated in cancer. Cervical cancer is strongly linked to the herpes virus.[4] Radiation from the sun, X-rays and nuclear particles can also alter the microscopic DNA and cause cancer. Safe levels of radiation have not yet been determined, which is why there is so much controversy surrounding the use of X-rays in diagnosing various diseases and in treating anything less serious than cancer.

Many researchers feel that our bodies are probably producing mutant cells, some of them cancerous, all of the time, but that our incredibly efficient immunological system is able to isolate and destroy these aberrant cells. People who have organ transplants and are given drugs to suppress the immunological system so that their bodies won't reject the transplants are particularly susceptible to cancer. Some scientists think that it is only when those errors in twinning occur *and* our immunological system is unable to cope that cancer occurs.

Cancer also seems to be related to aging. Although cancer can affect children and young adults, the overwhelming majority of cancer occurs in people over the age of 55. Some researchers attribute this to a decline in the efficiency of the immunological system with age.

667

You cannot catch cancer the way you can catch a cold, nor can you transmit cancer to someone else. (There is, however, some speculation that cervical cancer may be related to a sexually transmitted agent, perhaps the herpes virus; see the section on cervical cancer for details.)

Types of Abnormal Cell Growth

Not all of the irregularities in cell growth are so extreme as to be called cancerous, or malignant. Sometimes growth irregularities occur in which the cells, unlike cancerous cells, are not so abnormal, don't destroy the neighboring normal cells, don't grow as rapidly, don't spread into or invade the surrounding tissue and are not capable of metastasizing to other organs. These growths are called benign tumors, "benign" meaning "noncancerous" and "tumors" meaning simply "new growth." A wart or a uterine fibroid would be an example of a benign tumor.

Abnormal cells that do not or have not yet metastasized to other organs or invaded the surrounding tissue, yet do have the extreme abnormalities of cancer cells, are called carcinoma in situ ("carcinoma" being a medical term for a particular kind of cancer and "in situ" meaning "in place"). It is not known whether carcinoma in situ always progresses to cancer. We know that some carcinoma in situ does become true invasive, and eventually metastatic, cancer, but it may be that some carcinoma in situ remains dormant.

There is, then, some controversy about the term "carcinoma in situ." Some doctors object to calling something cancerous that does not actually invade the surrounding tissue.

There are also certain other abnormal cell growth patterns that are possibly precancerous. These include dysplasia and hyperplasia. Sometimes they will progress to carcinoma in situ (or, possibly, directly to invasive cancer), but other times they will revert to normal.

In routine autopsies of people who have died from other causes, these carcinomas in situ and other precancerous conditions are found in much higher numbers than are true cancers. In one series of autopsies of women over the age of 70, these sorts of precancerous conditions were found in the breast at a rate 19 times higher than the actual rate of cancer in this age group.[5] Thus, it is obvious that not all of these precancerous conditions and carcinomas in situ do become true cancer. It is thought that the body's efficient immune system prevents this. This, as we shall see, raises some questions about the value of early detection and may have important implications for the treatment of cancer.

Another lesser form of cancer is microinvasive cancer. This is true cancer that is actually invading the neighboring tissue, but that has been diagnosed while the spread is still quite minimal. Precise definitions of what exactly constitutes microinvasion have not been established, so different doctors will use different definitions.

Types of Cancer

There are many different types of cancer, and cancers may be classified in a number of different ways. They may be classified as to the organ in which they arise, which is how this book classifies them. They include:

☐ Preinvasive cancer of the vulva
☐ Vulvar cancer
☐ Clear cell adenocarcinoma of the vagina and cervix
☐ Vaginal cancer
☐ Cervical dysplasia
☐ Carcinoma in situ of the cervix
☐ Cervical cancer
☐ Endometrial hyperplasia
☐ Uterine cancer
☐ Cancer of the Fallopian tube
☐ Cancer of the ovary
☐ Breast cancer
☐ Choriocarcinoma (cancer of fetal tissue)

Most of the cancers discussed in this book are carcinomas, cancers that arise from tissues that cover the surface or line the interior of internal organs and passageways of the body. A few sarcomas, cancers that arise from the connective or muscle tissue, are discussed, but in less detail since carcinoma is far more common.

Cancers are also classified by the type of cell. This is known as histological classification. An adenocarcinoma would be composed of glandular (*adeno*) cells, whereas an epithelial carcinoma would be composed of epithelial, or skin, cells. These may be further broken down into subcategories. A squamous cell carcinoma would be one that arose from the particular type of epithelial tissue known as squamous cell epithelium that lines the vaginal cavity. Sometimes the histological type will greatly influence the choice of treatment, as well as the chances of surviving.

Cancerous tumors are generally solid, but they may become fluid-filled, either because the tumor itself secretes fluid or because it breaks down in its center. In either case, they are referred to as cystic. A mucinous cystadenocarcinoma of the ovary, then, is a fluid-filled cancer of a specific type of epithelial gland tissue that produces a mucus-type secretion.

Incidence

Incidence rates are given in terms of the number of people per 100,000 who contract the disease each year. Most of the time incidence rates for cancer are age-adjusted so that people too young to develop the disease have been eliminated from the figuring. For many types of gynecological cancer, the incidence rates are adjusted to include only women in their reproductive and postmenopausal years since gynecologic cancers are rare in prepubertal girls.

Incidence rates are valuable for two reasons. Differences in incidence rates among certain groups may help isolate causes related to difference in diet, behavior, environment or other factors. Incidence rates can also help us identify women who are at high risk. If a woman knows she is at high risk, she can take extra precautions and undergo more frequent routine tests, so that the disease, should she develop it, can be detected in its earlier stages. For example, women with a history of herpes have higher rates of cervical cancer, so such women might decide to have more frequent Pap smears.

Risk Factors

Being at "high risk" means that your chances of getting the disease are, statistically speaking, greater than those of the general population. But this high risk does not necessarily mean that you will get the disease. Conversely, not having any of the high-risk characteristics doesn't mean that you won't develop the disease. Epidemiologists—scientists who study the kinds of people who get certain diseases—have been able to identify risk factors for some forms of cancer, but not for all.

Symptoms

The symptoms of cancer vary according to the organ in which the cancer arises and the stage of the cancer. The particular location within the organ may have an influence on the symptoms. Sometimes the particular cell type of the tumor will play a role in determining the symptoms.

The American Cancer Society lists these warning signs or symptoms.

☐ Unusual bleeding or discharge
☐ A lump that does not go away
☐ A sore that does not heal within two weeks
☐ Change in bowel or bladder habits
☐ Persistent hoarseness or cough
☐ Indigestion or difficulty in swallowing
☐ Change in a wart or mole

These symptoms can, of course, be produced by other, noncancerous conditions. Cancer is frequently asymptomatic until it is fairly advanced, although some cancers will produce symptoms fairly early. The specific symptoms associated with the female cancers are discussed under the appropriate headings.

Diagnosis

A suspicious symptom may be discovered by the woman herself or by her doctor in the course of a routine physical.

Screening Tests

For some forms of cancers, there are tests that can detect cancer even before there are obvious symptoms. These tests may be used to screen asymptomatic women for cancer. For example, the Pap smear, which can detect cervical cancer in its earliest stages, has been used to screen large numbers of women. Mammograms, X-ray studies of the breast, can detect breast tumors before they are large enough to be felt, but X-rays carry some risk and there has been considerable controversy about the routine use of mammography to screen women for breast cancer. The endometrial biopsy can be used to screen women who are at high risk for uterine cancer, but since the endometrial biopsy is not a simple, painless, inexpensive procedure like the Pap smear—indeed, it can be quite painful—it is not used routinely on all women.

Biopsy

Screening tests and symptoms are not usually enough to confirm a diagnosis. A biopsy, which involves removing all or part of the suspicious tissue and examining sections of it microscopically, is the most reliable method of determining whether or not cancer is actually present. If only a portion of the tumor is removed, the term "incisional biopsy" is used. If

671

the entire tumor is removed, the term "excisional biopsy" is used. Sometimes a needle is used to get a tissue sample, and this is termed a "needle biopsy."

One-Step and Two-Step Biopsies: Frozen and Permanent Sections

Different types of biopsies are done for different types of cancer. Sometimes a one-step procedure is done. In one-step procedures, the woman is prepared for major surgery and given a general anesthetic. The surgeon then performs the biopsy and, while the woman remains on the operating table, the biopsied tissue is sent to a laboratory in the hospital, where it is examined by a pathologist, a specially trained doctor. The pathologist carefully cuts the tumor into sections. One or more of these tissue sections are then placed on a slide, quick-frozen and examined microscopically. The whole process, which is called a frozen section, takes about 10−15 minutes. The pathologist then reports back to the surgeon in the operating room. If the pathologist's diagnosis is "benign" the woman is "closed up" and taken to the recovery room. If a malignancy is diagnosed, the doctor will usually proceed with a cancer operation.

In the two-step procedure, the biopsy and the treatment are done at separate times. The biopsy may be done in the doctor's office or on an outpatient basis at the hospital, depending on the type of cancer the woman is being tested for. Generally, only a local anesthetic is needed. The biopsied specimen is again sent to the pathologist, but in the two-step procedure the pathologist performs a permanent section, rather than a frozen section. It takes longer to get the results from a permanent section, generally a few days, but the results are easier to "read" than a frozen section, for the freezing process may distort the cells and make it more difficult to tell if the cells are normal.

Whenever possible, a two-step procedure should be done. If the biopsy indicates cancer, the two-step procedure allows for further testing, second opinions and time for the woman to make important decisions before the cancer operation. The permanent section is also more accurate than the frozen section. However, as long as she is being treated at a good hospital with a good pathology department (see below), a woman need not be overly concerned about inaccuracy in frozen sections, for a good pathologist will realize when the frozen section is too distorted for conclusive diagnosis. If there is any doubt in the pathologist's mind, s/he will tell the surgeon that the case is borderline and that it is necessary to wait for the results of the permanent section. Even in one-step procedures where surgical decisions are based on frozen sections, permanent sections are always done afterwards as a double check.

Most biopsies can be done as two-step procedures; however, in certain types of cancer, when the suspicious mass is located deep inside the body, it may not be possible to do a two-step procedure. If, for example, a woman had a suspicious ovarian mass, a two-step procedure would not be done. Major surgery is already necessary in order to get at the ovary for the biopsy, and there would be no point in doing a two-step procedure and subjecting the woman who did turn out to have cancer to a second major surgery. In breast cancer, one-step procedures are sometimes done, even though it is generally possible to do two-step procedures. This is one of the important consumer issues that women with breast lumps should be aware of, and it is discussed more fully in the section on breast cancer.

Biopsies may also be done at the time of the cancer surgery to detect the possibility of microscopic spread to other organs, adjacent tissues and lymph nodes and are a common part of cancer treatment. These may be analyzed via frozen section so that more extensive surgery can be done right away. If the doctor plans to use radiation therapy to treat any further spread should the biopsies be positive, a permanent section will be done. Here again, even when frozen sections are done, permanent sections will also be done to "double-check" the results.

Pathology

Regardless of how or when the biopsy is done, its accuracy will depend on the skill and experience of the doctor doing the biopsy, the skill and experience of the pathologist, and good communication between the doctor and pathologist. Mistakes can happen and may have tragic consequences. A woman's reproductive organs or breast could be removed unnecessarily, or, conversely, necessary, lifesaving surgery could be neglected. No one knows for sure how frequently this happens. It is probably rather rare, but since on at least some occasions it does happen, a woman should be aware of the possibility and take proper precautions.

One type of mistake that could lead to misdiagnosis is insufficient medical history. If, for instance, a doctor sends the pathologist a tissue sample from a uterine tumor that is actually a benign fibroid but neglects to tell the pathologist that the woman is pregnant or taking some form of hormone treatment, the benign fibroid could be misinterpreted as a sarcoma, a cancerous condition. Such a woman could end up having her uterus removed or her pregnancy terminated unnecessarily. Similarly, a woman with genital warts who had been treated a few days prior to biopsy with a medication called podophyllin might get a pathology report of dysplasia or even carcinoma in situ if her doctor failed to tell the pathologist about the podophyllin treatment. One way that women can protect themselves from these sorts of problems is to make sure that the doctor doing the biopsy is board-certified. Although board-certification doesn't guarantee that mistakes won't happen, it is a valuable indicator of a doctor's competency.

Good communication between the doctor and the pathologist is of utmost importance. First of all, because the same terms can be used differently by different doctors, the woman's doctor and the pathologist must be aware of each other's use of terminology. It is a good idea then to find out whether or not the doctor has consulted personally with the pathologist on your case rather than merely having read the report and, if not, to request that s/he do so, because failures of communication are more likely to be detected in discussion between them than via written report.

It is also a good idea for a woman to request a second pathology opinion. This may already have been done, for some doctors do it as a matter of routine. But not all doctors are this conscientious, so by all means, women should ask about this and should seek second opinions if necessary. If a one-step biopsy is done or if further biopsies are done at the time of surgery it isn't possible to get a second opinion prior to treatment. Obviously, an anesthetized woman flat out on an operating table cannot run down to the pathology lab and request a second opinion on her frozen section. There are, however, things she can do prior to surgery to assure an accurate diagnosis.

First of all, she can find out how many pathologists will be on duty. If only one pathologist will be on hand at the time of her operation, the woman might choose to have her surgery done at another time when more pathologists will be available or at another hospital with a larger pathology staff. Secondly, she can find out whether the pathologist in charge of her case is board-certified. Pathologists are certified by the American Board of Pathology. In order to be certified, the pathologist must first complete basic medical training and then must complete four years of training in pathology in general and three years of specialized training in either clinical or anatomical pathology, or have eight years of practical experience. In addition, the pathologist must pass certain oral and written examinations. Although many good pathologists are not board-certified and although board-certification doesn't guarantee competency, it is nonetheless a reliable guide to judging the skill and experience of your pathologist.

Pathology is not a hard-and-fast science: Equally skilled, board-certified pathologists can sometimes disagree. There are certain gray areas, where what one doctor calls benign, another may call malignant. This is most likely to happen in very early-stage cancers. In such cases, more than two pathology opinions may be in order, and, if necessary, they can be obtained long-distance—the slides being mailed to expert pathologists for review. Some doctors do this as a matter of routine, especially if there is disagreement within their own pathology department. However, women should realize that they may not be informed about differences in opinion. Sometimes the doctor may say something along the lines of "You have a borderline case and we're not sure if you have a malignant or benign disease, so we'll have to follow this closely," which may be a completely accurate description of the situation. All the pathologists may have looked at your slide and been unable to determine whether it was benign or malignant.

On the other hand, this kind of statement may actually be a subtle variation on the truth of the matter. A "borderline case" in which the doctor is "not sure" may also be one in which three experts thought the slide revealed a malignancy and three others read it as benign. You should know the doctors' opinions so that you can, if you wish, play a part in choosing the treatment.

Suppose there was this sort of disagreement among the experts and that a woman possibly had breast cancer. One woman might decide to "play it safe" and have herself treated as if she actually did have breast cancer, for fear that the three experts who said "malignant" were right and that some tumor cells might break away and spread to other locations, thus greatly reducing her chances of surviving, before the follow-up program revealed that it actually was cancer; another woman might not want to take the chance of losing a breast unnecessarily and might decide to go with the pathologists who said the disease was benign and hope that if they were wrong, the follow-up program would catch it before it metastasized. Still others might decide to have treatment, but to have minimal surgery or radiation therapy, which is less likely to disfigure the breast but which has not been totally proven to be as effective as surgical removal of the breast.

Such a decision would certainly be a tough one for a woman to make. Some doctors would hesitate to confront a woman with such a decision, perhaps for fear of overburdening her or perhaps because they felt their judgment was superior to hers (the old M.D.eity syndrome). Hospital politics may sometimes come into play, too, especially at a large teaching hospital or cancer center where a woman is being treated by a doctor who is on staff rather than by a private doctor. If the official diagnosis of the pathology department was benign disease, a doctor who operated on such a woman would be in serious trouble, indeed would risk his or her career if s/he went ahead and performed a mastectomy in the face of an official diagnosis of benign disease.

Regardless of the motivation that would lead a doctor to give a woman less than accurate information, we feel it is wrong to withhold such information. The decision, no matter how difficult, is hers and hers alone. Women should be alert to the possibilities of conflicting pathology reports; they should ask the doctor whether there were any conflicting opinions or whether their cancer is one of the debatable types. If questioned directly, most doctors will have to answer frankly or risk a possible malpractice suit. Once again, it's all a matter of knowing the right questions to ask.

Staging

The stage of the cancer—Stage I, Stage II, Stage III and Stage IV—gives an indication of how far the disease has spread and how serious a particular case of cancer is. The stage will influence the type of treatment and the chances of survival. Staging is also helpful because it allows doctors to compare the results of various treatments in order to determine which is most effective.

There are two basic types of staging, clinical staging and surgical staging. Clinical staging is done prior to treatment and is based on careful physical exam, symptoms and palpation (feeling) of the pelvic organs, breasts and lymph nodes. Certain X-ray studies and other laboratory tests may be used as well. Clinical staging is generally an estimate, the doctor's considered opinion as to how far the disease has spread. It is often inaccurate. Mistakes in clinical staging are not necessarily a reflection on the doctor's ability. Sometimes lymph nodes are enlarged, which leads the doctor to believe that the cancer has already spread to the lymph nodes and therefore to assign the case to a higher stage. But lymph nodes may become enlarged due to infection and there may not be any cancer in the nodes at all. On the other hand, lymph nodes may appear completely normal, yet contain cancer.

Moreover, the spreading cancer may be located in an area that cannot be reached by the doctor's examining fingers. Or the metastasized cancer may be too small to be detected by even the most sensitive type of X-rays or tests.

Surgical staging is based on the doctor's inspection of the abdominal cavity during surgery and/or on the results of the pathologist's analysis of biopsies and tissue removed during surgery. In ovarian cancer, for example, the doctor carefully inspects the entire abdominal cavity for signs of spread. The ovarian tumor is removed. Cell samples and biopsies are also taken at the time of the operation. The removed tissue is examined by the pathologist. On the basis of this information, along with the results of tests to detect metastasis, the disease is assigned to a particular stage.

Tests to Detect Metastasis and Evaluate the Extent of the Spread of Disease

Doctors are often accused of ordering too many tests, but in the diagnosis of cancer, such tests are generally necessary. If anything, there may be too few tests. The testing required will depend on the type of cancer and what the doctor finds from the physical exam and palpation. Women have a right to a full explanation of the tests that may be used, exactly what will be done and why it is necessary . Any of the procedures listed below may be used in the staging work-up:

☐ Basic blood tests
☐ Urinalysis
☐ Liver-function tests
☐ Chest X-rays
☐ Cystograms
☐ Hysterograms
☐ Lymphangiogram
☐ Barium enema
☐ Intravenous pyelogram
☐ Bone scans
☐ Liver scans
☐ Tomograms
☐ CAT Scans
☐ Ultrasound examinations
☐ Cystoscopy
☐ Hysteroscopy
☐ Colposcopy
☐ Culdoscopy
☐ Laparoscopy
☐ Proctosigmoidoscopy
☐ Colonoscopy

TNM Code

In addition to staging, doctors sometimes use a TNM code to classify a particular case of cancer. The *T* stands for *tumor, N* for *lymph nodes* and *M* for *metastasis.*

The T is accompanied by a number or letter. The number generally refers to the size of the tumor, T1 being a small tumor while T4 is a larger one. In some cases, for example, in endometrial cancer, the number may indicate the depth of invasion of the tumor. The particular size or depth represented by the various numbers varies from cancer to cancer. A T1 designation in breast cancer, for instance, would mean a tumor that was 2 cm or less in diameter.

TIS means carcinoma in situ; TX means the size of the tumor cannot be determined or even estimated, and TO means that there is no evidence of the primary tumor. A TO classification might, for instance, be used for a cancer that obviously did not originate at the site in which it was found when either its cells were too abnormal to determine its original site or the tumor in the primary site was still too small to be detected.

The N, which designates lymph node involvement, may be accompanied by an O, (NO) meaning no lymph node involvement, or an X, (NX) meaning nodal involvement cannot, for some reason, be assessed. Numbers 1-4 may also be used to indicate the number of lymph nodes involved or the size of the involved nodes. The exact manner in which the numbers are used will vary from cancer to cancer.

In a similar vein, MO means no known metastases; MX means this has not been assessed; M+ indicates that evidence of metastasis is present. Numerals may be used to indicate the amount or extent of the spread and letters might be used to indicate the organ to which the disease is spread. A P might, for instance, indicate pulmonary metastasis, or spread to the lungs.

Grade

Confusion sometimes exists between the grade of the tumor, which depends on the individual cell characteristics, and the stage of the disease, which refers to how widely the disease has spread. Generally speaking, the stage of the disease has more influence on the type of treatment selected and the chances of survival, but grade too may play a role, especially in certain forms of cancer like cancer of the ovary or uterus.

Grade refers to how well differentiated the cells are, that is, the degree of immaturity or abnormality. High-grade cancers are those that are poorly differentiated, immature and quite abnormal. Low-grade cancers are well differentiated, less abnormal and generally less serious. Various grading schemes have been devised. One commonly used scheme uses three numerical grades, ranging from Grade 1 for low-grade, less serious tumors, to Grade 3 for the more abnormal tumors.

Treatment

The type of treatment you receive will depend on many factors, including the type of cancer you have, the extent and location of the disease and your general physical condition. There are basically five types of treatment available: surgery, which involves cutting away the affected tissue; radiation, which involves destroying or disabling the cancer cells by the use of high-energy rays; chemotherapy, which involves the use of drugs that cripple or destroy cancer cells; hormones, which alter the growth of the cancer; and immunotherapy, which makes use of the body's immune system. Often different therapies are used in combination with each other.

The various specialists involved in cancer treatment are discussed in the following pages and in Chapter Seven. You may be referred to one of these specialists by your own doctor. Sometimes there is a choice of treatments. You should discuss this with your referring doctor and ask to be referred to doctors who are specialists in the various treatment options available to you. Second opinions and consultations (*see* p. 226) are always a good idea.

Where you are treated is very important. The National Cancer Institute has designated 20 comprehensive cancer-care centers across the country. These hospitals provide the finest and most up-to-date treatment. If you live near one of these centers, which are listed in the appendix of this book, you should by all means take advantage of them.

The NCI also supports programs known as clinical and nonclinical centers. The nonclinical centers conduct research, but the clinical centers treat patients and can offer most of the same services as a comprehensive care center. These are also listed in the appendix. In addition, there are cancer clinical cooperative groups sponsored by NCI. Each of these groups specializes in a particular type of cancer and conducts studies to determine the most effective forms of treatment. Either you or your doctor can call the Cancer Information Service Hotline for the names, locations and phone numbers of the national directors of each of the various clinical cooperative groups. It doesn't matter where the national directors are located, because they will be able to give you the names and phone numbers of those doctors in your area who are participating in these groups.

Being treated by cancer specialists at one of these special cancer-care facilities has several advantages. First of all, it assures you that a team approach will be used in treating you. Doctors from all the various specialties will confer and consult on your case. Doctors who are part of these programs are more apt to be up-to-date on the latest treatment advances. Sometimes it takes quite a while for these developments to percolate through the rank and file of the medical profession. There are doctors using forms of treatment that have been abandoned by the experts, and you will want to make sure that you have the advantage of the latest knowledge and most effective treatments. Moreover, doctors at these major centers and those participating in these groups are likely to have more experience in the operations and other forms of therapy used in the treatment of cancer, for they receive referrals from many doctors.

If you can take advantage of one of the NCI-sponsored cancer programs, by all means do so. If you have an early-stage cancer, seeking treatment at one of these centers is not as critical. Still, you will want to make sure that your doctor and the hospital* in which you are treated are top-notch.

The American College of Surgeons' Commission on Cancer operates a voluntary surveillance program whereby hospitals are approved if they meet certain criteria which, if properly used, will promote a high level of care for the patient with cancer. It does not judge the actual care given to the patient. In order to be approved the hospital must meet certain basic standards: It must have a cancer registry, a cancer committee, an educational program for doctors, and a system for evaluating the quality of the care in that institution.

Approved cancer programs are listed in a directory entitled *Cancer Programs Approved by the Commission on Cancer of the American College of Surgeons* which is updated twice yearly. Most medical libraries have one, or it can be obtained by writing to the Director, Cancer Department, American College of Surgeons, 55 East Erie Street, Chicago, Illinois 60611.

Surgery:

Surgery is the most widely used form of therapy employed in the treatment of cancer. The nature of the surgery will depend on the type of cancer and the extent of its spread. A number of different surgical procedures may be used, and these are discussed in more detail in the sections on the specific types of cancer and in the chapter on procedures, tests and operations.

Extent of Surgery:

Generally, the more extensive the cancer, the more radical the surgery. In conservative therapy the tumor itself and perhaps the organ in which it is located are removed. In more radical surgery, the adjacent tissues and lymph nodes in the area may be removed as well. Sometimes this more extensive surgery is done because there is clear evidence that the cancer has spread to these areas, but at other times the tissue is removed even though cancer cells have not actually been detected, for experience has shown that there is a high likelihood that tumors too small to be detected, which could grow and metastasize before they *were* detected, may be lurking in these tissues.

Surgery is performed with the idea of removing all the obvious, visible cancer. A margin of surrounding, apparently healthy tissue may be

*Additional information on hospitals is included in Chapter Seven.

removed as a safeguard. However, it is not always possible to surgically remove all of the cancer. If it is obvious that the disease has already metastasized, there may be no point in performing surgery. Yet even in these cases, surgery may be performed, to relieve symptoms and to prolong life. Sometimes, surgery is used in combination with radiation therapy, or chemotherapy, which will shrink the tumor to the point where it can be removed by subsequent surgery.

Since it is not always possible to determine the extent of the disease prior to surgery, sometimes more extensive surgery than was originally planned will be necessary. There are also instances in which there is a choice between conservative and more radical surgery. Unfortunately, a number of doctors fail to discuss the options with their clients. Anyone considering cancer surgery should ask the questions listed in Chapter Seven before consenting to surgery.

Cancer Surgeons

Cancer surgery may be performed by a gynecologist, a general surgeon, a surgical oncologist or a gynecological oncologist. Any of these doctors may be qualified to perform surgery for early cancers, but for more advanced cancers you may want to seek out a surgical or gynecological oncologist, for these doctors have specialized training and concentrate on the treatment of cancer.

No matter what type of doctor you choose, you will want to check his or her credentials and, preferably, you will have a board-certified doctor perform your surgery. The board-certification process for gynecologists is discussed in Chapter Six and board-certification for general surgeons in Chapter Seven. Gynecologic oncology is a board-certifiable subspecialty of gynecology. Additional years of training in the treatment of cancer of the female reproductive organs is required for certification in this subspecialty. Rigorous written and oral examinations are also required. Unfortunately, surgical oncology is not yet a board-certifiable subspecialty of surgery, so it is a bit more difficult to check the credentials of a surgical oncologist. At a minimum, the surgical oncologist should be a board-certified general surgeon. You might also ask where the surgical oncologist received special training in cancer surgery and whether s/he is a member of the Society of Surgical Oncologists. Be suspicious of any doctor who claims to be a surgical oncologist who is not a board-certified general surgeon.

It is sometimes difficult for a layperson to know when to seek out a specialist, and if your doctor is not a specialist, s/he may not readily refer you to one. If, for example, a general surgeon has performed your breast biopsy, s/he may want to also perform your mastectomy. While many general surgeons do excellent mastectomies, our preference is to seek out an oncologist who has specialized in this field. S/he is much more likely to be skilled and experienced in the operation than a doctor who performs this surgery only a few times a year. It is always a good idea to have a second opinion before any type of surgery, and in the case of cancer, having a second opinion from a surgical oncologist or a gynecological oncologist is especially wise.

Radiation Therapy

Radiation is caused by electromagnetic waves similar to light and heat waves. Radiation therapy uses these high-energy rays to destroy cancer cells or to alter them in such a way that they can no longer reproduce. The rays destroy the malignant cells when they are most vulnerable, during their twinning phase, when the chromosome strips are replicating themselves. As the cells die, they break down, are carried away in the bloodstream and excreted from the body, so the tumor shrinks in size.

These rays also destroy normal healthy cells, but since cancer cells are reproducing at a faster rate than normal cells, a greater number of cancer cells will be twinning at any given time. This is why radiation therapy can sometimes be effective against malignant cells without causing undue damage to normal cells.

Not all of the cancer cells in a tumor are reproducing at the same time. Since only those in the process of twinning will be affected by the radiation, only a certain percentage of cells will be destroyed in a single therapy session. This is why radiation therapy involves either constant low doses of radiation or a number of short, higher-intensity exposures spread out over a period of time.

Radiation therapy is used in a number of different ways in the treatment of cancer. Sometimes it is used alone and can successfully destroy all the cancer cells. This is known as curative therapy.

Sometimes the cancer is so large that radiation cannot hope to destroy all the cancer cells without undue damage to the surrounding tissue. In these cases, lower doses of radiation designed to shrink the tumor may be given, for shrinking the tumor may provide relief of symptoms. If, for example, the tumor is pressing on a vital organ, the radiation may succeed in shrinking the tumor, providing relief from the pressure effects of the tumor. Or if metastatic cancer is growing in a weight-bearing bone, radiation therapy may be used to shrink the tumor and prevent fractures. When radiation therapy is used in this manner, the term "palliative treatment" is used.

At other times, radiation therapy is used in combination with other forms of therapy. Sometimes radiation is given prior to surgery to shrink the tumor to the point where it is small enough to be removed surgically. Radiation may be used after surgery to "dry up" any microscopic areas of cancer that may have been left behind. This is known as adjuvant radiation therapy.

Radiation therapy is given in one of two ways, externally or internally.

External Radiation

External radiation involves a machine that produces a high-energy beam that is directed at the cancerous area. This is known as external beam therapy. External beam therapy makes use either of X-rays from a machine known as a linear accelerator or gamma rays from a cobalt machine. External beam therapy is sometimes used alone. For example, a woman too sick to undergo surgery or even to withstand the use of the local anesthetic that is sometimes used for internal radiation therapy may be treated by external therapy alone. Generally speaking, however, external beam therapy is used in conjunction with surgery or internal radiation. A number of treatments may be required, for external beam therapy only kills a certain percentage of the cells at a single therapy session.

Internal Radiation

Internal radiation involves placing a radioactive substance such as radium or cesium inside the body as close to the tumor as possible. If the radioactive source is placed in special containers and inserted into a body cavity, the term "intracavity implant" is used. If special needles or hollow plastic tubes are inserted into the tumor area, the terms "interstitial implant" or "needle implant" may be used. Sometimes, a radioactive substance is mixed with a fluid and circulated through a body cavity and this is called radioactive colloid therapy.

Internal radiation requires the use of either a local or general anesthetic so that the containers or needles can be inserted near the tumor. Since the containers are inserted into a hollow body cavity (the uterus or vagina) or the needles are inserted into the tumor area, a surgical incision is not required. X-rays are usually taken to assure that the containers are properly placed. Then the radioactive substance is loaded into the needles or containers and is left in place until the specified dose of radiation is achieved. This may take a few hours or several days, and since certain of these substances put out rays that could be harmful to others, the woman may be isolated in a special room of the hospital. If the containers or needles create discomfort, painkillers may be used.

Since the radioactive substance is left in place for some time, many cancer cells will come into the twinning phase during treatment and will be destroyed. Internal radiation is limited and can only affect cancer fairly close to the source. The effect of the rays decreases dramatically as the distance from the source increases. It is often combined with external beam therapy, which can affect cancer cells that have spread beyond the initial tumors to the adjacent tissues or lymph nodes. More than one internal treatment session may be necessary, but once the radioactive source is removed from the body, the woman is no longer radioactive and can continue her normal routine.

Side Effects

There may be some side effects from radiation therapy. These side effects usually develop after one or two weeks. In some cases they may persist from four to six weeks following treatment. The intensity of the side effects depends on the location of the cancer, the intensity of the therapy, the woman's tolerance to radiation and her general health. Some women experience little or nothing in the way of side effects. For some the effects are quite severe.

Most women experience some degree of fatigue. Some women experience nausea and vomiting. If this happens, antinausea medication may be prescribed. There may be some hair loss in the area being treated, for instance, pubic or armpit hair may be lost, but unless the head is being treated, the woman should not experience hair loss there from the radiation therapy.

In addition, any of the following side effects may occur: dizziness, sore throat, diarrhea, constipation, skin irritation and difficulty in swallowing. Although most of these symptoms are not serious and are generally short-lived, they should be reported to the doctor, for they may be signs of something more serious.

Complications

Just as a surgical wound can heal improperly, causing an unsightly scar, so radiation can cause scarring. Different women's tissues react differently to radiation. For example, one woman's breast may be changed only slightly after radiation therapy while another's may become misshapen and distorted. There is no way to predict how a woman will react.

Since the bowels, rectum, bladder and other parts of the urinary tract are especially sensitive to radiation, exposure to high doses of radiation can cause permanent damage to these tissues. Fistulas, which are abnormal holes connecting the bladder and the vagina, the vagina and rectum or other areas, may occur. The bowels, intestines or urinary tract may become obstructed, which can cause serious, even fatal problems.

A possible long-term complication is radiation-induced cancer. We know that exposure to radiation can increase a person's chance of developing cancer in future years, but we actually know very little about how radiation affects the development of cancer in the human body. There has been a great deal of concern in recent years about radiation risks from diagnostic X-rays, which involve only a fraction of the exposure that radiation therapy does. It may be that women treated with radiation will develop radiation-induced cancer in 15-20 years, but this risk is considered worthwhile since the radiation can cure the existing cancer.

Radiation Oncologist

A specially trained doctor called a radiation therapist, therapeutic radiologist, radiotherapist or radiation oncologist plans and administers radiation therapy. Women are usually referred to such specialists by their doctors, and since radiation oncologists have varying levels of skill, women should make sure the one recommended by their doctor is a good one. Often, your doctor may make a recommendation based on location, not necessarily on quality. If you need radiation therapy, you may have to balance the convenience of being treated at a small nearby community hospital or private facility against the advantages associated with being treated at a major medical center or large hospital more likely to have the latest equipment and the most highly skilled doctors.

One way to evaluate the skill of your doctor is to find out whether he or she is board-certified. The American Board of Radiology certifies doctors in two radiation specialties, diagnostic radiology and therapeutic radiology. A diagnostic radiologist is skilled in interpreting X-rays taken to diagnose a disease. A therapeutic radiologist is skilled in treating disease with radiation and is the specialist that women being treated for cancer will want to be treated by. It should be noted, however, that this separation of the two specialties by the American Board of Radiology is fairly recent. Before the mid 60s, the two fields were not separated, so doctors certified prior to that time may not have certificates saying "therapeutic radiology." Such a doctor may, however, be as skilled in therapeutic radiology as a younger doctor who is certified as a therapeutic radiologist.

685

Of course, being board-certified doesn't assure competence, and there are many good doctors who are not board-certified. But board-certification is an indication that the doctor's colleagues have evaluated his or her training and skill and have found it to be of the highest quality.

For certain types of cancer, there may be a choice between radiation therapy and surgery. If a woman is treated at a large hospital or a cancer center, consultations between surgeons and radiologists as to which method of treatment is best for her may be a matter of routine. But at smaller hospitals, such consultations may not take place and women would do well to seek consultations with specialists in both fields.

Chemotherapy

Chemotherapy involves the use of drugs to kill cancer cells. Most of these drugs work by interfering with the growth of the cancer cells or by preventing them from reproducing. Chemotherapy is generally used in combination with other forms of treatment.

Unlike surgery or radiation, which can be effective in dealing with local disease, chemotherapy, which enters the bloodstream, can be effective in treating disease that has spread throughout the body. It is used in the treatment of metastatic or recurrent cancer. It may also be used as preventive, or adjuvant, therapy in cases where there is a high likelihood that the undetected microscopic cancer has already spread to other parts of the body. For instance, women with breast cancer whose lymph nodes are found to have cancer are given adjuvant chemotherapy since there is a significant chance that undetected cancer is already lurking elsewhere in the body.

Chemotherapy used to be a last resort, but great strides have been made in this field. When the first studies were done, the drugs were used only on women with advanced incurable disease. Although these women were not cured, the drugs were sometimes effective in reducing the size of the tumor, prolonging life and relieving symptoms. Experiments with laboratory animals suggested that if the chemotherapy were administered earlier, before the cancer had grown too large, it might be able to provide a cure as well.

Like radiation, chemotherapy is most effective at certain points in a cell's life cycle. Only a certain portion of the tumor's cells will be in this vulnerable situation at any given time, so repeated courses of the drug are necessary. The drug may be given orally or by injection. The particular dosage, drug, schedule and length of treatment will vary according to the individual woman and her particular type of cancer. In some cases, only one drug is given, but many times a combination of drugs is used, for this has been shown to be more effective in certain instances.

Not all types of cancer are responsive to chemotherapy and not all women are suitable candidates for this form of therapy, for it carries certain risks that may outweigh any anticipated benefits.

Side Effects and Complications

Chemotherapy has its problems. The drugs used are powerful cell poisons, which affect the normal cells as well as the cancerous ones.

The side effects may last from a few hours to several days. The type and severity of the side effects will vary according to the drugs used and the woman's personal body chemistry. Any of the following effects may be noted, and if so, should be reported to the doctor:

Nausea
Vomiting
Diarrhea
Constipation
Hair loss
Pain
Loss of appetite
Weight gain
Fluid retention
Flulike symptoms
Fatigue
Male hair patterns
Headaches
Darkening of fingernails
Cough
Fever
Chills

Swelling of veins
Cramps
Absence of menstrual periods
Prolonged and excessive menstrual
  periods
Blood in urine or stools
Abscesses or pain at injection site
Mouth sores
Tingling and numbness in feet and
  hands
Pale skin
Dry skin
Tendency to feel cold
Mental depression
Skin rashes tending toward infec-
  tions
Excessive bleeding from cuts

In some cases these symptoms can be controlled by medications. For example, antinausea medicines may be given for nausea and vomiting. It may be necessary to alter your diet. Most of these side effects are relieved once chemotherapy is discontinued. Lost hair grows back, appetite returns, and so forth; however, sometimes chemotherapy causes permanent damage to the liver, kidneys, lungs, heart and other organs. Chemotherapy has not been in use long enough for us to say with certainty what all the long-term risks and complications will be; only time will tell. We do know that chemotherapy can cause as well as cure cancer. Women who have been on certain forms of chemotherapy have a higher incidence of leukemia, a cancer of the blood-forming cells.

The Chemotherapist

Chemotherapy involves the use of potent drugs that have many potential side effects and complications. They are too risky to be administered by a general physician and should be administered by a chemotherapist, who may also be called a hematologist (blood specialist) or medical oncologist. The chemotherapist is a doctor of internal medicine who has specialized in the administration of drugs used to treat cancer. As with other specialists, a chemotherapist may be board-certified, which indicates that s/he has received special training and has passed rigorous oral and written exams.

The field of chemotherapy is always changing. There are new developments all the time. Women will want to be treated by doctors who are knowledgeable about the latest and most effective drugs. If there is no chemotherapist in your community, make sure your doctor takes advantage of the consultations offered to doctors by cancer centers. That way, you will receive the most effective drugs in the proper dose and will be properly monitored for side effects.

Experimental Drugs

New drugs are constantly being tested. Many of the newer drugs are available only at large cancer centers where careful studies are being done to test their effectiveness. Programs sponsored by the National Cancer Institute to encourage the development of new cancer drugs are carefully controlled. In order to become approved for use, a drug must first be shown to be effective against tumors in mice and rats and then in larger animals. Then, if the drug looks promising, it is tested on people with many different types of advanced cancer who have failed to respond to other forms of treatment. Side effects as well as tumor response are carefully noted. This is referred to as phase I. Phase II also involves people with advanced disease who are not responding to other drugs. Only those with types of cancers that have responded in phase I studies are tested. Again, side effects and effectiveness are carefully noted. Next, in phase III, the new drug is compared to the standard therapy to determine whether it can produce superior results.

Experimental or investigational drugs should be administered only by cancer specialists chosen to participate in these experiments. Supposedly, no woman can be treated with an experimental drug without her knowledge. Everyone receiving an experimental drug must sign an informed consent form, which indicates that what is known about the risks and benefits of this form of therapy has been thoroughly explained to the woman (*see* p.   ). Not everyone can receive these experimental drugs. In order to be eligible, certain specific criteria must be met. For patients with advanced disease, being treated at a major hospital where these studies are being done may be the only way to be included in such studies.

Hormone Therapy

Hormone therapy involves controlling the output of certain substances produced by your body—hormones—to treat cancer. Hormone therapy is only rarely curative. Generally, it is given in hopes of relieving symptoms and temporarily stopping or slowing the growth of the cancer. Hormone therapy may require the introduction of additional amounts of hormones into your body or, alternatively, the reduction of the amounts of those hormones via surgical removal or radiation of hormone-producing glands or administration of a drug that blocks hormone production. Hormone therapy, regardless of whether it involves the introduction of hormones or hormone-blocking drugs or the destruction of hormone-producing glands, may produce side effects, including a permanent or temporary absence of menstrual periods, infertility, sterility, premature menopause, menopausal symptoms, male hair growth patterns, a deepening of the voice and other masculinization symptoms.

Of the cancers described in this book, hormone therapy has its widest application in the treatment of recurrent breast cancer, carcinoma in situ of the uterus and advanced uterine cancer and is discussed in more detail under these headings.

Immunotherapy

Immunotherapy is one of the newest types of cancer treatment and is still largely experimental. Immunotherapy makes use of the body's own defense system to fight cancer. Any time a foreign invader or something abnormal is detected by our immune systems, special substances called antibodies are produced to defend the body. Some doctors feel that cancerous cells are constantly being produced by the body and are normally dealt with by this incredibly efficient immune system. Only when there are too many cancerous cells or when the immune sysem is too weak to handle these cells do we develop cancers. Other doctors think that cancer cells have some way of tricking the immune system or camouflaging their abnormalities so that they are not detected and destroyed.

The fact that some tumors undergo a partial or complete spontaneous regression—that is, they disappear on their own without treatment—has stimulated interest in immunotherapy. Actually, less than 500 well-documented cases of complete spontaneous remission have been reported in world-wide medical literature; however, it is not uncommon for a tumor to get smaller and even to disappear for a while and then to grow larger or to reappear at a later time. Some scientists think that the body's immune system may be responsible for these temporary remissions.

Most of us are familiar with immunotherapy in the form of vaccines. Small amounts of a weakened strain of a disease-causing organism or an antibody-stimulating substance are injected into the body in order to trigger antibody production that will protect the person from the disease in the future. In cancer, the aim of immunotherapy is to bolster the person's own immune system. Vaccines may be prepared from the person's own tumor or from another person's tumor, or deactivated cancer cells incapable of reproducing may be used to trigger antibody reactions. Another type of immunotherapy involves transferring immune factors from one person to another person. Yet another type involves the use of agents known to be strong stimulators of the immune system.

Immunotherapy is still in its infancy; however, it is being used experimentally to treat certain advanced cancers. For instance, one substance made from human blood, interferon, is being used on a small group of women with breast cancer. Initial results have not shown cures, but significant regressions have been noted. Immunotherapy is not without risks and complications, some of them fatal ones. There is still much work to be done, but in the future interferon and other immunotherapeutic agents may play a role in the treatment of cancer.

Laetrile and Other Alternative Therapies

Because of the high mortality rates for many kinds of cancer and the suspicion and distrust that many people feel for the medical establishment, alternative treatments for cancer have received a good deal of attention, at least in the popular press.

Laetrile is perhaps the most widely known of these alternative cancer treatments. It is derived from apricot pits and contains cyanide. Although there is little in the way of sound scientific data to support its effectiveness, Laetrile has many passionate supporters.

Proponents of Laetrile and other alternative therapies usually offer case histories of cancer victims who have been cured by the alternative as proof of the treatment's effectiveness. Anyone considering these forms of therapy should be very skeptical of this type of proof. Many times, the people treated never had cancer in the first place. Breast cancer is a particularly good example of this. We know that 80 percent of all breast lumps are benign. The only way to tell for certain whether a lump is benign or malignant is to remove it and examine it microscopically. We also know that many of these benign lumps will disappear without treatment. Sometimes proper diet, avoiding coffee, tea, colas, chocolate and cigarettes will cause these benign lumps to disappear.[6] If a woman has a breast lump and has not had a biopsy to prove that it is actually cancerous, any claim of cure must be disregarded, for in all probability the woman never had breast cancer in the first place. If you are investigating these alternative treatments and talking to or reading about people who have been "cured" by these methods, be sure to find out how the diagnosis of cancer was made. Were the proper diagnostic tests and biopsies done? Were the diagnostic procedures done by the person or the clinic offering the alternative form of treatment or were they done elsewhere, by a member of the traditional medical establishment? Were there second opinions on the diagnostic tests from recognized, establishment doctors? Be skeptical if the tests and biopsies were done by the person offering the alternative treatment and if they were not confirmed in second opinions from doctors not affiliated with the clinic or person offering the alternative therapy.

As far as scientific proof for Laetrile's effectiveness, there is very little. Since the 1950s more than 23 experiments with Laetrile have been done with laboratory animals. None of these tests demonstrated any antitumor effects; however these early tests have been criticized by Laetrile supporters, who claim that the Laetrile used in the testing was impure, lacked certain essential enzymes and was not employed in sufficient quantity.

Despite the lack of laboratory evidence, the NCI has continued research in Laetrile because of pressure from Laetrile proponents. The NCI launched a nationwide search for cancer patients who had benefited from Laetrile.[7] Letters were sent to more than 835,000 doctors. In addition, some 70,000 health groups and professionals who supported Laetrile were contacted and the research effort was publicized nationally.

It was hoped that some 200-300 cases would be collected for study, but only 90 such patients signed consent forms allowing NCI to study their medical records. One problem was that the major groups advocating Laetrile refused to participate because they felt this was not a good way to determine the drug's effectiveness. Only 67 of these cases had enough information in their medical files to allow for a review. A panel of experts from NCI eliminated 11 cases that had insufficient data and 35 others that were "non-evaluable" (because, for instance, chemotherapy had been given as well). Of the remaining 22 cases, 7 showed progressive disease; 9

showed stable disease (no change); 4 showed shrinkage of tumor by 50 percent or more; and 2 showed complete remission.

Those who support Laetrile saw the results as a victory; those opposing it saw it as evidence that the drug has no value, pointing out that it is not uncommon for tumors to go into remission, only to flare up later. Thus, the study that it was hoped would resolve the long-standing Laetrile controversy only served to fuel it. Still, in the wake of this study the Decision Network Committee of the National Cancer Institute voted (14 to 11) to recommend that sound, scientific studies of Laetrile effectiveness should be undertaken.[8] Results from these tests are not yet available.

Follow-Up, Cures and Survival Rates

All cancer patients must be followed for life. The extent and timing of the follow-up program will depend on the type and seriousness of the cancer.

Survival rates for cancer are usually given in terms of five years, for if the disease has not recurred in that period it is not likely to; however, for certain types of cancer, survival rates may be given in terms of ten years, and certain cancers can recur many, many years later. It is difficult, then, to think of some cancers as ever being cured. A cancer may regress or get smaller, but it may eventually begin to grow again. A remission is a regression of the disease, which means that the symptoms have disappeared and the doctor can no longer discover any signs of the disease. A partial remission means that the symptoms and signs have partially disappeared. Cancer may be in remission for many years, but if there are still cancer cells in the body, it may flare up again at a later date.

Survival rates for the various cancers in this book are listed under the appropriate headings. The prognosis (outcome) of your case may depend on many factors and your doctor may be able to give you more accurate survival rates for your case.

Services for Cancer Patients

There are two major organizations that provide services for cancer patients: the American Cancer Society (ACS) and the Cancer Information Service (CIS).

The American Cancer Society is a national organization of volunteers that sponsors research and education and provides patient service and rehabilitation programs. There are local chapters throughout the country that provide information about various forms of treatment, assistance in obtaining social security, medicare and other benefits and counseling in regard to the problems and concerns of cancer patients. They can provide transportation to and from medical treatments for people unable to make other arrangements, dressings (bandages), bed jackets, gowns and other items, rental or loan of wheelchairs, hospital beds, commodes and other equipment, household assistance according to the physical and financial needs of the patient and emotional and physical rehabilitation, which may be especially helpful to women who have had breast cancer operations or pelvic exenterations. They also sponsor Reach to Recovery, a program designed to meet the physical, emotional, and cosmetic needs of women who have had mastectomies. Their services are often free of charge. They are usually listed in the phone book, or contact the national office, ACS, 777 Third Avenue, New York, New York 10017, for the name of the office nearest you.

The Cancer Information Service, sponsored by the National Cancer Institute, has a nationwide telephone hot-line for both patients and doctors. They can provide information on the medical aspects of cancer, rehabilitation assistance, medical facilities, home-care assistance programs, financial aid, emotional counseling and referrals to cancer specialists in the area. They also provide written materials about various forms of cancer. The phone numbers of the CIS hotlines are listed in the appendix of this book.

7

Gynecological Operations, Tests, Procedures and Drugs

This chapter deals with surgery, tests, procedures and drugs used in gynecological medicine.

Surgery

Anyone faced with the prospect of surgery is apt to feel somewhat nervous or anxious about it. This is perfectly normal. Many people find that a detailed understanding of what exactly is wrong, why the surgery is necessary and what the operation entails helps to relieve their anxiety. It is often easier to cope with clear-cut information about the risks and possible complications than to deal with vague, uninformed fears. Some doctors don't discuss operations with their patients ahead of time for fear of upsetting them, so you may have to press your doctor for details. Remember, though, that it's your body and you have a right to know.

Unnecessary Surgery

American doctors are often criticized for performing unnecessary surgery. Hysterectomies are one of the most flagrant examples of the unnecessary surgical procedures done in this country each year. In fact, the operation is jokingly referred to as "hip-pocket surgery." In case you have trouble, as we did, getting this "joke," it's called hip-pocket surgery because that's where doctors keep their wallets. Since so many hysterectomies are done when there is no medical necessity, the motivation for doing them is presumably financial, for hysterectomies are quite lucrative, netting the surgeon anywhere from about $1,000 to $3,000 or more per operation.

Surgery in general is quite a lucrative business. In 1978 the average gross income for surgeons in this country was about $75,000.[1] This average is undoubtedly distorted by the superspecialists, who earn from $500,000 to a million dollars a year. There is probably a sizable group of surgeons earning $30,000-$50,000 a year to counterbalance these six-figure incomes. Still, $30,000 to $50,000 is hardly chicken feed. In order to keep all these higher earners gainfully employed, a fair amount of surgery must be done. Doctors who specialize in obstetrics and gynecology and are therefore qualified to perform certain types of surgery have been accused of drumming up business, often in the form of hysterectomies, to bolster the falling income from the obstetrics side of their practice, which, with the decreasing birth rate, has declined considerably.

There is some objective evidence to support this. In 1977 approximately 794,000 hysterectomies were performed, and as many as 30-40 percent of them may have been unnecessary.[2] Women who have medical insurance are twice as likely to undergo hysterectomy as those who don't.[3] The rate of hysterectomies in countries with socialized medical care systems is considerably lower. The American rate of hysterectomies is twice that of England and four times that of many other European countries.[4]

Overly Extensive Surgery

American surgeons have a reputation for being "knife-happy." Not only do they sometimes perform unnecessary surgery, but they also are said to perform more extensive surgery than necessary. For instance, healthy ovaries are routinely removed by some surgeons every time they do a hysterectomy. Radical mastectomies, operations that involve removal of the breast, the lymph nodes in the armpit area and the muscles of the chest wall, are still performed in many cases where this more extensive and disfiguring operation is not necessary.

How to Avoid Unnecessary or Overly Extensive Surgery

How does a woman protect herself from unnecessary or overly extensive surgery? Well, first of all, never consent to surgery unless it has been made clear to you, in plain and simple terms, exactly what the doctor plans to remove and why. Don't allow yourself to be intimidated by medical terminology. Your doctor's explanation of what is planned may not be clear to you. If it's not, insist on clarification. The doctor may, for instance, tell you that it is necessary to remove the uterus, tubes, ovaries and parametrial tissues. Not even the most educated woman could be expected to know what parametrial tissues are, and the sad truth of the matter is that a whole lot of us, well educated or not, may not have a clear understanding of what even the uterus, tubes and ovaries are. There is an overwhelming ignorance about our bodies imposed on women in this culture. Don't hesitate to ask questions about anything you don't understand.

When the doctor answers your questions, it may be done with an of-course-you-know-about-*that* air. Doctors use medical terminology every day and often assume that women are familiar with it. And if the terms the doctor uses *are* over our heads, many of us are too embarrassed to let on that we don't understand. We may feel rather like a naive girl at a cocktail party full of sophisticates, who dumbly nods agreement when someone says, "Don't you just love ... " (the latest novel that we haven't read, the work of a painter we've never heard of). Embarrassed by our ignorance, we may feign knowledge and understanding when in reality we haven't the faintest idea of what's being said. Don't allow yourself to be intimidated. It's your body that's going to be cut, and you have the right to know what's happening. Ask the doctor to draw you a picture so that you are entirely sure you understand the procedure.

You should also ask the doctor why this surgery is necessary. Other questions you should ask include:

- [ ] What are the chances of success?
- [ ] What are the possible side effects and complications?
- [ ] How great are the risks?
- [ ] What will happen if I don't have surgery?
- [ ] Can the surgery be delayed?
- [ ] What will be the effects of delaying surgery?
- [ ] Are there any possible benefits from delaying surgery?
- [ ] Are there any less extensive, less deforming, less painful or less risky operations that are ever done in the treatment of cases like mine?
- [ ] Are there forms of treatment other than surgery that are ever used in cases like mine?
- [ ] Do you consider the other form of treatment to be as effective?
- [ ] Are there other doctors who feel it is as effective?
- [ ] What are the risks of the other form of therapy?
- [ ] How do they compare to the risks of the surgery you are suggesting?
- [ ] Why do you feel the form of treatment you are recommending is best?
- [ ] What will this operation cost? Will my insurance cover the costs? How will I be billed?

We encourage women to seek second opinions (*see* p. 226) before submitting to any form of surgery. In the reference section on diseases, we have tried to indicate those instances in which alternative forms of treatment are available. Try to get second opinions from doctors who are advocates of the other form of therapy. If your doctor has recommended a hysterectomy to treat carcinoma in situ of the cervix, for example, call the Cancer Information Service (*see* p. 859) for names of doctors who perform cryosurgery, that being an alternative form of treatment for carcinoma in situ.

Choosing a Surgeon

Once you've determined that the surgery planned is neither unnecessary nor too extensive and that surgery is, indeed, the best choice of treatment, the next important factor to consider is the skill of the doctor performing the surgery. We have discussed how to go about finding a good gynecologist in Chapter Six, and much of that information applies here as well. But perhaps a word or two about surgeons is in order.

Gynecologists are qualified to perform certain types of surgery. (Those gynecologists who specialize in gynecological surgery used to treat cancer are called gynecologic oncologists and are discussed in the section on cancer.) Other types of surgeons also perform "female surgery." A general surgeon is qualified to perform operations in the abdominal and chest cavities. (General surgeons who specialize in cancer treatment are called surgical oncologists and are also discussed in the section on cancer.) Although the general practitioner/surgeon—the family doctor who performs surgery—is a dying breed, there are some older doctors who've been around so long that they've managed to establish certain operating privileges at the hospital with which they are associated. Don't have your operation performed by one of these general practitioners; seek out a specialist, a gynecologist or a general surgeon.

Regardless of whether your surgery is done by a gynecologist or general surgeon, make sure that your doctor is board-certified. Surgery is risky business. One out of every 1,600 patients operated on dies as a result of anesthesia complications.[5] Sloppy operating procedures can cost you your life or can have crippling consequences, so it is vital that you find both a good surgeon and a board-certified anesthesiologist.

Board-certification does not guarantee that a doctor is top-notch, but it does tell you that his or her qualifications and experience have been carefully reviewed by colleagues and been judged outstanding. Board-certification requirements for a gynecologist are discussed in Chapter Six. In order to be certified by the American Board of Surgery a doctor must first be a licensed M.D. and must have a minimum of four years of residency training in general surgery. Then s/he must successfully complete writen and oral exams. In addition, general surgeons must be recertified periodically to assure that they are keeping up-to-date in their fields.

Another important credential to check for is membership in the American College of Surgeons. In order to become a member, the surgeon must be board-certified and must have been in practice for two years. His or her performance is then evaluated and if it is satisfactory, the surgeon is inducted into the college. If a doctor has the initials F.A.C.S. after his or her name, this indicates the doctor is a Fellow of the College and has received special training and been judged as extremely competent by his peers.

Besides checking these criteria, you can find out about your surgeon's qualifications by doing a bit of detective work. Try to find a scrub nurse, an anesthesiologist (a doctor who specializes in anesthesia), an anesthetist sspecially trained nurses who administer anesthesia) or any member of the nursing staff who assists in operations. These people have insider's information and can provide the most valuable recommendations.

Another important factor to consider is the experience the surgeon has in performing the operation you need. A doctor who performs an operation once or twice a year is not going to be as skilled as one who performs it two or three times a week.

Yet another consideration is the hospital in which the surgery will be done. Just as there are good surgeons and poor surgeons, so there are good hospitals and poor hospitals. There are more than 7,000 hospitals in this country, and of these, about 4,700 are accredited by the Joint Commission on Accreditation of Hospitals (JCAH). This organization carefully evaluates a hospital's performance before extending accreditation. One thing they will evaluate is the surgical tissue committee, which reviews the operations done in the hospital. In a good hospital, a doctor must first submit a preoperative diagnosis; then the removed tissue is examined by the hospital's pathology laboratory. If the preoperative diagnosis doesn't line up with the pathology report, then the doctor is called before the tissue committee. If, for instance, a surgeon removed a woman's uterus as a treatment for endometriosis and the pathology department found no evidence of endometriosis, then that doctor would be called before the tissue committee. (Note: In the case of unnecessary hysterectomy, the preoperative diagnosis could be nonspecific, indicating that the doctor is not removing the uterus for any specific medical reason. Thus, even though the pathology department finds that a healthy uterus has been removed, there is no tissue committee review, for there is no discrepancy between the pre- and postoperative diagnosis.)

In addition to reviewing the workings of the tissue committee the JCAH considers many other factors. They audit the surgical charts and investigate patient care, record-keeping, administration, staff qualifications, facilities and equipment. JCAH accreditation does not guarantee that every doctor who operates in that hospital is top-notch, but these hospitals do have larger proportions of board-certified doctors on their staffs. Just as there are many excellent doctors who are not board-certified, so there are excellent hospitals that are not accredited, but JCAH accreditation is a valuable guideline in helping you assess the quality of a hospital. Women who are being treated for cancer should read the discussion of cancer-care hospitals in the general section on cancer. A list of JCAH-accredited hospitals in your area may be obtained by writing to JCAH, 645 North Michigan Avenue, Chicago, Illinois.

Prior to Surgery

Prior to surgery, you will be asked to sign a consent form giving the doctor permission to perform the required surgery. READ IT CAREFULLY! Do not sign any "blanket permission" forms or anything you don't understand. Ask to see a copy of the form before you go to the hospital so that you will be able to read it and ask questions and make changes before the day of surgery.

The doctor will usually order certain tests before surgery. The type of tests ordered will depend on the nature of the surgery and the type of anesthesia being used. At a minimum, a blood count and urinalysis will be done. If a general anesthetic is being used, tests to determine blood-clotting time may be done as well as blood-typing and cross-matching tests in case blood transfusions are necessary. If you are over 40 or have had previous medical problems, chest X-rays and/or cardiograms may be done.

It is important that you arrive at the hospital on time, since your doctor has scheduled use of the operating room for a certain time and if you are late, there might not be time to perform all the necessary preoperative tests. Follow any preoperative instructions carefully. You will probably be asked not to eat or drink anything for about 12 hours prior to the operation, because food or liquids in your stomach could be regurgitated while you were under the anesthetic and cause choking. Even if only a local anesthetic is planned, this fasting is necessary, for if complications should develop, a general anesthetic might be required.

If you have forgotten your doctor's instructions and have had anything to eat or drink, tell the doctor before the operation. It might mean rescheduling the operation, but this would be preferable to taking the risk of having anesthesia problems.

In some cases you may be given a sleeping pill the night before the operation. An hour or two before the operation an injection is generally given so that you will be in a calm, semiconscious state. An injection of a drug designed to dry up secretions in the mouth and throat is sometimes given preoperatively.

Being "prepped" (prepared) for surgery may include having the skin shaved and the area around the incision site cleansed with an antiseptic solution. This is done to cut down on the chances of infection. An enema may be given the night before major surgery. A tube called a catheter may be inserted through the urinary opening and into the bladder so that the bladder will be empty and there will be less danger of injuring it during the operation. This may be done in your hospital room or in the operating room. If it is done before you are anesthetized, you may experience a brief stinging feeling as the tube is inserted.

If you are wearing jewelry or false teeth, these must be removed. Fingernail polish must be removed so that the anesthesiologist will be able to see the skin beneath your nails and monitor you for signs of oxygen deprivation. You are usually required to wear a sterile surgical gown and cap. Then you are placed on a wheeled cot or bed and taken to the operating room.

In the Operating Room

Once you are in the operating room, you will be transferred to the operating table. The position in which you are placed will depend on the type of surgery you are having. If, for instance, you are having vaginal surgery, your feet may be placed in stirrups similar to those used during a gynecological exam. A needle attached to a tube and to a hanging bottle called an IV (intravenous) may be inserted into your hand or arm. This may contain special medications or sugar water. The anesthetic may be administered through the IV. You may feel a slight pinprick when the IV needle is inserted, but once it is in place you shouldn't feel any pain.

If you are having a general anesthetic, you will be unconscious within a few moments of the injection of the drug. If you are having a local anesthetic, you might feel a slight pinprick or a tingling or numbness when the anesthetic is injected, but this generally passes within a few moments.

You should discuss the operating room procedures and any questions you have with the doctor prior to surgery. Once you have been sedated and wheeled into the operating room, you may not be able to get clear answers to your questions. First of all, you are apt to be feeling a little fuzzy from the sedative. Secondly, your doctor may not be there yet, and the assistant doctors or nurses may not be willing or able to answer your questions.

After the Operation

Following the operation, you will go to the recovery room, where your temperature, pulse, respiration and blood pressure will be carefully monitored until you recover from the effects of the anesthesia. The amount of time you spend in the recovery room will depend on the nature and extent of your surgery and the type of anesthesia used. Then you will be returned to your hospital room.

If you have had minor surgery requiring only a local anesthetic, you may leave within an hour or two after surgery, but you should not try to get home by yourself, for reflexes and reaction time may be slow for 24—48 hours. If you have had a general anesthesia, you may still be able to leave the hospital the same day after most minor forms of surgery, but if complications develop, you may have to remain in the hospital overnight or longer.

After major surgery, you will usually have to stay in the hospital for at least five or six days. Bed rest is usually required, although you will be encouraged to change position and move your arms and legs to stimulate your circulation and to get you to breathe deeply so you will not form blood clots or develop pneumonia. After most types of major surgery, you will be made to get out of bed and walk a bit the next day. Getting out of bed as soon as possible speeds recovery time and cuts down on the possibility of complications.

You may be allowed some fluids within a few hours and a bland diet on the following day. Depending on the nature of your surgery, pain medications, antibiotics, IVs, enemas or blood transfusions may be ordered. Ask your doctor what to expect postoperatively so that you are not shocked by waking up and finding various tubes and needles stuck in you.

Nausea and vomiting are not unusual following operations. You may feel dizzy and rather weak. Expect some soreness around the incision, gas pains and other discomfort. You may be given injections of a narcotic immediately after surgery. Later on you may be switched to pain pills.

Any form of surgery involves risks. In addition to the risks involved in the use of anesthesia there may be bleeding problems, infection or injury to adjacent organs during surgery. Before you leave the hospital, make sure you have a *written* list of possible danger signs, an emergency phone number and careful postoperative instructions. The list of postoperative instructions should tell you when you can shower, bathe, use tampons and have intercourse. If you have specific questions about certain activities—for example, When can I drive a car? Go back to work? Play tennis?—be sure to ask the doctor. A follow-up appointment should be scheduled before you leave the hospital.

In the reference section following, the various types of surgery mentioned in other sections of this book are described in greater detail. Descriptions of various diagnostic tests and other routine procedures are also included.

Diagnostic Tests and Procedures

Doctors are often accused of practicing defensive medicine—of ordering too many tests to protect themselves from malpractice suits. To protect yourself from unnecessary or overly extensive tests, ask the following questions.

- ☐ What is the purpose of this test and what will the test results tell you about my condition?
- ☐ Are there other tests that could be done instead? If so, are these other tests less expensive, less risky, less time-consuming or less painful?
- ☐ What are the risks involved in this test?
- ☐ Do I need to be hospitalized? For how long? Could this test be done on an outpatient basis? Why not?
- ☐ What exactly will happen to me during the test?
- ☐ How long will it take to get test results?
- ☐ What could the test results possibly indicate and what decisions might I be faced with if the test results are positive?
- ☐ What type of doctor will be performing the tests or analyzing the results of the test? Are these doctors board-certified?
- ☐ What will the test cost? Will my insurance cover the costs? How will I be billed?

Only by asking questions and insisting on complete answers and explanations can women assure themselves of getting top-notch medical care.

Routine Exams

While it is true that many tests are done unnecessarily, it is also true that many women don't have physical exams and routine screening tests, many of them simple office procedures, that could detect diseases and abnormalities in their earliest stages. The following routine examinations and screening tests are important to your health:

General physical exam: These should be done at regular intervals, but there is considerable controversy as to how often they should be done on healthy people with no symptoms. Many authorities feel that a general physical should be done by an internist or family practitioner rather than by a gynecologist, since gynecologists are trained to deal with problems affecting the reproductive tract, not with the body as a whole.

Blood pressure (BP): Women under 40 should have their BP checked once a year, and, according to some doctors, those over 40, every six months. Hypertension (high blood pressure), which is a common problem for women, can have serious consequences and often can be detected only by a BP check. Women on birth control pills, who may be especially susceptible, may want to have their BP checked every six months regardless of their age.

Urine tests: According to some experts, urine tests to determine protein and urine levels should be done once a year; others recommend once every three to five years. These tests can detect kidney and bladder disease, diabetes and other medical problems.

Breast exam: Every woman should practice monthly breast self-exam. Women under 40 should have a doctor examine their breasts once a year; women over 40, every six months.

Mammography: A single mammogram at the age of 35 will serve as a baseline to which to compare results from subsequent testing, which should be done once a year after the age of 50. Younger women at high risk for breast cancer (*see* p. 492) may want to have more frequent mammograms and doctor exams.

Complete Blood Count (CBC): This blood test can detect anemia. Some experts feel it should be done on a yearly basis, while others recommend every three to five years.

Stool analysis: This should be done once every year or two after the age of 40.

Pelvic and rectal exam: This should be done once a year from the age of about 16-18 or before if sexual activity is begun and twice a year after the age of 40.

Pap smear: Although there is some debate as to how frequently this simple screening test for cervical cancer should be done, we recommend it on a yearly basis. Women at high risk for cervical cancer (*see* p. 349) may want to have a Pap smear twice a year.

VD tests: Tests for venereal disease should be done on a yearly basis for sexually active, heterosexual women.

Multiple blood screening tests: Tests to measure cholesterol, blood sugar and blood urea, nitrogen and calcium are done by some doctors on a yearly basis, but most feel once every five years is sufficient. Some feel cholesterol levels should be done once a year after the age of 50.

Proctosigmoidoscopy: Some doctors recommend this on a yearly basis for all women over 60; others recommend every three years after the age of 40.

Endometrial biopsy: Some doctors recommend this test for postmenopausal women who are using estrogen replacement therapy or who are otherwise at high risk for endometrial cancer (*see* p. 419).

Skin test for tuberculosis: This should be done once every five years until the age of 35.

Screening for vision and hearing: This should be done every five years after the age of 60.

Tonometry: This test can detect glaucoma, an eye disease that can cause blindness, in its earliest stages. Women over the age of 40 should have this test every two or three years or annually if there is a family history of glaucoma.

Electrocardiogram (ECG): The "resting" ECG is not as accurate as the "exercise" ECG. A single ECG at the age of 35 will serve as a baseline to which to compare results from subsequent testing, which should be done once every ten years.

Chest X-ray: In the absence of symptoms the chest X-ray is not valuable as a periodic screening test. Lung cancer is rarely detected by chest X-ray early enough to affect the eventual outcome.

Drugs

Some of the most heated controversies in medicine today revolve around drugs, in particular, around the use of hormones. DES, a synthetic estrogen given to millions of pregnant women in this country between 1940 and 1971, has caused cancer[6] and other serious problems[7] in the offspring of those women who took the drug and may increase the chances of developing cancer in the DES mothers.[8] Estrogen products used to treat menopausal symptoms have been implicated in an increased risk for cancer of the endometrial lining of the uterus[9] and may play a role in the development of breast cancer.[10] Estrogen and synthetic progesterone used in birth control pills have caused the deaths of some women, and more than 50 side effects and complications have now been attributed to Pill usage.

Hormones have a definite role in gynecological medicine, but they should be used with caution. Women who are considering the use of hormones should read the information on side effects and complications given in the section on birth control. These risks have been determined as the result of studies of women using birth control pills containing estrogen and progestin (synthetic progesterone). It is not known whether women using hormone preparations that contain only estrogen or only progestin face the same risks as those associated with Pill usage. For instance, women given progestin for the treatment of abnormal bleeding and other problems may not face the same risks as women who are using progestin in combination with estrogen, but until the risks are clearly delineated, women using progestin-only preparations should consider themselves at similar risk and should watch for the same danger signs.

We know a bit more about the risks associated with estrogen-only preparations, for these drugs have been widely used in the treatment of women with menopausal symptoms. These women have been studied, although not as extensively as Pill users. In some cases, the use of estrogen in menopausal women (called estrogen replacement therapy, or ERT) has resulted in problems similar to those experienced by Pill users. Larger doses of estrogen may be used in the treatment of menopausal symptoms than in birth control pills. This may account for the fact that some effects, such as increased risk for endometrial cancer and possibly for breast cancer, that are seen in studies of menopausal estrogen users have not been seen in Pill users. Menopausal women have not been studied for all the Pill effects. Here again, until these risks have been more clearly identified, women using estrogen-only preparations should consider themselves at similar risk to women using estrogen in birth control pills and should watch for the same danger signs.

Getting Information About Drugs

In the reference section that accompanies this chapter, we have provided detailed information on some of the more common and some of the more controversial drugs used in gynecological medicine. In addition, certain drugs used to treat a specific condition are described in the section on that disease. You can locate information on these drugs by referring to the index.

Hormone preparations are required by law to include printed package inserts; be sure to read them carefully. Another way to obtain information about a drug is to use a reference book called the *Physician's Desk Reference*, or the *PDR*, for short. Most medical libraries and hospitals have a copy, and it can also be purchased at or ordered from large bookstores. While only those drug manufacturers that pay a fee are included in this book, most companies do pay and so are in it. Products are listed by manufacturer, with cross-references by brand name, generic name and uses. The *PDR* also includes detailed information on dosage, ingredients, uses, side effects, complications and contraindications for the drugs listed, as well as pictures of many of them. While the *PDR* is a valuable source of information, it is essentially an advertising tool for the drug industry and not surprisingly tends to downplay adverse effects of drugs. For example, the side effects and complications associated with hormones are presented in the most restrained way. The *PDR*, by law, must reveal that estrogen replacement therapy has been implicated in the development of breast cancer, but it tosses this fact off in one sentence:[11]

> At the present time there is no satisfactory evidence that estrogens given to postmenopausal women increase the risk of cancer of the breast, although recent long-term follow-up of a single physician's practice has raised this possibility.

The *PDR* does not tell you that this was the first and only long-term study of breast cancer risk and ERT or that the single physician happened to be Dr. Robert Hoover of the National Cancer Institute or that the study was published in the *New England Journal of Medicine*, the foremost medical journal in this country.[12]

706

The point of all this is that while the *PDR* is a valuable source of information, it will never be accused of muckraking or sensationalism. As mentioned, it tends to downplay negative aspects. If the *PDR* lists something as a possible negative effect of a manufacturer's product, you can be sure there is significant and respected scientific opinion to back it up.

General Considerations

All drugs involve some risk, so before a drug is prescribed or taken, you should observe certain precautions. First of all, be sure that the doctor knows about any allergic reactions you have had to drugs or to foods in the past. It is especially important to let the doctor know if you are pregnant, are breastfeeding or have a history of kidney or liver disease or any other special medical condition, such as diabetes. Also tell the doctor if you are on a special diet or are taking vitamins or other over-the-counter or prescription drugs, including birth control pills or insulin. Ask your doctor what side effects are associated with the use of the drug and what to do if such side effects occur, and find out if there are any foods you should avoid while taking the drug. Some antibiotics, for instance, won't work if you drink milk or eat dairy products; other drugs should not be taken in combination with alcoholic beverages.

It should also be clear to you exactly how the drug is to be taken. If you are told to take it "three times a day," does this mean morning, noon and night? Before or after meals? If it is to be taken "every six hours," does this mean only while you're awake or should you wake up to take the medicine? Should you take the medicine until it is all gone or just until you feel better? With some medications, it is important to take all the medicine or the disease is apt to recur. You should always read labels carefully for storing instructions. Some drugs must be refrigerated or stored in special ways. Discard medicines that are outdated. Ask for child-proof caps on medicines if there are children around your home.

You should ask whether the drug being prescribed has been approved by the FDA *for the specific condition that you have.* It is important to take this precaution because doctors can and do prescribe drugs to treat conditions even though the FDA has not approved the drug for that particular condition. In order for a drug to become available for a doctor to prescribe, it must be tested for safety and effectiveness. But the FDA's job is to regulate the pharmaceutical industry, not the medical profession. Once a drug is approved, a doctor may prescribe it for any condition.

For example, consider the drug Depo-Provera. This drug has been associated with a number of serious side effects, including cancer in studies involving laboratory animals.[13] The FDA, however, approved it as a treatment for advanced uterine cancer because in these cases it was felt that the proven benefits outweighed the possible risks.[14] Depo-Provera also works as a contraceptive, but since it is associated with cervical cancer in women[15] and with other serious complications, the FDA has not given its approval for use of the drug as a contraceptive.[16] This has not stopped doctors from prescribing it for that use. According to the Ralph Nader-affiliated Health Research Group, Depo-Provera was prescribed as a contraceptive for some 10,000 American women in 1975.[17]

Be sure to ask whether the drug being prescribed has been clearly proven to be effective for the condition for which it is being prescribed. It was not until 1962 that the FDA required that effectiveness as well as safety be proven before a drug could be approved. Some doctors still prescribe drugs for conditions for which they have not been proven effective. Consider, for example, sulfanilamide, sold under brand names like AVC Cream, Sufamal and Vagitrol. This drug is widely used to treat vaginitis, but a review of the drug by the National Academy of Science/National Research Council found that it was only "possibly" effective for the treatment of trich, candidiasis and hemophilus.[18]

If your doctor cannot assure you that the drug is approved for the condition you have or has been proven effective for that condition, then your use of the drug is "investigational" or "experimental" and you should be given a consent form to sign that explains the possible risks and benefits. In some cases, a woman may be acting wisely in her decision to take a drug on this basis. If, for example, you are being treated for breast cancer, it might be worthwhile to take an experimental drug. In other instances, where the disease is not a serious one, you may decide that you are not interested in the risks of experimentation.

One way to check on whether or not a drug is approved for and effective in treating your condition is to look it up in the *PDR*; however, it is possible for a drug to have been proven effective for a condition and not be so listed in the *PDR* since some drugs (penicillin, for instance) are effective for so many conditions that it is impractical to list all the indications. You may also call your local FDA office (look in the phone book for the nearest major city under: U.S. Government, Department of Health and Human Services, Food and Drug Administration). If you suspect you have been given a drug for an unapproved use, you can contact the Institute for the Study of Medical Ethics, P. O. Box 17307, Los Angeles, California 90017, (213) 413-4997.

Buying Drugs

The cost of the same drug may vary considerably from one pharmacy to another. Do a little comparison shopping by phone and you may find that you save yourself quite a bit of money. Also, ask your doctor if it is possible to prescribe the drug by a generic name rather than by a brand name. A generic name is the chemical name for a substance, while a brand name is the name used for this same substance by a particular company. For example, aspirin is the generic term for a product that may be sold under various brand names, such as Bayer or Bufferin. There is no difference in the painkilling quality of these drugs, for any drug that claims to be aspirin must meet the Food and Drug Administration standards set for that drug.

There may, however, be differences between products with the same generic name that are manufactured by different companies. To use aspirin as an example again, certain brands of aspirin may contain additional substances that aid in the breakdown and absorption of the aspirin so that it gets out of your stomach faster. With aspirin, which has detrimental effects on the lining of the stomach, these additional substances may make a crucial difference. In most instances, however, there is no difference between generic and brand name drugs. Indeed, many times the generic product is manufactured and sold by one company that also sells it in bulk to another company that then prints its own brand-name label and sells the identical product to you at a higher price. For example, consider ampicillin, a widely used antibiotic that is sold under 224 brand names but is made by only 24 manufacturers, or conjugated estrogens, sold under 219 different names but made by only 45 manufacturers.

Many doctors are not aware that the differences in price between brand-name and generic drugs can be quite hefty. They are used to prescribing a particular brand or have been wooed by drug salesmen, who are liberally supplied with expense accounts for just this purpose, and so they don't consider writing prescriptions for the less expensive, generic drugs. In some states there are now laws that allow pharmacists, after informing patients, to substitute generic drugs for brand names when the substances are equivalent. However, this is not true in all states, so women should ask their doctors about the generic alternatives.

Reference Section:
Operations, Tests, Procedures
and Drugs

VULVECTOMY

AKA: removal of the vulvar tissue

Types: "skinning" vulvectomy
simple, or total, vulvectomy
radical vulvectomy

A vulvectomy is an operation in which all or part of the vulva is removed. A "skinning" vulvectomy involves removal of the outer layers of the vulvar skin. It is used to treat certain deep-seated vulvar infections, in severe cases of condyloma acuminata and for precancerous vulvar conditions. It is sometimes used to treat vulvar dystrophies, but many experts feel it is ineffective in these cases and should not be used.

A simple, or total, vulvectomy involves the removal of the skin of the vulvar area, as well as the skin of the vaginal lips and the skin of the clitoris. It is more extensive than a skinning vulvectomy, but in both of these procedures, new skin will usually grow back to replace the skin that has been removed.

A radical vulvectomy is used to treat invasive vulvar cancer. In this operation the vaginal lips, clitoris and the skin surrounding the vulva are removed. A pelvic lymphadenectomy—removal of the pelvic lymph nodes—is usually done at the same time. Skin grafts may be required to close the wound.

Illustration 59 *Simple Vulvectomy*

A general anesthetic is required, and the woman is usually confined to bed for at least two days. For a simple vulvectomy, the hospital stay is generally two weeks or less. To cut down on infections and other complications, the wound is frequently irrigated with salt water. Heat lamps, whirlpool baths and hot sitz baths may be ordered. Honey may be applied to the wound to promote healing.

Women who have had vulvectomies can become pregnant, although it may be necessary to perform a Caesarean rather than to use a vaginal delivery; however, most women who have vulvectomies are well past the childbearing years. Intercourse is still possible but, depending on the extensiveness of the vulvectomy, sexual responsiveness may be diminished. If a radical vulvectomy is done, the nerve endings of the clitoris may be so damaged that orgasm is not possible. Since vulvectomies are usually done in older women, doctors tend to ignore the importance of retaining the ability to experience orgasm, for they assume that this is not

711

important to older women. If you need to have a vulvectomy, be sure to discuss this with your doctor. It may be possible to perform the operation in such a way that sexual functioning will not be impaired. If you don't discuss this issue with your doctor, s/he may rely on assumptions about older women and sexuality and perform a more extensive procedure as a matter of routine.

VAGINECTOMY

AKA: removal of all or part of the vagina

Types: partial vaginectomy
total vaginectomy

Vaginectomy is a removal of all or part of the vagina. This operation is used in the treatment of certain forms of cancer. It is usually part of another operative procedure, such as a radical hysterectomy or a pelvic exenteration. Vaginectomies have been used to treat women with vaginal adenosis, but the operation is no longer recommended for this purpose.

If the entire vagina is removed, it may be possible to reconstruct a new vagina using plastic surgery techniques. If only a part of the vagina, generally the upper third, is removed, there may not be any problems; however, many women experience pain on intercourse or vaginal stenosis following such surgery. The risks and complications are similar to those of any major form of surgery.

HYSTERECTOMY

AKA: removal of the uterus

Types: subtotal hysterectomy
total, or simple, abdominal hysterectomy
total, or simple, abdominal hysterectomy with bilateral
salpingo-oophorectomy, or complete hysterectomy

radical abdominal, or Wertheim, hysterectomy
vaginal hysterectomy
radical vaginal hysterectomy, or Schauta procedure

In Chapter One we discussed the well-documented fact that many hysterectomies are performed unnecessarily. Of course, a woman's doctor does not say, "How would you like to have an unnecessary hysterectomy?" It's done with a good deal more subtlety than that. Consider, for example, what might happen to a woman who, although she has no symptoms, happens to have a small fibroid tumor in her uterus that is discovered by her doctor in the course of a routine physical. This doctor could push all her panic buttons by telling her that she has a tumor in her uterus that might be cancer. S/he might further tell her that although in all probability the tumor is benign, there's always the chance that it's cancer, so "just to make sure," s/he recommends an operation. Another doctor, dealing with the same woman, might tell her that she has a tumor that in all probability is a benign one that may well get smaller after menopause, and although it should be watched carefully, unless it starts to grow larger or cause problems there is no need to subject her to the risk and expense of major surgery. Most of us are so frightened of cancer that had we seen the doctor who suggested the possibility of cancer, we might well have panicked and agreed to an unnecessary operation, without investigating the alternatives and seeking second opinions. This is just one of the many ways in which unnecessary hysterectomies are foisted on women.

Indications

The only times that a hysterectomy is absolutely necessary are:

- ☐ To remove cancer of the vagina, cervix, uterus, Fallopian tubes or ovaries. In the early stages of these diseases, it is sometimes possible to avoid hysterectomy.
- ☐ To stop severe, uncontrollable infection.
- ☐ To stop severe, uncontrollable bleeding.
- ☐ As part of surgery for life-threatening problems affecting other organs when it is technically impossible to treat the other problem without removing the uterus.

Hysterectomy may be a wise choice in certain other cases as well, but if it is proposed, make sure you understand why. Read the section of this book that relates to your particular problem so that you will understand your options and alternatives. Get your doctor to answer the questions

713

listed in Chapter Seven, and by all means get a second opinion (*see* p. 226) before consenting to surgery.

Risks and Complications

In many of the cases where hysterectomy is not an absolute medical necessity, you will have to weigh the risks versus the benefits before making your decision.

Hysterectomy is a major surgical procedure requiring the use of a general anesthetic and can have serious complications, including death. The risks depend on your age, general health, the competence of the surgeon, the quality of the hospital and the specific type of hysterectomy you are having. For a relatively healthy woman under the age of 45, the mortality rate for hysterectomy is about 50 per 100,000 operations performed.[1] For a woman over 50 with high blood pressure the mortality rate is 15 times higher. The more extensive the type of hysterectomy, the greater the risks.

Although deaths from hysterectomies are relatively rare, complications are not. The most common complication is infection.[2] These infections are usually mild or moderate and can be controlled with oral antibiotics. Bleeding during the operation is also common, with about 15 percent of patients requiring blood transfusions.[3] Bleeding may also occur following the operation, although less than 1 percent of women having hysterectomies require transfusions or readmission to the hospital because of postsurgical bleeding complications.

Urinary tract problems are also rather common but are usually not serious. A portion of the women will have a bladder or kidney infection following the operation. However, damage to the bladder or tubes that carry urine from the kidney occurs in about one out of every 200 operations. Bowel problems caused by damage to the intestines during surgery or scar tissue that prevents the intestines from contracting properly are relatively rare, but about 2 percent of all hysterectomy patients require a second surgery to remove scar tissue on the bowels. Blood clots occur in 1 percent of the women having hysterectomies and may be fatal. Some women experience a loss of pelvic support and problems such as cystoceles and rectoceles following hysterectomy.

If the ovaries are also removed in a premenopausal woman, she will probably experience premature menopause. Even if the ovaries are spared, a woman may still experience a premature menopause, for at times the blood supply to the ovaries is disrupted and they gradually lose their ability to produce hormones. At other times the disruption to the ovaries during

714

surgery leads to the subsequent formation of ovarian cysts that require a second operation and removal of the cysts and ovaries, again causing premature menopause. Loss of ovarian function following removal of the uterus alone is not a common complication, but it does happen.

Hysterectomy and Your Sex Life

One area that has received little attention is the effect of hysterectomy on a woman's sex life. For women who have had hysterectomies for conditions that were causing pain, their sex lives may be greatly improved. For some women freedom from the fear of pregnancy and the hassles of birth control may have beneficial effects on their sex lives. For others, the fact that they can no longer bear children may make sex less enjoyable. These are psychological effects and vary from woman to woman depending on her own personal attitudes about sex and her role as a woman.

Following certain types of hysterectomies, the vagina may be shortened somewhat, which can make intercourse more difficult. Scar tissue may also form in the pelvis or at the top of the vagina following any type of hysterectomy, and this can cause painful intercourse.

The ability to achieve orgasm is not lost when your uterus and ovaries are removed. Many women don't notice any change in their orgasms at all, but some do. Some women find that their orgasms are less intense. Until recently, the observations of such women were dismissed as psychological. We now know from the pioneering work of the well-known sex researchers Masters and Johnson that the uterus becomes congested with blood prior to orgasm and participates in the general release of congestion at the time of orgasm. This is yet another example of the discovery of a physiological basis for a phenomenon formerly considered to be of the "it's-all-in-your-head" variety. There has been little research done in this area, and doctors rarely mention it to their patients. Not all women have this reaction, but some do, and we feel that women should be made aware of this possibility.

Types

There are several different types of hysterectomies (Illustration 60), including:

The subtotal hysterectomy: This operation involves removal of the body of the uterus but not the lower cervical portion. Since the cervix has no function once the uterus is removed and since the cervix may be the site of cancer in the future, this operation is rarely done anymore. No surgeon

715

Illustration 60 *Subtotal Hysterectomy (A), Total, or Simple, Hysterectomy (B), and Total, or Simple, Hysterectomy with Bilateral Salpingo-Oophorectomy (C).*

does it deliberately. It is done only when circumstances force it, if, for instance, removal of the uterus has been difficult and time-consuming and taking extra time to remove the cervix would prolong the woman's time under anesthesia and subject her to undue risks.

The total, or simple, abdominal hysterectomy: Both the body of the uterus and the cervix are removed through an abdominal incision.

The complete hysterectomy (total, or simple, abdominal hysterectomy plus bilateral salpingo-oophorectomy): Same as the above except that the ovaries and tubes are also removed.

The radical abdominal, or Wertheim, hysterectomy: Same as above except that the upper third of the vagina and the parametrial tissues (the tissues adjacent to the uterus and cervix) are also removed. This operation is used to treat certain types of cancer.

Vaginal hysterectomy: This operation involves removal of the entire uterus, the cervix and the body of the uterus, through a vaginal incision. It is also possible to remove the ovaries and tubes through a vaginal incision—to do a vaginal hysterectomy plus bilateral salpingo-oophorectomy—but this is often technically difficult and is not usually done.

Radical vaginal hysterectomy, or Schauta procedure: The same tissues are removed as in the radical abdominal hysterectomy, but the incision is vaginal. This operation is done only in the treatment of cancer and then only rarely, for it doesn't allow the doctor to inspect the pelvic lymph nodes for cancer. If your doctor recommends this procedure, be sure you understand why, and get a second opinion before consenting to it.

Vaginal vs. Abdominal Hysterectomy

Most hysterectomies are done through an abdominal incision that may be either vertical or horizontal. If you have had previous pelvic surgery, the incision may be made along the lines of your previous scar. The horizontal incision is preferred by many women since it is less noticeable in a two-piece bathing suit. If you are concerned about this, ask your doctor what type of incision is planned and whether it would be possible for you to have a horizontal incision.

Sometimes hysterectomies are done through an incision in the vagina. This has both advantages and disadvantages. The incision is made in the vagina, so there is no scar. The vaginal incision also heals faster, requires less recuperation time and is less painful than an abdominal incision. Some surgeons feel that the vaginal hysterectomy is less likely to produce adhesions, or bands of internal scar tissue. On the other hand, there is

717

more likely to be bleeding and infection following a vaginal hysterectomy than following an abdominal operation. The vagina has a greater chance of being shortened following a vaginal hysterectomy, which can cause pain on intercourse. Some doctors feel the complication rate is higher for vaginal hysterectomies. It is certainly easier for the surgeon to see what s/he is doing if an abdominal incision has been made, which may mean fewer complications.

The vaginal hysterectomy calls for a greater involvement on the part of the assisting surgeon than an abdominal hysterectomy does. It is especially important that women who are having vaginal hysterectomies carefully investigate the credentials of the assisting surgeon.

Sometimes it is not possible to do a vaginal hysterectomy. If a woman has a particularly large uterus, extensive scar tissue from previous operations or from pelvic infection or a large fibroid tumor in her uterus, vaginal hysterectomy is probably not in order. If a woman is having a hysterectomy for cancer, an abdominal operation is often necessary since it allows the doctor to get a complete view of the abdominal cavity. Although it is possible to remove the ovaries as well as the uterus through a vaginal incision, it is more difficult to do so. The main indication for a vaginal hysterectomy is for prolapse of the uterus when there is associated prolapse of the other pelvic organs. The vaginal repair of the other prolapses can be done through the same approach.

You should ask your doctor what type of hysterectomy is planned and why. Women who are being operated on in teaching hospitals should realize that since vaginal hysterectomies are done less frequently, doctors may sometimes push this form of surgery so that students have a chance to learn how to do it. If your ovaries are being removed or you require a radical operation for cancer and your doctor recommends a vaginal hysterectomy, you would do well to question the reasoning behind this and to seek a second opinion.

Removal of the Ovaries

Sometimes the ovaries must be removed because of the nature of the disease, but at times doctors performing hysterectomies will remove healthy ovaries as well, even though this is not strictly necessary to cure the disease. Some doctors routinely remove the ovaries in all their women patients over the age of 35 who are having hysterectomies; others use 40 as the cut-off point, and still others use 45. Most doctors will remove the ovaries in postmenopausal women having hysterectomies.

Those who argue for removal of the ovaries have three points to make.

First, they argue that removing the ovaries precludes the development of ovarian cancer. Secondly, they point out that the hysterectomy interferes with the blood supply to the ovaries. In a small number of women, this results in cystic ovaries and pelvic pain, requiring a second operation to remove the ovaries. Even though the number of women to whom this happens is small, these doctors feel that it is foolish to take the risk. Thirdly, they point out that in a number of women—again, a small percentage—the ovaries cease functioning within a few years after the hysterectomy. Thus, they say, it is better to remove the ovaries and prevent possible cancer than to leave them in when they may function for only a few years anyway.

Those who prefer to leave the ovaries in point out that removing the ovaries will usually cause premature menopause. Premature menopause increases a woman's risk of developing hypertension, a disease characterized by high blood pressure, and osteoporosis, a disease associated with loss of bone density. Since both of these diseases can have serious, even fatal, consequences, they favor preserving the ovaries. Moreover, with removal of the ovaries there is an abrupt cessation of hormone production rather than the gradual tapering off that occurs in a natural menopause, so that menopausal symptoms are likely to be more severe. In the past, those who favored removal of the ovaries countered these arguments by pointing out that a woman who has a surgical menopause can be given estrogen replacement therapy (ERT). The fact that ERT can cause uterine cancer[4] would not be a problem for such a woman since she no longer has her uterus. However, a recent study, while not conclusive, has indicated that women on ERT may be at increased risk for the development of breast cancer.[5] Thus, posthysterectomy women can no longer take ERT with complete assurance that it is safe to do so.

A doctor's decision to remove or preserve the ovaries may depend on his or her personal experience. For instance, a surgeon who treats many ovarian cancer patients might be more apt to remove the ovaries in younger women than a doctor who doesn't deal with these sorts of cases. As one doctor put it, "Sometimes whether or not I remove the ovaries depends on what has happened to me in the last few weeks. If I've watched a patient die from cancer of the ovary, I often remove them. But if I've been free of this experience for a while, I'm more inclined to leave them in."[6]

While this doctor's attitude is understandable, it is hardly scientific. Women should realize that doctors' decisions on this issue are often made on the basis of personal beliefs and attitudes rather than scientific facts. Moreover, women should realize that many doctors don't even discuss this issue with their patients. Women should take the initiative and ask their doctors the appropriate questions—does s/he plan to remove one or both ovaries or to leave one or both of them intact and why or why not? —prior to surgery. It should be noted that it is not always possible for the doctor to preserve the ovaries although s/he may intend to. Upon operation, the doctor may discover some unsuspected condition that requires that the ovaries be removed, but women should nonetheless discuss the doctor's intent prior to surgery.

Women should also make sure that they understand the doctor's terminology, for one doctor may use the term "total hysterectomy" to include removal of the ovaries while another uses the term to refer to an operation in which the ovaries are not removed.

Our personal preference is to leave the ovaries intact in a younger woman, but different doctors can in good faith and for sound reasons disagree. Furthermore, while this is our recommendation, it is the patient's decision, and if she wants her ovaries removed, we will respect her wishes. In postmenopausal women we recommend removal of the ovaries, for there is nothing to be gained by leaving them in and there is a possibility of cancer developing later on. While there is some new evidence that the postmenopausal ovaries are not the functionless organs we once thought,[7] there is no evidence that the value of leaving them in outweighs the possible risks. We therefore would not perform a hysterectomy on a postmenopausal woman without removing her ovaries.

Following Hysterectomy

The majority of women who have hysterectomies leave the hospital within seven to ten days. Recovery times vary greatly. Most women return to work in about six weeks, but some women take nine weeks or longer, especially those over the age of 36. It was not uncommon for women to say that they didn't really feel back to normal for an entire year. Many women experience severe fatigue in the first few days at home, and some find they must spend an entire week in bed.

Women often have feelings of depression following hysterectomy. This is quite natural, and these feelings do not usually last for too long. Try to arrange with loved ones and friends for support so that you can have someone to talk to if you're feeling blue.

Many women experience hot flashes following hysterectomy even if their ovaries have not been removed. This may be due to a disruption in the blood supply of the ovaries during surgery. For most women these are relatively short-lived.

You will probably have some vaginal bleeding that may be rather brownish in color, but this should taper off in a few days. You are also likely to experience some pain and discomfort, for hysterectomy is a major operation.

Women are usually told not to have sex for six to eight weeks because of the possibility of infection or of jarring the stitches. Most doctors recommend a two to three month wait before returning to active sports like tennis. You should use your common sense and consult with your doctor about postoperative activities.

If you have any of the following symptoms following surgery, call your doctor, for they might be signs of complication.

* Fever over 100.4°F
* Pain that is not relieved by the painkillers the doctor gave you
* More than 3 days without a normal bowel movement
* Persistent pain in the bladder, burning sensation on urination, blood in the urine or an inability to urinate
* Pain, swelling, tenderness or redness in your leg
* Chest pain, cough, difficulty in breathing and coughing up blood
* Bright red vaginal bleeding that soaks two or more pads in an hour or forms large clots.

OOPHORECTOMY

AKA: removal of one or both ovaries, salpingo-oophorectomy, ovariectomy

Types: bilateral oophorectomy
unilateral oophorectomy

A bilateral oophorectomy (Illustration 61) is a procedure in which the ovaries are removed. Actually, the correct term for this operation is "bilateral salpingo-oophorectomy," since the Fallopian tubes (*salpingo*) as well as the ovaries (*oophoro*) are removed. A unilateral oophorectomy is the removal of one ovary or a portion of the ovary and may also be accompanied by salpingectomy, or removal of the Fallopian tube. Bilateral salpingo-oophorectomy is generally accompanied by a hysterectomy since without the ovaries, the uterus has no function and may be the site of future problems. Sometimes both ovaries are removed because of a problem in the ovaries themselves, but some doctors routinely remove healthy ovaries in women having hysterectomies. This is discussed in more detail under the heading Hysterectomy above.

Oophorectomies may be done to treat a number of conditions, including ectopic pregnancy, benign and malignant ovarian cysts and tumors and pelvic inflammatory disease.

A unilateral oophorectomy, in which only one ovary is removed, is

721

Illustration 61   *Unilateral Oophorectomy (A) and Bilateral Oophorectomy (B)*

sometimes possible. With a unilateral oophorectomy, a woman is not subject to premature menopause and she preserves her ability to bear children, for even a small nub of ovarian tissue can continue to produce hormones. Women who have had a unilateral oophorectomy are still fertile.

Oophorectomy is a major operation and involves the same risks and potential complications as any form of major surgery. If both the ovaries are removed in a premenopausal woman, she will have a premature menopause. The doctor may recommend estrogen replacement therapy (ERT) in such cases; however, women should read the section on ERT and carefully weigh the risks and benefits before making a decision about ERT.

PELVIC EXENTERATION

AKA: removal of the pelvic organs

Types: total exenteration
partial exenteration
anterior exenteration
posterior exenteration

Pelvic exenteration (Illustration 62) is an ultraradical form of surgery used in the treatment of cancer. A total exenteration involves removal of the uterus, tubes, ovaries, vagina, the tissues adjacent to these organs, the bladder, the urethra and the rectum. Sometimes a partial exenteration, either anterior or posterior, is done. An anterior exenteration involves removal of all the pelvic tissues except the rectum. A posterior exenteration spares the bladder and urethra.

If a total exenteration is done, urinary and fecal wastes are collected in plastic bags attached to the outside of the body. If an anterior exenteration is done, it may be possible to divert urinary wastes to the bowels and thereby avoid the external collection bag. If a posterior exeneration is done, the urinary tract may function normally, but fecal wastes must be collected in a bag.

Understandably, many women find the idea of having to empty the bags that collect the waste materials distasteful. Anyone who has grown up in this culture is apt to have intensely negative associations with the natural bodily processes of elimination. Yet, many people who have this operation do learn to adjust. Moreover, the operation need not affect a woman's sexual responsiveness, and for women who desire it, plastic surgery techniques can be used to reconstruct the vagina. One way of finding out about the effects of this operation is by talking to people who have gone through it. The United Ostomy Association, at 1111 Wilshire Boulevard, Los Angeles, California 90017, telephone (213) 481-2811, is a support group for people who have had this type of surgery, and they can be very helpful in answering questions and helping you to adjust.

The survival rates for women having this procedure are often high enough to justify the risks and complications involved. Women with

723

Illustration 62 *Anterior Pelvic Exenteration (A), Posterior Pelvic Exenteration (B), and Total Pelvic Exenteration (C)*

advanced cancer who are candidates for this radical procedure (and not everyone is) are entitled to a frank discussion of risks and benefits with their doctors prior to making a decision.

CONIZATION

AKA: cold-knife conization, or cone; surgical conization, or cone;
cone biopsy

Conization (Illustration 63) is a surgical procedure whereby a cone of tissue is removed from the center of the cervix, a process somewhat akin to paring out the core of an apple. It is considered a major surgical procedure and must be done in a hospital using a general anesthetic. Although it sounds like a fairly simple procedure, it actually requires a good deal of skill. The tissue should be removed in one piece rather than whittled out in little bits so that the pathologist can study the architecture of the cells.

Indications

Conization is used both as a diagnostic procedure for cervical cancer and as a form of treatment for cervical dysplasia and carcinoma in situ of the cervix. In the past, conization was used as a treatment for chronic cervicitis, but cryosurgery, which is less expensive and less risky, has pretty much replaced conization for this purpose.

Before colposcopy was available, conization was used to do biopsies of the cervix. But since colposcopy is painless, has no complications, is less expensive and is less risky, it is now the preferred method in most cases. If, however, a woman has an abnormal Pap smear but the colposcopic examination fails to reveal any abnormalities on the surface of the cervix, if the abnormal area is quite large or if the abnormality that is seen leads into the cervical canal, then conization must still be done. But whenever possible, colposcopy should be done instead of conization. Not all doctors are skilled colposcopists, and some might be tempted to go ahead and do a conization rather than refer you to a doctor who is. If conization is recommended, always ask why conization, rather than colposcopy and biopsy, is being done.

Conization plays a vital role in establishing the diagnosis of microinvasive (Stage IA) cervical cancer. No woman should accept a diagnosis of microinvasive cancer unless a conization has been done.

Illustration 63   *Conization: An incision is made in the cervix (A), and a cone-shaped wedge of tissue is removed (B).*

Procedure

The woman is taken to the operating room and placed in stirrups as if she were having a routine gynecological exam. A speculum is placed in the vagina and the cervix and vagina are washed with an antiseptic solution. A general anesthetic is given and the doctor places sutures (stitches) on either side of the cervix to steady it and to diminish bleeding. A circular incision large enough to include the entire affected area is made on the surface of the cervix and is extended deep into the cervix so that the lower part of the cervix that opens into the uterus is also removed. The cut edges of the cervix are then sutured together.

Complications

Heavy bleeding is a common complication and may occur immediately after surgery or about ten days later, when the stitches are absorbed. One woman in ten requires transfusion, further surgery or readmission to the hospital because of bleeding problems. Infection and perforation of the uterus, although uncommon, are other complications that can result from conization.

Conization is apt to have a negative affect on fertility, depending on how much tissue has to be removed. If the cervical mucus glands, which produce the secretions that help the sperm swim up into the uterus, are destroyed, the woman may not be able to get pregnant. Cervical stenosis and incompetent cervix may also follow conization and affect fertility. About 25 percent of women who have conizations are not able to get pregnant. About 25 percent of those who do get pregnant will miscarry.

DILATION AND CURETTAGE

AKA: D&C, uterine scraping

The D&C (Illustration 64), a simple operation in which the endometrial lining of the uterus is surgically removed, is one of the most commonly performed surgical procedures and takes only about 10-15 minutes. It can be done using either a local or a general anesthetic. Most doctors prefer to use a general. First of all, the local doesn't fully eliminate the pain:

Illustration 64   *Dilation and Curettage: The cervix is dilated with a dilating rod (A), and the uterine lining is removed with a curette (B).*

Secondly, often the point of doing a D&C is to allow the doctor to make a careful examination of the uterine cavity, and patient discomfort under a local might cause him or her to hurry, resulting in a less thorough procedure. It is possible, however, to use a local. Regardless of the anesthetic used, the D&C, a hospital procedure, can usually be done on an outpatient basis.

Procedure

The woman is taken to the operating room, given a general (or local) anesthetic and put on a table with stirrups in a position similar to that used in the routine gynecological examination. The vagina, vulva and cervix are carefully cleaned with an antiseptic solution. Although some doctors shave the pubic hair to reduce the chances of infection, most do not. The doctor does a careful bimanual pelvic exam. Under the anesthetic the muscles are completely relaxed and this allows the doctor to feel the pelvic organs more readily than is possible if the woman is not anesthetized. A speculum is inserted into the vagina. The cervix is gently grasped with a clamplike instrument called a tenaculum to hold it steady. If a local anesthetic is used, it is usually injected into the cervix and the ligaments that support the uterus at this point.

A thin metal rod called a uterine sound is used to measure the depth and position of the uterus. It resembles the device used to check the oil level in a car's engine and is introduced into the uterus through the cervical opening. Then a tapered rod is inserted into the cervical opening to widen (dilate) it. A series of graduated rods of varying widths are inserted until the cervix is dilated about a half inch. An instrument called a curette, a thin rod with a sharp spoon-shaped tip, is inserted into the uterus and the uterine lining is gently scraped out. A curette may be used to take samples of the tissue lining the cervical canal as well. The doctor will carefully explore the entire uterine cavity with the curette.

The tissue removed through curettage is carefully collected and sent to the lab for analysis. In 24 to 48 hours, the pathologist will know whether or not cancer is present. The pathologist's final report should be ready within a week.

The curette, clamp and speculum are removed and the woman is taken to the recovery room, where her blood pressure and temperature are carefully monitored until the anesthetic wears off. Then she is usually asked to remain at the hospital for a few hours in case there are any serious complications or delayed reactions to the anesthetic.

Postoperative Care and Complications

It is common for a woman to have some bleeding after a D&C, and sometimes staining continues for a week. Small clots may be passed. Some women do not bleed at all afterward. Some have backache or mild cramps for a day or two.

The cervical opening remains slightly dilated for a week or two after a D&C. To cut down on the possibility of introducing disease-causing organisms into the uterus through the dilated opening, tampons and douches should be avoided for ten days to two weeks. Some doctors will allow intercourse during the first ten days if the woman is not bleeding and if the man uses a condom (a rubber); however, we personally recommend avoiding sexual intercourse for the first ten days since infection, should it occur, can have very serious consequences.

After a D&C, it is impossible to predict when the next menstrual period will take place. It may be early or late. For some women, the first couple of menstrual periods following a D&C may be unusually profuse, so women who have had a D&C because of heavy bleeding problems should not be too quick to judge the results.

The D&C is a relatively safe procedure. The death rate for D&Cs performed on healthy women under the age of 50 is about two per 10,000.[8] In addition to complications from the use of anesthesia, infection, hemorrhage, perforation of the uterus or other organs and the formation of scar tissue within the uterus can follow a D&C.

Pelvic inflammatory disease is the most common of the serious complications. Any time instruments are inserted into the uterus, the possibility of germs being carried from the cervix or vagina up into the uterus exists. Most of these infections are readily cured by antibiotics; however, in some cases, they may be serious enough to require hysterectomy and can even be fatal. Perforation (puncture) of the uterus, nearby blood vessels, bladder or bowel can occur, although this is rare. If only the uterus is punctured, chances are that it will heal itself. If other organs are damaged, immediate reparative surgery may be necessary. If puncture is suspected, the woman is asked to remain in the hospital and laparoscopy may be recommended to assess the possible damage. Heavy bleeding may occur if the walls of the uterus or the cervix are injured or if a polyp or fibroid tumor is only partially removed, but in general, heavy bleeding is a rare complication, more likely to occur in women who have certain blood disorders. Another rare complication, known as Asherman's syndrome, a condition in which scar tissue forms in the uterus, causing an absence of menstrual periods and infertility, may also follow a D&C.

A checkup is usually done two weeks after the D&C. At that time the doctor will check for tenderness in the uterus and tubes which could indicate infection and to see that the cervix is normal. If, however, any of the following signs or symptoms occur, the woman should contact her doctor *immediately*:

* A fever of 100.4°F or higher
* Persistent abdominal pain or cramps
* Faintness, weakness or dizziness
* A foul-smelling vaginal discharge
* Heavy bleeding (more than three pads soaked in one hour)

Indications

The D&C is a diagnostic tool and sometimes a cure for certain conditions. It is used to diagnose uterine cancer and is sometimes part of the diagnostic work-up in cervical cancer. It may be used to diagnose abnormal uterine bleeding. Endometritis, which is an infection of the uterine lining that can cause abnormal bleeding, may be cured by a D&C if the infected lining is totally removed. Fibroid tumors that distort the endometrial cavity, causing abnormal bleeding, can be diagnosed by a D&C, for the doctor will feel a "bump" as the curette moves over the surface of the uterine cavity. On occasion, small, protruding fibroids can be removed during a D&C, but most of the time more extensive surgery is needed. Endometrial polyps, another source of abnormal bleeding, can be diagnosed and treated by a D&C. Cervical polyps will at times require a D&C. Endometrial hyperplasia, yet another source of abnormal bleeding, can also be diagnosed and cured by a D&C. It may also be used to treat Asherman's syndrome.

Sometimes a D&C will allow a woman nearing menopause who has been experiencing abnormal bleeding to avoid a hysterectomy. Sometimes the D&C itself can be avoided by the use of hormone treatment. This is discussed in more detail under the headings Abnormal Uterine Bleeding and Endometrial Hyperplasia. It should be mentioned that the D&C should be a last resort in young girls with abnormal bleeding problems, for in this age group such problems often revert to normal by themselves or can be handled with hormone therapy. If a doctor suggests a D&C as the first step in the treatment of abnormal bleeding in this age group, it would probably be wise to seek a second medical opinion (*see* p. 226).

A D&C is not a treatment for infertility or menstrual cramps. On occasion, the D&C may be part of the diagnostic work-up for these conditions but not until other, less drastic diagnostic procedures such as endometrial biopsy and certain X-ray or ultrasound techniques have been used. Although the D&C was once used for abortions, the newer, safer suction methods are now preferred.

If the first D&C is not successful in controlling abnormal bleeding, a second or even a third one may be in order; however, after that, a woman may begin to consider a hysterectomy as an alternative to repeated D&Cs. Factors like the number of years until menopause, whether or not the abnormal bleeding is getting progressively worse and whether or not the hyperplasia (if it exists) is getting progressively more serious in nature will influence this decision. Some women choose to undergo a number of D&Cs rather than have a hysterectomy.

CAUTERY

AKA: electric or heat cautery, cauterization, burning

Cauterization (Illustration 65) involves destroying tissues by means of a controlled electric current. A pointed instrument is electrically heated until the tip becomes red-hot. The instrument is then applied to the affected area. The heat destroys the surface layers of tissue, allowing new and unaffected cell growth to replace the burned-off tissue. A scab forms as the tissue heals. The scab sloughs off in a week or two, leaving new, healthy tissue.

Indications

Cautery is used to treat conditions such as chronic cervicitis, dysplasia, carcinoma in situ and vaginal or vulvar warts. It may also be used to close off the tubes in certain sterilization procedures and to destroy areas of endometriosis.

Procedure

If, as is often the case, it is the cervix that is to be treated, a speculum is first inserted into the vagina. The vagina and cervix are cleaned and the cautery tip is applied to the affected area. A grayish, greenish scab forms and falls off in a week or two. Underneath the scab, new, healthy tissue will

732

Illustration 65 *Cautery*

have formed. Complete healing usually takes seven to eight weeks, and some doctors prescribe antiseptic creams and jellies during this time to promote healing.

The procedure can usually be done in a doctor's office without an anesthetic although if the area to be treated is up inside the cervical canal, hospitalization and a general anesthetic may be necessary.

Since cauterization causes temporary swelling of the cervix and narrowing of the cervical canal, it is usually performed just after a woman's menstrual period so that the swelling and narrowing will have subsided by the next period and there won't be any blockage of the menstrual flow. The next menstrual period following treatment may, however, be heavier than usual.

There is apt to be a profuse discharge, sometimes with blood in it, for two to three weeks following treatment, and this is quite normal. If, however, the discharge turns yellow or develops a foul odor, this may be a sign of infection and your doctor should be notified.

Sanitary napkins may be used to catch the discharge, but tampons cannot be used. In fact, most doctors recommend that nothing be inserted in the vagina for two to three weeks, which means that intercourse and douching are also prohibited.

After the scab falls away, the discharge subsides. There may still be some bleeding since the new tissue on the cervix is still rather raw and may bleed easily.

Complications

Complications are relatively rare but may include infection, bleeding, cervical stenosis and infertility. The risks of infection can be minimized by refraining from intercourse or from inserting anything into the vagina for two weeks. Antibiotic vaginal creams or jellies may also help in preventing or curing infection.

Some spotting or even bleeding is normal; however, accidental damage to deeper cervical tissues can cause excessive bleeding. Cervical stenosis, a more permanent narrowing of the cervical canal, can occur if there is tissue damage that causes adhesions, or bands of scar tissue, in the canal. This complication may be treated by gentle dilation of the cervical canal over a period of weeks.

If the glands in the cervical canal are damaged, this may impair their function, which may in turn cause infertility because it is the secretions from these glands that help nourish the sperm and aid them on their journey into the uterus.

Some doctors fear that electric cautery may cause such scarring that subsequent Pap smears may be difficult to interpret. Certainly, the Pap smear will not be accurate until the healing process is complete.

Cautery vs. Cryosurgery

Cryosurgery (see below) can often be used instead of cautery. Cryosurgery has several advantages. First of all, it is less painful. Although the textbooks say that cautery causes only mild to moderate discomfort and point out that the treatment takes just a short time, many women we have talked to have found the treatment quite painful.

Moreover, the doctor is better able to control the depth of tissue destruction with cryosurgery, which accounts for the fact that cryosurgery has a lower complication rate than cautery. There are certain instances in which cryosurgery is inappropriate and cautery must be used, but these are rare.

Unfortunately, many doctors do not have cryosurgery equipment in their offices. If your doctor suggests cautery, ask whether cryosurgery could be done instead. If so, request cryosurgery or referral to a cryosurgeon if your doctor does not have the necessary equipment.

CRYOSURGERY

AKA: freezing, cold cautery

Cryosurgery (Illustration 66) is a new technique that is replacing cautery (described above) in many instances. It involves the use of nitrogen or carbon dioxide to quick-freeze the affected areas, killing the abnormal tissue and allowing new, unaffected tissue to take its place. It can be used to treat the same conditions as cautery. Much of the information given in the above description of cautery applies to cryosurgery, so be sure to read that section as well.

Procedure

Cryosurgery is an office procedure and does not require an anesthetic. If the cervix is to be treated, a speculum is placed in the vagina. An instrument that looks like a miniature spear gun is attached to a tank of compressed gas. The gas is released into the gun and expands rapidly to

Illustration 66   *Cryosurgery*

produce intense cold. The tip of the gun is then applied to the area to be treated. The treatment takes about two minutes. You may experience a feeling of intense cold and a mild cramp. Since some women experience dizziness and lightheadedness afterward, you will be asked to remain lying down for 15 minutes to a half hour after treatment.

Immediately following treatment the cervix is like a block of ice. Within 24 hours the cervix turns a deep purple-blue color and is so swollen that it is impossible to distinguish the cervical os (opening).

Most women have a profuse discharge for a week or two following treatment. The discharge is occasionally bloody, and this is normal. The next period may be heavier than usual, and this is also normal. If, however, the discharge becomes yellowish or develops a foul odor, this may be a sign of infection and you should contact the doctor.

Douching, intercourse and the use of tampons are prohibited until the discharge subsides, in about two weeks.

Complications

Infection may occur but can usually be treated with antibiotics. Avoiding intercourse, douching and tampons will help prevent this complication. Vaginal creams or jellies may be prescribed to aid in healing and cut down on the chance of infection. Some bleeding is normal, but on occasion this may become excessive. Neither cervical stenosis, a narrowing or blockage of the cervical canal due to scar tissue, nor infertility, both of which may occur following cautery, have been reported in women treated with cryosurgery.[8] Pap smears may be inaccurate for three months following treatment.

BIOPSIES

Types: breast biopsy
vulvar biopsy
cervical biopsy
endocervical curettage, or ECC
endometrial biopsy

A biopsy (Illustration 67) involves the removal of a small piece of tissue for microscopic exam. Biopsies are done on lumps, warts or sores, when

Illustration 67   *Endometrial Biopsy (A), Vulvar Biopsy (B), and Cervical Biopsy (C)*

there is an abnormal Pap smear or anytime the doctor wants to rule out the possibility that cancer is present. General information about biopsies is given in the section on cancer. Breast biopsies are discussed in the section on breast cancer (*see* p. 505). Some of the more common types of biopsies are discussed below.

Types

Almost any tissue in the body can be biopsied. The following biopsies are frequently performed in gynecological medicine:

Vulvar biopsy: The vulvar biopsy is done to rule out the possibility that a persistent lump, sore or abnormality is a cancerous one. A special solution may be painted on the vulva to help the doctor detect abnormal areas that can't be seen with the naked eye. A colposcope or magnifying glass may also be used to detect abnormal areas. One or more tiny (quarter-inch) pieces of skin are taken from the edge of the sore where it joins the normal skin. The procedure can usually be done in the doctor's office with a local anesthetic, but some doctors do it in the hospital with a general anesthetic. If your doctor suggests this, read the information on vulvar biopsies in the introduction to the section on vulvar diseases.

After the biopsy specimen has been taken, it is sent to the lab for analysis by a pathologist. If you have been treated for vulvar warts with a drug called podophyllin prior to biopsy, make sure your doctor notes this on the lab specimen or the pathologist may mistakenly think that cancer is present.

After the tissue sample has been obtained, the doctor may stitch up the biopsied area since the vulva is richly supplied with blood vessels and may bleed profusely; if bleeding is not a problem, s/he may allow the cut to heal by itself. The biopsy wound can become infected, so proper hygiene is important. If redness, swelling or tenderness develops, contact the doctor.

Cervical biopsy: Important information about the value of using a colposcope in cervical biopsies is included in the section on cervical dysplasia. A cervical biopsy may be done because of an abnormal Pap smear when the doctor sees an abnormality on the cervix with the naked eye or with the use of a colposcope.

The biopsy can be done in the doctor's office. One or several tissue specimens may be taken with the aid of an instrument that looks like a paper punch. A special stain is painted on the cervix to help the doctor identify areas for biopsy and the colposcope is also useful for this purpose.

A local anesthetic is generally not necessary. Although some women experience a mild cramping, this is usually not too painful because the cervix has few nerve endings. There may be some spotting afterward but heavy bleeding is not normal and should be reported to the doctor. Pain, abnormal discharge or fever may be a sign of infection and should also be reported. To prevent infection, avoid intercourse, douching and the use of tampons for at least a week.

Endocervical curettage: Many times, the cervical biopsy will include an endocervical curettage (ECC). A thin instrument with a spoon-shaped tip is used to scrape cells from the cervical canal. ECC is recommended when the abnormal area on the cervix extends into the canal and in the follow-up of women with dysplasia or carcinoma in situ who have been treated by cryosurgery. Like the cervical biopsy, endocervical curettage is an office procedure that doesn't usually require an anesthetic, although it may cause mild cramping and, on occasion, infection.

Endometrial biopsy: An endometrial biopsy involves the use of a small scraping instrument, a curette, which is inserted through the cervix into the uterine cavity. The spoon-shaped tip of the curette is used to obtain a tissue sample of the endometrial lining of the uterus. The biopsy can be done in the doctor's office. Most women experience moderate to strong cramping, and a local anesthetic may relieve the pain somewhat.

The endometrial biopsy is often used in fertility work-ups to tell whether or not the woman is ovulating. It can also detect uterine cancer in women who have abnormal bleeding. If, however, the endometrial biopsy is negative, this does not rule out the possibility of cancer, for the cancer may exist in one area but not in another. A positive endometrial biopsy — one that shows cancerous cells — may eliminate the need for a diagnostic D&C, but a D&C is still necessary if the endometrial biopsy is negative.

Although the endometrial biopsy may fail to detect cancer that is actually present, it does have a high rate of accuracy (about 85 percent) and may be used to screen women at high risk for the development of uterine cancer. In particular, many doctors recommend yearly endometrial biopsies for women who use estrogen replacement therapy.

ENDOSCOPY

Types: cystoscopy
proctosigmoidoscopy
laparoscopy
culdoscopy
colposcopy

Endoscopic examination involves using lighted, magnifying instruments called endoscopes to view the interior of a body cavity.

Types

There are a number of different types of endoscopy, including:

Cystoscopy: Cystoscopy allows the doctor to inspect the interior of the bladder for fistulas, stones, tumors and other irregularities. It is often used in the diagnostic work-up of gynecological cancer and in the investigation of persistent and puzzling urinary tract problems or blood in the urine. The bladder is first filled with air or fluid and then the thin cystoscope is inserted through the urethra into the bladder. The cystoscope can collect cell samples and remove very small tumors.

Proctosigmoidoscopy: This procedure, in which an instrument is inserted through the rectum, allows the doctor to inspect the lower portion of the gastrointestinal tract, usually without an anesthetic. It is often used to detect cancer of the rectum and colon. Its main application in gynecology is in the staging of certain gynecological cancers.

Hysteroscopy: The hysteroscope is a fairly recent innovation and is not yet widely used. It allows the doctor to view the inside of the uterus and can be used to look for lost IUDs, and to detect the presence of certain fibroid tumors and other benign and malignant uterine tumors. It is also being used in fertility work-ups. The hysteroscope looks like a spear diver's gun and has a flexible tip and an eyepiece to allow for a full view of the uterus. The tube of the instrument is inserted into the vagina, through the cervix and into the uterine cavity. The procedure can usually be done on an outpatient basis using a local anesthetic.

Laparoscopy: Laparoscopy is a surgical procedure in which a tubelike lighted endoscope called a laparoscope is inserted into the pelvic cavity through a half- to one-inch incision just below the navel. The laparoscope works on the same principal as the periscope of a submarine and allows the doctor to look at the uterus, ovaries and tubes.

Although laparoscopy has been around for more than 60 years, it is only in the last few years that the newly refined instrument has been used widely in this country. It has proven to be a valuable diagnostic tool, enabling doctors to diagnose questionable cases without major exploratory surgery. In some instances, it can be used to treat certain diseases by means of special instruments inserted through the tube that holds the laparoscope. It is also used in sterilization procedures.

Laparoscopic examinations are done in the hospital using either local or general anesthetics, but unless complications occur, it isn't necessary for the woman to stay overnight. Some doctors prefer a local anesthetic, which involves less risk, while others prefer a general anesthetic, both because it is totally pain-free and because, should complications arise and emergency surgery be required, there won't be any time lost while the patient is put under a general. The procedure is described in more detail under the heading Laparoscopic Tubal Ligation.

Culdoscopy: Culdoscopy (Illustration 68) is similar to laparoscopy except that the incision is made in the vagina and the Culdoscope is inserted into the body through this incision. This allows the doctor to view the cul-de-sac, an area behind the uterus and between it and the rectum. Culdoscopy has many of the same applications and advantages as laparoscopy and may be used when scar tissue from previous operations or infections rules out laparoscopy. It, too, requires at least outpatient hospitalization and a local or general anesthetic.

Colposcopy: Unlike other forms of endoscopy, colposcopy (Illustration 69) does not require insertion of an instrument into the body. Instead, a speculum is placed in the vagina and a beam of light from the colposcope, which looks like a pair of binoculars mounted on a stand, is directed into the vaginal cavity. This form of endoscopy is completely painless, doesn't require an anesthetic and can be performed in the doctor's office in about 10-20 minutes.

Colposcopy is a fairly recent innovation and though its use is quite widespread, many doctors did not receive instruction in this technique in medical school. Unless a doctor has taken special training, s/he will not have the skill and expertise needed to interpret colposcopic findings, so be sure to ask whether or not your doctor has received this training.

The colposcope magnifies the doctor's view 10-20 times and is often used in the follow-up of abnormal Pap smears. With the use of special color filters, the doctor can see abnormalities on the cervix even before the Pap smear can detect them. In addition, the doctor can see changes in the blood vessels in the area that are associated with cancerous and precancerous conditions.

The colposcope is also used to identify areas for cervical biopsy. The importance of a colposcopic-directed biopsy is discussed in detail under the heading Cervical Dysplasia. Colposcopic exam is also recommended for DES daughters. The colposcope may also be used to investigate pain or bleeding associated with intercourse if the doctor feels the problems are due to a cervical abnormality. In addition, the colposcope may be used to examine sores or other abnormalities on the vulva or in the vagina.

741

Illustration 68   *Culdoscopy: The woman is placed on the operating table in a knee-chest position. The vagina is held open by means of vaginal retractors (A). The cervix is held down with a tenaculum (B). The Culdoscope (C) is inserted through an incision in the back of the vaginal wall.*

742

Illustration 69 *Colposcopy: A speculum is placed in the vagina. A beam of light from the colposcope is directed toward the cervix, and the doctor views the cervix and the interior of the vagina through the eyepiece of the colposcope.*

DIAGNOSTIC RADIATION

Types: plain film X-rays
contrast X-rays
radioactive scans

Radiation is used in the treatment of cancer and as a tool in the diagnostic work-up of a wide variety of diseases and abnormalities, including many gynecologic conditions. X-rays are the most widely used type of diagnostic radiation. They are taken by positioning the area of the body to be studied between an X-ray machine and a sheet of film. A short burst of rays is then emitted from the machine. The rays pass through the body and strike the film. As the rays pass through the body some of them are absorbed by denser tissue, such as the bone tissue, and don't make it all the way through the body with their full force. Other tissues, such as the soft tissues that make up your organs, don't absorb much radiation, so the rays pass through this type of tissue and strike the film at almost full force. The more rays the film has absorbed, the darker the film will be once it has been processed. Thus, the processed X-ray film will be a picture of contrasting shadows, with the most dense tissues, the bones, showing up as almost white and the least dense tissues dark in color. Fractures or other bone irregularities can be seen easily, and tumors, which are denser than normal tissues can often be seen.

For contrast X-rays, a dense substance called a dye, or contrast solution, is injected into an organ or body cavity prior to the X-ray so that tumors or irregularities in the outline of your organs can be seen more clearly. Yet another type of diagnostic radiation technique is the radioactive scan. This involves injecting a radioactive material into the bloodstream and following its progress through the body with a special cameralike machine that produces pictures that are then "read" by a specially trained doctor.

Types

There are a number of different types of radiation used in diagnostic work-ups of women with gynecological problems, including:

Plain film X-rays: These are the standard X-rays with which most of us are familiar. A chest X-ray is one example and is often used preoperatively in women undergoing major surgery, especially if the woman is over 40 or is suspected of having certain medical problems that might cause anesthesia complications. Chest X-rays are also used in the work-up of cancer patients to rule out the possibility that the cancer has spread to the lungs.

744

Mammograms: These are X-rays of the breast tissue used to diagnose and to follow-up women with breast abnormalities. Mammography is discussed in more detail in the section on breast cancer.

Barium enema, or BE: Barium, a very dense substance, is introduced into the body through the rectum prior to X-ray. This contrasting X-ray may be used in the diagnosis of various gynecological conditions, notably in the staging of certain forms of gynecological cancer.

Cystogram or cystourethrogram: The cystogram is a contrast-type X-ray used to visualize the bladder, while a cystourethrogram is used to visualize both the bladder and the urethra. Dye is placed in the bladder by means of a tube known as a urinary catheter. These X-rays are used in the work-up of gynecological cancer and other gynecologic and urinary diseases.

Hysterogram, or hysterosalpingogram: Again, this is a contrast-type X-ray in which a dye is injected into the uterus through a small tube. It outlines the interior of the uterus and Fallopian tubes. It is frequently used in the work-up of fertility patients.

Intravenous pyelogram (IVP): Yet another type of contrast X-ray, the IVP outlines the urinary tract, the kidneys, ureters and bladder. The dye is injected into a vein in the arm. It is often used in the work-up of cancer patients and prior to operations done to investigate or remove pelvic masses.

Lymphangiography: This contrast X-ray is used to visualize the lymph nodes. Dye is injected into the lymph system through an incision in the big toe. Since the lymph vessels are very small, it usually takes a couple of hours before the dye is fully distributed and the X-rays can be taken. The procedure is often used in the staging work-up of women with gynecologic cancer. It is not a totally reliable procedure, for even though the X-rays show some sort of obstruction to the flow of the dye, this may be due to infection and does not necessarily indicate that cancer is present in the lymph system. Conversely, cancer too small to be detected by lymphangiography may be present. Still, lymphangiogram techniques are being improved constantly and in many instances the results of the lymphangiogram can be correlated with other findings to yield information valuable in diagnosing and staging cancer. Moreover, the dye is usually retained in the body for some time and may be useful in helping the surgeon locate and identify lymph nodes if surgical removal of the nodes is required.

Radioactive scans: Radioactive scans, which are more sensitive than standard X-rays, are used in the work-up of cancer patients to determine whether or not the cancer has spread to other organs. They are also used in the follow-up of certain types of cancer. One type of scan that is frequently used in women with cancer, particularly those with breast cancer, is the bone scan. A liquid containing a mildly radioactive substance is injected

745

into the bloodstream and carried to the bones. Cancerous areas in the bone will usually absorb more radiation than other areas. The pictures taken by the scanning machines will show denser concentrations in this area. These concentrations, or "hot spots," as they are called, can be caused by infections, injuries, arthritis and other abnormal conditions as well as cancer, so having a hot spot does not necessarily mean that a woman has metastatic cancer.

Liver scans and brain scans, which work in similar fashion, may also be used in the diagnostic work-up and the follow-up program of women with female cancers.

The Diagnostic Radiologist

There are two types of doctors who specialize in radiation: therapeutic radiologists, who are involved in using radiation to treat diseases, and diagnostic radiologists, who are specialists in taking and interpreting the results of diagnostic radiation exams. The use of radiation involves certain risks (see below) and since accurate interpretation requires experience, judgment and skill, you might want to insist on a board-certified radiologist. In order to be board-certified as a diagnostic radiologist, a doctor must be a graduate of an approved medical school, have completed four years of postgraduate training in a department of radiology and have passed written and oral examinations administered by the board. Although there are many good radiologists who are not board-certified and certification is not an absolute assurance that a radiologist is competent, it does indicate that their training, skill and performance have been evaluated by their peers and judged to be of the highest quality.

Radiation Risks*

Radiation can cause as well as cure cancer. When radioactive rays pass through the body, they damage the cells of our bodies. Radiation can destroy these cells outright or can damage them so that they are unable to reproduce. Sometimes the cells are damaged but are still able to reproduce. However, the reproduced cells may be abnormal. As you may recall from the section on cancer, cancer results when damaged cells that do not have the proper "brakes" to tell them when to stop reproducing continue doing so at a wild pace. Even subtle damage to a single cell could increase the risk of cancer in a susceptible individual, although it may take many years for the damage to manifest itself. Of course, not everyone who is exposed to

*For more details, see the section on Mammography.

radiation will develop cancer. In most people, the damaged cells will simply die or the body's immune system will destroy the abnormal cells. But in some people, exposure to radiation can cause cancer.

Most of our knowledge of radiation-induced cancer comes from studies of people exposed to large amounts of radiation—more than 100 rads. Radiation doses are measured in rems and rads. A rem, or roentgen, is a unit of measurement of the amount *emitted* by the X-ray machine or source of radiation. A rad is a unit of measurement of radiation *absorbed* by the body. Terms like "millirem" (mrem) or "millirad" (mrad) are used to denote one-thousandth of a rem (.001 rem) or of a rad (.001 rad). We are all subject to a certain amount of natural radiation from the earth and the sun, about 130 millirems a year. It is not known whether or not this "natural" radiation is harmful.

We do know that people exposed to large amounts of radiation, for instance survivors of the atomic bomb dropped in World War II, have higher rates of cancer than would normally be expected. Until recently, it was thought that exposure to lower levels of radiation associated with medical diagnostic X-rays or on-the-job exposure would not be harmful. But now most experts feel that radiation risks are cumulative—they add up. Exposure to low levels over a period of time may be just as bad as exposure to a large amount in a single dose.

Part of the controversy about low-level radiation risks comes from the few studies that have been done. One study begun in 1964 involved workers in Hanford, Washington, who were exposed to very low doses, .5 rem a year, over a number of years.[9] A 6-7 percent increase in cancer was found in this group. These and other, similar studies have been sharply criticized. The Hanford study involved 35,000 workers, but many experts point out that in order to be statistically valid such a study would have to include millions of people; otherwise, the 6-7 percent increase could be a mere statistical fluke.

To those unfamiliar with statistics, 35,000 seems like a substantial enough number from which to draw conclusions, but actually it is not. Radiation-induced cancers are but a small fraction of the cancers expected to occur normally. In a group of 400,000 people we would expect 65,000 of them to die of cancer in any event. If such a group were exposed to low-level radiation and 50 cancers more than the 65,000 expected cancers were found, could we attribute this to radiation exposure or could it be a mere statistical fluke?

These questions are unanswered at this time. But the fact that this study and others have suggested that low-level radiation over a period of years may be harmful should make us cautious about the use of X-rays.[10] Since as many as 30 percent of the medical X-rays ordered in this country each year may be unnecessary,[11] you should take precautions.

☐ Never submit to an X-ray without understanding why.

☐ Always ask if other tests, for instance, ultrasound, (see below) could be done instead.

☐ Give careful consideration to a decision to visit a hospital emergency room for a bump on the head or a superficial wound. Fear of malpractice may lead the doctor to recommend an X-ray that may not be strictly necessary.

☐ Avoid repetitions by telling the doctor about similar X-rays you have had. If you have a chronic condition or are getting a second opinion, you can ask to have a second copy of your X-ray made for your own files for a nominal fee.

☐ Make sure that your X-ray machine is well-calibrated and is giving the lowest exposure possible. Ask what agency inspects the machine and with what frequency. Have your X-rays done in a hospital or radiologist's office. These machines usually give less exposure than those taken in a doctor's office or a mobile X-ray unit.

☐ Never submit to an X-ray if you think you might be pregnant unless it is *absolutely* necessary.

ULTRASOUND

AKA: sonograms, sonography, B-Scans

Ultrasound is a method of visualizing the interior of the body by means of high-frequency sound waves. Unlike X-rays, sonograms do not involve radiation and are therefore thought to be less risky. But sonography is a relatively new technique, and we do not yet know if there are any long-term effects. Many health-care activists are therefore questioning the routine use of sonography on pregnant women. While there may be a legitimate need in certain high-risk pregnancies and while ultrasound is probably preferable to X-rays in such instances, sonography may not be necessary in routine pregnancies.

Uses

Sonography is used to detect structural defects in pregnancy, to determine the size of the uterus, to estimate the length of the pregnancy, to monitor the fetal heartbeat and the strength and frequency of contractions during labor, to confirm the presence of twins or to determine the position of the fetus. It may also be used to locate a lost IUD or to detect an ectopic pregnancy. It is often useful in evaluating ovarian enlargements and pelvic masses and in planning radiation therapy for cancer.

Procedure

Ultrasound is completely painless. You will be asked to drink a glass of water about an hour before the examination so that your bladder will be full and will serve as a reference point for the technician performing the examination. Sound waves are directed toward your body by means of a microphone-type instrument that is passed over it. The sound waves bounce back to the microphone receiver and these "echo patterns" are translated into a picture.

You may be required to lie quite still and to hold your breath for part of the exam. The whole exam takes about half an hour and is usually done at a hospital or at a radiologist's office.

PAP SMEAR

AKA: Papanicolaou smear, Pap test, vaginal smear, cervical smear

The Pap smear is a simple completely painless office procedure that is used primarily to screen for cervical cancer. The doctor inserts a speculum into the vagina. The surface of the cervix is then gently scraped with a wooden spatula. The cells thus collected are smeared onto a slide that is then labeled and sent to a pathology laboratory for analysis.

How the Pap Smear Works

In order to understand how a Pap smear works, it is necessary to know a bit about the cellular make-up of the cervix. The cervix is covered by layers of tissue known as epithelial (skin) tissue, which grows from the bottom layer, known as the basal cell layer, outward toward the surface. The tissue constantly regenerates itself. New cells on the bottom layer are very active, dividing, growing and multiplying constantly. As they grow, they force the more mature cells upward, toward the surface layers.

As the cells mature and move upward they change character. At the bottom level, where the cells are very active and are reproducing constantly, they have large nuclei, or centers. At the middle level the cells themselves are larger, the nuclei are smaller, and they show less activity. They're getting older. By the time they get to the surface, they are flattened out, less active and nearly dead, about to be shed.

On our outer skin we recognize such cells as flaky scales or dandruff. The same continual process of shedding takes place in the skin tissue of the cervix, and it is these sloughed-off cells that are picked up in a Pap smear.

As long as the cells picked up in the Pap smear are all mature, flattened-out inactive cells, the smear is normal. But if immature cells that are still active and dividing constantly are seen on the surface, this abnormality may mean that a cancerous or precancerous change is taking place, for, as explained in the section on cancer, cancer is a disease that involves irregularities in the growth patterns of cells.

Classifying Pap Smear Results

If the pathologist looks at the slide and sees only mature, flattened-out, near dead cells, it will be labeled "normal," "benign" or "Class I."

Sometimes a woman will have an infection that has irritated the surface layers of the cervical tissue. In such cases, there may be inflammatory cells, disease-fighting white blood cells and perhaps infectious bacteria as well. Because the surface layer of the cervical epithelium has been disturbed, immature cells may reach the surface and may be picked up in the Pap smear. These are referred to as atypical cells. The pathologist may use terms such as "inflammatory," "atypical," "atypical metaplasia" or "Class II" to describe this type of smear. Although this smear is abnormal, it does not indicate that a cancerous or precancerous condition exists. It is a benign smear, and the cells can be expected to revert to normal once the infection has healed. There are occasional women who routinely have unexplained inflammatory cells in their Pap smear. While this is not serious, it's inconvenient, for such women must have frequent Pap smears.

If the pathologist looks at a slide and sees immature and abnormal cells, s/he will classify the Pap as abnormal. If the degree of abnormality is relatively mild, s/he will use terms such as "mild or moderate cervical intraepithelial neoplasia," "mild or moderate CIN," "mild or moderate dysplasia" or "Class III" to describe the smear. These changes are considered precancerous, meaning that a large portion of *untreated* cases would, over a period of years, progress to cervical cancer. However, these conditions are 100 percent curable. Diagnosis and treatment of these conditions is discussed in the section on the cervix under the heading Cervical Dysplasia.

If the pathologist looks at a smear and sees more severe abnormalities and a greater proportion of immature cells, s/he may use terms such as "cervical intraepithelial neoplasia, grade three," "carcinoma in situ" or "Class IV." Again, this is a precancerous condition that, if not treated, has a high likelihood of progressing to cervical cancer but with treatment is virtually 100 percent curable. Diagnostic steps and treatment are discussed in the section on the cervix under the heading Carcinoma in Situ.

If the pathologist looks at the slide and sees extremely abnormal, immature, cancerous cells, s/he will use terms such as "malignant," "invasive" or "Class V." This means that the pathologist thinks there is evidence of cervical cancer, and that further tests and treatment, which are discussed under the heading Cervical Cancer, will be needed. Table 26 summarizes Pap smear classifications.

Table 26
Pap Smear Results

Class	Terms Used to Describe
I	Normal, negative, benign
II	Benign, inflammatory, atypical, atypical metaplasia
III	Mild or moderate cervical intraepithelial neoplasia (CIN), mild or moderate dysplasia, CIN, grades I and II
IV	Severe cervical intraepithelial neoplasia (CIN), severe dysplasia, CIN, grade III, carcinoma in situ
V	Malignant, invasive cancer

Accuracy

The Pap smear is not 100 percent accurate. Sometimes it fails to detect cancer that is actually there. At other times, it may suggest a cancerous or precancerous condition when in fact everything is normal. The smear may be inaccurate for a number of reasons. Faulty technique in collecting the cells from the cervix or improper preparation or handling of the slides can cause inaccurate results, but many times no one is at fault. For example, precancerous cells may be present but may not be among those picked when the cervix is scraped. Still, the Pap smear is about 95 percent accurate in detecting cancerous and precancerous cell changes. The fact that it is sometimes inaccurate is not too disturbing, for cervical cancer is usually a slowly progressing disease. It generally takes about five years for dysplasia to progress to invasive cancer, so even if the cancerous or precancerous cells are missed one time, they will probably be picked up on the next smear.

While the Pap smear is 95 percent accurate in determining whether or not abnormal cancerous or precancerous cells are present, it is considerably less accurate in detecting the degree of abnormality. It is not uncommon for Pap smears to be "off" by one or more steps. Thus, a smear that indicates carcinoma in situ may, in reality, be invasive cancer, or a smear that indicates moderate dysplasia may actually be carcinoma in situ.

Pathology is not a hard-and-fast science. Classifying a Pap smear is a matter of judgment. One pathologist may look at a slide and call it dysplasia, while another might classify it as carcinoma in situ. Then, too, the smear may only have picked up dysplastic cells when, in reality, the more abnormal carcinoma in situ cells were present but just didn't happen to be picked up. Other noncancerous conditions may fool the pathologist into thinking cancerous cells are present when they are not.

Because of this lack of accuracy, cancerous and precancerous smears must be followed up with cervical biopsies, preferably biopsies done with the aid of a colposcope. This is discussed in detail under the heading Cervical Dysplasia.

Frequency

Once a young woman begins sexual activity or reaches the age of 16 or 18, she should have periodic Pap smears. Until recently, it was recommended that women have a Pap smear once a year unless they were at high risk for cervical cancer, had abnormal Pap results in the past, had a history of herpes or were DES daughters, in which case more frequent Pap smears might be called for. However, the American Cancer Society recently changed this and now recommends that all women age 20 and over and those under 20 who are sexually active have a Pap smear annually for two negative examinations and then one at least every three years until the age of 65. There is some controversy about the new recommendation, and many doctors still recommend annual Pap smears.

Those who favor the once-every-three-years schedule argue that cervical cancer is a slowly progressing disease that usually takes at least five to seven years to become invasive cancer, so once every three years should be sufficient to detect it. Those who favor the once-a-year schedule argue that while the precancerous conditions usually take several years to develop into cancer, this may not always be the case. Moreover, since the Pap smear is not 100 percent accurate, getting a yearly Pap smear can minimize the risk of inaccurate results, as it would be very rare to get a false negative two years in a row. Otherwise a false negative that wasn't corrected for three years could mean that invasive cervical cancer was allowed to develop in the interim. Invasive cervical cancer, unlike carcinoma in situ, is not 100 percent curable and may require more drastic treatment. Although the number of women who would be adversely affected by the once-every-three-year schedule is small, to be on the safe side we recommend once-a-year Pap smears.

Another reason we favor the once-a-year schedule is that it's easier to remember. Many of us would have a hard time recalling whether two or three years had gone by since our last smear. It would simply be too easy to let three years slide into four or even five. The Pap smear is a safe, simple, painless, relatively inexpensive, life-saving test, but one that too many women still ignore: There is no reason *not* to have it every year.

Other Uses

The Pap smear will sometimes pick up cancer of the uterus, Fallopian tubes or ovaries. In order for this to occur, the cancerous cells from the other organs would have to have made their way through the cervical canal and onto the slide. If this happened, it would be a lucky coincidence, for the Pap smear is not a reliable screening method for any of these other forms of cancer.

Theoretically, a Pap smear could be used to screen for vaginal cancer, but this would involve scraping all of the vaginal walls, which would be impractical since the surface area of the vagina is much greater than that of the cervix. Scrapings are taken of the vaginal wall when there is an abnormality on the vagina that can be seen with a naked eye or with a colposcope. These more extensive smears, which are sometimes called four-quadrant Pap smears, are also used in the follow-up of DES daughters.

Scrapings from the vaginal wall may also be used to evaluate the estrogen content of cells and to tell whether or not a woman has ovulated. This may be useful in fertility work-ups.

Pap smears may also reveal the presence of vaginal or cervical infections. Evidence of sexually transmitted diseases may also be an incidental finding in a Pap test report; however, the Pap is not used for diagnosing these, as other, simpler, more accurate tests are available.

PELVIC EXAM

AKA: gynecological exam, or checkup, bimanual pelvic

Associated Terms: bimanual vaginal exam, rectovaginal exam, digital rectal exam, speculum exam.

Pelvic exams are not most women's idea of a good time, but if you know what is happening and what to expect, the process becomes a lot more bearable—and perhaps even interesting. Pelvic exams should be done at least once a year, starting at the age of 16 or 18 or the onset of sexual activity, whichever comes first. They consist of three parts: the speculum exam, the bimanual pelvic and the rectal exam. (Incidentally, the doctor cannot tell whether or not you are a virgin, although s/he may be able to tell if you've had a child or an abortion.) You will be asked to lie on the examining table with your feet up in stirrups (Illustration 70).

Speculum Exam

Speculum self-exam has been explained in detail in Chapter Two. The process is essentially the same when the doctor does it. If you are tense, the exam may feel uncomfortable, but if you are relaxed and the doctor is skilled at it, you shouldn't feel any discomfort unless you have an infection or disease, in which case the vagina may be irritated and tender. The doctor will be looking for any obvious abnormalities or signs of infection. Once the speculum is in place, s/he may use a cotton-tipped applicator or a wooden spatula to take cell samples for a wet smear, a gonorrhea culture or a Pap smear.

Bimanual Pelvic

The doctor inserts two gloved fingers into the vagina and places the fingers of the other hand on the lower abdomen as shown in Illustration 70, in order to feel for enlargements or abnormalities in the shape and contour of the pelvic organs. If you are tense, your muscles will be rigid, which makes it hard for the doctor to feel for abnormalities, so try to relax. You might ask the doctor to place your hand on your abdomen and help you feel the outline of your uterus.

Rectovaginal Exam

The doctor inserts the index finger into the vagina and the middle finger into the rectum. The fingers of the opposite hand are placed on the lower

Illustration 70   *Bi-Manual Pelvic Exam (A) and Rectovaginal Exam (B)*

abdomen to help outline the organs and any enlargements or masses that may be present. This exam allows the doctor to feel areas not accessible by bimanual vaginal exam. Again, you will be more comfortable and the doctor's job will be that much easier if you can relax.

PREGNANCY TESTS

Types: urine tests
blood tests
progesterone-challenge, or progesterone-withdrawal, tests

Most women first become aware of pregnancy because their menstrual period does not begin on time; however, pregnant women may have menstrual-type bleeding, and missed periods are not necessarily an indication of pregnancy. Certain other signs may suggest pregnancy, including: breast swelling and tenderness, nausea and vomiting, frequent urination, slightly increased body temperature, weight gain, unusual food cravings, mood swings and possibly an increase in sex drive. Women who practice self-exam may notice a bluish tinge or hue to the cervix that may appear as early as a few days following conception, but this sign is not obvious in all women. The doctor may be able to feel an enlarged uterus once the pregnancy has progressed to a certain point. But none of these signs or symptoms is entirely reliable. The only reliable tests to detect pregnancy measure levels of the pregnancy hormone, human chorionic gonadotropin, or HCG, for short.

Urine tests: Urine tests are the most widely used pregnancy tests. They are not, however, completely accurate. The tests may give false negative results, that is, they may indicate that you are not pregnant even though you really are. False negative results may be caused by faulty technique in performing the test, urine that is too dilute or has been allowed to sit at room temperature for too long, an ectopic pregnancy or a threatened or incomplete miscarriage. If the urine tests are given too early in the course of the pregnancy (before six weeks from the first day of your last menstrual period) or too late (after five months), there may be false negative results. False positive results, that is, results indicating that a woman is pregnant when she really isn't, may be caused by faulty technique, blood or protein in the urine sample, chemical residue in the urine container, thyroid disorders, large doses of aspirin and the use of marijuana, methadone, certain anticonvulsant drugs, psychoactive drugs such as tranquilizers and antidepressants, drugs used to treat Parkinson's disease and some drugs used to treat hypertension. A test performed within ten days of a miscarriage, abortion or childbirth may give false positive results since levels of HCG may remain high for a period of time following pregnancy. The urine of menopausal women contains high levels of luteinizing hormone, as does the urine of women in their reproductive years for a period of 24 hours around the time of ovulation each month, so these women, too, may have false positive results.

Urine tests are more likely to be accurate if the test is made on the first urine of the morning, when the concentration of HCG is highest.

There are two types of urine tests: the two-minute urine slide test and the two-hour tube test. The urine slide test is the most widely used pregnancy test and is 95 percent accurate if used 42 days, or six weeks, after the first day of your last menstrual period (that is, once your period is about two weeks late). One drawback to this test is the fact that you may have already been pregnant for six weeks by the time this test confirms the pregnancy.

The two-hour urine tube test can be accurate once your period is one to one and a half weeks late. Many of the do-it-yourself pregnancy test kits now on the market are tube tests. No one should rely on these home tests, and if you do use one, make sure it measures HCG and not estrogen or progesterone levels, which are not very accurate indicators of pregnancy.

Blood tests: New, highly sensitive blood tests can give accurate results within about a week after conception, that is, about a week before your period is due. The original blood tests, called radioimmune assays, were very expensive lab tests, but a newer blood test called a radioreceptor assay, or a Bio-Cept G Test, is less expensive, about $15-$20, and 97-98 percent accurate eight to ten days after conception. It is 100 percent accurate if you wait until four weeks from the first day of your last menstrual period or within about one day of your missed period. The test is not available everywhere but can usually be obtained at large hospital labs. It is often used in women who have diabetes, hypertension, heart disease, kidney disease or other health problems that can adversely affect pregnancy.

Progesterone-challenge, or progesterone-withdrawal, test: Progestins are given either orally or by injection if a woman's period is late. As the progestin is gradually excreted by the body, the uterine lining will break down and be shed. If, however, you are pregnant, your period will not begin. This test does not stop pregnancy; it merely indicates whether or not pregnancy has occurred. In fact, it is not even a reliable indicator of that, for failure to bleed following this test may be caused by conditions other than pregnancy. Given the availability of other, more reliable tests,

757

we can hardly recommend this procedure for pregnancy testing. Women who do not plan to have an abortion if they discover that they are pregnant should definitely not take this test, for the use of hormones in early pregnancy has been linked to birth defects.[12]

BASIC BLOOD AND URINE TESTS

AKA: complete blood counts (CBC), serum factors test (SMA 12), urinalysis

Blood Tests

These blood tests, which are also called complete blood counts (CBCs) and serum factor tests (SMA 12s), can usualy be done in the doctor's office or lab. Blood is taken from a vein with a needle, and a pinprick is also made on the finger and the blood from there smeared on a slide as well. The blood samples are then subjected to various laboratory analyses. These tests can yield much basic information about your health, including whether or not you are anemic and if there is an infection present. They also can tell the doctor what your clotting time is, which is especially important if you are going to have surgery. The blood tests currently in use cannot indicate whether or not you have cancer, but experimental work is now being done in an effort to devise blood tests that could do so.

Urine Tests

Urinalysis (UA) can also provide a great deal of information. The urine sample is usually collected by simply having you void into a cup. At other times in order to collect the urine the doctor will need to insert a tube called a catheter through the urethra and into the bladder. Urinalysis can detect urinary-tract infection, diabetes, kidney damage and urinary obstruction. It can be especially valuable in staging certain forms of gynecological cancer since it can help the doctor to determine whether or not the cancer has spread to kidneys, ureters, bladder and so forth.

ANESTHESIA

Types: general anesthesia
local anesthesia

Associated terms: regional anesthetics; spinal, saddle, epidural or caudal block; paracervical block

Anesthetics are drugs used to prevent pain during surgery. Basically there are two types of anesthesia, local and general. General anesthetics put you to sleep or completely block the nerve passageways in large areas of the body (regional anesthetic). Local anesthetics temporarily numb a small area of the body so that you feel little or no pain.

General Anesthetics

General anesthetics are used for operations such as hysterectomy or laparoscopy. A light anesthetic or a deeper one may be used, depending on the nature of the surgery. The drug may be administered intravenously, by means of a needle that is usually attached to a tube and a hanging bottle called an IV bottle. A drug called sodium pentothal is frequently given in this way. A mask may be placed over your face and a mixture of anesthetic gas and oxygen may be administered through a tube attached to the mask. Sometimes sodium pentothal is given first, and once you are out the gas mask is applied. In any case, once you are asleep, a tube may be inserted into your windpipe to allow the doctor to control your respiration.

Regional anesthetics are used in childbirth, for D&Cs and for other relatively minor procedures. Terms such as "spinal," "saddle," "epidural" and "caudal block" may be used to specify the various types of regionals. Basically, all regionals involve injection of a drug into the space surrounding the spinal column or the area around a major nerve. The drug blocks nerve messages from the area and causes numbness and temporary paralysis. Since only the area to be operated on is affected, you will not be asleep if a regional is used; however, you may not be fully alert, since a sedative is often given prior to surgery so that you will not be anxious or feel discomfort.

Most people recover from general anesthesia fairly rapidly, within a period of several hours. It takes about 24 hours before the drugs are fully excreted from the body. Overweight people may take longer to recover since the drugs are absorbed by fat tissue. The mortality (death) rate for women who are given anesthetics is about 2.7 per 10,000 operations.[13] Serious problems like stroke and stopping of the heart or lung activity are

759

rare in young, healthy women but are higher for women with such medical problems as heart or lung disease. The longer the anesthesia time, the greater the chances of serious complications. Other complications, including headaches, which may persist for days or even weeks, can occur, especially with a spinal. In rare cases injury to or infection of the spinal cord can cause permanent paralysis. Both during and after anesthesia, blood pressure and heart rate must be carefully monitored so that drugs or other measures can be used if problems occur.

Local Anesthetics

Local anesthetics are used for minor operations that are short and technically simple. A drug similar to the novocaine used by dentists is injected into the area and is usually effective for a half-hour to an hour. When the drug is injected into the area around the cervix, the term "paracervical block" is used.

Although locals are less risky than generals, there may be allergic reactions including rashes, hives, swelling and asthma symptoms. On rare occasions allergic reactions are so severe that they cause seizures, strokes, heart attacks and death.

ANTIBIOTICS

Types: penicillin
tetracycline
erythromycin
sulfa drugs

Antibiotics are drugs that act against bacteria. They are used in the treatment of infections of the gynecological tract, including vaginitis and sexually transmitted diseases. Antibiotics can kill disease-causing organisms but may also destroy the friendly bacteria that help maintain the body's health. Women taking antibiotics may be more susceptible to vaginal infections, particularly yeast infections, and may want to take certain precautions (*see* p. 274).

Types

There are four major families of antibiotics: penicillin, tetracycline, erythromycin and sulfa drugs.

Penicillin: This widely used antibiotic can cause serious allergic reactions, but fortunately these are rather rare (1.5-2 per 100,000 users).[14] If you have an allergic reaction, discontinue use and contact the doctor immediately. If you have a reaction to one penicillin drug, you may be allergic to all drugs in this family and should not use any of them.

Ampicillin is a member of the penicillin family, so if you have had a reaction to penicillin, do not use ampicillin. You should also avoid ampicillin if you are using birth control pills since the drug may diminish the effectiveness of the pills. Diarrhea, which with other antibiotics may be a sign of a serious allergic reaction, is a fairly common side effect with ampicillin. Yeast infections are a common complication.

Tetracycline: Tetracycline may be prescribed for gynecological infections, particularly for women allergic to penicillin. Tetracycline should be avoided by pregnant women, infants and preteens since it can cause permanent tooth discoloration and, sometimes, bone abnormalities in the fetus. Yeast infections and gastrointestinal upsets may also occur, as can skin rashes if you're not careful to avoid prolonged exposure to sunlight (sunbathing). Food, particularly dairy products, may interfere with the absorption of the drug, so it shoud be taken one to two hours prior to eating and should not be taken with milk.

Erythromycin: This drug is used for people who are allergic to penicillin but cannot take tetracycline. The side effects are relatively few, but safe usage in pregnancy has not been determined.

Sulfa drugs: Sulfa drugs are often used in cream form to treat vaginal infections. Safe use of these drugs during pregnancy has not been established, and since abnormalities in the offspring of laboratory animals treated with those drugs have been noted, they are not recommended for pregnant women. People with a certain hereditary form of anemia that occurs mostly in black people should not use sulfa drugs.

Preparations containing one sulfa drug, sulfonamide, are still widely used to treat vaginitis, but their effectiveness has been seriously questioned. The FDA rates them as only "probably effective in the treatment of trich, hemophilus and yeast infections."[15] There are other, more effective medications for treating these conditions, and women should question their doctors about the choice of drugs if a sulfonamide is prescribed.

DEPO-PROVERA

AKA: the birth control shot, injectable Provera

Depo-Provera is a progestin, a synthetic (man-made) form of pro-gesterone, the hormone produced during the second half of the menstrual cycle. The drug comes in an oral form (Provera) and in an injectable form, which is Depo-Provera. While the use of Provera carries certain risks—the same risks associated with the use of any progestin compound—it is the drug in its injectable form that has been the center of a great deal of controversy.

Originally, the drug was developed as a treatment for endometriosis, threatened miscarriage and repeated miscarriage. It was approved by the FDA (Food and Drug Administration) for these uses in 1960 on the basis of its supposed safety but without an assessment of effectiveness.[16] In 1974 the FDA withdrew its approval, both because the drug had not been shown to be effective and because it had been shown to cause birth defects in children of women who took it while pregnant.[17] In 1972 the FDA approved the drug for use in the treatment of advanced cancer of the endometrial lining. Currently, this is the only approved use of the drug.

Depo-Provera has several effects on the body, including:

☐ Inhibiting ovulation in many women
☐ Increasing the thickness of cervical mucus, so that sperm cannot pass into the uterus
☐ Speeding up the time that the egg spends in Fallopian tubes, making fertilization less likely
☐ Changing the endometrial lining of the uterus, so that a fertilized egg cannot implant

These effects suggested that Depo-Provera might be used as a contraceptive. Studies of Depo-Provera as a "birth-control shot" given once every three months were begun in 1963.[18] In 1967, Upjohn, the company that manufactures the drug, applied for permission to market the drug as a contraceptive.

Permission was denied because of problems with the drug. Some of the women injected with the drug have menstrual irregularities and may even stop menstruating altogether.[19] Even after use is discontinued some women do not regain their periods for quite some time. Fertility may be impaired, perhaps permanently. Those women who do manage to conceive while on the drug, or who take it without realizing they are pregnant, may unknowingly damage their babies, since the drug is transmitted through breast milk and its effects on infants are unknown. In addition, some statistics suggest, but do not prove, that cervical carcinoma in situ, an early stage of cervical cancer, may occur more often among Depo-Provera users than among nonusers.[20] Beagle dogs treated with both low doses and high doses developed diseases of the endometrial lining of the uterus and malignant breast lumps.[21] The significance of these findings for humans has not been established.

Although the drug is not approved as a contraceptive, some family-planning clinics and private physicians are prescribing the drug for this purpose. In addition, the drug is being given to women in Third World countries despite the fact that Upjohn is restricted from marketing the drug in this country. Many health-care activists are working to prevent its use on Third World women. In addition, the National Women's Health Network has established a registry to investigate the use of the drug in this country. Women who received contraceptives by injection can register by writing to Depo-Provera Registry, National Women's Health Network, 2025 I Street NW, Washington, D.C. 20006.

ESTROGEN REPLACEMENT THERAPY

AKA: ERT

Estrogen replacement therapy (ERT) as the name implies involves the administration of estrogen to replace estrogen that for one reason or another is no longer being made by the body.

Uses

ERT is used most widely in menopausal and postmenopausal women, who may no longer be producing large amounts of estrogen in their bodies. It is also given to women who have premature menopause, insufficient amounts of pituitary hormones or congenital abnormalities of the ovary, all of which prevent them from producing the normal ovarian hormones.

ERT is a dangerously misused form of therapy. It first became popular in the late 50s and early 60s as a cure for a wide variety of menopausal symptoms and changes that women of this age are apt to experience. Actually, the only menopausal symptoms on which ERT has any effect are hot flashes and the drying and thinning of vaginal, vulvar and urinary tissues that occur in postmenopausal women as estrogen levels decline. Its effectiveness in treating osteoporosis, a condition that involves loss of bone density and increases a woman's chances of bone fractures, has been hotly debated. As the result of a clever and well-financed advertising campaign, many women and doctors came to believe that ERT was a sort of magic cure-all that would prevent wrinkles, weight gain and psychological problems and that would keep women "forever young." The stereotyped image of the menopausal woman as an emotionally unstable harpy and the insecurities caused by our youth-worshipping culture made it possible to convince millions of women to use this drug even if they didn't have any of the problems for which it is in fact useful.

Although some studies have indicated that menopausal women have a slightly higher percentage of serious emotional problems—a 7 percent incidence as compared to 6 percent for other age groups[22]—and a somewhat higher rate of complaints about nervousness, irritability, "feeling blue" and other symptoms of psychological tension,[23] there is no evidence that lack of estrogen per se causes these symptoms or that taking ERT will relieve them.

Still, many women feel that estrogen relieves their depression. This erroneous impression is the result of several factors.[24] First of all, many ERT products also contain antidepressants, tranquilizers or sedatives. It is these added drugs and not the estrogen that have the psychological effects. Secondly, depression is often self-limiting, which means that it goes away by itself in time. Women suffering from depression who started ERT and found that their depression lifted may mistakenly attribute the relief of their symptoms to the estrogen.

A third reason that women may attribute relief of psychological problems to ERT has to do with hot flashes. Some women have frequent and severe flashes during the night, which causes insomnia. Not surprisingly, these are the women who are most likely to complain of irritability, nervousness and so forth. ERT may eliminate or reduce the flashes, which in turn solves the insomnia and psychological tensions, but it is the reduction of hot flashes, not the estrogen per se, that is responsible for relief of tensions. ERT should not be taken for psychological problems.

ERT is also supposed to prevent skin wrinkling, weight gain and other effects of aging. There is no evidence that any of these conditions are caused by lack of estrogen or that they can be relieved by use of estrogen. In fact, there is some evidence that estrogen can cause drying and wrinkling of the skin.[25]

ERT *is* effective in preventing hot flashes, but once the estrogen is discontinued the hot flashes may come back and may be more severe. Using estrogen may merely delay the occurrence of hot flashes rather than prevent or cure them. Hot flashes normally don't continue for more than a year. There are also alternative treatments that don't involve the serious risks that ERT does. Some doctors have been experimenting with progesterone, clonidine (Catapres) and propanolal (Indral).[26] Vitamin therapy has proven successful for some women.[27] Vitamins E and C and the B-complex vitamins seem to be particularly helpful. Ginseng, an oriental herb, is also effective for some women.[28] These herbal and vitamin therapies seem to take four to six weeks to become effective. We suggest that women investigate these alternative therapies. ERT should not be used unless the flashes are so severe that the sufferer is willing to risk developing cancer or the other problems associated with ERT. If ERT is used, it should be taken in the lowest possible effective dose and for the shortest possible time. Women who have premature menopause and are therefore likely to suffer more severe hot flashes due to the abrupt transition should also avoid ERT, but if it is absolutely necessary, they should taper the dose off gradually and should also use the smallest dose for the shortest amount of time.

Osteoporosis, a condition in which bone mass is lost, can apparently be prevented by ERT.[29] Osteoporosis can lead to fractures. Some women have fairly extensive osteoporosis without any apparent problems; others suffer greatly and are prone to multiple bone fractures. This can be serious in elderly women in whom hip fractures can have fatal complications.

Although ERT has been shown to prevent osteoporosis, it has not been proven that it actually reduces the number of fractures. Other factors like exercise and nutrition, in particular sufficient amounts of calcium, apparently play a role in osteoporosis, so it is not clear that estrogen alone, in the form of ERT, will prevent fractures. At this time ERT is rated "probably effective" for this purpose.[30]

There has been a great deal of controversy surrounding ERT and osteoporosis. Some doctors, those who feel that osteoporosis can indeed reduce the incidence of fractures, recommend small daily doses of ERT for their postmenopausal patients.[31] While they recognize that ERT increases the risk of endometrial cancer, they point out that such cancers are caught in the early stages when they are curable. Since osteoporosis can have fatal consequences, they feel the benefits of ERT in preventing osteoporosis outweigh the risks.

Other doctors are hesitant to prescribe ERT merely to prevent the possible development of osteoporosis. Even if they were certain that ERT would reduce the incidence of fractures, they are not convinced that the risks of developing cancer are outweighed by the possible benefits. (We tend to agree with the latter group.)

The question of osteoporosis and ERT is a difficult one. Large women, tall women and black women, who are less susceptible to osteoporosis and bone fracture, probably do not need preventative ERT. Women who are delicate and small boned and/or have a family history of osteoporosis or women who have a surgically-induced menopause are at higher risk and would be more likely to benefit from a program of preventative ERT. Such women may want to investigate some of the alternative preventative treatments for osteoporosis. One study showed that large amounts of calcium carbonate was effective in preventing osteoporosis.[32] Some doctors feel these large amounts are too toxic. Others feel that smaller amounts may be effective. (Certainly, a calcium supplement is a good idea for all postmenopausal women since their bodies don't use calcium as effectively.) Experiments with injections of calcitonan given three times a week have also proven effective.[33] A long-acting progestational agent given by injection once a month has likewise been studied and appears to be effective.[34]

At this time, it is impossible to clearly evaluate these alternatives or the risks and benefits of ERT for osteoporosis. Women should watch for developments in this area and should seek second opinions before accepting ERT treatment. ERT is also effective in treating conditions related to the thinning and drying out of vulvar, vaginal and urinary tissues. It may be used to treat postmenopausal vulvitis and vaginitis and vaginal stenosis, as well as cystoceles and rectoceles. The addition of estrogen will return these tissues to the premenopausal state, so that symptoms like leaking of urine, vaginal dryness, painful intercourse and vulvar itching may be relieved. The estrogen may be given orally or in the form of creams and lotions applied to the area. At first it was thought that the creams might not be as dangerous, but there is now evidence that the estrogen is absorbed into the bloodstream, so creams must also be considered risky, although the amount of estrogen absorbed by the body may be lower and therefore the creams may be preferable to oral therapy. Once again, given the risks of ERT, we suggest that women investigate the alternative forms of therapy for these condition, which are discussed under the headings Menopausal Problems, Postmenopausal Vulvitis, Postmenopausal Vaginitis and Cystoceles and Rectoceles, before considering ERT.

Younger women with certain rare congenital abnormalities of the ovary may also be given ERT to stimulate the development of secondary sex characteristics. Such women and their parents should discuss the risk and benefits with the doctor before using this form of therapy for the prolonged periods required. They should also use the lowest possible dose of estrogen. Sometimes when these young girls see the effect of estrogen on their breasts, they will decide to take extra pills, in hopes of developing larger breasts. Extra estrogen will not further increase their breast size, however, for that is determined by heredity. (It should also be noted that only in those rare instances of young girls whose bodies are not capable of producing estrogen does ERT have any effect on breast development. It will not have any permanent effect on the size of older women's breasts and cannot—and should not—be used, either orally or in the form of creams, for that purpose.)

Risks

The risks of ERT have not been fully studied. Most of our information about the risks of estrogen itself has come from studies of women using the birth control pill. It has not always been clear whether the risks associated with Pill use have been due to the progestins or to the estrogens in the Pill. Since ERT doesn't involve the use of progestins and because it involves higher doses of estrogen, the risks associated with the Pill may not be the same as those associated with ERT. Every woman considering ERT should, however, realize that the risks associated with the Pill (*see* p. 103) may also be associated with ERT. Moreover, there are some Pill-associated side effects and risks that studies have demonstrated are also associated with ERT. For example, there is a two-fold increase in the incidence of gall bladder disease requiring surgery among Pill users, and a recent study has confirmed a two- to three-fold increase for postmenopausal women using ERT.[35] Moreover, the use of oral contraceptives is associated with high blood pressure, which may have fatal consequences, and recent studies have shown that ERT can also increase blood pressure.[36] As further studies are done, further correlations between Pill effects, especially those known or suspected to be estrogen-related, and ERT may be discovered.

Just as there are Pill effects that may also turn out to be risks for ERT users, so there are ERT risks that may have implications for Pill users. Perhaps the most disturbing of the studies on ERT users are those linking ERT to endometrial cancer. Several studies have reported that postmenopausal women on ERT have a higher rate, anywhere from 4.5 to 13.9 times higher than nonusers. This means that about one woman out of every nine on ERT could expect to develop endometrial cancer.

ERT has also been associated with breast cancer. The association is by no means conclusive, but one study reported alarming findings.[37] In this study it was found that for the first five years, breast cancer incidence does not increase; it may even occur more frequently in women not taking hormones. But after five years the risks of ERT start increasing. Fifteen years after ERT use, the breast cancer incidence was double that of women who had never used it. Women who develop benign breast disease while on ERT seem to be especially susceptible to developing cancer. A particularly alarming aspect of this study was that although the dosage was related to increased incidence, the length of time the women took the drug was not. So, even taking ERT for a relatively short time may increase the incidence of breast cancer. It must be emphasized that this study involved only a small number of women. However, there are also studies of laboratory animals indicating that estrogen can induce tumors.[38] Caution must be used in applying the results of animal studies to women, for cancer is species-specific (is caused by different factors and behaves differently in different species). Also, large doses are often administered in animal studies. Still, we do know that 50-60 percent of all breast tumors are estrogen-sensitive and that estrogen may act as a fertilizer to stimulate the growth of existing breast tumors. While none of these facts "proves" that use of ERT increases a woman's chances of breast cancer, it is certainly a possibility that must be considered. And since this possibility exists, we can no longer assume that ERT is safe for women who have had their uteri removed and are therefore not at risk for endometrial cancer, as some ERT proponents have argued.

Contraindications

A contraindication is a condition that makes a form of therapy inadvisable. Since ERT risks have not been clearly defined, contraindications are a subject of some debate, but there are certain, absolute contraindications that everyone accepts, including:

- ☐ Current or past blood-clotting disorders
- ☐ Stroke
- ☐ Cardiovascular disease
- ☐ Undiagnosed abnormal vaginal bleeding
- ☐ Cancer of the breast, reproductive organs or skin
- ☐ Pregnancy

Most doctors would agree that the following are also contraindications:

- ☐ Impaired liver function
- ☐ High blood pressure
- ☐ Diabetes
- ☐ Fibrocystic disease or fibroadenoma of the breast
- ☐ Sickle cell disease
- ☐ High levels of factors called serum lipid levels
- ☐ Surgery planned in the next four weeks

Some doctors would also include the following contraindications, while others would prescribe ERT for such women. All would agree that if women with the following conditions take ERT, they must be monitored very closely.

- ☐ Fibroid tumors of the uterus
- ☐ Family history of diabetes
- ☐ Epilepsy
- ☐ Asthma
- ☐ Varicose veins

Since estrogens can interact with certain other medications, such as anticoagulants, insulin, promazine hydrochloride, meperidine hydrochloride and tuberculin skin tests, estrogen use may be modified or contraindicated if these are being used. Women on ERT should discuss this issue with their doctors.

Monitoring

Women on ERT therapy should be followed closely. Any vaginal bleeding, chest pain, difficulty in breathing, coughing, headaches, dizziness, faintness, leg pain, breast lumps, vision changes or yellowing of the skin should be reported to the doctor immediately. Should vaginal bleeding occur, a D&C is mandatory to rule out the possibility of cancer. Some doctors recommend that women on ERT have an endometrial biopsy prior to beginning treatment and that this procedure be repeated annually.

DES

AKA: diethylstilbestrol, stilbestrol

Diethylstilbestrol, or DES, for short, was the first man-made estrogen. Beginning in 1940, DES and similar drugs were given to pregnant women who had a history of premature birth, miscarriage, diabetes, hypertension or who showed signs of bleeding in the early stages of pregnancy. Upwards of a million women were given the drug, for it was thought that DES could help prevent miscarriage. DES was apparently also given to healthy women who had none of these problems.[39]

DES Effects

The tragic consequences of DES usage in pregnant women did not become apparent until 1970, when an alert physician, Dr. Arthur Herbst, and his colleagues reported seven cases of a rare form of vaginal cancer, clear cell adenocarcinoma, in women 15 to 22 years of age.[40] Until this time, there had only been three cases of this disease in women under the age of 35 reported in the entire world-wide medical literature. As the result of a careful investigation, the link between DES exposure and the cancers was established. This led to the creation of a world-wide tumor registry to which such cases could be reported. Thus far, over 400 cases have been reported.[41] The peak incidence seems to occur at about the age of 19, although DES-related cancer has been reported in girls as young as 7 and women as old as 29. Only a small proportion of DES daughters have actually developed vaginal cancer. Currently, it is estimated that about one out of 1,000 DES daughters will develop clear cell adenocarcinoma. Some doctors feel this estimate is too high; others feel that it is too low and fear that DES daughters are at higher risk for vaginal cancer and other types of cancer as well. For example, some researchers have reported a higher incidence, as much as a five-fold increase, of cervical dysplasia, a possible precursor to cervical cancer, in DES daughters.[42] They fear that as more women reach the age when cervical cancer is most common, 35-50 years of age, more cancer will be seen in DES daughters. Other experts do not believe that there is an increased risk for dysplasia in DES daughters. These issues are discussed more fully under the heading Vaginal Adenosis.

While only a small portion of DES daughters have developed vaginal cancer, a much higher number, as many as 90 percent in some studies, have a condition known as vaginal adenosis, in which the glandular-type tissue that normally lines the cervical canal is found growing on the vaginal surface of the cervix and on the walls of the vagina.[43] This abnormal tissue growth can be likened to growth of the tissue that is found inside the mouth and cheeks on the lips and face.

Until DES, vaginal adenosis was a rare condition. In most instances, it is not thought to have any serious consequences. However, the majority of DES daughters who have vaginal cancer also have had vaginal adenosis, and so it is feared that in a small number of women, adenosis may be a precursor to cancer.

In addition to cancer and adenosis, DES daughters may be more likely to have congenital abnormalities of the cervix, including a peculiarly shaped or strange-looking cervix, ridged cervical or vaginal tissues, a condition called incompetent cervix, in which the cervix dilates prematurely during pregnancy, causing miscarriage, and cervical eversion, a less extensive form of vaginal adenosis.[44] An unusual, T-shaped uterus has been found in the course of fertility work-ups in some DES daughters.[45] Studies comparing DES daughters to unexposed women of the same age group indicate that DES daughters may be more likely to have irregular or infrequent menstrual periods and a lower level of fertility.[46] There have not been any studies indicating that the children of DES daughters or DES sons will have any abnormalities. However, DES sons and daughters may have infertility problems, and DES daughters may have more difficulty in carrying a pregnancy to term.[47] Any DES daughter who becomes pregnant should let her doctor know that she is a DES daughter and should look for a doctor experienced in DES cases (see below).

DES sons have not been studied as extensively as DES daughters, so it is only recently that male problems have been identified. Because of the publicity surrounding DES daughters and vaginal cancer, DES sons seeking medical treatment are often quite worried about the possibility of developing cancer. Thus far, there have been no studies linking DES exposure in males to cancer. However, there are studies that indicate that DES sons may have a higher incidence of hypoplastic (small) testicles and undescended testicles, a condition in which one or, less frequently, both of the sperm-producing testicles fail to descend into the scrotal sac.[48] These two conditions also occur in males who have not been exposed to DES and may predispose such men to cancer of the testicle. Whether these conditions, when they occur in DES sons, may similarly predispose these men to testicular cancer is not known; however, it is suggested that DES sons practice monthly testicular self-examination to detect any lumps or abnormalities.

In addition to the abnormalities stated above, studies have indicated that as many as 40 percent of all DES sons have low sperm counts or abnormally shaped sperm cells.[49] It is not yet known how this will affect the fertility of such men. Moreover, DES sons have a higher incidence of testicular cysts and abnormal placements of the urinary opening. In addition to being examined for abnormalities, DES sons should keep in touch with their doctors and DES Action (see below) to keep abreast of new developments.

Sources and Uses of DES

DES and two similar synthetic estrogens, dienestrol and hexestrol, were the main drugs used. All of these drugs are referred to as DES, or DES-type drugs, and all are thought to have similar harmful effects. Table 27 lists some of the names under which DES and similar drugs have been sold.

DES was also given to cattle in this country to fatten them up before slaughter. This use of DES was the subject of a lengthy battle between drug companies, consumer groups and the Food and Drug Administration (FDA).[50] The drug was first approved for use in animal feed and as pellet implants in 1947. But in 1958, further tests showed that DES caused cancer in laboratory animals. In 1959, newly developed techniques to detect relatively low levels of residues of DES in the tissue of animals that had been given the hormones revealed that the amount of hormone left in poultry was too high, and the FDA withdrew approval of its use with poultry. More sensitive tests to detect DES residue in beef and lamb were developed later, and the use of DES on cows and sheep was banned in

Table 27
DES-Type Drugs That May Have Been Prescribed to Pregnant Women*

Nonsteroidal Estrogens

AVC cream with dienestrol	Estrobene	Pabestrol D.
Benzestrol	Estrobene (DP)	Palestrol
Chlorotrianisene	Estrosyn	Restrol
Comestrol	Fonatol	Stilbal
Cyren A.	Gynben	Stilbestrol
Cyren B.	Gynegen	Stilbestronate
Delvinal	H-Bestrol	Stilbetin
DES	Hexestrol	Stilbinol
DesPlex	Hexoestrol	Stilboestroform
Dibestil	Menocrin	Stilboestrol
Diestryl	Meprane	Stilboestrol (DP)
Dienestrol	Methallenestril	Stilestrate
Dienestrol cream	Microest	Stilpalmitate
Dienoestrol	Mikarol	Stilphostrol
Diethylstilbenediol	Mikarol forti	Stil-Rol
Diethylstilbestrol Dipalmitate	Milestrol	Stilronate
	Monomestrol	Stilrone
Diethylstilbestrol Diphosphate	Neo-Oestranol I	Stils
	Neo-Oestranol II	Synestrin
Diethylstilbestrol Dipropionate	Nulabort	Synestrol
	Oestrogenine	Synthoestrin
Digestil	Oestromenin	Tace
Domestrol	Oestromon	Vallestril
Estilben	Orestol	Willestrol

Nonsteroidal Estrogen — Androgen Combinations

Amperone	Teserene
Di-Erone	Tylandril
Estan	Tylosterone
Metystil	

Nonsteroidal Estrogen — Progesterone Combination

Progravidium

*SOURCE: This listing is adapted from the US Department of Health, Education and Welfare's *Information for Physicians: DES Exposure in Utero*, Publication No. (NIH) 76-1119, pp. 10−11.

November of 1979. However, anyone who included meat in their diet prior to that time may have been exposed to DES.

DES is also used as a method of birth control, as described under the heading Morning-After Pill. Some doctors still prescribe DES to dry up a woman's milk after childbirth if she does not plan to breastfeed.

Determining DES Exposure

Any woman who became pregnant between the years 1941 and 1971* should consider the possibility of DES exposure. Women who had a previous history of miscarriage, premature birth, hypertension, toxemia during pregnancy or diabetes or who had bleeding problems during their pregnancies are more likely to have received this drug. However, even apparently healthy women were given this drug, sometimes without their consent. Some women were apparently told that it was "just a vitamin pill."[51]

Those born during these years should ask their mothers if they remember taking any drug during pregnancy. DES was usually given as a pill but may have been given as a shot. Even small doses of the drug, given for only a few days, have been associated with subsequent cancer. Understandably, a mother may not recall if she took anything, especially if a number of years have passed, the medication was given for only a few days or she was told that it was just a vitamin pill. Anyone born during the period from 1941 to 1971 should talk with his or her mother about a previous medical history or any complications with pregnancy that may have made her a likely candidate for DES therapy.

Another way to find out about DES exposure is by checking with the doctor or hospital involved. Unfortunately, it may be impossible to get such records since they may not have been kept properly or may have been destroyed. Additional difficulty arises from the fact that the medical profession, perhaps from fear of legal problems, has been, by and large, uncooperative about informing DES-exposed women. Details about how to obtain medical records are discussed in Chapter Six.

Medical Care and Follow-Up of DES Daughters

If there is any reason for a woman to think she may have been exposed, she should go to a doctor or clinic experienced in DES screening. It is important to find experienced doctors, for inexperienced ones may not know how to do the proper tests, may miss important signs or may mistreat or dismiss the condition. Table 28 lists DES centers sponsored by the National Cancer Institute that can provide information on proper DES follow-up. Table 29 lists DES Action groups, consumers' groups that can direct women to doctors or clinics experienced in DES exposure.

Females with known or suspected DES exposure should have the diagnostic exam if they have started their first period, if they are 14 years

---

*Some say 1975, since despite the FDA's 1971 recommendation that DES not be given to pregnant women, some doctors continued to do so.

Table 28
DESAD Project Centers and Project Directors

Dr. Duane E. Townsend
DESAD Project
California Hospital Medical Center
1414 South Hope Street
Los Angeles, California 90015
(213) 747-5666

Dr. Robert Bowser
Director, DESAD Project
Division of Cancer Control and
  Rehabilitation
National Cancer Institute
Blair Building
8300 Colesville Road
Silver Spring, Maryland 20910
(301) 427-4477

Dr. Ann Barnes and Dr. Stanley J. Robboy
DESAD Project

Massachusetts General Hospital
32 Fruit Street
Boston, Massachusetts 02114
(617) 726-2780

Dr. David G. Decker
DESAD Project
Mayo Clinic
Rochester, Minnesota 55901
(507) 284-3288

Dr. Raymond H. Kaufman
DESAD Project
Baylor College of Medicine
1200 Moursand Avenue
Houston, Texas
(713) 790-4405

of age or older or if, at any age, they show any unusual vaginal discharge or irregular bleeding. A few experts feel that even younger females known to have been exposed should be examined, since girls as young as seven years of age have developed associated cancer. Some of these doctors have developed special techniques for examining young girls whose vaginal canals may be too small to allow for insertion of the speculum used for diagnosis. A general anesthetic has been used by some doctors, but, of course, general anesthesia involves risks of its own. Most doctors, pointing to the fact that 90 percent of the exposed daughters who developed cancer were 14 years or older, feel that age 14 is young enough. It is true that it is highly unlikely that a girl under the age of 14 would develop this cancer. Anyone who decides to have a young daughter examined (and if symptoms like excessive vaginal discharge or abnormal vaginal bleeding appear, she *must* be examined, regardless of age) should read the section on psychological aspects below. Even girls 14 years of age may have vaginal canals too small for comfortable examination. Many doctors suggest that they use tampons for a few months prior to examination.

DES changes may not show up in the routine pelvic exam and Pap smear. Special techniques that are quick and usually involve little discomfort are required. First, the doctor will do a very careful examination of the vagina by palpating (feeling) the cervix and vagina for rough, sandy

Table 29
DES Action Groups

DES Action National
Long Island Jewish — Hillside
  Medical Center
New Hyde Park, New York 1104
(516) 775-3450

Regional Offices:
DES Action/Massachusetts
P. O. Box 117
Brookline, Massachusetts 0214

DES Action/New York
Long Island Jewish — Hillside
  Medical Center
New Hyde Park, New York 1104
(516) 775-3450

DES Action/Northern Californi
16388 Haight Street
San Francisco, California 94117
(415) 621-8032

DES Action/Oregon
P. O. Box 12092
Portland, Oregon 97212
(503) 282-8868

DES Action/Pennsylvania
Pennsylvania Women's Center
Houston Hall
University of Pennsylvania
Philadelphia, Pennsylvania 19104

DES Action/Sacramento
707 45th Street
Sacramento, California 95819

DES Action/Washington
P. O. Box 5311
Rockville, Maryland 20851
(301) 468-2170

DES Action/Michigan
9146 Greensboro
Detroit, Michigan 48224

DES Action/Connecticut
P. O. Box 49
Mansfield Depot, Connecticut 06251

DES Action/Florida
9586 Portside Drive
Seminole, Florida 33542

or nodular areas. A careful speculum exam of the vaginal walls and cervix to detect red areas or physical abnormalities is also done. The exam should also include the special Pap smear known as a four-sided (quadrant) Pap test, in which the vaginal walls as well as the cervix are lightly scraped for cell samples, which should be sent to a lab for analysis by a pathologist familiar with DES-type changes. The walls of the vagina and the cervix are then painted with a special iodine stain (called Schiller's, or Lugol's, stain) that turns the normal tissue a dark brown color. Abnormal tissue will not absorb the stain. If there are areas that do not stain, they must be biopsied. The biopsy, which involves cutting away a bit of the suspicious tissue, does not cause too much pain since there are few nerve endings in the upper vagina but it may cause some bleeding. The tissue samples are then studied in the lab to eliminate the possibility of cancer.

A special magnifying instrument called a colposcope that allows the doctor to see changes not visible to the naked eye can also be used in diagnosing DES daughters. Colposcopic exam is a simple, safe office procedure; however, there is some controversy about the use of colposcopy to detect DES changes.

There is no doubt that the colposcope is a valuable tool when used by a trained and skilled doctor. The problem lies in interpretation of what is seen. Many private doctors, although they own or have access to colposcopes, may not see enough DES patients to be able to correctly interpret what they see. Another problem is that colposcopes are relatively expensive. A doctor, especially one who sees relatively few DES cases or other conditions requiring a colposcope, may have to charge quite a bit to recover his or her investment in equipment and training. The cost of a colposcopic exam may run as high as $100. Not all insurance plans completely cover these costs. Then, too, colposcopes are not always available, especially to women who live in rural areas without easy access to medical facilities.

Medical opinion as to the role colposcopy should play in DES follow-up is divided. Some doctors feel that the special Pap smear, palpation and visual inspection, staining and, if necessary, biopsy are sufficient. Some feel that if the staining indicates abnormality, colposcopy, which will make the biopsy more accurate, should then be done, but that unless abnormalities are revealed by staining, colposcopic examination is unnecessary. Others feel the initial exam of a DES daughter should be done with a colposcope, but if there are no abnormalities, it should not be required in follow-up. Some of the doctors who express these viewpoints feel that more extensive use of the colposcope is just to make money for the doctor. Still other doctors feel that a colposcope exam should be done on an annual (or even biannual) basis, with careful charts or photos being kept to follow the progress of the disease, since little is known about it. Recently, one doctor reported a case of cancer in a woman who had shown no abnormality during two years of routine examination.[52] This doctor felt that without colposcopic examination this woman's cancer would not have been detected as early as it was.

It will probably be some time before the proper role of colposcopic examination of DES women can be determined. Until more research is done, the decision about colposcopy lies with the consumer — the daughter or her parents. Availability (either financial or geographic) and age (the incidence of clear cell adenocarcinoma seems to drop dramatically after the age of 22, although other types of cancer, as noted earlier, may occur later) may influence this decision.

Furthermore, as more information is compiled about uterine abnormalities in DES daughters, hysterograms, special X-ray studies of the uterus, or sonograms, pictures of internal organs taken by means of high-frequency sound waves, may also become part of the medical evaluation.

Here again, women can keep abreast of the latest development through DES Action (see below).

After the initial examination, follow-up exams in which all or some of the procedures done in the initial exam are repeated, are scheduled every three or six months, depending on whether any abnormalities, such as vaginal adenosis, are found and on their extent. If no abnormalities are found, many doctors recommend follow-up exams once a year.

DES Women and the Pill

Many DES daughters and mothers have questions about the advisability of using birth control pills. Medical opinion on this issue is divided. Some doctors point out there is no evidence to date that these women should avoid the Pill or that Pill risks for DES women are higher than they are for other women. Some doctors even use the Pill to treat the menstrual irregularities that may occur in DES daughters. Other doctors feel strongly that DES women should not be given birth control pills or estrogen replacement therapy. They point out that little is known about the long-term effects of the Pill or DES. Adding another hormone to an already complex hormonal situation may have serious effects. We feel that other forms of birth control are preferable for DES mothers and daughters. Indeed, some doctors feel that the diaphragm or spermicidal foams may actually improve DES-related conditions.

Psychological Aspects

One important but often ignored aspect of DES exposure is the psychological impact it may have on both mothers and children. DES mothers are likely to be fearful about the effects on their own health and on their children's health. They may be angry with the medical profession and may also feel terribly guilty. Children may be fearful and angry both at the mother and the medical profession.

The need for a DES exam may come at a time in a young girl's life when she is feeling self-conscious about her genitals. Having a gynecological examination can be a physically and emotionally uncomfortable procedure for a woman of any age and may be especially difficult for a young girl, particularly if she is having her first exam because of possible DES exposure. The fear that some abnormality, perhaps even cancer, might be found makes the situation even more frightening.

Some DES centers have psychological counseling available, and women should take advantage of this if it is offered. DES Action (see below) has local groups across the country where women can receive support and advice from other DES mothers and daughters who have faced these problems. Some DES clinics and doctors use videotapes and mirrors so that parents and daughters can actually see what the inside of the vagina looks like. DES-type changes don't as a rule produce the striking abnormalities that some people imagine, so actually "taking a look" can be reassuring. We suggest that DES mothers practice self-exam and, once they are comfortable with the procedure, include their daughters in the process. Young girls who watch their mothers practice speculum exam are more likely to be comfortable with the procedure.

Legal Aspects

Individual DES mothers and daughters have filed lawsuits against drug manufacturers and against their doctors.[53] There have been some legal difficulties with these suits revolving around problems in identifying exactly which company manufactured the DES pills any given woman may have taken (since there were so many manufacturers) and around the fact that, at the time most DES was given, the use of DES was acceptable medical practice and thus not an instance of medical malpractice. However, one lawsuit in New York filed by a DES daughter who developed cancer resulted in a $500,000 award against Eli Lilly Co., as representative of all manufacturers of the drug.

Class-action suits aimed at trying to get the drug companies or the government to pay for the medical care and follow-up of DES daughters have also been filed. For more legal information, contact DES Action (see below) or the National Women's Health Network, 2025 I Street, NW, Washington, D.C. 20006.

DES Action

DES Action is a national organization of DES-exposed women and of health-care activitists and medical personnel. It has chapters throughout the country. It is available to help people with questions and concerns about DES. DES Action teaches doctors and nurses about DES, encourages needed medical research, sponsors legislation mandating public information campaigns and the establishment of DES screening clinics and provides referrals and emotional support for those exposed to DES. They have training materials available and information on how to set up a local group. In addition, they publish a quarterly newsletter *DES Action Voice*, which keeps people up to date on medical and legal developments and other news of interest to anyone concerned about DES exposure. To find out more about DES Action groups or to subscribe to their excellent newsletter (yearly subscription, four issues, costs $15), contact them at the locations listed in Table 29.

FERTILITY DRUGS

Types: estrogen
human chorionic gonadotropin, or HGC
clomiphene citrate, or Clomid
human menopausal gonadotropin, HMG, or Pergonal

Throughout history humankind has been looking for magic brews—love potions, youth elixirs and fertility concoctions. Thus far, we haven't had much luck with the first two, but we now have drugs that can help an infertile woman become pregnant. Although they can't help every woman, they are often effective for women who are unable to conceive because they are not ovulating. Women who are not ovulating regularly are said to have anovulatory cycles. These women may also have a variety of menstrual irregularities, including abnormal uterine bleeding, no menstrual periods (a condition known as amenorrhea) or irregular periods. Certain fertility drugs may be used to treat women who have a luteal phase defect, a condition in which the corpus luteum regresses too soon, depriving the fertilized egg of the necessary support of the rich uterine lining.

Since use of these drugs involves some risk, a woman should first have a complete fertility work-up (*see* p. 630) to make sure that her infertility is actually due to failure to ovulate and not to some other problem. If a woman with an infertility problem also has amenorrhea, she should similarly have a complete diagnostic work-up (*see* p. 592) to determine that her amenorrhea is due to failure to ovulate and that it and her particular infertility problem are of the type that will be responsive to fertility drugs. Moreover, women using these drugs must be monitored carefully for side effects and for the return of ovulation. Frequent pelvic exams must be done. The woman will be asked to keep a basal body temperature chart (BBT). (*see* p. 163) because once she ovulates, her temperature will rise, due to the progesterone that is produced following ovulation. However, a BBT is not always entirely accurate; a vaginal smear can also be used to detect ovulation, as can an endometrial biopsy, but the latter should not be used on a woman who might be pregnant. Urine and

779

blood tests to measure hormone levels may be necessary in some cases. Pregnancy tests (*see* p. 756) of the most sensitive type must be done before a course of therapy is repeated, because some fertility drugs may be dangerous to a developing fetus and should be discontinued as soon as a woman becomes pregnant.

Estrogen

If the woman's vaginal smear or endometrial biopsy indicates a lack of estrogen, then some doctors will prescribe small amounts of this hormone.[54] Too much estrogen may prevent ovulation, so only small amounts are given orally. Premarin, an estrogen taken from the urine of pregnant horses, may be prescribed on days 6 through 15 of the menstrual cycle. If this doesn't cause ovulation, the treatment may be repeated the next month and perhaps again the third month. If ovulation does occur, the woman continues treatment each month, timing intercourse so that it occurs just before or during the expected time of ovulation.

Many doctors are hesitant to use estrogen as a fertility drug. First of all, they find that it is rarely effective, especially in women with amenorrhea. Moreover, they are concerned about the possibility that a woman might ovulate and conceive while taking the estrogen. If, for instance, the woman ovulated on Day 10 or 12, she could still be taking estrogen when conception took place. Or, should a woman get pregnant and still have what appears to be a menstrual period, as occasionally happens, the doctor might inadvertently prescribe another round of estrogen. We know that certain synthetic estrogens, like DES, taken during pregnancy have resulted in a rare form of vaginal cancer in some of the daughters, as well as other abnormalities in both the sons and daughters of the women who took them.[55] Whether Premarin would have similar tragic consequences is not known. However, no one wants to find out the hard way, as we did with DES; so the woman must be given pregnancy tests of the most sensitive type before each course of estrogen.

HCG

Some doctors use HCG, human chorionic gonadotropin, a hormone that is normally produced by the placenta within a few days of conception. HCG behaves very much like luteinizing hormone, which is the pituitary hormone whose midcycle surge triggers ovulation. A high-dose injection of HCG, which is obtained from the urine of pregnant women, is given at midcycle. If this does not produce ovulation, then a higher-dose injection may be tried the following month. If this is not effective, a third course of treatment may be prescribed.

Many doctors are reluctant to use this form of treatment, for they feel that HCG by itself is rarely effective. Instead, they may use HCG in combination with Clomid or with the more powerful Pergonal (see below).

Clomid

Clomiphene citrate, sold under the brand name Clomid, is also used to treat infertility. The drug is similar in structure to a synthetic estrogen but has only a few weak estrogen effects. It works on the hypothalamus, which in turn stimulates the pituitary to produce luteinizing hormone (LH) and follicle-stimulating hormone (FSH). These hormones cause an egg in the ovary to ripen and to be released at the time of ovulation. Clomid is used, then, in cases where the pituitary gland is normal and capable of producing its hormones but the hypothalamus is not functioning properly. It is frequently used to treat women with Stein-Leventhal disease of the ovaries.

The drug is given on days 5 through 10 of the menstrual cycle. (The period may have to be induced by using progesterone if the woman also has amenorrhea.) It is then continued for five days. Most women will ovulate within the next several days. If the woman's basal body temperature chart does not indicate that she has ovulated, treatment may be attempted again the following month, using higher doses of Clomid. Most women are started with doses of 50-100 mg a day in successive months. Some doctors will use higher doses, but this is controversial.[56] Some doctors feel that if laparoscopic examination has not been done as part of the diagnostic work-up, the woman should have one before 200-mg doses are used. Also, it is recommended that women who have Stein-Leventhal disease not receive more than 600 mg of Clomid a month, for they may already have elevated levels of one of these hormones.

HCG may be used in combination with Clomid. It is generally given after Clomid therapy, to trigger ovulation. Estrogen may also be given if the cervical mucus of the woman taking Clomid does not seem to be the proper consistency to allow the sperm to penetrate the cervix, but it should be given only in the early days of the cycle, prior to ovulation, to eliminate the possibility of its being taken after the woman becomes pregnant.

The most serious complication with Clomid therapy is the formation of multiple ovarian cysts that may rupture and then lead to destruction of the ovary or even death. About 10 percent of the women using Clomid will have twins, but other multiple births (triplets, etc.) are rare.[57] There may be hot flashes, abdominal pain, soreness, bloating, breast tenderness, nausea, vomiting, headaches and vision problems including blurring, spots and flashes. These symptoms should be reported to the doctor. If vision problems occur, the medication should be discontinued and the doctor called immediately. Most of these side effects can be prevented if the woman is started on low doses and followed carefully.

Women should be monitored carefully before each course of Clomid to rule out the possibility of pregnancy and the formation of multiple cysts. Careful pelvic exams and the most sensitive pregnancy tests should be done. Pregnancies conceived after Clomid treatment have not shown an increased incidence of birth defects. However, pregnancies conceived during treatment may have problems. There is no direct evidence that Clomid taken during pregnancy can cause abnormalities in humans, but studies have shown that doses given in early pregnancy can cause birth defects in laboratory animals.[58] Because Clomid is similar in its chemical structure to DES, a synthetic hormone that caused birth defects in the children of the women who took it, most medical personnel are extremely careful to rule out the possibility of pregnancy before giving a second course of the drug. Furthermore, Clomid has been in wide use for only 15 years, and, as with DES, it could be that possible carcinogenic effects will begin to show only after 15 years or more.

Because of these considerations and the fact that Clomid has caused precancerous conditions in the reproductive tract of the mother rats[59] as well as in the offspring exposed during pregnancy, in our opinion a doctor should administer Clomid only to a woman who wants to become pregnant. The doctor who gives it should be experienced in its use and know how to monitor the woman carefully.

About 70 percent of the women treated will actually ovulate, and of these, about 40 percent will become pregnant.[60] If a woman is going to ovulate with Clomid, she will usually do so within the first three courses of treatment. Most women who ovulate with Clomid will continue to do so with each repeated course. In some cases, the response will be erratic. If Clomid is unsuccessful, Pergonal may be used.

Pergonal

Pergonal is used to treat infertility in women who have some sort of problem in the pituitary gland that is preventing the pituitary from producing LH and FSH, but pituitary tumors must first be ruled out. It is also used to treat women who have failed to respond to Clomid. A very expensive drug, Pergonal is extracted from the urine of postmenopausal women, and is known as HMB, human menopausal gonadotropin. The urine of these women contains high levels of LH and FSH. Since Pergonal involves greater risks than Clomid, Clomid may be used along with Pergonal so that lower doses of Pergonal can be used. HCG may also be used in combination with Pergonal to trigger ovulation. The major complications with Pergonal therapy, due to possible overstimulation of the ovary by the drug, are multiple ovulations, the formation of multiple cysts on the ovary and subsequent multiple pregnancies.[61] These complications have lead to death through rupture of the cysts or rupture of the uterus during pregnancy. In less severe cases, the rupture of the cysts may still necessitate surgery to remove the ovary. Even where the overstimulation of the ovary by Pergonal doesn't cause these drastic complications, a woman must still be hospitalized and monitored carefully.

About 50 percent of the women given Pergonal treatment will actually ovulate.[62] About half of these will get pregnant and about one-fourth of these will have multiple births, usually twins. About 10 percent of the women will develop enlarged cystic ovaries. The severe complications occur in about 1 percent of the women using this drug; if the doctor administering the drug is inexperienced, however, the complication rate may be higher.

A woman being treated with Pergonal must be monitored carefully with daily tests to measure the amount of estrogen in the blood, and frequent pelvic exams must be done to make sure that more than one egg follicle isn't forming. If more than one follicle forms and the estrogen levels rise too high, treatment must be discontinued for that month and the HCG must not be given. Withholding the HCG will usually prevent ovulation.

The trick is in knowing when to stop the Pergonal and when to give the HCG. If too little Pergonal is given and the HCG is given too early, the woman won't ovulate. If too much Pergonal is given, the woman may face serious complications. For this reason, it is important that women use Pergonal only under the guidance of an expert who is experienced in the use of this drug. The best place to find such a specialist is through your gynecologist or a fertility clinic connected with a large university hospital or medical center.

Notes

Chapter One: HOW THIS BOOK CAME TO BE WRITTEN

1. Nancy Friday, *My Mother, My Self* (New York: Dell, 1977), p. 141.
2. Friday, p. 141.
3. Friday, p. 141.
4. National Center for Health Statistics, "Surgical Operations, Short-Stay Hospitals, U.S.," *Vital Health Statistics*, Series 13, no. 21, Washington DC, 1976.
5. Based on a mortality rate of 0.2 percent.
6. Frank J. Dyck et al., "Effects of Surveillance on the Numbers of Hysterectomies in the Province of Saskatchewan," *New England Journal of Medicine* 296 (1977), pp. 1326–28. Note: The actual rates quoted in this study range from 17 to 59 percent. We have used an average figure of 30–40 percent, which is the figure generally quoted in the literature and by consumer groups.

Chapter Three: BREAST SELF-EXAM

1. P. Greenwald, M.D., et al., "Estimated Effect of Breast Self-Examination on Breast Cancer Mortality," *New England Journal of Medicine* 299 (1978), pp. 271–73.
2. American Cancer Society, *Facts and Figures* (New York: ACS, 1975).

Chapter Four: THE MONTHLY MIRACLE: MENSTRUATION

1. Nancy Friday, *My Mother, My Self* (New York: Dell, 1977) Note: Friday is quoting here from a book review by Anatole Broyard that appeared in the *New York Times* on Sept. 21, 1976.

2. Barbara Seaman and Gideon Seaman, M.D., *Women and the Crisis in Sex Hormones* (New York: Rawson Assoc., Inc., 1977), p. 298.

3. There are a number of case-control studies that report increased risk for endometrial cancer in women using menopausal estrogens. The three most widely cited studies are:

H. K. Ziel and W. D. Finkle, "Increased Risk of Endometrial Carcinoma Among Users of Conjugated Estrogens," *New England Journal of Medicine* 293 (1975), pp. 1167—70;

D. C. Smith et al., "Association of Exogenous Estrogen and Endometrial Carcinoma," *New England Journal of Medicine* 293 (1975), pp. 1164—67; and

T. M. Mack et al., "Estrogens and Endometrial Cancer in a Retirement Community," *New England Journal of Medicine* 294 (1976), pp. 1262—67.

These findings are further supported by the fact that incidence rates of endometrial cancer have increased sharply since 1969, which may be related to the rapidly expanding use of estrogens in the last decade.

4. M. K. McClintock, "Menstrual Syncrony and Suppression," *Nature* 299 (1971), pp. 244—45.

5. James Hassett, "Sex and Smell," *Psychology Today* (March 1978), pp. 40—45.

6. T. A. Holding and K. Minkoff, "Parasuicide and the Menstrual Cycle," *Journal of Psychosomatic Research* 17(5—6), (Dec. 1973), pp. 365—68.

Chapter Five: BIRTH CONTROL: THE STATISTICAL LIE

1. "Sequential Pills Being Withdrawn," *New York Times*, Feb. 26, 1976.

2. There are a number of case-control studies that report increased risk for endometrial cancer in women using menopausal estrogens. The three most widely cited studies are:

H. K. Ziel and W. D. Finkle, "Increased Risk of Endometrial Carcinoma Among Users of Conjugated Estrogens," *New England Journal of Medicine* 293 (1975), pp. 1167—70;

D. C. Smith et al., "Association of Exogenous Estrogen and Endometrial Carcinoma," *New England Journal of Medicine* 293 (1975), pp. 1164—67; and

T. M. Mack et al., "Estrogens and Endometrial Cancer in a Retirement Community," *New England Journal of Medicine* 294 (1976), pp. 1262—67.

These findings are further suppported by the fact that incidence rates of endometrial cancer have increased sharply since 1969, which may be related to the rapidly expanding use of estrogens in the last decade. See the FDA-approved package insert for all products containing estrogens for more details.

3. A. L. Herbst, H. Ulfedler and D. C. Poskanzer, "Adenocarcinoma of the Vagina," *New England Journal of Medicine* 284 (1971), pp. 878—81;

P. Greenwood et al, "Vaginal Cancer After Maternal Treatment With Synthetic Estrogens," *New England Journal of Medicine* 285 (1971), pp. 390—92.

4. A number of different abnormalities have been found in DES daughters, including alterations in the shape of the cervix, vaginal adenosis, lowered fertility and irregular menstrual periods. DES sons have been reported as having testicle cysts, underdeveloped or undescended testes, abnormally placed urinary openings, low sperm counts, abnormally shaped sperm cells and impaired fertility. For further information see:

R. Mattingly and A. Stafl, "Cancer Risk in DES-Exposed Offspring," *Journal of Obstetrics and Gynecology* 128 (1977), pp. 43—50; R. Kaufman et al., "Upper Genital Tract Changes Associated With Exposure in Utero to Diethylstilbestrol," *Journal of Obstetrics and Gynecology* 128 (1977), pp. 51—59.

M. Bibbo et al., "Follow-up Study of Male and Female Offspring of DES-Exposed Mothers," *Obstetrics and Gynecology* 49:1 (1977), pp. 1—8.

5. US Dept. of Health, Education and Welfare, Food and Drug Administration, "DES and Breast Cancer," *FDA Drug Bulletin* 8 (March-April 1978), p. 2.

6. Mattingly and Stafl, pp. 43—50.

7. Ward Rinehart and Judy C. Felt, "Debate on Oral Contraceptives and Neoplasia

Continues; Answers Remain Elusive," *Population Reports*, Series A, no. 4 (May 1977), p. A-80.

8. Elizabeth Stern et al., "Steroid Contraceptive Use and Cervical Dysplasia: Increase in the Risk of Progression," *Science* 196 (1977), p. 1460.

9. Several studies have looked for, but failed to find, a link between use of birth control pills and breast cancer, including:

Boston Collaborative Drug Surveillance Program, "Oral Contraceptive Use and Venous Thromboembolic Disease, Surgically Confirmed Gallbladder Disease and Breast Tumors," *Lancet* 1 (1973), pp. 1399—404;

M. P. Vessey, R. Dall and P. M. Sutton, "Oral Contraceptives and Breast Neoplasia: A Retrospective Study," *British Medical Journal* 3 (1972), pp. 719—24; and

F. G. Arthes, P. E. Sartwell and E. F. Lewison, "The Pill, Estrogens and the Breast: Epidemiologic Aspects," *Cancer* 28 (1971), pp. 1391—94.

10. Several studies have reported this finding, including:

Boston Collaborative Drug Surveillance Program, pp. 1399—404;

Vessey, Dall and Sutton, pp. 719—24; and

E. Fasal and R. S. Paffenbarger, "Oral Contraceptives as Related to Cancer and Benign Lesions of the Breast," *Journal of the National Cancer Institute* 55 (1975), pp. 767—73.

11. Fasal and Paffenbarger, pp. 767—73.

12. R. Hoover et al., "Menopausal Estrogens and Cancer," *New England Journal of Medicine* 295 (1976), pp. 401—5.

13. FDA-approved package insert included with all estrogen products.

14. V. J. Wynn, J. W. H. Doar and G. L. Mills, "Some Effects of Oral Contraceptives on Serum Lipid and Lipoprotein Levels," *Lancet* 2 (1966), pp. 720—23.

15. W. N. Spellacy, "Metabolic Effects of Oral Contraceptives," *Clinical Obstetrics and Gynecology* 17 (March 1974), pp. 53—63.

16. A. M. Shojania, "Effect of Oral Contraceptives on Vitamin B_{12} Metabolism," *Lancet* 2 (1971), p. 932;

A. S. Prasad et al., "Effect of Oral Contraceptive Agents on Nutriments: II, Vitamins," *American Journal of Clinical Nutrition* 28 (1975), pp. 385—91;

M. K. Horwitt, C. C. Harvey and C. H. Dahm, "Relationship Between Levels of Blood Lipids, Vitamins C, A and E, Serum Copper Compound and Urinary Excretions of Tryptophan Metabolites in Women Taking Oral Contraceptive Therapy," *American Journal of Clinical Nutrition* 28 (1975), pp. 403—12.

17. FDA-approved package insert included with all estrogen products.

18. C. J. Levinson and D. C. Richardson, "The Dalkon Shield Story," *Advances in Planned Parenthood* 11:2 (1976), pp. 53—63.

19. P. T. Piotrow et al., "IUD's Update on Safety, Effectiveness and Research," *Population Reports*, Series B, no. 3 (May 1979), p. B-57 (table).

20. US Dept. of Health, Education and Welfare, "IUD Safety: Report of a Nationwide Physician Survey," *Morbidity and Mortality* 23 (1974), pp. 226—31.

21. J. Balog et al., "Recent Trend in Preference of Contraceptive Methods—Pills Down, Diaphragm on Rise," *Obstetrics and Gynecology Survey* 33:4 (April 1978), pp. 282—83.

22. T. J. Trussell, R. Faden and R. A. Hatcher, "Efficacy and Information in Contraceptive Counseling: Those Little White Lies," *American Journal of Public Health* 66 (1976), pp. 761—67.

23. Robert Hatcher et al., *Contraceptive Technology, 1978—1979,* 9th rev. ed. (New York: Irvington Pub., Inc., 1978), p. 20 (table).

24. G. Carpenter and J. Martin, "Clinical Evaluation of a Contraceptive Foam," *Advances in Planned Parenthood* (New York: Excerpta Medical Foundation, 1970), p. 170—78.

25. US Dept. of Health, Education and Welfare, *Contraception: Comparing the Options,* HEW Publication no. (FDA) 78,3069.

26. G. W. Beebe, *Contraception and Fertility in the Southern Appalachians* (Baltimore: Williams and Wilkins, 1974), p. 274.

27. Hatcher et al., p. 26 (table)

28. L. J. Latz and E. Reiner, "Failures in Natural Contraception Control and their Causes," *Illinois Medical Journal* 71 (March 1937), pp. 210—16.

29. Elizabeth B. Connell, M.D., "Contraception," *Current Therapy, 1973* (Philadelphia: W. B. Saunders, 1973), p. 813.

30. US House Select Committee on Population, "Domestic Consequences of United States Population Change," Report to the 95th Congress, Second Session Serial E (Washington, DC: US Govt. Printing Office, Dec. 1978), p. 16 (table).

31. Barbara Seaman and Gideon Seaman, M.D., *Women and the Crisis in Sex Hormones* (New York: Rawson Assoc., Inc., 1977), p. 202. Note: The authors are quoting from a personal communication with Drs. Howard and Joy Osofsky, authorities on abortion and birth control.

32. Ward Rinehart and Phyllis Piotrow, "OC's—Update on Usage, Safety and Side Effects," *Population Reports*, Series A, no. 5 (Jan. 1979), p. A-137 (table).

33. Seaman and Seaman, p. 14.

34. Seaman and Seaman, p. 14.

35. Planned Parenthood Federation of America, Medical Committee, *Methods of Birth Control in the United States* (New York: Planned Parenthood Federation of America, 1972), p. 41.

36. Personal communication with Dr. Robert Goeppe.

37. Personal communication with Dr. Milos Chapvil and Dr. James Heine.

38. Robert A. Hatcher et al., p. 126.

39. Judith Wortman, "Vasectomy: What are the Problems?" *Population Reports*, Series D, no. 2 (Jan. 1975), p. D—31.

40. J. R. Neil et al., "Late Complications of Sterilization by Laparoscopy and Tubal Ligation," *Lancet* 1 (Oct. 11, 1975), p. 699.

Reference Section: BIRTH CONTROL METHODS

Note to readers: Most of the facts about birth control pills in the text are taken from the FDA-approved package insert that comes with each package of pills and that includes complete reference citations. These facts are given in the text without any specific references. In cases where we have included information that is not from the package insert, we provide specific citations.

1. Ward Rinehart, "Minipill—A Limited Alternative for Certain Women," *Population Reports*, Series A, no. 3 (Sept. 1975), p. A-56.

2. Robert A. Hatcher et al., *Contraceptive Technology, 1978—1979,* 9th rev. ed. (New York: Irvington Pub., Inc., 1978), p. 20 (table).

3. Elizabeth B. Connell, M.D., "Contraception," *Current Therapy, 1973* (Philadelphia: W. B. Saunders, 1973), p. 813.

4. M. P. Vessey, et al., "A Long-Term Follow-up Study of Women Using Different Methods of Contraception: An Interim Report," *Journal of Biosocial Science* 8 (Oct. 1976), pp. 375—427.

5. Royal College of General Practitioners, *Oral Contraceptives and Health: An Interim Report* (London: Pitman, 1974).

6. K. J. Rothman and C. Louick, "Oral Contraceptives and Birth Defects," *New England Journal of Medicine* 299 (Sept. 7, 1978), pp. 522—24.

7. Royal College of General Practitioners, "The Outcome of Pregnancy in Former Oral Contraceptive Users," *British Journal of Obstetrics and Gynecology* 83 (Aug. 1976), pp. 608—16.

8. Vessey, et al., pp. 375—427.

9. M. P. Vessey, et al., "Fertility After Stopping Different Methods of Contraception," *British Medical Journal* 1 (Feb. 4, 1978), pp. 265—67.

10. B. M. Sherman et al., "Pathogenesis of Prolactin-Secreting Pituitary Adenomas," *Lancet* 2 (1978), pp. 1019—21.

11. A. M. Shojania, "Effect of Oral Contraceptives on Vitamin B_{12} Metabolism," *Lancet* 2 (1971), p. 932.

12. A. S. Prasad et al., "Effect of Oral Contraceptive Agents on Nutrients: II, Vitamins," *American Journal of Clinical Nutrition* 28 (1975), pp. 385—91.

13. M. K. Horwitt, C. C. Harvey and C. H. Dahm, "Relationship Between Levels of Blood

Lipids, Vitamins C, A and E, Serum Copper Compound and Urinary Excretions of Tryptophan Metabolites in Women Taking Oral Contraceptive Therapy," *American Journal of Clinical Nutrition* 28 (1975), pp. 403—12.

14. V. Beral, S. Ramcharan and R. Faris, "Malignant Melanoma and Oral Contraceptive Use Among Women in California," *British Journal of Cancer* 36 (Dec. 1977), p. 804—9.

15. Elizabeth Stern et al., "Steroid Contraceptive Use and Cervical Dysplasia: Increase in the Risk of Progression," *Science* 196 (1977), p. 1460.

16. R. Hoover et al., "Menopausal Estrogens and Cancer," *New England Journal of Medicine* 295 (1976), pp. 401—5.

17. US Dept. of Health, Education and Welfare, Food and Drug Administration, "DES and Breast Cancer," *FDA Drug Bulletin* 8 (March-April 1978), p. 2.

18. E. Fasal and R. S. Paffenbarger, "Oral Contraceptives as Related to Cancer and Benign Lesions of the Breast," *Journal of the National Cancer Institute* 55 (March 1975), pp. 767—73.

19. C. J. Levinson and D. C. Richardson, "The Dalkon Shield Story," *Advances in Planned Parenthood* 11:2 (1976), pp. 53—63.

20. M. Dowie and M. Johnson, "A Case of Corporate Malpractice," *Mother Jones*, Nov. 1976, p. 36.

21. US Dept. of Health, Education and Welfare, Food and Drug Administration, 'Progestasert IUD and Ectopic Pregnancy," *FDA Drug Bulletin* 8 (Dec. 1978—Jan. 1979), p. 37.

22. J. Jennings, "Report of the Safety and Efficacy of the Dalkon Shield and Other IUDs," FDA Ad Hoc Obstetric—Gynecology Advisory Committee, Oct. 1974.

23. US Dept. of Health, Education and Welfare, Food and Drug Administration, Medical Device and Drug Advisory Committee on Obstetrics and Gynecology, *Second Report on Intrauterine Contraceptive Devices* (Washington, DC: Govt. Printing Office, Dec. 1978), p. 102.

24. P. T. Piotrow et al., "IUDs—Update on Safety, Effectiveness and Research," *Population Reports*, Series B, no. 3 (May 1979), p. B-57 (table).

25. US Dept. of Health Education and Welfare, *Second Report . . .*, p. 102.

26. US Dept. of Health, Education and Welfare, Center for Disease Control, "IUD Safety: Report of a Nationwide Physician Survey," *Morbidity and Mortality Weekly Report* 23 (July 5, 1974), pp. 226—31.

27. Piotrow et al., pp. B-57 (table) and B-64.

28. Piotrow et al., pp. B-64—67.

29. Piotrow et al., p. B-65.

30. Piotrow et al., p. B-68 (table).

31. C. Tietze and S. Lewit, "Evaluation of Intrauterine Devices: Ninth Progress Report of the Cooperative Statistical Program," *Studies in Family Planning* 55 (July, 1970), pp. 1—40.

32. Piotrow et al., pp. B-57 (table) and B-62.

33. Piotrow et al., p. B-62.

34. Piotrow et al., p. B-62.

35. Piotrow et al., p. B-62.

36. Tietze and Lewit, pp. 1—40.

37. Tietze and Lewit, pp. 1—40.

38. Piotrow et al, p. B-70 (table).

39. Piotrow et al., pp. B-70—72.

40. US Dept. of Health, Education and Welfare, "Progestasert . . .," p. 37.

41. H. J. Tatum et al., "Management and Outcome of Pregnancies Associated With the Copper-T Intrauterine Contraceptive Device," *American Journal of Obstetrics and Gynecology* 126 (Dec. 1, 1976), pp. 869—79.

42. Jennings, p. 19.

43. W. Cates et al., "The Intrauterine Device and Deaths From Spontaneous Abortion," *New England Journal of Medicine* 295 (Nov. 18, 1976), pp. 1155—59.

44. Piotrow et al., p. B-69.

45. G. T. Alvior, Jr., "Pregnancy Outcome with Removal of the Intrauterine Device," *Obstetrics and Gynecology* 41:6 (June 1973), pp. 894—96.

46. R. M. Shine and J. F. Thompson, "The In Situ IUD and Pregnancy Outcome," *American Journal of Obstetrics and Gynecology* 119:1 (May 1, 1974), pp. 124—30.

47. J. F. Permutter, "Pregnancy and the IUD," *Journal of Reproductive Medicine* 20:3 (March 1978), pp. 133—37.

48. H. Barrie, "Congenital Malformation Associated with Intrauterine Contraceptive Device," *British Medical Journal* 1 (1976), pp. 488–90.

49. Tatum et al., pp. 869–79.

50. Tietze and Lewit, pp. 1–40, and S. J. Segal and C. Tietze, "Contraceptive Technology: Current and Prospective Methods," *Reports on Population/Family Planning*, no. 1 (July 1971), pp. 1–24.

51. M. P. Vessey, et al., "Fertility . . .," pp. 265–67.

52. A. K. Jain and B. Moots, "Fecundability Following the Discontinuation of IUD Use Among Taiwanese Women," *Journal of Biosocial Science* 9(2) (1977), pp. 135–51.

53. V. E. Johnson and W. H. Masters, "Intravaginal Contraceptive Study, Phase II: Physiology," *Western Journal of Surgery, Obstetrics and Gynecology* 71 (May-June 1963), pp. 144–53.

54. US Dept. of Health, Education and Welfare, Food and Drug Administration, "Comparing the Options," HEW Publication no. (FDA) 78–3069.

55. M. Vessey and P. Wiggins, "Use-Effectiveness of the Diaphragm in a Selected Family-Planning Clinic Population in the United Kingdom," *Contraception* 9:1 (Jan. 1974), pp. 15–21.

56. M. Lane, R. Arleo and A. J. Soberero, "Successful Use of the Diaphragm and Jelly by a Young Population: Report of a Clinical Study," *Family Planning Perspectives* 8:2 (1976), pp. 81–86.

57. Lane, Arleo and Soberero, pp. 81–86.

58. D. W. Beacham and W. D. Beacham, *Synopsis of Gynecology* (St. Louis: C. V. Mosby, 1972), pp. 351–66.

59. M. R. Melamed et al., "Prevalence Rates of Uterine Cervical Carcinoma in Situ for Women Using the Diaphragm or Contraceptive Steroids," *British Medical Journal* 3 (1969), pp. 195–200; and

N. H. Wright et al., "Neoplasia and Dysplasia of the Cervix Uteri and Contraception: A Possible Protective Effect of the Diaphragm," *British Journal of Cancer* 38:2 (August 1978), pp. 273–79.

60. "Seven Year Prospective Study of 17,000 Women Using the Pill, IUD and Diaphragm," *Family Planning Perspectives* 8:5 (1976), pp. 241–48.

61. B. Singh et al., "Studies on the Development of a Vaginal Preparation Providing Both Prophylaxis Against Venereal Disease and Other Genital Infections and Contraception II: Effect in Vitro of Vaginal Contraceptive and Noncontraceptive Preparations on Treponema Pallidum and Neisseria gonorrhoeae," *British Journal of Venereal Diseases* 48 (1972), pp. 51–64.

62. Masters and Johnson, pp. 144–53.

63. Masters and Johnson, pp. 144–53.

64. Hatcher et al.; see addendum in front of book.

65. M. E. Panragua, "Field Trial of a Contraceptive Foam in Puerto Rico," *Journal of the American Medical Association* 177 (1961), p. 125.

66. G. Carpenter and J. Martin, "Clinical Evaluation of a Contraceptive Foam," *Advances in Planned Parenthood* (New York: Excerpta Medical Foundation, 1970), pp. 170–78.

67. Seaman and Seaman, p. 202. Note: The authors are quoting from a personal communication with Drs. Howard and Joy Osofsky.

68. G. S. Bernstein, "Clinical Effectiveness of an Aerosol Contraceptive Foam," *Contraception* 3 (1971), pp. 37–43.

69. B. Vaughan et al., "Contraceptive Failure Among Married Women in the United States, 1970–73," *Family Planning Perspectives* 9:6 (Nov.-Dec. 1977), pp. 251–58.

70. N. B. Ryder, "Contraceptive Failure in the United States," *Family Planning Perspectives* 5 (1973), pp. 133–42.

71. S. Coleman and P. Piotrow, "Spermicides—Simplicity and Safety Are Major Assets," *Population Reports*, Series H, no. 5 (Sept. 1979), p. H-95 (table).

72. Singh et al., pp. 57–64.

73. B. Postic et al., "Inactivation of Clinical Isolites of Herpes Virus hominis, Types 1 and 2, by Chemical Contraceptives," *Sexually Transmitted Diseases* 5 (Jan.-Mar. 1978), pp. 22–24.

74. G. W. Beebe, *Contraception and Fertility in the Southern Appalachians* (Baltimore: Williams and Wilkins, 1974), p. 274.

75. J. Peel, "A Male-Oriented Fertility-Control Experiment," *Practitioner* 202 (1969), pp. 677−81.

76. M. Potts and J. McDevitt, "A Use-Effectiveness Trial of Spermicidally Lubricated Condoms" *Contraception* 11:6 (1975), pp. 701−10.

77. US Supreme Court, Decision of June 6, 1977.

78. Press release, Young Drug Products Corporation, Oct. 5, 1978.

79. D. Barlow, "The Condom and Gonorrhea," *Lancet* 2:8042 (Oct. 15, 1977), pp. 811−13.

80. "Condom Sales Rise in Sweden, VD Falls," *Obstetrics and Gynecology News* 8:15 (August 1, 1973), p. 9.

81. Planned Parenthood Federation of America, Medical Committee, *Methods of Birth Control in the United States* (New York: Planned Parenthood Federation of America, 1972), p. 41.

82. C. Tietze et al., "The Effectiveness of the Cervical Cap as a Contraceptive Method," *American Journal of Obstetrics and Gynecology* 66 (1953), pp. 904−8.

83. Renee Potick, "Informed Consent," patient handout on the cervical cap.

84. Clara Ross and P. T. Piotrow, "Birth Control Without Contraceptives," *Population Reports*, Series I, no. 1 (June 1974), p. I-11 (table).

85. Ross and Piotrow, p. I-12.

86. Ross and Piotrow, p. I-33.

87. Piet H. Jongbloet and Johanna H. J. Van Erkelens-Zwets, "Rhythm Methods: Are There Risks to Progeny," in *Controversies in Fertility Control* ed. J. Sciarra, G. Zatuchni and J. Speidel (New York: Harper and Row, 1978) p. 520−33.

88. Lois Bradshaw, "Vasectomy Reversibility: A Status Report," *Population Reports*, Series D, no. 3 (May 1976), p. D-49 (table).

89. Bradshaw, p. D-159.

90. Judith Wortman, "Vasectomy: What Are the Problems?" *Population Reports*, Series D, no. 2, (Jan. 1975), p. D-32.

91. Wortman, p. D-31.

92. Wortman, p. D-27.

93. Wortman, p. D-27.

94. Wortman, p. D-25.

95. Wortman, p. D-31, and Hatcher et al., p. 132.

96. Wortman, p. D-33. 97.

97. Seaman and Seaman, p. 229. Note: The authors are quoting from an article written by Judith Herman, M.D., entitled "Controlling Third World Populations: Forced Sterilization," which appeared in *Sister Courage*, Feb. 1976. Similar statistics are found in literature from the Committee to End Sterilization Abuse, P.O. Box A 244−Cooper Station, NY, NY 10003.

98. Seaman and Seaman, p. 229. Note: The authors are quoting from an article sponsored by the Fund for Investigative Journalism that was written by Claudia Dreifus entitled "Sterilizing the Poor," which appeared in *The Progressive* 39:13−18, 1975.

99. Seaman and Seaman, p. 234.

100. Hatcher et al., p. 20 (table).

101. Alice M. Rothchild, M.D., testimony given at public hearings on proposed HEW Sterilization Regulations, Jan. 17, 1978.

102. R. Roe et al., "Female Sterilization: 1. Vaginal Approach," *American Journal of Obstetrics and Gynecology* 112 (1972), pp. 1031−36.

103. J. Philips et al., "Laparoscopic Procedures: A National Survey for 1975," *Journal of Reproductive Medicine* 18 (1977), pp. 219−26.

104. J. R. Neil et al., "Late Complications of Sterilization by Laparoscopy and Tubal Ligation," *Lancet* 1 (Oct. 11, 1975), p. 699.

105. Supreme Court of the United States, *June Roe et al., Appelants, v. Henry Wade*, Jan. 22, 1973.

106. National Women's Health Network, *Abortion* (Washington, DC: NWHN, 1980), p. 8.

107. Supreme Court of the United States, *Planned Parenthood of Missouri* v. *Danforth*, July 1, 1976.

108. D.T. Liu et al., "Dilation of the Parous Non-Pregnant Cervix," *British Journal of Obstetrics and Gynecology* 82 (1975), p. 246.

109. Emiline Royco Ott, "Cervical Dilation—A Review," *Population Reports*, Series F, no. 6 (Sept. 1977), p. F-92.

110. B. N. Nathanson, "Ambulatory Abortion: Experience with 26,000 Cases," *New England Journal of Medicine* 286 (1972), pp. 403—7.

111. Hatcher et al., p. 119.

112. Center for Disease Control, *Abortion Surveillance 1976*, HEW Publication no. (CDC) 78-8205, 1978.

113. Ott, p. F-94.

114. Susan L. Chaudry, "Pregnancy Termination in Midtrimester—A Review of the Major Methods," *Population Reports*, Series F, no. 5 (Sept. 1976), p. F-69.

115. Chaudry, pp. F-69—70.

116. Chaudry, pp. F-72—74.

117. Chaudry, pp. F-77—79.

118. Chaudry, pp. F-76.

119. Y. Moriyama and O. Hirokawa, "The Relationship Between Artificial Termination of Pregnancy and Abortion of Premature Birth," *Harmful Effects of Induced Abortion*, The Family Planning Federation of Japan, 1966, and L. H. Roht and H. Aoyama, "Induced Abortions and Its Sequels: Prematurity and Spontaneous Abortion," *American Journal of Obstetrics and Gynecology* 120, 1974, pp. 868—74.

120. Hatcher et al., p. 103.

121. Hatcher et al., p. 103.

122. Ward Rinehart, "Postcoital Contraception—An Appraisal," *Population Reports*, Series J, no. 9, Jan. 1976, p. J-147.

123. Rinehart, p. J-147.

124. Rinehart, p. J-144.

125. Seaman and Seaman, p. 42.

126. Rinehart, p. J-150.

Chapter Six: DEALING WITH DOCTORS

1. This bill was signed into law in November 1979. Copies are available from the State House Bookstore, Commonwealth of Massachusetts, Boston, Massachusetts 02133.

2. See Chapter One, notes 4 and 6.

THE VULVA

1. J. R. Willson, C. T. Beacham and E. R. Carrington, *Obstetrics and Gynecology*, 4th ed. (St. Louis: C. V. Mosby Company, 1971), p. 544.

2. There are a number of case-control studies that report increased risk for endometrial cancer in women using estrogen replacement therapy. The three most widely cited studies are:

H. K. Ziel and W. D. Finkle, "Increased Risk of Endometrial Carcinoma Among Users of Conjugated Estrogens," *New England Journal of Medicine* 293 (1975), pp. 1167—70;

D. C. Smith et al., "Association of Exogenous Estrogen and Endometrial Carcinoma," *New England Journal of Medicine* 293 (1975), pp. 1164—67; and

T. M. Mack et al., "Estrogens and Endometrial Cancer in a Retirement Community," *New England Journal of Medicine* 294 (1976), pp. 1262—67.

These findings are further supported by the fact that incidence rates of endometrial cancer have increased sharply since 1969, which may be related to the rapidly expanding use of estrogens in the last decade. See the FDA-approved package insert for all products containing estrogens for more details.

In addition, one study has indicated that women who used estrogen replacement therapy may be at increased risk for the development of breast cancer; see:

R. Hoover et al., "Menopausal Estrogens and Cancer," *New England Journal of Medicine* 295 (1976), pp. 401—5.

3. Raymond H. Kaufman, "The Management of Benign and Malignant Vulvar Lesions," *Audio-Digest, Obstetrics and Gynecology*, 23:18 (Sept. 14, 1976).
4. Kaufman, *Audio-Digest*.
5. Kaufman, *Audio-Digest*.
6. Personal communication, Dr. Raymond H. Kaufman.
7. Kaufman, *Audio-Digest*.
8. Duane E. Townsend, "Cryosurgery," *Surgical Clinics of North America* 58:1 (Feb. 1978), pp. 97−108.
9. Ernest W. Franklin, III, M.D., "Malignancy of the Vulva." In *Gynecologic Oncology* (Larry McGowan, ed.), (New York: Appleton-Century-Crofts, 1978), pp. 148−68.
10. Phillip J. Krupp, M.D., "Cancer of the Vulva," *Surgical Clinics of North America* 58:1 (Feb. 1978), pp. 19−38.
11. Franklin, pp. 148−68.
12. Franklin, pp. 148−68.
13. E. W. Franklin and F. D. Rutledge, "Epidemiology of Epidermal Carcinoma of the Vulva," *Obstetrics and Gynecology* 39 (1972), p. 165.
14. Franklin and Rutledge, p. 165.
15. Franklin, pp. 148−68.
16. The following discussion is based primarily on two sources: Franklin, pp. 148−68, and Krupp, pp. 19−38.
17. Franklin, pp. 148−68.
18. Franklin, pp. 148−68.
19. Julian P. Smith, "Chemotherapy in Gynecologic Cancer," *Surgical Clinics of North America* 58:1 (Feb. 1978), pp. 202−15.

THE VAGINA

1. K. D. Gunston and P. F. Fairbrother, "Treatment of Vaginal Discharge with Yoghurt," *South African Journal of Medicine* 49:16 (Apr. 12, 1975), pp. 675−76.
2. *Physician's Desk Reference*, 32nd ed., Charles Baker, ed. (New Jersey: Litton Industries, 1978), pp. 1547−48.
3. Mario Rustia and Philippe Shubik, "Induction of Lung Tumors and Malignant Lymphomas in Mice by Metronidazole," *Journal of the National Cancer Institute* 48 (1972), pp. 721−29.
4. *Physician's Desk Reference*, pp. 1547−48.
5. *Physician's Desk Reference*, pp. 1547−48.
6. Lamon E. V. Ekbladh, "The Expanding Use of Metronidazole (Flagyl)," *Audio-Digest, Obstetrics and Gynecology* 26:11 (June 5, 1979).
7. Herman L. Gardner, M.D., and W. Graham Guerriero, M.D., "Should the Male Sexual Partner Be Treated for Haemophilus or Trichomonas?" *Audio-Digest, Obstetrics and Gynecology*, 26:22 (Nov. 20, 1979).
8. Gerald Bernstein, M.D., "Diagnosis and Treatment of Vaginitis," *Audio-Digest, Obstetrics and Gynecology*, 26:16 (Aug. 21, 1979).
9. Bernstein, *Audio-Digest*.
10. W. Gifford-Jones, *What Every Woman Should Know About Hysterectomy*, (New York: Funk & Wagnalls, 1977), pp. 41−42.
11. J. H. Ferguson, "Effects of Stilbestrol on Pregnancy Compared to the Effect of a Placebo," *American Journal of Obstetrics and Gynecology* 65 (1953), pp. 592−601.
12. A. L. Herbst, H. Ulfedler and D. C. Poskanzer, "Adenocarcinoma of the Vagina," *New England Journal of Medicine* 284 (1971), pp. 878−81; P. Greenwood et al., "Vaginal Cancer After Maternal Treatment With Synthetic Estrogens," *New England Journal of Medicine* 285 (1971), pp. 390−92.
13. A number of different abnormalities have been found in DES daughters, including alterations in the shape of the cervix, lowered fertility and irregular menstrual periods. Testicle cysts, underdeveloped or undescended testes, abnormally placed urinary openings,

low sperm counts, abnormally shaped sperm cells and impaired fertility have been reported in DES sons. For further information, see:

R. Mattingly and A. Stafl, "Cancer Risk in DES-Exposed Offspring," *Journal of Obstetrics and Gynecology* 128 (1977), pp. 43–50;

R. Kaufman et al., "Upper Genital Tract Changes Associated with Exposure in Utero to Diethylstilbestrol," *American Journal of Obstetrics and Gynecology* 128 (1977), pp. 51–59; and

M. Bibbo et al., "Follow-up Study of Male and Female Offspring of DES-Exposed Mothers," *Obstetrics and Gynecology* 49:1 (1977), pp. 1–8.

14. US Dept. of Health, Education and Welfare, Food and Drug Administration, "DES and Breast Cancer," *FDA Drug Bulletin* 8 (Mar.-Apr. 1978), p. 10.

15. Registry for Clear Cell Adenocarcinoma of the Genital Tract in Young Women, Boston, Massachusetts, 1977 Report.

16. Anne P. Lanier et al., "Cancer and Stilbestrol, A Follow-up of 1,719 Persons Exposed to Estrogens in Utero 1943–1959," *Mayo Clinic Proceedings* 48 (1973), p. 793;

A. Stafl et al., "Clinical Diagnosis of Vaginal Adenosis," *Journal of Obstetrics and Gynecology* 43 (1974), pp. 118–28;

Sherman et al., "Cervical and Vaginal Adenosis After in Utero Exposure to Synthetic Estrogens," *Journal of Obstetrics and Gynecology* 44 (1974), pp. 531–45; and

A. L. Herbst et al., "Pre-natal Exposure to Stilbestrol," *New England Journal of Medicine* 292 (1975), pp. 334–39.

17. Herbst et al., pp. 334–39.

18. M. S. Singer et al., "Incompetent Cervix in a Hormone-Exposed Offspring," *Obstetrics and Gynecology* 51:5 (May 1978), pp. 625–26.

19. Kaufman et al., pp. 51–59.

20. Bibbo et al., pp. 1–8, and Singer et al., pp. 51–59.

21. Herbst, Ulfedler and Poskanzer, pp. 878–81.

22. Registry for Clear Cell Adenocarcinoma, 1977 Report.

23. H. Ulfedler, "Stilbestrol, Adenosis and Adenocarcinoma," *American Journal of Obstetrics and Gynecology* 117 (1973), p. 795.

24. P. C. O'Brien et al., "Vaginal Epithelial Changes in Young Women Enrolled in the National Cooperative Diethylstilbestrol Adenosis (DESAD) Project," *Obstetrics and Gynecology*, vol. 53:3 (Mar. 1979), pp. 300–8.

25. William C. Fetherston, "Squamous Neoplasia Related to DES Syndrome," *American Journal of Obstetrics and Gynecology* 122 (May 15, 1975), pp. 176–80;

Mattingly and Stafl, p. 543; and

Sherman et al., pp. 531–45.

26. Mattingly and Stafl, p. 543.

27. A. B. P. Ng et al., "Natural History of Vaginal Adenosis in Women Exposed to Diethylstilbestrol in Utero," *Journal of Reproductive Medicine* 18:1 (1977), pp. 1–13.

28. Registry for Clear Cell Adenocarcinoma, 1977 Report.

29. Herbst, Ulfedler and Poskanzer, pp. 878–81.

30. S. N. Hajj and A. L. Herbst, "Evaluation and Management of Diethylstilbestrol Exposed Offspring," *Surgical Clinics of North America* 58:1 (Feb. 1978), pp. 87–96.

31. A case can be made for radiation over surgery in some instances. When the tumor is small, some doctors will remove only the tumor itself. A section of the cervix is usually removed as well, via an operation known as conization, a process somewhat akin to removing the core of an apple. The tissue is then examined microscopically. If the lab report indicates that there is no cervical invasion, these doctors will then treat the remaining, hidden disease with a special needle-type of internal radiation, which is less destructive. The ovaries may, in some cases, be preserved. In one case, a pregnant woman so treated delivered a baby by Caesarean section and also completed two more pregnancies in which apparently normal babies were delivered. However, the radiation damage to the ovaries can produce birth defects, including retardation, so many experts are wary of pregnancy following radiation to the ovaries.

Since less radiation is involved, the risk of radiation-induced cancer should be less, and in some cases the vagina may be able to function normally. The main risk that a woman takes in selecting this form of treatment is that the cancer may have already spread to areas beyond the scope of this more restricted type of treatment. Thus, some experts are hesitant about using it.

32. Robert C. Park and Tim H. Parmley, "Vaginal Cancer." In *Gynecologic Oncology* (Larry McGowan, ed.), (New York: Appleton-Century-Crofts, 1978), pp. 174−84.
33. Robert D. Hilgers, M.D., "Squamous Cell Carcinoma of the Vagina," *Surgical Clinics of North America* 58:1 (Feb. 1978), pp. 25−38.
34. Hilgers, pp. 25−38.
35. Hilgers, pp. 25−38.
36. Hilgers, pp. 25−38.
37. Park and Parmley, pp. 174−84.
38. Luther W. Brady, M.D., "Radiation Therapy for Carcinoma of the Vagina." In *Gynecologic Oncology* (Larry McGowan, ed.), (New York: Appleton-Century-Crofts, 1978), pp. 185−90.
39. Duane E. Townsend, M.D., "Cryosurgery," *Surgical Clinics of North America* 58:1 (Feb. 1978), pp. 97−108.
40. Helmut F. Schellhas, "Laser Surgery in Gynecology," *Surgical Clinics of North America* 58:1 (Feb. 1978), pp. 97−108.
41. Park and Parmley, pp. 174−84; and
Julian P. Smith, "Chemotherapy in Gynecologic Cancer," *Surgical Clinics of North America* 58:1 (Feb. 1978), pp. 201−15.

THE CERVIX

1. William L. Benson and Henry J. Norris, "Current Problems in Gynecologic Pathology." In *Gynecologic Oncology* (Larry McGowan, ed.), (New York: Appleton-Century-Crofts, 1978), pp. 7−36; and
Richard A. Malmgren, "Cytopathology." In *Gynecologic Oncology*, pp. 37−69.
2. In addition to the standard texts used as sources throughout this book (see Chapter Six), the following sources were used in the preparation of this discussion:
William T. Creasman, "Outpatient Management of CIN," *Audio-Digest, Obstetrics and Gynecology*, 26:11 (June 5, 1979), (Side B);
Henry Clay Frick, II, M.D., "Management of Non-Invasive Carcinoma of the Cervix," *Surgical Clinics of North America* 58:1 (Feb. 1978), pp. 55−60;
Raymond H. Kaufman and John F. Irwin, "The Cryosurgical Therapy of Cervical Intraepithelial Neoplasia," *American Journal of Obstetrics and Gynecology* 131 (1978), p. 381 (Note: This same study is reported in Irwin, *Audio-Digest* 25:1 (Jan. 10, 1978);
John Irwin, "Cryosurgical Therapy of CIN," *Audio-Digest, Obstetrics and Gynecology*, 25:1 (Jan. 10, 1978);
George W. Morely et al., "Diagnosis and Treatment of Vulvar and Cervical Lesions," *Audio-Digest, Obstetrics and Gynecology*, 23:18 (Sept. 14, 1976), (Side B); and
Duane E. Townsend, "Cryosurgery," *Surgical Clinics of North America* 58:1 (Feb. 1978), pp. 97−108.
3. See Note 2 above.
4. David M. Mumford, Raymond H. Kaufman and Nancy McCormick, "Immunity, Herpes Simplex Virus and Cervical Carcinoma," *Surgical Clinics of North America* 58:1 (Feb. 1978), pp. 39−54.
5. Mumford, Kaufman and McCormick, pp. 39−54.
6. Mumford, Kaufman, McCormick, pp. 39−54. Note: The authors provide an excellent summary of the evidence regarding herpes virus and cervical cancer. Specific citations are included in the article.
7. Elizabeth Stern et al., "Steroid Contraceptive Use and Cervical Dysplasia: Increase in Risk of Progression," *Science* 196 (1977), p. 1460.
8. Howard W. Jones, "Recurrent Cervical Cancer," *Audio-Digest, Obstetrics and Gynecology*, vol. 26, no. 18 (Sept. 18, 1979).

9. John B. Schlaerth, "Early Invasive Cervical Cancer," *Audio-Digest, Obstetrics and Gynecology* 26:18 (Sept. 18, 1979).

10. Luther W. Brady, "Radiotherapy Treatment of Cervical Cancer." In *Gynecologic Oncology* (Larry McGowan, ed.), (New York: Appleton-Century-Crofts, 1978), pp. 217–33.

11. Schlaerth, *Audio-Digest.*

12. Schlaerth, *Audio-Digest.*

13. J. R. van Nagell, Jr., E. S. Donaldson and E. C. Gay, "Evaluation and Treatment of Patients with Invasive Cervical Cancer," *Surgical Clinics of North America* 58:1 (Feb. 1978), pp. 67–86; and

Schlaerth, *Audio-Digest.*

14. Hugh R. K. Barber, "Cervical Cancer." In *Gynecologic Oncology* (Larry McGowan, ed.), (New York: Appleton-Century-Crofts, 1978), pp. 202–16; and

van Nagell, Donaldson and Gay, pp. 67–89.

15. E. Burghardt and E. Holzer, "Diagnosis and Treatment of Microinvasive Carcinoma of the Cervix Uteri," *Journal of the American College of Obstetricians and Gynecologists* 49:6 (June 1977), pp. 641–52;

Barber, pp. 202–16; and

van Nagell, Donaldson, Gay, pp. 67–89.

16. van Nagell, Donaldson and Gay, pp. 67–89.

17. Burghardt and Holzer, pp. 641–52.

18. The discussion of treatment is based upon the discussions in Barber, pp. 202–16; and van Nagell, Donaldson and Gay, pp. 67–89.

19. Barber, pp. 67–89.

THE UTERUS AND THE FALLOPIAN TUBES

1. In addition to the standard medical texts used as references throughout this book (see Chapter Six), the information about the treatment of endometriosis given here is derived primarily from three sources:

1. A roundtable discussion that involved a number of experts, including John A. Berger (assistant clinical professor, University of California School of Medicine), L. Russell Malinak (associate professor, Baylor College of Medicine), Jaroslav J. Marik (director of the Tyler Medical Clinic and assistant professor, University of California, Los Angeles), George T. Schneider (associate chairman, Ochsner Medical Center, and professor, Louisiana State University School of Medicine) and Samuel B. Ganz (editorial board of *Patient Care*). A version of this discussion, edited by Marion E. Prilook, and entitled "Endometriosis: New Views, New Therapies" appeared in *Patient Care,* Nov. 15, 1978, pp. 24–96. (Specific citations are included at the end of this article.)

2. A talk on infertility problems and endometriosis given by Dr. L. Russell Malinak and recorded on *Audio-Digest, Obstetrics and Gynecology,* 26:8 (Apr. 1979).

3. Product information supplied by the manufacturers of Danocrin that appears in *Physician's Desk Reference,* 32nd ed. (New Jersey: Litton Industries, 1978), p. 1782.

2. J. Phillips et al., "Laparoscopic Procedures: A National Survey for 1975," *Journal of Reproductive Medicine* 18 (1977), pp. 219–26.

3. W. P. Donowski and M. R. Cohen, "Antigonadotropin (danazol) in the Treatment of Endometriosis—Evaluation of Post-Treatment Fertility and Three Year Follow-up Data," *American Journal of Obstetrics and Gynecology* 130 (1978), pp. 41-48.

4. R. S. Schenken and L. R. Malinak, "Reoperation After Initial Treatment of Endometriosis With Conservative Surgery," *American Journal of Gynecology* 131 (1978), pp. 416–21.

5. William Benson and Henry Norris, "Current Problems in Gynecologic Pathology." In *Gynecologic Oncology* (Larry McGowan, ed.) (New York: Appleton-Century-Crofts, 1978), p. 20.

6. P. Greenwald, T. A. Caputo, P. E. Wolfgang, "Endometrial Cancer After the Menopausal Use of Estrogens," *Obstetrics and Gynecology* 50 (1977), pp. 239–43.

7. D. W. Cramer and S. J. Cutler, "Incidence and Histopathology of Malignancies of the Female Genital Organs in the United States," *American Journal of Obstetrics and Gynecology* 118 (1974), p. 443.

8. P. K. Silteri, B. E. Schwarz and P. C. MacDonald, "Estrogen Receptors and Estrone Hypothesis in Relation to Endometrial and Breast Cancer," *Gynecologic Oncology* 2 (1974), p. 228.

9. US Department of Health, Education and Welfare, Federal Drug Administration, "Sequential Oral Contraceptives Removed From the Market," *FDA Drug Bulletin* 6 (1976), p. 26, and

H. W. Kelley et al., "Adenocarcinoma of the Endometrium in Women Taking Sequential Oral Contraceptives," *Obstetrics and Gynecology* 47 (1976), p. 200.

10. There are a number of case-control studies that report increased risk for endometrial cancer in women using menopausal estrogens. The three most widely cited studies are:

H. K. Ziel and W. D. Finkle, "Increased Risk of Endometrial Carcinoma Among Users of Conjugated Estrogens," *New England Journal of Medicine* 293 (1975), pp. 1167—70.

D. C. Smith et al., "Association of Exogenous Estrogen and Endometrial Carcinoma," *New England Journal of Medicine* 293 (1975), pp. 1164—67; and

T. M. Mack et al., "Estrogens and Endometrial Cancer in a Retirement Community," *New England Journal of Medicine* 294 (1976), pp. 1262—67.

These findings are further supported by the fact that incidence rates of endometrial cancer have increased sharply since 1969, which may be related to the rapidly expanding use of estrogens in the last decade. See the FDA-approved package insert for all products containing estrogens for more details.

11. B. MacMahon, "Risk Factors for Endometrial Cancer," *Gynecologic Oncology* 2 (1974), p. 239; and

S. B. Gosberg, "The Individual at High Risk for Endometrial Carcinoma," *American Journal of Obstetrics and Gynecology* 126 (1976), p. 535.

12. The staging scheme here is an adaptation of the classification and staging of malignant tumors from the International Federation of Gynaecology and Obstetrics, 1971, which is accepted by the American College of Obstetricians and Gynecologists.

13. J. Taylor Warton and Gilbert H. Fletcher, "The Principle of Radiation Therapy for Malignant Pelvic Lesions," *Surgical Clinics of North America* 58:1 (Feb. 1978), pp. 181—200.

14. G. Malkasian, T. W. McDonald and J. H. Pratt, "Carcinoma of the Endometrium," *Mayo Clinic Proceedings* 52 (1977), p. 175.

15. Larry McGowan, M.D., "Endometrial Cancer." In *Gynecologic Oncology* (Larry McGowan, ed.), (New York: Appleton-Century-Crofts, 1978) pp. 238—57.

16. McGowan, pp. 238—57.

17. John G. Maier, "Radiotherapy Treatment of Endometrial Cancer." In *Gynecologic Oncology* (Larry McGowan, ed.), (New York: Appleton-Century-Crofts, 1978), pp. 258—65.

18. Maier, pp. 258—65.

19. John G. Boutselis, "Endometrial Carcinoma: Prognostic Factors and Treatment," *Surgical Clinics of North America* 58:1 (Feb. 1958), pp. 109—19.

20. In addition to the standard medical texts used as references throughout this book (see Chapter Six), the information about the treatment of Stage IA, Grade 2 and 3, Stage IB and Stage II is derived from:

Boutselis, p. 109—119;

Maier, p. 258—255; and

McGowan, p. 238—257.

21. In addition to the standard medical texts used as references throughout this book (see Chapter Six), the information about the treatment of Stage III and IV is derived from:

Boutselis, pp. 109—19;

Maier, pp. 258—55;

McGowan, pp. 238—57; and

Staffan R. B. Nodquist, "Advanced Endometrial Carcinoma," *Audio-Digest, Obstetrics and Gynecology,* 26:18 (Sept. 18, 1979).

22. Richard H. Nalick, "Recurrent Endometrial Cancer," *Audio-Digest, Obstetrics and Gynecology* , 26:18 (Sept. 18, 1979).

23. Nalick, *Audio-Digest.*
24. Alexander Sedlis, M. D., "Carcinoma of the Fallopian Tube," *Surgical Clinics of North America* 58:1 (Feb. 1978), pp. 121–29.
25. Robert C. Park, M.D., and Tim H. Parmley, M.D., "Fallopian Tube Cancer." In *Gynecologic Oncology* (Larry McGowan, etc.), (New York: Appleton-Century-Crofts, 1978), pp. 274–80.
26. Sedlis, pp. 121–29.
27. Sedlis, pp. 121–29.
28. Sedlis, pp. 121–29.

THE OVARIES

1. Richard H. Nalick, "The Pelvic Mass: Diagnosis," *Audio-Digest, Obstetrics and Gynecology*, 26:1 (Jan. 23, 1979).
2. John J. Mikuta, "Primary Ovarian Cancer," *Audio-Digest, Obstetrics and Gynecology,* 24:22 (Nov. 15, 1977).
3. Richard K. Kleppinger, "Ovarian Cyst Fenestration by Laparoscopy," *Audio-Digest, Obstetrics and Gynecology,* 26:11 (June 5, 1979).
4. Larry McGowan, "Ovarian Cancer." In *Gynecological Oncology* (Larry McGowan, ed.), (New York: Appleton-Century-Crofts, 1978), pp. 283–331.
5. D. W. Cramer and S. J. Cutler, "Incidence and Histopathology of Malignancies of the Female Genital Organs in the United States," *American Journal of Obstetrics and Gynecology* 118 (1974), p. 443.
6. Brian MacMahon, M.D., Philip Cole, M.D., and Jones Brown, Ph.D., "Etiology of Human Breast Cancer: A Review," *Journal of the National Cancer Institute* 50 (1973), pp. 21–42.
7. C. Paul Morrow, "Advanced Ovarian Cancer: Treatment," *Audio-Digest, Obstetrics and Gynecology*, 26:2 (Jan. 23, 1979).
8. C. Paul Morrow, *Audio-Digest.*
9. McGowan, pp. 283–331.
10. McGowan, pp. 283–331.
11. John B. Schlaerth, "Early Ovarian Cancer: Treatment," *Audio-Digest, Obstetrics and Gynecology*, 26:2 (Jan. 23, 1979).
12. Julian P. Smith, M.D., "Chemotherapy in Gynecological Cancer," *Surgical Clinics of North America* 58:1 (Feb. 1978), pp. 201–15.
13. Stephen J. Alderman et al., "Postoperative Use of Radioactive Phosphorus in Stage I Ovarian Carcinoma," *Obstetrics and Gynecology* 49:659 (1977), pp. 764–65.
14. Ronald R. Reimer et al., "Acute Leukemia After Alkylating Agent Therapy of Ovarian Carcinoma," *New England Journal of Medicine* 297 (July 28, 1977), pp. 177–81.
15. This study found that, overall, a woman with ovarian cancer has 21 times the normal risk of developing acute leukemia, a cancer of the blood-forming tissues. If a woman has ovarian cancer and is treated with an alkylating agent, the risk rises to 36 times normal. If she has ovarian cancer, is treated with an alkylating agent and survives for more than two years, her risk of developing acute leukemia jumps to 171 times normal. Women with those Stage I cancers who have adjuvant therapy are the ones who would have the best chance of surviving for longer than two years. They would, then, fall into this highest-risk group.
    There are, however, a couple of points to be made about this study. First of all, if the women studied had not received any radiotherapy, then they received the alkylating agent for long periods of time—46, 84, 90 months. If they had not received the alkylating agent for long periods of time, they had received radiation therapy. Thus, it is impossible to say from this data whether the alkylating agents used alone, without radiation therapy, for the shorter periods of 12–18 months would be as dangerous. Many doctors feel that the radiation more than the drug may be responsible for the increased rates of leukemia. The question of whether the risks are worth the benefits in Stage I cases cannot be answered at this time. In certain Stage I cases the risk may be worth the benefits. But, we know that about 10 percent of women with low-grade Stage IA(1) cancers arising inside a benign ovarian cyst will eventually die from ovarian cancer. In other words, unrecognized microscopic cancer had

spread prior to surgery. These women may have benefited from adjuvant therapy. But, according to this study, we could expect that somewhere between 5 and 10 percent of these women would develop leukemia as the result of therapy. Further studies may indicate that this form of chemotherapy is worth the risk, but for now, some institutions, in light of this information and preliminary studies showing no increased survival in these cases regardless of whether radiation, chemotherapy, or surgery alone was used, have discontinued the use of chemotherapy in Stage I cases.

16. Schlaerth, *Audio-Digest.*
17. McGowan, pp. 283—331.
18. C. Thomas Griffiths, M.D., and Arlan F. Fuller, M.D., "Intensive Surgical and Chemotherapeutic Management of Advanced Ovarian Cancer," *Surgical Clinics of North America* 58:1 (Feb. 1978), pp. 131—42.

Robert C. Young et al., "Advanced Ovarian Adenocarcinoma: A Prospective Clinical Trial of Melphalan (C-Pam) Versus Combination Chemotherapy," *New England Journal of Medicine* 299 (1978), p. 1261, and

J. Taylor Warton, "Advanced Ovarian Cancer," *Audio-Digest, Obstetrics and Gynecology,* 24:22 (Nov. 15, 1977).
19. Schlaerth, *Audio-Digest.*
20. Schlaerth, *Audio-Digest.*
21. Schlaerth, *Audio-Digest.*
22. Julian P. Smith, Gregorio Delgado and Felix Rutledge, "Second-Look Operations in Ovarian Carcinoma: Postchemotherapy," *Cancer* 38 (1976), p. 1438.
23. McGowan, pp. 283—331.
24. McGowan, pp. 283-331.

THE BREAST

1. Cancer Information Service, "Diagnosis and Treatment of Breast Cancer," Fact Sheet from CIS.
2. American Cancer Society, *1977 Facts and Figures* (New York: ACS, 1977).
3. P. Greenwald, M.D., et al., "Estimated Effect of Breast Self-Examination on Breast Cancer Mortality," *New England Journal of Medicine* 299 (1978), pp. 271-73.
4. V. K. Frantz et al., "Incidence of Chronic Cystic Disease in So-called Normal Breasts: A Study Based on 225 Postmortem Examinations," *Cancer* 4 (1951), pp. 762—82.
5. Oliver Cope, M.D., *The Breast: Its Problems—Benign and Malignant—and How to Deal with Them* (Boston: Houghton-Mifflin Co., 1977), p. 24.
6. Brian MacMahon, M.D., Philip Cole, M.D., and James Brown, Ph.D., "Etiology of Human Breast Cancer: A Review," *Journal of the National Cancer Institute* 50 (1973), pp. 21—42.
7. Personal Communication, Dr. Peter Schick.
8. Sarah Hainline et al., "Mammographic Patterns and Risk of Breast Cancer," *American Journal of Roentgenology* 130 (June 1978), pp. 1157—58; and

John N. Wolfe, M.D., "Breast Parenchymal Patterns: Prevalent and Incident Carcinomas," *Radiology* 131 (April 1979), pp. 267—68; and

John N. Wolfe, M.D., "Risk for Breast Cancer Development," *Cancer* 37:5 (May 1976), pp. 2486—92.
9. J. P. Minton et al., "Response of Fibrocystic Disease to Caffeine Withdrawal and the Correlation of Cystic Nucleotides with Breast Disease," *American Journal of Obstetrics and Gynecology* 135:1 (Sept. 1, 1979), p. 157—58.
10. M. Blichert-Toft, M.D., et al., "Treatment of Mastagia with Bromocriptive: A Double-Blind Cross-Over Study," *British Medical Journal* 1 (1979), p. 237.
11. Val Davajan, M.D., "Management of Amenorrheas and Galactorrhea," *Audio-Digest, Obstetrics and Gynecology* 26:20 (Oct. 23, 1979).
12. Davajan, *Audio-Digest.*
13. Davajan, *Audio-Digest.*
14. Davajan, *Audio-Digest.*
15. American Cancer Society, 1977 *Facts and Figures.*

16. US Department of Health, Education and Welfare, *The Breast Cancer Digest* (Washington, DC: US Govt. Printing Office, 1979), p. 4.

17. Henry P. Lease, "Breast Cancer," *Audio-Digest, Obstetrics and Gynecology* 22:7 (April 8, 1975).

18. Rose Kushner, *Why Me? What Every Woman Should Know About Breast Cancer to Save Her Life* (New York: Signet, 1977), p. 77–98.

19. MacMahon, Cole and Brown, p. 21–42. (Unless noted otherwise, the information on risk and cause is derived from this source.)

20. Personal communication, Dr. Peter Schick.

21. Hainline et al., pp. 1157–58;
Wolfe, pp. 267–68; and
Wolfe, pp. 2486–92.

22. R. Hoover et al., "Menopausal Estrogens and Cancer," *New England Journal of Medicine* 295 (1976), pp. 401–5.

23. US Dept. of Health, Education and Welfare, Public Health Service, National Institutes of Health, *Survival for Cancer of the Breast*, DHEW Publication no. (NIH) 78–1542, p. 5 (table).

24. Greenwald, pp. 271–73.

25. Kushner, p. 153.

26. S. Schwartz, *Textbook of Surgery,* Vol. I (New York: McGraw-Hill, 1974), p. 532.

27. Personal Communication, Dr. Peter Schick.

28. Oliver H. Beahrs, M.D., "Report of the Working Group to Review the National Cancer Institute–American Cancer Society Breast Cancer Demonstration Projects," *Journal of the National Cancer Institute* 62:3 (March 1979), pp. 640–709.

29. Sidney M. Wolfe, M.D., and Rebecca Warner, *Mammography: A Case for Informed Consent* (Washington, DC: Health Research Group, Nov. 1976).

30. Beahrs, pp. 640–709.

31. S. Shapiro, "Evidence on Screening for Breast Cancer in a Randomized Trial," *Cancer* 39 (1977), pp. 2772–82.

32. Advisory Committee on the Biological Effects of Ionizing Radiation, *Report on the Effects on Populations Exposed to Low Levels of Ionizing Radiation* (Washington, DC: Research Council of the National Academy of Sciences–National Research Council, 1977).

33. Beahrs, pp. 640–709.

34. John C. Bailer, M.D., "Mammography: A Contrary View," *Annals of Internal Medicine* 84 (1976), pp. 72–84.

35. Beahrs, pp. 640–709.

36. Beahrs, pp. 640–709.

37. George M. Walker, II, M.D., et al., "Breast Biopsy: A Comparison of Outpatient and Inpatient Experience," *Archives of Surgery* 113 (1978), pp. 942–46.

38. S. Schwartz, p. 443.

39. Several studies have supported this conclusion, including: C. D. Haagensen, "Role of the Detection of Breast Disease" in *Diseases of the Breast* (Philadelphia: W. B. Saunders Co., 1971), p. 99;
P. P. Jackson and H. H. Pitts, "Biopsy with Delayed Radical Mastectomy for Carcinoma of the Breast," *American Journal of Surgery* 98 (1959), pp. 184–89;
E. H. Pierce et al., "Biopsy of the Breast Followed by Delayed Radical Mastectomy," *Surgery, Gynecology and Obstetrics* 103 (1956), pp. 559–64; and
A. Scheel, "Some Prognostic Factors, Particularly Biopsy, in Carcinoma of the Breast," *Acta Radial* 39 (1953), pp. 249–54.

40. "Special Report: Treatment of Primary Breast Cancer," *New England Journal of Medicine* 301:6 (Aug. 9, 1979), p. 340.

41. Bernard Fisher, M.D., Carol Redmond, Sc.D., and Edwin R. Fisher, M.D., "Clinical Trials and the Surgical Treatment of Breast Cancer," *Surgical Clinics of North America* 58:4 (Aug. 1978), pp. 723–36.

42. Beahrs, pp. 640–709.

43. This figure is perhaps conservative, for it assumes that the other 86 cases (of the 592 minimal cancers) that were not reviewed by the board were diagnosed correctly. On the other hand, it may be a bit high. When it was discovered that 66 cases had been misdiagnosed, yet another pathology review was done. Additional pathology slides were obtained, and it was then decided that 11 of the 66 had been correctly diagnosed in the first place and were indeed cancerous. In 5 of the 66 cases, the experts said that they were now unable to decide whether or not the woman had cancer and that 2 of the 66 cases had been included by mistake, leaving only 48 mistaken diagnoses (*Washington Post*, Oct. 24, 1978). Thus, the percentage of misdiagnosed cases might have been as low as about 2.5 percent.

Unfortunately, the fact remains that at least 48 women diagnosed at BCDDP projects prior to June 30, 1976, were misdiagnosed. There are then some women who had unnecessary mastectomies, women who thought, and still think, that they have had breast cancer when in fact they haven't and believe that they and their female relatives—their sisters and daughters—are at higher risk for the development of cancer, when in fact they aren't. Moreover, the pathology review reviewed only minimal cases that had been detected at a BCDDP over a certain period. Since that time there may have been others misdiagnosed, both at the BCDDPs and at other places.

Lawyers at the Department of Health, Education and Welfare determined that legally the federal government could not notify these women that they did not have cancer. The BCDDPs were set up only as screening centers. If a woman's mammogram was suspicious, notification was sent to her doctor. From that time on, although the BCDDPs collected data on the cases, the NCI, sponsor of the BCDDPs, was out of the picture. The entire matter was seen as a doctor-patient relationship, and, of course, the government couldn't violate this sacred contract. So, the procedure decided upon was to inform the individual BCDDP that it had been discovered that Ms. So & So didn't really have cancer after all. Then the director of the center was to inform Ms. So & So's doctor that she had actually had benign disease and not cancer and therefore was not at high risk for recurrent cancer and did not need to have the lifetime follow-up visits. She was also to be told that her daughter and sisters were not at high risk and did not (depending on their age) need annual mammograms.

The NCI cannot, however, force the doctor to pass the word along to those women and thus invite a malpractice suit. (Whether or not such a woman would actually win a malpractice suit is a moot point, for some pathologists insist that all microscopic diagnoses are a matter of judgment and subject to personal interpretations.) Admittedly, it would take a special kind of courage to call up a woman, especially one who had been treated with a mastectomy, and tell her that she hadn't had cancer after all. As a result, most of those women who have had cancer surgery because of diagnoses from the BCDDPs still don't know whether they did indeed have cancer.

The National Women's Health Network attempted to learn the names of the women involved by way of the Freedom of Information Act, but the information cannot be released to an organization. To do so would be a violation of privacy laws. The individual woman herself may, however, obtain information on her own case. The person to contact is Richard Costlow, Chief, Division of Preventive Medicine, Division of Cancer Control and Rehabilitation, Blair Building/NCI, 8300 Colesville Road, Silver Spring, Maryland 20910.

44. Beahrs, pp. 640—709.

45. C. Kent Osborne, M.D., and William L. McGuire, M.D., "Current Use of Steroid Hormone Receptor Assays in the Treatment of Breast Cancer," *Surgical Clinics of North America* 58:4 (Aug. 1978), pp. 777—88.

46. Craig Henderson, M.D., and George D. Canellos, M.D., "Cancer of the Breast, the Past Decade, Part One," *New England Journal of Medicine* 302:1 (Jan. 3, 1980), pp. 17—30.

47. Cancer Information Service, *Diagnosis and Treatment of Breast Cancer* (training manual for volunteers), p. 14.

48. Henderson and Canellos, pp. 17—30.

49. Readers interested in a more detailed and academic discussion of the history of breast cancer treatments are referred to Hendersen and Canellos, pp. 17—30.

50. Robert E. Hermann, M.D., and Ezra Steiger, M.D., "Modified Radical Mastectomy," *Surgical Clinics of North America* 58:4 (Aug. 1978), pp. 743—54.

51. T. Nemato and T. Dao, "Is Modified Radical Mastectomy Adequate for Axillary Lymph Node Dissection?" *Annals of Surgery* 182 (1975), p. 722.

52. Hendersen and Canellos, pp. 17—30; and
Nemato and Dao, p. 722.

53. Fisher, Redmond and Fisher, pp. 723—36.

54. The study did not directly compare the radical and the modified radical. To do so would have been impractical because the study would have had to involve such large numbers of women. Finding small differences between treatments being compared requires large numbers of women. Setting up a protocol that could possibly have demonstrated a significant difference between the modified and the radical (if indeed such a difference existed) would require such large numbers of women and so many years to complete that it was simply not practical.

55. The study accomplished this by having women with negative nodes in one arm of the protocol receive only a simple mastectomy, removal of the breast. If the nodes subsequently became positive, they were removed. Since survival rates in these women were no worse than in the group as a whole it could be concluded that removing the pectorals did not enhance survival.

56. F. W. Foote, Jr., and F. W. Stewart, "Comparative Studies of Cancerous versus Noncancerous Breasts," *Annals of Surgery* 121 (1945), p. 197; and

R. Muir, "Evolution of Carcinoma of the Mammary Gland," *Journal of Pathol Bacteriology* 55 (1941), pp. 155–72.

57. Fisher, Redmond and Fisher, pp. 723–36.

58. Avram M. Cooperman, M.D., Janet M. Blanchard, M.D., and Caldwell Esselstyn, Jr., M.D., "Partial Mastectomy," *Surgical Clinics of North America* 58 (Aug. 1978), pp. 737–42.

59. Fisher, Redmond and Fisher, pp. 723–36.

60. Jay R. Harris, Martin B. Levere and Samuel Hellman, "Results of Treating Stage I and II Carcinoma of the Breast with Primary Radiation Therapy," *Cancer Treatment Reports* 62:7 (July 1978), pp. 985–91; and

Martin B. Levere, M.D., Jay R. Harris, M.D., and Samuel Hellnan, M.D., "Primary Radiation Therapy for Operable Carcinoma of the Breast," *Surgical Clinics of North America* 58:4 (Aug. 1978), pp. 767–76.

61. Vincent R. Pennises, M.D., Angelo Capozzi, M.D., and F. M. Perez, M.D., "Subcutaneous Mastectomy Data: An Interim Report," *Breast, Diseases of the Breast* 5:2 (1977).

62. Cope, p. 172.

63. Henderson and Canellos, pp. 17–30.

64. Beahrs, table, pg. 659.

65. Henderson and Canellos, pp. 17–30.

66. B. Fisher et al., "L-phenylalanine mustard (L-Pam) in the Management of Primary Breast Cancer: An Update of Earlier Findings and a Comparison with Those Utilizing L-Pam Plus 5-Fluorouracil (5-FU)," *Cancer* 39 (1977), pp. 2883–903; and

B. Fisher et al., "Adjuvant Chemotherapy in Breast Cancer," *International Journal of Radiat Oncol Biol Phys* 4 (1978), pp. 295–98.

67. Bernard Fisher and Norman Wolmark, "Systemic Adjuvant Therapy in Primary Breast Cancer." In *Breast Cancer, Advances in Research and Treatment*, vol. I (William McGuire, M.D., ed.), (New York: Plenum, 1977), pp. 125–63.

68. G. Bonadonna et al., "Are Surgical Adjuvant Trials Altering the Course of Breast Cancer," *Semin Oncology* 5 (1978), pp. 450–64; and

G. Bonadonna et al., "Combination Chemotherapy as an Adjuvant Treatment in Operable Breast Cancer," *New England Journal of Medicine* 294 (1976), pp. 405–10.

69. Fisher and Wolmark, pp. 125–163.

70. G. F. Robbins et al., "An Evaluation of Postoperative Prophylactic Radiation Therapy in Breast Cancer," *Surgery, Gynecology and Obstetrics* 122 (1966), pp. 979–82.

71. W. T. Bessler, "Radiotherapy of Metastatic Breast Cancer." In *Breast Cancer* (A. Montague, G. Stonesifer and E. Lewison, eds.), (New York: Alan R. Liss, Inc., 1977), pp. 493–504; and

Kushner, pp. 277–78.

72. Kushner, pp. 277–78.

73. Henderson and Canellos, pp. 17–30.

74. The information on breast reconstruction is drawn primarily from two sources:

a) a fact sheet, "Breast Reconstruction After Breast Cancer," available from the Cancer Information Service; and

b) a Pamphlet, "Breast Reconstruction After Breast Cancer: Some Questions and Answers," prepared by the American Society of Plastic and Reconstructive Surgeons, Inc.

SEXUALLY TRANSMITTED DISEASES

1. *V.D. Fact Sheet 1977* and *V.D. Fact Sheet 1978* (Joseph H. Blount, ed.), US Dept. of Health, Education and Welfare, Public Health Service, Center for Disease Control, Venereal Disease Control Division, 1978 and 1979 (respectively).
2. D. Barlow, "The Condom and Gonorrhea," *Lancet* 2:842 (Oct. 15, 1977), pp. 811–13.
3. "Condom Sales Rise in Sweden, VD Falls," *Obstetrics and Gynecology News* 8:15 (Aug. 1, 1973), p. 9.
4. B. Singh et al., "Studies on the Development of a Vaginal Preparation Providing Both Prophylaxis Against Veneral Disease and Other Genital Infections and Contraception II: Effect in Vitro of Vaginal Contraceptive and Noncontraceptive Preparations on Treponema pallidum and Neisseria gonorrhoeae," *British Journal of Venereal Disease* 48 (1972), pp. 51–64.
    B. Postic et al., "Inactivation of Clinical Isolites of Herpes Viris Hominis, Types 1 and 2, by Chemical Contraceptives," *Sexually Transmitted Diseases* 5 (Jan.-Mar. 1978), pp. 22–24.
5. Boston Women's Health Collective, *Our Bodies, Ourselves*, 2nd ed. (New York: Simon and Schuster, 1976), p. 168.
6. Herman L. Gardner, M.D., "Herpes Genitalis," *Audio-Digest, Obstetrics and Gynecology*, 26:3 (Feb. 6, 1979);
    Raymond H. Kaufman, "Herpes Genitalis, Clinical Features and Laboratory Diagnosis," *Audio-Digest, Obstetrics and Gynecology*, 26:3 (Feb. 6, 1979); and
    Erwin Adam, M.D., et al., "Asymptomatic Virus Shedding After Herpes Genitalis," *American Journal of Obstetrics and Gynecology*, 137:7 (Aug. 1, 1980), pp. 827–30.
7. Dr. William E. Josey, "Herpes Genitalis, Effects on Infants," *Audio-Digest, Obstetrics and Gynecology*, 26:3 (Feb. 6, 1979); and
    Anne S. Yeager, M.D., "Genital Herpes Simplex Virus (HSV), Infections and Pregnancy," *The Helper*, 1:2 (Oct. 1979), pp. 1–2.
8. *V.D. Fact Sheet, 1978.*
9. Center for Disease Control, "Herpes Genital Infection," Information Sheet.
10. Kaufman, *Audio-Digest.*
11. Adam et al., pp. 827–30.
12. Kaufman, *Audio-Digest.*
13. Kaufman, *Audio-Digest.*
14. David K. Mumford, Raymond H. Kaufman and Nancy McCormick, "Immunity, Herpes Simplex Virus and Cervical Carcinoma," *Surgical Clinics of North America* 58:1 (Feb. 1958), pp. 39–54.
15. A. J. Nahmias, "Significance of Herpes Simplex Virus During Pregnancy," *Clinical Obstetrics and Gynecology* 15:4 (1972), p. 929.
16. Josey, *Audio-Digest.*
17. Josey, *Audio-Digest.*
18. Yeager, pp. 1–2.
19. Kaufman, *Audio-Digest.*
20. Kaufman, *Audio-Digest.*
21. Kaufman, *Audio-Digest.*
22. *V.D. Fact Sheet, 1977.*
23. *V.D. Fact Sheet, 1977.*
24. *V.D. Fact Sheet, 1977.*
25. *V.D. Fact Sheet, 1977.*
26. US Department of Health, Education and Welfare, Public Health Service, National Institutes of Health, *Sexually Transmitted Diseases*, DHEW Publication no. (NIH) 76-909.

PROBLEMS RELATED TO THE MENSTRUAL CYCLE

1. Edmund R. Novak, M.D., Georgeanna Seegar Jones, M.D. and Howard W. Jones, Jr., M.D., *Novak's Textbook of Gynecology*, 9th ed. (Baltimore, Williams & Wilkins Co., 1975), p. 652.

2. Katherine Dalton, M.D., *The Premenstrual Syndrome* (Springfield, Ill.: Charles C. Thomas, 1964).

3. P. Adams, V. Wynn and D. Rose, "Effects of Pyridoxine Hydrochloride (Vitamin B6) Upon Depression Associated with Oral Contraception," *Lancet* 1 (1969), p. 897.

4. A. Schwartz et al., "Primary Dysmenorrhea, Alleviation by an Inhibitor of Prostaglandin Synthesis," *Obstetrics and Gynecology* 44 (1974), pp. 709—12.

5. F. H. Boehm and H. Sarralt, "Indomethacin for the Treatment of Dysmenorrhea, A Preliminary Report," *Journal of Reproductive Medicine* 15 (1975), pp. 84—86.

6. M. R. Henzl et al., "The Treatment of Dysmenorrhea with Naproxen Sodium: A Report on Two Independent Double-Blind Trials," *American Journal of Obstetrics and Gynecology*, 127 (1977), pp. 818—23.

7. P. W. Budoff, "Use of Mefenamic Acid in the Treatment of Primary Dysmenorrhea," *Journal of the American Medical Association* 241:25 (June 22, 1979), pp. 2713—16.

8. K. T. Witty et al., "Dysmenorhea, Quelling Severe Menstrual Cramps," *Patient Care*, April 15, 1978, pp. 198—216.

9. Witty, pp. 198—216.

10. Val Davajan, M.D., "Management of Amenorrheas and Galactorrhea," *Audio-Digest, Obstetrics and Gynecology*, 26:20 (Oct. 23, 1979).

11. Davajan, *Audio-Digest.*

12. Davajan, *Audio-Digest.*

13. Davajan, *Audio-Digest.*

14. Lorraine C. King, M.D., "Dysfunctional Uterine Bleeding: Medical vs. Surgical Treatment," *Audio-Digest, Obstetrics and Gynecology*, 26:21 (Nov. 6, 1979).

15. Gilbert S. Gordon, "Osteoporosis: Prevention of Bone Loss," *Audio-Digest, Obstetrics and Gynecology* 27:16 (Aug. 19, 1980).

16. G. Winokur, "Depression in the Menopause," *American Journal of Psychiatry* 130 (1973), pp. 92—93.

17. B. Neugarten and R. J. Kraines, "Menopausal Symptoms in Women of Various Ages," *Psychosomatic Medicine* 27 (1965) pp. 266—73.

18. Nancy Friedman, "The Truth About Tampons," *New West* (Oct. 20, 1980) pp. 33—42.

19. Friedman, pp. 33—42.

PROBLEMS RELATED TO PREGNANCY AND FERTILITY

1. Tracy Hotchner, *Pregnancy and Childbirth* (New York: Avon Books, 1979), p. 41.

2. Langdon Parsons, M.D. and Sheldon Sommers, M.D. *Gynecology*, 2nd ed. (Philadelphia: W. B. Saunders Co., 1978), p. 494.

3. A. L. Herbst, H. Ulfedler and D. C. Poskanzer, "Adenocarcinoma of the Vagina," *New England Journal of Medicine* 284 (1971), pp. 878—81.

4. Michael Leviton, Commentary, broadcast on KPFK, Nov. 7, 1979. NOVA, the public television show, also did an expose of the Agent Orange problem. Additional information on Agent Orange is available from the Citizen Soldier, Suite 1010, 175 Fifth Avenue, New York, NY 10160.

5. J. B. Van Dijk, M.D., et al., "The Treatment of Unexplained Fertility With Danazol," *Fertility and Sterility* 31 (May, 1979), pp. 481—85.

6. Hotchner, pp. 440—41.

7. Jennie Kline et al., "Smoking: A Risk Factor for Spontaneous Abortion," *New England Journal of Medicine* 297 (Oct. 13, 1977), pp. 793—96.

8. See Note 4 above.

9. I. Gal, B. Kirman and J. Stern, "Hormonal Pregnancy Tests and Congenital Malformation," *Nature* 216 (1967), p. 83;

E. P. Levy, A. Cohen and F. C. Fraser, "Hormone Treatment During Pregnancy and Congenital Heart Defects," *Lancet* 1 (1973), p. 611;

D. T. Janevich, J. M. Piper and D. M. Glebatis, "Oral Contraceptives and Congenital Limb-reduction Effects," *New England Journal of Medicine* 291 (1974), pp. 697−700; and

L. Wilkins, "Masculization of Female Fetus Due to Use of Orally Given Progestins," *Journal of the American Medical Association* 172 (1960), p. 1028.

10. See Note 9 above.

11. Kline et al., pp. 793−96.

12. Martin M. Quigley, "Trophoblastic Disease: Diagnosis and Treatment," *Audio-Digest, Obstetrics and Gynecology*, 24:5 (March 3, 1977).

13. Charles B. Hammond, M.D., Herbert J. Schmidt, M.D. and Roy T. Parker, M.D., "Gestational Trophoblastic Disease." In *Gynecologic Oncology* (Larry McGowan, ed.), (New York: Appleton-Century-Crofts, 1978), pp. 359−81.

14. Quigley, *Audio-Digest*.

15. Quigley, *Audio-Digest*.

16. Quigley, *Audio-Digest*.

17. Quigley, *Audio-Digest*.

18. Hammond, Schmidt and Parker, pp. 359−81; and

Walter B. Jones, M.D., "Gestational Trophoblastic Neoplasms," *Surgical Clinics of North America* 58:1 (Feb. 1978), pp. 167−79.

19. Quigley, *Audio-Digest*.

CANCER

1. A. L. Herbst, H. Ulfedler and D. C. Poskanzer, "Adenocarcinoma of the Vagina," *New England Journal of Medicine* 284 (1971), pp. 878−81.

2. B. MacMahon, "Risk Factors for Endometrial Cancer," *Gynecologic Oncology* 2 (1974), p. 239.

3. There are a number of case-control studies that report increased risk for endometrial cancer in women using menopausal estrogens. The three most widely cited studies are:

H. K. Ziel and W. D. Finkle, "Increased Risk of Endometrial Carcinoma Among Users of Conjugated Estrogens," *New England Journal of Medicine* 293 (1975), pp. 1167−70.

D. C. Smith et al., "Association of Exogenous Estrogen and Endometrial Carcinoma," *New England Journal of Medicine* 294 (1976), pp. 1164−67.

T. M. Mack et al., "Estrogens and Endometrial Cancer in a Retirement Community," *New England Journal of Medicine* 294 (1976), pp. 1262−67.

These findings are further supported by the fact that incidence rates of endometrial cancer have increased sharply since 1969, which may be related to the rapidly expanding use of estrogens in the last decade. See the FDA-approved package insert for all products containing estrogens or more details.

4. David M. Mumford, Raymond H. Kaufman and Nancy McCormick, "Immunity, Herpes Simplex Virus and Cervical Carcinoma," *Surgical Clinics of North America* 58:1 (Feb. 1978), pp. 39−54.

5. Bernard Fisher, M.D., Carol Redmond, Sc.D., and Edwin R. Fisher, M.D., "Clinical Trials and the Surgical Treatment of Breast Cancer," *Surgical Clinics of North America* 58:4 (Aug. 1978), pp. 723−36.

6. J. P. Minton et al., "Response of Fibrocystic Disease to Caffeine Withdrawal and the Correlation of Cystic Nucleotides with Breast Disease," *American Journal of Obstetrics and Gynecology* 135:1 (Sept. 1, 1979), pp. 157−58.

7. William L. Broad, "New Laetrile Study Leaves Cancer Institute in the Pits," *Science* 202:4363 (October 6, 1978), pp. 33−36; and

William L. Broad, "Upton OK's Laetrile Test on Humans," *Science* 202:4364 (Oct. 13, 1978), p. 196.

8. John Elliott, "Clinical Trials of Laetrile May Soon Be Under Way," *Journal of the American Medical Association* 243:6 (Feb. 8, 1980), pp. 505−6.

Chapter Seven: GYNECOLOGICAL OPERATIONS, TESTS, PROCEDURES AND DRUGS

1. William Nolen, M.D., "The Big Knives," *Esquire* 93:4 (April 1980), pp. 58—60.
2. See Notes 4 and 6 at the end of Chapter One.
3. Barbara Caress, "Womb Bomb," *Health/PAC Bulletin* (July-Aug. 1977).
4. Caress, *Health/PAC Bulletin.*
5. S. Schwartz, *Textbook of Surgery*, vol. I (New York: McGraw-Hill, 1974), p. 443.
6. A. L. Herbst, H. Ulfedler and D. C. Poskanzer, "Adenocarcinoma of the Vagina," *New England Journal of Medicine* 284 (1971), pp. 878—81.
7. A number of different abnormalities have been found in DES daughters, including alterations in the shape of the cervix, vaginal adenosis, lowered fertility and irregular menstrual periods. Testicle cysts, underdeveloped or undescended testes, abnormally placed urinary openings, low sperm counts, abnormally shaped sperm cells and impaired fertility have been reported in DES sons.
For further information, see:
R. Mattingly and A. Stafl, "Cancer Risk in DES-exposed Offspring," *Journal of Obstetrics and Gynecology* 128 (1977), pp. 43—50;
R. Kaufman et al., "Upper Genital Tract Changes Associated with Exposure in Utero to Diethylstilbestrol," *American Journal of Obstetrics and Gynecology* 128 (1977), pp. 51—59; and
M. Bibbo et al., "Follow-up Study of Male and Female Offspring of DES-exposed Mothers," *Obstetrics and Gynecology* 49:1 (1977), pp. 1—8.
8. Food and Drug Administration, Department of Health, Education and Welfare, "DES and Breast Cancer," *FDA Drug Bulletin* 8 (March-April 1978), p. 2.
9. There are a number of case-control studies that report increased risk for endometrial cancer in women using menopausal estrogens. The three most widely cited studies are:
H. K. Ziel and W. D. Finkle, "Increased Risk of Endometrial Carcinoma Among Users of Conjugated Estrogens," *New England Journal of Medicine* 293 (1975), pp. 1167—70;
D. C. Smith et al., "Association of Exogenous Estrogen and Endometrial Carcinoma," *New England Journal of Medicine* 293 (1975), pp. 1164—67; and
T. M. Mack et al., "Estrogens and Endometrial Cancer in a Retirement Community," *New England Journal of Medicine* 294 (1976), pp. 1262—67.
These findings are further supported by the fact that incidence rates of endometrial cancer have increased sharply since 1969, which may be related to the rapidly expanding use of estrogens in the last decade. See the FDA-approved package insert for all products containing estrogens for more details.
10. R. Hoover et al., "Menopausal Estrogens and Cancer," *New England Journal of Medicine* 295 (1976), pp. 401—5.
11. *Physician's Desk Reference*, 32nd ed., Charles Baker, ed., (New Jersey: Litton Industries, 1978), p. 624.
12. Hoover et al., pp. 401—5.
13. Ward Rinehart and Jane Winter, "Injectable Progestogens—Officials Debate, But Use Increases," *Population Reports*, Series K. no. 1 (March 1975), p. K1-K9.
14. Rinehart and Winter, p. K1-K9.
15. Rinehart and Winter, p. K1-K9.
16. Rinehart and Winter, p. K1-K9.
17. Center for Medical Consumers and Health Care Information "Informed Consent," vol. IV, no. 22 (July-Aug. 1980) pp. 1—8.
18. *Physician's Desk Reference*, p. 1661.

Reference Section: OPERATIONS, TESTS, PROCEDURES AND DRUGS

1. J. P. Bunker, K. McPherson and P. C. Henneman, "Elective Hysterectomy." In *Costs, Risks and Benefits of Surgery* (New York: Oxford University Press, 1977), pp. 262—76.

2. W. Ledger and M. Child, "The Hospital Care of Patients Undergoing Hysterectomy: An Analysis of 12,026 Patients from the Professional Activity Study," *American Journal of Obstetrics and Gynecology* 117 (1973), pp. 423–33.

3. Ledger and Child, pp. 423–33.

4. There are a number of case-control studies that report increased risk for endometrial cancer in women using menopausal estrogens. The three most widely cited studies are:

H. K. Ziel and W. D. Finkle, "Increased Risk of Endometrial Carcinoma Among Users of Conjugated Estrogens," *New England Journal of Medicine* 293 (1975); pp. 1167–70;

D. C. Smith et al., "Association of Exogenous Estrogen and Endometrial Carcinoma," *New England Journal of Medicine* 293 (1975); pp. 1164–67; and

T. M. Mack et al., "Estrogens and Endometrial Cancer in a Retirement Community," *New England Journal of Medicine* 294 (1976); pp. 1262–67.

These findings are further supported by the fact that incidence rates of endometrial cancer have increased sharply since 1969, which may be related to the rapidly expanding use of estrogens in the last decade. See the FDA-approved package insert for all products containing estrogens for more details.

5. Robert Hoover et al., "Menopausal Estrogens and Cancer," *New England Journal of Medicine* 295 (1976); pp. 401–5.

6. W. Gifford Jones, *What Every Woman Should Know About Hysterectomy* (New York: Funk & Wagnalls, 1977), p. 175.

7. H. Judd et al., "Endrocrine Function of the Post-Menopausal Ovary," *Journal of Clinical Endocrinology and Metabolism* 39 (1974), p. 1020.

8. L. Moses, "Comparison of Crude and Standardized Anesthetic Death Rates." In *The National Halothane Study: Report of the Subcommittee on the National Halothane Study* (J. P. Bunker et al., eds.) (Washington, DC: US Government Printing Office, 1969), Chapter IV-2.

9. Barbara J. Culliton and Walter K. Waterfall, "Low-Dose Radiation," *British Medical Journal* 1:6177 (June 9, 1979), pp. 1545–46.

10. Culliton and Waterfall, pp. 1545–46.

11. "The X-Raying of America," *FDA Consumer* (Dec. 1979-Jan. 1980), pp. 13–17.

12. I. Gal, B. Kirman and J. Stern, "Hormonal Pregnancy Tests and Congenital Malformation," *Nature* 216 (1967), p. 83;

E. P. Levy, A. Cohen and F. C. Fraser, "Hormone Treatment During Pregnancy and Congenital Heart Defects," *Lancet* 1 (1973), p. 611.

D. T. Janevich, J. M. Piper and D. M. Glebatis, "Oral Contraceptives and Congenital Limb-reduction Effects," *New England Journal of Medicine* 291 (1974), pp. 697–700; and

L. Wilkins, "Masculization of Female Fetus Due to Use of Orally Given Progestins," *Journal of the American Medical Association* 172 (1960), p. 1028.

13. J. C. Phillips, "Public Health Aspects of Critical Care Medicine: Anesthesia Mortality," *Clinical Anesthesia* 10 (1974), pp. 220–44.

14. O. Idose, "Nature and Extent of Penicillin Side Reactions With Particular Reference to the Fatalistic Form: Anaphylatic Shock," *World Health Organization Bulletin* 38 (1968), p. 159.

15. *Physician's Desk Reference*, 32nd ed., Charles Baker, ed. (New Jersey: Litton Industries, 1978), p. 1166.

16. Ward Rinehart and Jane Winter, "Injectable Progestogens—Officials Debate, But Use Increases," *Population Reports*, Series K, no. 1 (March 1975), p. K1-K16.

17. Rinehart and Winter, p. K1-K16.

18. Rinehart and Winter, p. K1-K16.

19. Rinehart and Winter, p. K1-K16.

20. Rinehart and Winter, p. K1-K16.

21. Rinehart and Winter, p. K1-K16.

22. G. Winokur, "Depression in the Menopause," *American Journal of Psychiatry* 130 (1973), pp. 92–93.

23. B. Neugarten and R. J. Kraines, "Menopausal Symptoms in Women of Various Ages," *Psychosomatic Medicine* 27 (1965), pp. 266–73.

24. Barbara Seaman and Gideon Seaman, M.D., *Women and the Crisis in Sex Hormones* (New York: Rawson Associates, 1977), pp. 283–84.

25. Seaman and Seaman, pp. 300–2.

26. "Progesterone Therapy for Hot Flashes?" *Medical World News* (July 23, 1979), pp. 18—19.
27. Seaman and Seaman, pp. 363—70.
28. Seaman and Seaman, pp. 351—62.
29. Gilbert S. Gordon, "Osteoporosis: Prevention of Bone Loss," *Audio-Digest, Obstetrics and Gynecology* 27:16 (Aug. 19, 1980).
30. *Physician's Desk Reference*, p. 623.
31. Gordon, *Audio-Digest.*
32. Gordon, *Audio-Digest.*
33. Gordon, *Audio-Digest.*
34. Gordon, *Audio-Digest.*
35. Boston Collaborative Drug Surveillance Program, "Surgically Confirmed Gall Bladder Disease, Venous Thromboembolism and Breast Tumors in Relation to Post Menopausal Estrogen Therapy," *New England Journal of Medicine* 290 (1974), pp. 15—19.
36. R. I. Pfeiffer and S. Van Den Noort, "Estrogen Use and Stroke Risk in Postmenopausal Women," *American Journal of Epidemiology* 103 (1976), p. 445—56.
37. R. Hoover et al., "Menopausal Estrogens and Breast Cancer," *New England Journal of Medicine* 295 (1976), pp. 401—5.
38. *Physician's Desk Reference*, p. 623.
39. Seaman and Seaman, p. 34.
40. A. L. Herbst, H. Ulfedler and D. C. Poskanzer, "Adenocarcinoma of the Vagina," *New England Journal of Medicine* 284 (1971), pp. 878—81.
41. Registry for Clear Cell Adenocarcinoma of the Genital Tract in Young Women, Boston, Massachusetts, 1977 Report.
42. R. Mattingly and A. Stafl, "Cancer Risk in DES-Exposed Offspring," *Journal of Obstetrics and Gynecology* 128 (1977), pp. 43—50.
43. Anne P. Lanier et al., "Cancer and Stilbestrol, a Follow-Up of 1,719 Persons Exposed to Estrogens in Utero, 1943-1959," *Mayo Clinic Proceedings* 48 (1973), p. 793;
 A. Stafl et al., "Clinical Diagnosis of Vaginal Adenosis," *Journal of Obstetrics and Gynecology* 43 (1974), pp. 118—28; and
 Sherman et al., "Cervical Vaginal Adenosis After in Utero Exposure to Synthetic Estrogens," *Journal of Obstetrics and Gynecology* 44 (1974), pp. 531—45.
44. R. Kaufman et al., "Upper Genital Tract Changes Associated With Exposure in Utero to Diethylstilbestrol," *American Journal of Obstetrics and Gynecology* 128 (1977), pp. 51—59; and
 M. S. Singer et al., "Incompetent Cervix in Hormone-Exposed Offspring," *Obstetrics and Gynecology* 51:5 (May 1978), pp. 625—26.
46. Kaufman et al., pp. 51—59.
47. M. Bibbo et al., "Follow-Up Study of Male and Female Offspring of DES-Exposed Mothers," *Obstetrics and Gynecology* 49:1 (1977), pp. 1—8; and
 Singer et al, pp. 625—26.
48. Bibbo et al., pp. 1—8; and
 W. Gill, G. Schumacher and M. Bibbo, "Genital and Semen Abnormalities in Adult Males Two and One Half Decades After in Utero Exposure to Diethylstilbestrol." In *Intrauterine Exposure to Diethylstilbestrol in the Human* (A. Herbst, ed.), Proceedings of Symposium on DES, Chicago (Feb. 1977), American College of Obstetricians and Gynecologists (Monograph).
49. Bibbo et al., pp. 1—8; and Gill, Schumacher and Bibbo, Monograph.
50. Seaman and Seaman, pp. 49—59.
51. Seaman and Seaman, p. 6.
52. Personal communication, Nancy Adess, DES Action.
53. Fay A. Saber, "The DES Problem Revisited: On Whose Shoulders Should The Legal Responsibility Fall?," *DES Action Voice*, 1:2 (Spring 1979).
54. Abraham E. Rakoff, "Ovarian Failure," *Audio-Digest, Obstetrics and Gynecology* 24:10 (May 17, 1977).
55. See Notes 40, 42, and 43 through 47 above.
56. Rakoff, *Audio-Digest.*

57. Rakoff, *Audio-Digest.*
58. Shirley McCormack and James H. Clark, "Clomid Administration to Pregnant Rats Causes Abnormalities of the Reproductive Tract in Offspring and Mothers," *Science* 204 (May 11, 1979), pp. 629–31.
59. McCormack and Clark, pp. 629–31.
60. Rakoff, *Audio-Digest.*
61. Rakoff, *Audio-Digest.*
62. Rakoff, *Audio-Digest.*

Table of Measurements

Measurements in medicine are given in terms of centimeters. A doctor might, for instance, refer to a tumor as being 2 cm, which means that it is 2 cm in diameter at its greatest width. One inch equals 2.54 centimeters (cm). The following table will help you understand the measurements used in this book.

Centimeters	Inches	Approximate Diameter
1 cm	.3937 inch, or about 1/3″	Slightly larger than a pea
2 cm	.7874 inch, or about 3/4″	About the same as a cherry or a nickel
3 cm	1.811 inch, or about 1-1/5″	About the same as a Ping-Pong ball or a half-dollar
4 cm	1.5748 inch, or about 1-1/2″	About the same as a golf ball
5 cm	1.9685 inch, or about 2″	About the same as a chicken's egg
6 cm	2.3622 inch, or about 2-1/3″	About the same as a plum
7 cm	2.7559 inch, or about 2-3/4″	About the same as a peach
8 cm	3.1496 inch, or about 3-1/6″	About the same as a tomato
9 cm	3.5432 inch, or about 3-1/2″	About the same as a baseball
10 cm	3.937 inch, or about 4″	About the same as a navel orange
11 cm	4.3307 inch, or about 4-1/3″	About the same as a softball
12 cm	4.7244 inch, or about 4-3/4″	About the same as a grapefruit

Women's Clinics Where You Can Obtain a Speculum*

CALIFORNIA

Berkeley Women's Health Collective
2908 Ellsworth
Berkeley, CA 94705
(415) 843-6194 or 843-6195

Chico Feminist Women's Health Center
330 Flume Street
Chico, CA 95926
(916) 891-1911

Oakland Feminist Women's Health Center
2930 McClure Street
Oakland, CA 94609
(415) 444-5676

Our Health Center
270 Grant Avenue
Palo Alto, CA 94306
(415) 327-8717

Everywoman's Clinic
1936 Linda Drive
Pleasant Hill, CA 94532
(415) 825-7900

Womancare, A Feminist Women's Health
Center
424 Pennsylvania Avenue
San Diego, CA 92103
(714) 298-9352

Buena Vista Women's Medical Services
Buena Vista Counseling Center
2000 Van Ness Avenue
San Francisco, CA 94109
(415) 771-5000 or (415) 441-1204

San Francisco Women's Health Center
3789 24th Street
San Francisco, CA 94114
(415) 282-6999

Women's Needs Center
1698 Haight Street
San Francisco, CA 94117
(415) 621-1003

Women's Community Clinic
696 East Santa Clara Street
San Jose, CA 95112
(408) 287-4322

*Some of these organizations have self-help groups; some provide instruction on an individual basis; still others will refer you to local sources.

Santa Cruz Women's Health Collective
250 Locust Street
Santa Cruz, CA 95060
(408) 427-3500

COLORADO

Women's Health Service Clinic
111 East Dale
Colorado Springs, CO 80903
(303) 471-9492

FLORIDA

Gainesville Women's Health Center
805 South West 4th Avenue
Gainesville, FL 32601
(904) 377-5055

Feminist Women's Health Center
540 West Brevard Street, Suite C
Tallahassee, FL 32301
(904) 224-9600

GEORGIA

Feminist Women's Health Center
580 14th Street, North West
Atlanta, GA 30318
(404) 874-7551

HAWAII

Women's Health Center of Hawaii, Inc.
2500 Pali Highway
Honolulu, HI 96815
(808) 595-2506

Mailing address:
P. O. Box 17652
Honolulu, HI 96817

ILLINOIS

Chicago Women's Health Center
3435 North Sheffield
Chicago, IL 60657
(312) 935-6126

Emma Goldman Women's Health Center
1628 West Belmont
Chicago, IL 60657
(313) 528-4310

IOWA

Cedar Rapids Clinic for Women
86½ 16th Avenue, South West
Cedar Rapids, IA 52404
(319) 365-9527

Emma Goldman Clinic for Women
715 North Dodge
Iowa City, IA 52240
(319) 337-2111

MASSACHUSETTS

Everywoman's Center
Wilder Hall
University of Massachusetts
Amherst, MA 01003
(413) 545-0883

Women's Health Project
73 Union Avenue
Framingham, MA 01701
(617) 872-0711

Women's Community Health Center, Inc.
639 Massachusetts Avenue
Cambridge, MA 02139
(617) 547-2302

Family Planning of Hyannis
Cape Cod Medical Center
Hyannis, MA 02601
(617) 771-8010

Health Information Referral Service, Inc.
(H.I.R.S.)
P. O. Box 160
Marlboro, MA 01752
(617) 481-8290

New Bedford Women's Center
—Health Project
252 County Street
New Bedford, MA 02740
(617) 996-3341

814

MICHIGAN

Woman's Health and Information Project
Box 110 Warriner Hall
Central Michigan University
Mt. Pleasant, MI 48858
(517) 774-3151

MONTANA

Blue Mountain Women's Clinic
218 East Front
Missoula, MT 59801
(406) 542-0029

NEW HAMPSHIRE

New Hampshire Feminist Health Center
38 South Main Street
Concord, NH 03301
(603) 225-2739

and

232 Court Street
Portsmouth, NH 03801
(603) 436-7588

NEW JERSEY

Livingston Self-Help Group
Livingston College
Rutgers University
New Brunswick, NJ 08903
(201) 932-4333

NEW MEXICO

Women's Health Services
316 East Marcy Street
Santa Fe, NM 87501
(505) 988-8869

NEW YORK

Binghamton Women's Health Care Project
c/o Women's Center
P. O. Box 354
Binghamton, NY 13902
(607) 723-3200

Ithaca Women's Resource Center
112 The Commons
Ithaca, NY 14850
(607) 272-6922

Feminist Health Works
487-A Hudson Street
New York, NY 10014
(212) 929-7886

The Lesbian Health Collective
St. Marks Clinic
44 St. Marks Place
New York, NY 10003
(212) 533-9500/9501

Women's Health Alliance
of Long Island, Inc.
Health House
555 North Country Road
St. James, NY 11780
(516) 862-6743

OREGON

Ashland Community Health Center
295 East Main Street, No. 15
Ashland, OR 97520
(503) 482-9741

Portland Women's Health Center
6510 South East Foster
Portland, OR 97206
(503) 777-7044

PENNSYLVANIA

Elizabeth Blackwell Health Center
for Women
112 South 16th Street
Philadelphia, PA 19102
(215) 563-7577

Cindy Goldstein
258 Toftrees, No. 213
State College, PA 16801
(814) 234-8430

RHODE ISLAND

The Rhode Island Health Collective
2 Stimson Avenue
Providence, RI 02906
(401) 274-9264

TEXAS

Brookside Women's Medical Center
1902 South I H 35
Austin, TX 78704
(512) 443-9595

Houston Women's Health Collective
c/o Nancy Kern
2804 Morrison Street
Houston, TX 77009
(713) 523-6494

VERMONT

Planned Parenthood of Vermont
—Barre Center
24 Spauling Street
Barre, VT 05641
(802) 476-6696

Vermont Women's Health Center
P. O. Box 29
336 North Avenue
Burlington, VT 05401
(802) 863-1388

WASHINGTON

Blackwell Women's Health Resource Center
1520 North State Street
Bellingham, WA 98225
(206) 734-8592

Aradia Women's Health Center
1827 12th Avenue
Seattle, WA 98122
(206) 323-9388

Abortion and Birth Control Referral Service
4224 University Way, North East
Seattle, WA 98105
(206) 634-3460

Freemont Women's Clinic
6817 Greenwood Avenue North
Seattle, WA 98103
(206) 789-0773

WASHINGTON, D.C.

Washington Free Clinic
16th and Newton Streets, North West
Washington, DC 20010
(202) 667-1106

WISCONSIN

Bread & Roses Women's Health Center
238 West Wisconsin Avenue, No. 700
Milwaukee, WI 53203
(414) 278-0260

Cervical Cap Providers

CALIFORNIA

*Berkeley Women's Health Collective
2908 Ellsworth Street
Berkeley, CA 94705
(415) 843-6194 or 843-6195

Wholistic Health and Nutrition Institute
Nurse Practitioner—Sandy Stallinga, FPNP
150 Shoreline Hwy.
Mill Valley, CA 94901
(415) 332-2933

*Feminist Women's Health Center
6411 Hollywood Blvd.
Los Angeles, CA 90028
(213) 469-4844

*Renee Potik, RNNP
6333 Wilshire Blvd., Suite 101
Los Angeles, CA 90048
(213) 658-8224

Women's Needs Center
1698 Haight St.
San Francisco, CA 94117
(415) 621-1003

FLORIDA

Gainesville Women's Health Center
805 S.W. 4th Ave.
Gainesville, FL 32601

*Feminist Women's Health Center
540 W. Brevard St., Suite C
Tallahassee, FL 32301
(904) 224-9600

GEORGIA

Feminist Women's Health Center
580 14th Street, N.W.
Atlanta, GA 30318
(404) 874-7551

HAWAII

Women's Health Center of Hawaii
2500 Pali Highway
Honolulu, HI 96815
(808) 595-2506

*The asterisk indicates that these groups or individuals also provide training in fitting caps.

ILLINOIS

Chicago Women's Health Center
3435 N. Sheffield
Chicago, IL 60657
(312) 935-6126

IOWA

*Emma Goldman Clinic for Women
715 N. Dodge Street
Iowa City, IA 52240
(319) 337-2111

Cedar Rapids Clinic for Women
86½ 16th Ave., S.W.
Cedar Rapids, IA 52404
(319) 365-9527

MASSACHUSETTS

James P. Koch, M.D., and Associates
1037 Beacon Street
Boston, MA 02146
(617) 277-2151

*Family Practice Group
2464 Massachusetts Ave.
Cambridge, MA 02140
(617) 661-0951

Joan E. Richards, C.N.M.
8 East St.
Ipswich, MA 01938
(617) 356-0447

*Fran Ventre, C.N.M.
16 Summit Place
Newburyport, MA 01950
(617) 462-3169

Phyllis H. Smith, RNC-NP
Hampshire Obstetrical and Gynecological
   Associates, Inc.
264 Elm St.
Northampton, MA 01060
(413) 584-2303

NEW HAMPSHIRE

*Carol Leonard, Midwife
114 S. State St.
Concord, NH 03301
(603) 225-9586

Kenneth L. McKinney, Jr., M.D.
Deborah A. Black, CNM
33 Warren St.
Concord, NH 03301
(603) 228-0134

New Hampshire Feminist Health Center
38 South Main Street
Concord, NH 03301

Gerald T. Hamilton, M.D.
Christine F. Kuhlman, C.N.M.
OB-GYN Unlimited, Prof. Assn.
35 West St.
Concord, NH 03301
(603) 224-0000

*Marilyn Grainger-Harrison, Certified
   Nurse Midwife
271 Washington St.
Dover, NH 03820
(603) 749-4737

Strafford County Prenatal and Family
   Planning Program
791 Central Ave.
Dover, NH 03820
(603) 749-2346

Gary W. Lamphere, M.D.
Exeter Clinic
Exeter, NH 03833
(603) 772-4791

Barbara Brungot, PA-C
Gorham Medical Center
Gorham, NH 03581
(603) 466-2741

*Irene C. Snair, R.N.N.P.
New England College Health Center
Henniker, NH 03242
(603) 428-2253

*Jane N. Spragg, M.D.
Mill and Bridge Streets
Hillsborough, NH 03244
(603) 464-3327

Brian A. Beattie, M.D.
Box 32, North Road
Lancaster, NH 03584
(603) 788-2521

Ammonoosuc Family Planning Program,
  Inc.
19 Cottage St.
Littleton, NH 03561
(603) 444-2464

John M. Lewis, M.D.
93 Cottage St.
Littleton, NH 03561
(603) 444-6742

Newmarket Regional Health Center
14 Elm St.
Newmarket, NH 03857
(603) 659-3106

NEW MEXICO

*Women's Health Services
316 E. Marcy St.
Santa Fe, NM 87501
(505) 988-8869

NEW YORK

*Dr. Hans Lehfeldt
Clinical Professor, Dept. of Obstetrics and
  Gynecology
New York University School of Medicine
784 Park Ave.
New York, NY 10021
(212) 744-6880

OREGON

Sarah Hendrickson, M.D.
132 E. Broadway, No. 337
Euguene, OR 97401

*Dr. Barbara Rassow, Chiropractor
3339 NE Wasco St.
Portland, OR 97232
(503) 231-7586

PENNSYLVANIA

Elizabeth Blackwell Health Center for
  Women
112 S. 16th Street
Philadelphia, PA 19102
(215) 563-7577

VERMONT

*Vermont Women's Health Center, Inc.
P. O. Box 29
Burlington, VT 05402
(802) 863-1386

*The Holistic Health Center
A. August Burns, P.A./Gyn.
15 Pitkin Ct.
Montpelier, VT 05602
(802) 229-4636

Emma Wennberg, M.D./
A. August Burns, P.A.
55 So. Main Street
Waterbury, VT 05676
(802) 229-4636

WASHINGTON

Freemont Women's Clinic
6817 Creenwood Avenue
Seattle, WA 98103
(206) 789-0773

WISCONSIN

*Bread & Roses Women's Health Center,
  Inc.
238 W. Wisconsin Ave., Suite 700
Milwaukee, WI 53203
(414) 278-0260

Planned Parenthood Chapters

ALABAMA

BIRMINGHAM
Planned Parenthood of Alabama
1108 South 20th St. *(M)* (35256)
(205) 933-8444

ALASKA

ANCHORAGE
(See Rocky Mt. Planned Parenthood,
Denver, Colorado)

ARIZONA

PHOENIX
Planned Parenthood of Central & Northern
Arizona
1301 South Seventh Ave. *(M)* (85007)
(602) 257-1515

TUCSON
Planned Parenthood of Southern Arizona,
Inc.
127 South Fifth Ave. *(M)* (85701)
(602) 624-1761

CALIFORNIA

DAVIS
Planned Parenthood Assn. of Yolo County
116 B St., Suite B *(M)* 95616)
(916) 758-4592

EUREKA
Planned Parenthood of Humboldt County
2316 Harrison Ave. *(M)* (95501)
(707) 442-5709

FRESNO
Planned Parenthood of Fresno
633 No. Van Ness *(M)* (93728)
(209) 486-2411

LOS ANGELES
Planned Parenthood—World Population/Los
Angeles
3100 West Eighth St. *(M)* (90005)
(213) 380-9300

MONTEREY
Planned Parenthood of Monterey County,
Inc.
5 Via Joaquin *(M)* (93940)
(408) 373-1691 or 373-1709

(M) Medical   (E) Educational   (P) Provisional

PASADENA
Pasadena Planned Parenthood Committee, Inc.
1045 North Lake Ave. *(M)* (91104)
(213) 798-0708

SACRAMENTO
Planned Parenthood Assn. of Sacramento
Midtown Building, Suite 100
1507 21st St. *(M)* (95814)
(916) 446-5034

SAN DIEGO
Planned Parenthood of San Diego County
2100 Fifth Ave. *(M)* (92101)
(714) 231-1282

SAN FRANCISCO
Planned Parenthood Alameda—San Francisco
1660 Bush St. *(M)* (94109)
(415) 441-5454

SAN JOSE
Planned Parenthood Assn. of Santa Clara County
17 North San Pedro *(M)* (95110)
(408) 287-7526 or 287-7532

SAN MATEO
Planned Parenthood Assn. of San Mateo County
2211—2215 Palm Ave. *(M)* (94403)
(415) 574-2622

SAN RAFAEL
Planned Parenthood Assn. of Marin County
20 H St. *(M)* (94901)
(415) 454-0471

SANTA ANA
Planned Parenthood Assn. of Orange County
1801 N. Broadway *(M)* (92706)
(714) 973-1727

SANTA BARBARA
Planned Parenthood of Santa Barbara County, Inc.
518 Garden St. *(M)* (93101)
(805) 963-5801

SANTA CRUZ
Planned Parenthood of Santa Cruz County
212 Laurel St. *(M)* (95060)
(408) 426-5550

STOCKTON
Planned Parenthood of San Joaquin County
19 N. Pilgrim St. *(M)* (95205)
(209) 466-2081

WALNUT CREEK
Planned Parenthood of Contra Costa County, Inc.
1291 Oakland Blvd. *(M)* (94596)
(415) 935-3010

COLORADO

DENVER
Rocky Mountain Planned Parenthood
1525 Josephine *(M)* (80206)
(303) 321-2400

Anchorage, Alaska (Associate)
Planned Parenthood of Alaska *(M)*
2820 C St., Suite 3, Anchorage 99503
(907) 279-2576/7

Springfield, Missouri (Associate)
The Greater Springfield Planned Parenthood Assn., Inc. *(M)*
1918 E. Meadowmere, Springfield 65804
(417) 869-6471

CONNECTICUT

NEW HAVEN
Planned Parenthood League of Connecticut, Inc.
129 Whitney Ave. *(M)* (06510)
(203) 865-0595

Bridgeport Chapter
Planned Parenthood League of Connecticut, Inc.
Bridgeport Chapter *(M)*
1067 Park Ave., Bridgeport 06604
(203) 366-0664

(M) Medical   (E) Educational   (P) Provisional

Danbury Chapter
Planned Parenthood League of Connecticut,
  Inc.
Danbury Chapter *(M)*
44 Main St., Danbury 06810
(203) 743-2446

Greater Hartford Chapter
Planned Parenthood League of Connecticut,
  Inc.
Greater Hartford Chapter *(M)*
297 Farmington Ave., Hartford 06105
(203) 522-6201

Middlesex Chapter
Planned Parenthood League of Connecticut,
  Inc.
Middlesex Chapter *(M)*
45 Broad St., Middletown 06457
(203) 347-5255

Greater New Haven Chapter
Planned Parenthood League of Connecticut,
  Inc.
Greater New Haven Chapter *(M)*
129 Whitney Ave., New Haven 06510
(203) 865-0595

Northeast Chapter
Planned Parenthood League of Connecticut,
  Inc.
Northeast Chapter *(M)*
791 Main St., Willimantic 06226
(203) 423-8426

Northwest Chapter
Planned Parenthood League of Connecticut,
  Inc.
Northwest Chapter *(M)*
27 Pearl St., Torrington 06790
(203) 489-5500

Southeast Chapter
Planned Parenthood League of Connecticut,
  Inc.
Southeast Chapter *(M)*
420 Williams St., New London 06320
(203) 443-5820

Southern Fairfield Chapter
Planned Parenthood League of Connecticut,
  Inc.
Southern Fairfield Chapter *(M)*
80 Lincoln Ave., Stamford 06902
(203) 327-2722

Waterbury Chapter
Planned Parenthood League of Connecticut,
  Inc.
Waterbury Chapter *(M)*
125 Grove St., Waterbury 06702
(203) 753-2110

DELAWARE

WILMINGTON
Delaware League for Planned Parenthood
825 Washington St. *(M)* (19801)
(302) 655-7293 or 652-3948

DISTRICT OF COLUMBIA

WASHINGTON
Planned Parenthood of Metropolitan
  Washington, D.C.
1108 16th St., N.W. *(M)* (20036)
(202) 347-8500

Washington, D.C. Chapter
Planned Parenthood—Washington, D.C.
  Chapter *(M)*
1108 16th St., N.W.
Washington, D.C. 20036

Montgomery County Chapter
Planned Parenthood of Metropolitan
  Washington, D.C., Montgomery Co.
  Chapter *(M)*
Randolph Medical Center, Suite 209
4701 Randolph Road
Rockville, Maryland 20852
(301) 468-7676

(M) Medical   *(E) Educational*   *(P) Provisional*

823

Prince George's County Chapter
Planned Parenthood of Prince George
  County *(M)*
Landover Mall, East Tower Building No. 203
Landover, Maryland 20785
(301) 773-5601

Northern Virginia Chapter
Planned Parenthood of Northern Virginia
  (M)
5622 Columbia Pike
Falls Church, Virginia 22041
(703) 820-3335

FLORIDA

BOCA RATON
Planned Parenthood of South Palm Beach &
  Broward Counties, Inc.
160 N.W. 4th St. *(P) (M)*
(33432)
(305) 368-1023

GAINESVILLE
Planned Parenthood of North Central
  Florida, Inc.
P. O. Box 12385 *(E)* (32604)
(904) 377-0881

JACKSONVILLE
Planned Parenthood of Northeast Florida,
  Inc.
828 San Marco Boulevard *(M)* (32207)
(904) 398-2618

LAKELAND
Planned Parenthood of Central Florida, Inc.
1104 N. Dakota Ave. *(P) (M)* (33805)
(813) 688-2646

OPA LOCKA
Planned Parenthood Assn. of South Florida
3400 N.W. 135th St. *(M)* (33054)
(305) 685-7571

SARASOTA
Planned Parenthood of Southwest Florida
1958 Prospect St. *(M)* (33579)
(813) 953-4060/1 or 365-3913/4

Naples Chapter
Planned Parenthood—Naples Center *(M)*
482 Tamiami Trail N., Naples 33940
(813) 262-0301

TALLAHASSEE
Planned Parenthood of Tallahassee, Inc.
1834 Mahan Drive *(P) (E)* (32308)
(904) 877-1766

WEST PALM BEACH
Planned Parenthood Palm Beach Area
800 N. Olive *(M)* (33401)
(305) 655-7984

GEORGIA

ATLANTA
Planned Parenthood Assn. of Atlanta Area
15 Peachtree St. N.E., Suite 909 *(M)* (30303)
(404) 688-9300

AUGUSTA
Planned Parenthood of East Central
  Georgia, Inc.
1289 Broad St. *(M)* (30902)
(404) 724-5557

HAWAII

HONOLULU
Hawaii Planned Parenthood, Inc.
1164 Bishop St., 12th Floor *(M)* (96813)
(808) 521-6991

IDAHO

BOISE
Planned Parenthood Assn. of Idaho, Inc.
214 E. Jefferson St. *(M)* (83702)
(208) 345-0760

(M) Medical   *(E) Educational*   *(P) Provisional*

ILLINOIS

BLOOMINGTON
Planned Parenthood of Mid Central Illinois, Inc.
McBarnes Memorial Building
201 E. Grove St., 2nd Floor *(M)* (61701)
(309) 827-8025

CHAMPAIGN
Planned Parenthood of Champaign County
314 S. Neil St. *(M)* (61820)
(217) 359-8022

CHICAGO
Planned Parenthood Assn.—Chicago Area
55 East Jackson Blvd. *(M)* (60604)
(312) 322-4200

DECATUR
Planned Parenthood of Decatur, Inc.
988—990 S. Main St. *(M)* (62521)
(217) 429-9211

PEORIA
Planned Parenthood Assn. of Peoria Area
530 Fulton St. *(M)* (61602)
(309) 673-0907

SPRINGFIELD
Planned Parenthood—Springfield Area
500 E. Capitol, 3rd Floor *(M)* (62701)
(217) 544-2744

INDIANA

BLOOMINGTON
Planned Parenthood of South Central Indiana
421 South College Ave. *(M)* (47401)
(812) 336-0219

EVANSVILLE
Planned Parenthood of Southwestern Indiana
1610 South Weinbach Ave. *(M)* (47714)
(812) 479-1466

FORT WAYNE
Planned Parenthood of Northeastern Indiana
347 W. Berry, Suite 300 *(M)* (46802)
(219) 423-1322

INDIANAPOLIS
Planned Parenthood Assn. of Indianapolis, Inc.
615 North Alabama St., Room 332 *(M)* (46204)
(317) 637-8230

LAFAYETTE
Tecumseh Area Planned Parenthood Assn., Inc.
P. O. Box 1159
1016 E. Main *(M)* (47902)
(317) 742-9073

MERRILLVILLE
Planned Parenthood of Northwest Indiana, Inc.
8645 Connecticut *(M)* (46410)
(219) 769-3500

MUNCIE
Planned Parenthood of East Central Indiana, Inc.
110 N. Cherry at West Main *(M)* (47305)
(317) 282-8011

SOUTH BEND
Planned Parenthood of North Central Indiana
201 South Chapin *(M)* (46625)
(219) 289-7062

TERRE HAUTE
Planned Parenthood Assn. of Wabash Valley, Inc.
330 South 6th St. *(M)* (47808)
(812) 238-2636 or 232-0183

IOWA

CEDAR RAPIDS
Planned Parenthood of Linn County
212 Paramount Building
305 Second St., S.E. *(P) (M)* (52401)
(319) 363-8572

(M) Medical   (E) Educational   (P) Provisional

825

DES MOINES
Planned Parenthood of Mid Iowa
P. O. Box 4557 *(M)* (50306)
(515) 280-7000

MT. PLEASANT
Planned Parenthood of Southeast Iowa
125-½ W. Monroe *(M)* (52641)
(319) 385-8744

Burlington Chapter
Planned Parenthood of Des Moines County
 (M)
521 N. 5th, Burlington 52601
(319) 753-2281

Fort Madison Chapter
Planned Parenthood of North Lee County
 (M)
631 Avenue H, Fort Madison 52627
(319) 372-1130

Keokuk Chapter
Planned Parenthood of South Lee County
 (M)
927 Exchange St., Keokuk 52632
(319) 524-2759

Mt. Pleasant Chapter
Planned Parenthood of Henry County *(M)*
125-½ W. Monroe, Mt. Pleasant 52641
(319) 385-4310

Washington Chapter
Planned Parenthood of Washington County
 (E)
P. O. Box 44,
Clara Barton & 4th, Washington 52353
(319) 653-3525

SIOUX CITY
Planned Parenthood Committee of Sioux
 City
2825 Douglas St. *(M)* (51104)
(712) 277-3332

KANSAS

WICHITA
Planned Parenthood of Kansas
2226 E. Central *(M)* (67214)
(316) 263-7575

Hays Chapter
Planned Parenthood—Hays Chapter *(M)*
1012 Cody, Hays 67601
(913) 628-2434

KENTUCKY

BEREA
Mountain Maternal Health League
P. O. Box 429 *(M)* (40403)
(606) 986-4677

LEXINGTON
Lexington Planned Parenthood Center, Inc.
508 West Second St. *(M)* (40507)
(606) 252-8494

LOUISVILLE
Planned Parenthood of Louisville, Inc.
834 E. Broadway, Suite 506 *(M)* (40204)
(502) 584-2471

MARYLAND

BALTIMORE
Planned Parenthood Assn. of Maryland, Inc.
610 North Howard St. *(M)* (21201)
(301) 752-0131

Montgomery County Chapter
(See District of Columbia)

Prince George's County Chapter
(See District of Columbia)

MASSACHUSETTS

CAMBRIDGE
Planned Parenthood League of
 Massachusetts
99 Bishop Richard Allen Dr. *(E)* (02139)
(617) 492-0518

MICHIGAN

ANN ARBOR
Washtenaw County League for Planned
 Parenthood
912 N. Main St. *(M)* (48104)
(313) 769-8530

(M) Medical   (E) Educational   (P) Provisional

BENTON HARBOR
Planned Parenthood Assn. of Southwestern
  Michigan
785 Pipestone *(M)* (49022)
(616) 925-1306

DETROIT
Planned Parenthood League, Inc.
13100 Puritan *(M)* (48227)
(313) 861-6700

FLINT
Flint Community Planned Parenthood Assn.
310 E. Third St., Y.W.C.A. *(M)* (48503)
(313) 238-3631

Owosso Chapter
Shiawassee County Planned Parenthood
  Assn. *(E)*
P. O. Box 542, Owosso (48867)
(517) 723-6420

GRAND RAPIDS
Planned Parenthood Centers of West
  Michigan
425 Cherry, S.E. *(M)* (49503)
(616) 774-7005

Ionia Chapter
Planned Parenthood of Ionia County *(M)*
111 Kidd St., Ionia 48846
(616) 527-3250

KALAMAZOO
Reproductive Health Care Center of South
  Central Michigan, An Affiliate of PPFA,
  Inc.
4201 W. Michigan Ave. *(M)* (49007)
(616) 372-1200

MARQUETTE
Marquette-Alger Planned Parenthood
102 Harlow Block *(P) (M)* (49855)
(906) 225-5070

MUSKEGON
Muskegon Area Planned Parenthood Assn.,
  Inc.
1642 Peck *(M)* (49441)
(616) 722-2928

PETOSKEY
Northern Michigan Planned Parenthood
  Assn.
Lockwood Division, N.M.H.
820 Arlington *(M)* (49770)
(616) 347-9692

MINNESOTA

ST. PAUL
Planned Parenthood of Minnesota, Inc.
1965 Ford Parkway *(M)* (55116)
(612) 698-2401 or 646-9603

Bemidji Chapter
Planned Parenthood of Bemidji Area *(E)*
411-½ Beltrami, Bemidji (56601)
(218) 751-8683

Brainerd Chapter
Central Minnesota Planned Parenthood *(M)*
507 Washington, Brainerd (56401)
(218) 829-1469

Duluth Chapter
Planned Parenthood of Northeast Minnesota
  (M)
Arrowhead Place
211 West 2nd, 4th Floor, Duluth 55802
(218) 722-0833

Mankato Chapter
South Central Planned Parenthood *(E)*
104 E. Liberty, Room 203, Mankato 56001
(507) 378-5581

Minneapolis Chapter
Planned Parenthood of Metropolitan
  Minneapolis *(M)*
127 South 10th Street
Minneapolis, Minnesota 55403
(612) 336-8931

Rochester Chapter
Planned Parenthood of Rochester Area *(M)*
3-½ South Broadway, Rochester 55901
(507) 288-5186

(M) Medical   (E) Educational   (P) Provisional

St. Paul Chapter
Planned Parenthood of St. Paul Metro Area
   (M)
110 Hamm Building
408 St. Peter St., St. Paul 55102
(612) 224-1361

Willmar Chapter
Planned Parenthood of Western Minnesota
   (M)
Bonde Building, 2nd Floor
Fourth St. & Litchfield Ave., Willmar 56201
(612) 235-9150

MISSOURI

COLUMBIA
Planned Parenthood of Central Missouri
800 North Providence Rd., Suite 5 *(M)*
   (65201)
(314) 449-2475

KANSAS CITY
Planned Parenthood Assn. of Western
   Missouri/Kansas
1001 E. 47th St. *(M)* (64110)
(816) 756-2277

KIRKSVILLE
Planned Parenthood of Northeast Missouri
   Inc.
P. O. Box 763 *(M)* (63501)
(816) 665-5674

ROLLA
Planned Parenthood of the Central Ozarks
Box 359, 1032B Kings Highway *(M)* (65401)
(314) 364-1509

SPRINGFIELD
(See Rocky Mt. Planned Parenthood
Denver, Colorado)

ST. LOUIS
Planned Parenthood Assn. of St. Louis
2202 South Hanley Rd. *(M)* (63144)
(314) 781-3800

MONTANA

BILLINGS
Planned Parenthood of Billings
2722 Montana Ave. *(M)* (59101)
(406) 248-3636

MISSOULA
Missoula Planned Parenthood
235 E. Pine *(M)* (59801)
(406) 728-5490

NEBRASKA

LINCOLN
Planned Parenthood of Lincoln
3830 Adams St. *(M)* (68504)
(402) 467-4691

OMAHA
Planned Parenthood of Omaha-Council
   Bluffs
4610 Dodge *(M)* (68132)
(402) 554-1045

NEVADA

LAS VEGAS
Planned Parenthood of Southern Nevada,
   Inc.
601 S, 13th St. *(M)* (89101)
(702) 385-3451

RENO
Planned Parenthood of Northern Nevada
406 Elm St. *(M)* (89503)
(702) 329-1781

NEW HAMPSHIRE

LEBANON
Planned Parenthood Assn. of Upper Valley
127 Mascoma St. *(M)* (03766)
(603) 448-1214

(M) Medical   *(E) Educational*   *(P) Provisional*

NEW JERSEY

CAMDEN
Planned Parenthood-Greater Camden Area
590 Benson St. *(M)* (08103)
(609) 365-3519

HACKENSACK
Planned Parenthood Center of Bergen
  County
575 Main St. *(M)* (07601)
(201) 489-1140

MORRISTOWN
Planned Parenthood of Northwest New
  Jersey, Inc.
197 Speedwell Ave. *(M)* (07960)
(201) 539-9580

NEWARK
Planned Parenthood-Essex County
15 William St. *(M)* (07102)
(201) 622-3900

NEW BRUNSWICK
Planned Parenthood League of Middlesex
  County
84 Carroll Pl. *(M)* (08901)
(201) 246-2411

PATERSON
Passaic County Planned Parenthood Center
175 Market St. *(M)* (07505)
(201) 274-3883

PLAINFIELD
Planned Parenthood of Union County Area,
  Inc.
234 Park Avenue *(M)* (07060)
(201) 756-3736

SHREWSBURY
Planned Parenthood of Monmouth County,
  Inc.
69 Newman Springs Rd. *(M)* (07701)
(201) 842-9300

TRENTON
Planned Parenthood Assn. of the Mercer
  Area
437 E. State St. *(M)* (08608)
(609) 599-3736 or 599-4881

NEW MEXICO

ALBUQUERQUE
Rio Grande Planned Parenthood
113 Montclaire, S.E. *(M)* (87108)
(505) 265-5976

LAS CRUCES
Planned Parenthood of South Central New
  Mexico
302 West Griggs Avenue *(M)* (88001)
(505) 524-8516

SILVER CITY
Planned Parenthood of Southwest New
  Mexico
110 East 11th *(M)* (88061)
(505) 388-1553

NEW YORK

ALBANY
Planned Parenthood of Albany & Rensselaer
  Counties, Inc.
259 Lark St. *(M)* (12210)
(518) 434-2182

BINGHAMTON
Planned Parenthood of Broome & Chenango
  Counties, Inc.
710 O'Neill Bldg. *(M)* (13901)
(607) 723-8306

BUFFALO
Planned Parenthood Center of Buffalo
210 Franklin St. *(M)* (14202)
(716) 853-1771

ELMIRA
Planned Parenthood of the Southern Tier
200 East Market St. *(M)* (14901)
(607) 734-3313

GENEVA
Planned Parenthood of the Finger Lakes,
  Inc.
435 Exchange St. *(M)* (14456)
(315) 781-1092

(M) Medical   (E) Educational   (P) Provisional

829

GLENS FALLS
Southern Adirondack Planned Parenthood
  Assn.
144 Ridge St. *(M)* (12801)
(518) 798-8999

HUNTINGTON
Planned Parenthood of Suffolk County
17 East Carver St. *(M)* (11743)
(516) 427-7154

ITHACA
Planned Parenthood of Tompkins County
512 East State St. *(M)* (14850)
(607) 273-1513

MINEOLA
Planned Parenthood of Nassau County
107 Mineola Boulevard *(M)* (11501)
(516) 742-0144

NEWBURGH
Planned Parenthood of Orange-Sullivan, In.
91 DuBois St. *(M)* (12550)
(914) 562-5748

NEW YORK
Planned Parenthood of New York City, Inc.
380 Second Ave., Third Floor *(M)* (10010)
(212) 777-2002

NIAGARA FALLS
Planned Parenthood of Niagara County
906 Michigan Ave. *(M)* (14305)
(716) 282-1223/4

ONEONTA
Planned Parenthood Assn. of Delaware &
  Otsego Counties, Inc.
48 Market St. *(M)* (13820)
(607) 432-2250

PLATTSBURGH
Planned Parenthood of Clinton County
66 Brinkerhoff St. *(M)* (12901)
(518) 561-4430

POUGHKEEPSIE
Planned Parenthood of Dutchess—Ulster,
  Inc.
85 Market St. *(M)* (12601)
(914) 471-1540

ROCHESTER
Planned Parenthood of Rochester & Monroe
  Counties, Inc.
24 Windsor St. *(M)* (14605)
(716) 546-2595

SCHENECTADY
Planned Parenthood of Schenectady &
  Affiliated Counties, Inc.
414 Union St. *(M)* (12305)
(518) 374-5353

SYRACUSE
Planned Parenthood Center of Syracuse, Inc.
1120 E. Genesee St. *(M)* (13210)
(315) 424-8260

UTICA
Planned Parenthood Assn. of Mohawk
  Valley, Inc.
1424 Genesee St. *(M)* (13502)
(315) 724-6146

WATERTOWN
Planned Parenthood of Northern New York,
  Inc.
161 Stone St. *(M)* (13601)
(315) 782-1818

Canton Chapter
St. Lawrence County Planned Parenthood
  (M)
E. J. Noble Medical Center
80 E. Main St., Canton 13617
(315) 386-2441

Lowville Chapter
Lewis County Planned Parenthood *(M)*
7552 State St., Lowville (13367)
(315) 376-2741

Malone Chapter
Franklin County Planned Parenthood *(M)*
109 East Main St., Malone (12953)
(518) 483-7150

Watertown Chapter
Jefferson County Planned Parenthood *(M)*
161 Stone St., Watertown (13601)
(315) 788-8065

(M) Medical   (E) Educational   (P) Provisional

WEST NYACK
Planned Parenthood of Rockland County
37 Village Square *(M)* (10994)
(914) 358-1145

WHITE PLAINS
Planned Parenthood of Westchester, Inc.
Administrative Offices—Upper Level
88 East Post Road *(M)* (10601)
(914) 428-7876

NORTH CAROLINA

ASHEVILLE
Planned Parenthood of Asheville/Buncombe
County
P. O. Box 1348 *(E)* (28802)
(704) 252-7928

CHARLOTTE

Planned Parenthood of Greater Charlotte
East Independence Plaza Bldg.
951 S. Independence Blvd., Ste. 430 *(M)*
(28202)
(704) 377-0841

WINSTON-SALEM
Planned Parenthood of Greater Winston-
Salem
129 Fayette St. *(P) (M)* (27101)
(919) 761-1052

OHIO

AKRON
Planned Parenthood Assn. of Summit
County, Inc.
39 East Market St. *(M)* (44308)
(216) 535-2671

ATHENS
Planned Parenthood of Southeast Ohio
306 Security Bldg.
8 North Court St. *(M)* (45701)
(614) 593-3375

CANTON
Planned Parenthood of Stark County
626 Walnut Ave., N.E. *(M)* (44702)
(216) 456-7191

CINCINNATI
Planned Parenthood Assn. of Cincinnati
2406 Auburn Ave. *(M)* (45219)
(513) 721-7993

CLEVELAND
Planned Parenthood of Cleveland, Inc.
2027 Cornell Road *(M)* (44106)
(216) 721-4700

Elyria Chapter
Maternal Health Assn. of Lorain County
(M)
266 Washington Ave., Elyria 44035
(216) 322-9874

COLUMBUS
Planned Parenthood of Central Ohio, Inc.
206 East State St. *(M)* (43215)
(614) 224-2235

Circleville Chapter
Pickaway Family Planning Assn. *(M)*
Berger Hospital
600 N. Pickaway, Circleville (43113)
(614) 374-5143

DAYTON
Planned Parenthood Assn. of Miami Valley
224 N. Wilkinson St. *(M)* (45402)
(513) 226-0780

HAMILTON
Planned Parenthood Assn. of Butler Co., Inc.
P. O. Box 631, 11 Ludlow St. *(M)* (45012)
(513) 894-3875

MANSFIELD
Planned Parenthood Assn. of Mansfield
Area
35 North Park St. *(M)* (44902)
(419) 525-3075

Galion Chapter
Planned Parenthood Assn. of Crawford
County *(M)*
270 Portland Way South, Galion 44833
(419) 468-9926

(M) Medical   *(E) Educational*   *(P) Provisional*

831

Wooster Chapter
Planned Parenthood of Wayne County *(M)*
2680-½ Cleveland Road, Wooster 44691
(216) 345-7798

NEWARK
Planned Parenthood Assn. of East Central
  Ohio
Newark Medical Center
843 N. 21st St. *(M)* (43055)
(614) 366-3377

SPRINGFIELD
Planned Parenthood of West Central Ohio
Arcue Building, 5th Floor
6 W. High St. *(M)* (45504)
(513) 325-6417

TOLEDO
Planned Parenthood of Greater Toledo, Inc.
1301 Jefferson *(M)* (43624)
(419) 255-1115

YOUNGSTOWN
Planned Parenthood of Mahoning Valley
105 East Boardman St. *(M)* (44503)
(216) 746-5662

OKLAHOMA

OKLAHOMA CITY
Planned Parenthood Assn. of Oklahoma City
10 N.E. 23rd St. *(M)* (73105)
(405) 528-2157

TULSA
Planned Parenthood of Northeastern
  Oklahoma
1007 S. Peoria *(M)* (74120)
(918) 587-1101

OREGON

CORVALLIS
Planned Parenthood of Benton County, Inc.
530 N.W. 27th St. *(E)* (97330)
(503) 757-1629

EUGENE
Planned Parenthood Assn. of Lane County
134 East 13th Ave. *(M)* (97401)
(503) 344-9411 or 344-1611

MEDFORD
Planned Parenthood of Jackson County
650 Royal Ave., Suite 18 *(M)* (97501)
(503) 773-8285

PORTLAND
Planned Parenthood Assn., Inc.
1200 S.E. Morrison *(M)* (97214)
(503) 234-5411

PENNSYLVANIA

ALLENTOWN
Planned Parenthood Assn. of Lehigh County
112 N. 13th St. *(M)* (18102)
(215) 439-1033

BRISTOL
Planned Parenthood Assn. of Bucks County
721 New Rodgers Rd. *(M)* (19007)
(215) 785-4591

EASTON
Planned Parenthood of Northampton
  County, Inc.
275 S. 21st St. *(M)* (18042)
(215) 253-7195

EAST STROUDSBURG
Monroe County Planned Parenthood Assn.
162 E. Brown St. *(M)* (18301)
(717) 424-8306

JOHNSTOWN
Planned Parenthood Cambria/Somerset
502 Main St. *(M)* (15901)
(814) 535-5545

LANCASTER
Planned Parenthood of Lancaster
37 S. Lime St. *(M)* (17602)
(717) 299-2891

(M) Medical   *(E) Educational*   *(P) Provisional*

PHILADELPHIA
Planned Parenthood Assn. of Southeastern
  Pennsylvania
1220 Sansom St. *(M)* (19107)
(215) 629-2800

PITTSBURGH
Planned Parenthood Center of Pittsburgh,
  Inc.
102 9th St. *(M)* (15222)
(412) 434-8950

READING
Planned Parenthood Center of Berks County
48 South 4th St. *(M)* (19602)
(215) 376-8061

SCRANTON
Planned Parenthood Organization of
  Lackawanna County
207 Wyoming Ave., Suite 322 *(M)* (18503)
(717) 344-2626

WEST CHESTER
Planned Parenthood of Chester County
113 West Chestnut St. *(M)* (19380)
(215) 692-8080

WILKES—BARRE
Planned Parenthood of Luzerne County
63 North Franklin St. *(M)* (18701)
(717) 824-8921

YORK
Planned Parenthood of Central Pennsylvania
710 S. George St. *(M)* (17403)
(717) 845-9681

RHODE ISLAND

PROVIDENCE
Planned Parenthood of Rhode Island
187 Westminster Mall *(M)* (02903)
(401) 421-9620

SOUTH CAROLINA

COLUMBIA
Planned Parenthood of Central South
  Carolina
Kittrell Center
2711 Middleburg Dr., Suite 109 *(M)* (29204)
(803) 256-4908

TENNESSEE

KNOXVILLE
Planned Parenthood Assn. of Knox County
Lincoln American Insurance Building
2611 Magnolia Ave. *(M)* (37914)
(615) 522-0191

MEMPHIS
Memphis Planned Parenthood Assn., Inc.
1407 Union Ave. *(M)* (38104)
(901) 725-1717

NASHVILLE
Planned Parenthood Assn. of Nashville
University Plaza
112 21st Ave. South *(M)* (37203)
(615) 327-1066 or 327-1095

OAK RIDGE
Planned Parenthood Assn. of the Southern
  Mountains, Inc.
162 Ridgeway Center *(M)* (37830)
(615) 482-3406

TEXAS

AMARILLO
Panhandle Planned Parenthood Assn.
604 West Eighth St. *(M)* (79101)
(806) 372-8731

AUSTIN
Planned Parenthood Center of Austin
1823 E. 7th St. *(M)* (78702)
(512) 477-7050

(M) Medical   *(E) Educational*   *(P) Provisional*

833

BROWNSVILLE
Planned Parenthood of Cameron & Willacy
 Counties
15 E. Levee St. *(M)* (78520)
(512) 546-4571

CORPUS CHRISTI
South Texas Planned Parenthood Center
801 Elizabeth *(M)* (78404)
(512) 884-4352

EL PASO
Planned Parenthood Center of El Paso
214 West Franklin St. *(M)* (79901)
(915) 542-1919

FORT WORTH
Planned Parenthood of North Texas
327 S. Adams *(M)* (76104)
(817) 332-7966

HOUSTON
Planned Parenthood of Houston & Southeast
 Texas
3601 Fannin *(M)* (77004)
(713) 522-3976

KINGSVILLE
Planned Parenthood Assn. of Chaparral
 County
529 E. King
P. O. Box 1070 *(M)* (78363)
(512) 592-2201

LUBBOCK
Planned Parenthood Center of Lubbock
3821 22nd St.
P. O. Box 6193 *(M)* (79413)
(806) 795-7123

McALLEN
Planned Parenthood Assn. of Hidalgo
 County
1017 Pecan *(M)* (78501)
(512) 686-0585

ODESSA
Permian Basin Planned Parenthood, Inc.
910-B S. Grant St. *(M)* (79763)
(915) 563-2530

SAN ANGELO
Planned Parenthood Center of San Angelo
122 West Second St. *(M)* (76901)
(915) 655-9141

SAN ANTONIO
Planned Parenthood Center of San Antonio
106 Warren St. *(M)* (78212)
(512) 227-2227

WACO
The Central Texas Planned Parenthood
 Assn.
P. O. Box 6308, 1121 Ross Ave. *(M)* (76706)
(817) 754-2392

UTAH

SALT LAKE CITY
Planned Parenthood Assn. of Utah
Chapman Bldg.
28 East 2100 South *(M)* (84115)
(801) 487-8914

VERMONT

BURLINGTON
Planned Parenthood of Vermont
State Office
23 Mansfield Ave. *(M)* (05401)
(802) 862-9637

VIRGINIA

FALLS CHURCH
(See District of Columbia)

HAMPTON
Peninsula Planned Parenthood
1520 Aberdeen Rd., Room 304 *(M)* (23666)
(804) 826-2079

NORFOLK
Planned Parenthood of Tidewater Virginia,
 Inc.
712 Botetourt St. *(M)* (23507)
(804) 625-5591

(M) Medical　　*(E) Educational*　　*(P) Provisional*

RICHMOND
Virginia League for Planned Parenthood
1218 W. Franklin St. *(M)* (23220)
(804) 353-5516/18

Suffolk Chapter
Tri-County Area Planned Parenthood *(E)*
P. O. Box 1400, Suffolk 23434
(804) 539-3456

ROANOKE
Planned Parenthood of Roanoke Valley, In
309 Luck Ave. *(M)* (24016)
(703) 342-6741

WASHINGTON

BELLINGHAM
Mt. Baker Planned Parenthood
500 Grand Ave. *(M)* (98225)
(206) 734-9095

EVERETT
Planned Parenthood of Snohomish County
2730 Hoyt Ave. *(M)* (98201)
(206) 259-0096

KENNEWICK
Planned Parenthood of Benton-Franklin
Counties
P. O. Box 6842 *(M)* (99336)
(509) 586-2164

SEATTLE
Planned Parenthood of Seattle-King County
2211 East Madison *(M)* (98112)
(206) 447-2350 or 447-2364

SPOKANE
Planned Parenthood of Spokane
N. 507 Howard St. *(M)* (99201)
(509) 624-3271

TACOMA
Planned Parenthood of Pierce County
312 Broadway Terrace Bldg. *(M)* (98402)
(206) 572-6955

WALLA WALLA
Planned Parenthood of Walla Walla
136 E. Birch St. *(M)* (99362)
(509) 529-3570

(M) Medical   (E) Educational   (P) Provisional

YAKIMA
Planned Parenthood Assn. of Yakima
County
208 N. 3rd Ave. *(M)* (98902)
(509) 248-3625

WEST VIRGINIA

PARKERSBURG
Planned Parenthood Assn. of Parkersburg
1132 Market St., P. O. Box 1095 *(M)* (26101)
(304) 485-1144

WISCONSIN

MILWAUKEE

Planned Parenthood Assn. of Milwaukee
1135 West State St. *(M)* (53233)
(414) 271-8116

Appleton Chapter
Planned Parenthood Assn. of Fox Valley *(M)*
508 Wisconsin Ave., Appleton 54911
(414) 731-6304

Beaver Dam Chapter
Planned Parenthood Dodge-Jefferson Cos.
(M)
138 Front Street, Beaver Dam 53916
(414) 885-3528

Fond du Lac Chapter
Planned Parenthood Fond du Lac County
(M)
Empire Building, Room 305
20 Forest Avenue, Fond du Lac 54935
(414) 922-9884

Green Bay Chapter
Planned Parenthood of Green Bay *(M)*
Bellin Bldg., Rm. 801
130 East Walnut St., Green Bay 54301
(414) 432-0031

Kenosha Chapter
Planned Parenthood of Kenosha *(M)*
2002 63rd St., Kenosha 53140
(414) 645-0491

Madison Chapter
Planned Parenthood of Dane County *(M)*
1050 Regent St., Madison 53715
(608) 256-7257

Manitowoc Chapter
Planned Parenthood of Manitowoc—Two
    Rivers *(M)*
818 Washington St., Manitowoc 54220
(414) 684-1332

Sheboygan Chapter
Planned Parenthood of Sheboygan *(M)*
528A North 8th, Sheboygan 53081
(414) 458-9401

Sturgeon Bay Chapter
Planned Parenthood of Door County *(M)*
236 Michigan, Sturgeon Bay 54235
(414) 743-6211

West Bend Chapter
Planned Parenthood of Washington County
    (M)
P. O. Box 933, West Bend 53095
(414) 338-1303

Wild Rose Chapter
Lakeland Central Planned Parenthood *(M)*
P. O. Box 253, Wild Rose 54984
(414) 622-3867

Wisconsin Rapids Chapter
Central Wisconsin Planned Parenthood *(M)*
130 2nd Street North, Wisconsin Rapids
    54494
(715) 423-9610

WYOMING

(For information, Call Rocky Mt.
Planned Parenthood—See Denver,
    Colorado)

This list reprinted courtesy of:
The Planned Parenthood® Federation of America, Inc.

(M) Medical   *(E) Educational*   *(P) Provisional*

Breast Cancer Detection Demonstration Projects*
(BCDDP)

The Breast Cancer Detection Demonstration Projects (BCDDP) have not accepted any more women into the National Cancer Institute/American Cancer Society study since 1975. However, the centers provide breast examinations on a fee basis or refer women to the nearest facility where breast examinations and mammograms can be obtained free or at low cost. The machines at these centers are now monitored to insure lowest doses (this was not always true).

ALABAMA

Alabama Breast Cancer Project
UAB P. O. Box 193—University Station
Birmingham, AL 35294
(205) 934-3376 or 934-5070

ARIZONA

Breast Cancer Detection Project
2231 East Speedway Boulevard
Tucson, AZ 85719
(602) 626-7492

CALIFORNIA

Breast Screening Center
384-34th Street
Oakland, CA 94609
(415) 658-8525

Breast Cancer Detection Program
John Wesley County Hospital
2826 South Hope Street
Room 123
Los Angeles, CA 90007
(213) 748-3111

West Coast Cancer Foundation
50 Francisco Street
Suite 200
San Francisco, CA 94133
(415) 563-5213

DELAWARE

Breast Screening Project
1200 Jefferson Street
Wilmington, DE 19001
(302) 428-2113

*See section on breast cancer.

Delaware Breast Cancer Management
  Program—Executive Offices
Wilmington Medical Center
P. O. Box 1668
Wilmington, DE 19899
(302) 656-5740

DISTRICT OF COLUMBIA

Medical Center Cancer Screening
5125 MacArthur Boulevard NW
Washington, DC 20016
(202) 625-2181

FLORIDA

Breast Cancer Detection Center
St. Vincent's Medical Center
Barr Street at St. Johns Avenue
Jacksonville, FL 32204
(904) 338-3243

GEORGIA

Breast Cancer Screening Project
Georgia Baptist Hospital
Professional Building East
315 Boulevard, N.E.
Suite 516
Atlanta, GA 31312
(404) 481-3733

Georgia Cancer Management Network,
  Inc.—Freeway Office Park
1645 Tulle Circle, N.E.
Suite 126
Atlanta, GA 30329
(404) 329-7016

HAWAII

Breast Cancer Detection Center
Alexander Young Building, Pacific
  Health Research Institute, Inc.
Bishop and Hotel Streets
Honolulu, HI 96813
(808) 524-4411

IDAHO

Breast Cancer Detection Center
215 Avenue B
Boise, ID 50316
(208) 345-3590

IOWA

Breast Cancer Demonstration Project
Iowa Lutheran Hospital
University and Penn Avenue
Des Moines, IA 50316
(515) 283-5202

KANSAS

Breast Cancer Detection Center
Department of Surgery
University of Kansas Medical Center
39th and Rainbow Boulevard
Kansas City, KA 66103
(913) 588-6184

KENTUCKY

Cancer Center—University of Louisville
  Foundation, Inc.
Health Sciences Center
Walnut and Preston Streets
Louisville, KY 40202
(502) 582-2211, Ext. 510

Breast Cancer Demonstration Project
601 South Floyd Street
Louisville, KY 40202
(502) 588-5261, Ext. 64

MASSACHUSETTS

New England Medical Center Hospital
171 Harrison Avenue
Boston, MA 02111
(617) 956-5000

MICHIGAN

Breast Cancer Detection Center
396 West Washington Street
Ann Arbor, MI 48109
(313) 764-1474

MISSOURI

Breast Cancer Detection Project Cancer
  Research Center
Business Loop 70 and Garth Avenue
Columbia, MO 65201
(314) 449-3945

NEW HAMPSHIRE

Hitchock Clinic
Hanover, NH 03755
(603) 643-4000, Ext. 2467

NEW JERSEY

Breast Cancer Detection Project
Department of Surgery
Room 852
65 Bergen Street
Newark, NJ 07107
(201) 456-4128

NEW YORK

Breast Cancer Demonstration Project
Guttman Institute
200 Madison Avenue
New York, NY 10016
(212) 830-4000

Brooklyn Breast Cancer Demonstration
  Network
Downstate Medical Center
P. O. Box 1214
450 Clarkson Avenue
Brooklyn, NY 11203
(212) 270-1000

Regional Breast Cancer Program
Albany Medical College
47 New Scotland Avenue
Albany, NY 12208
(518) 445-5107

NORTH CAROLINA

Breast Cancer Detection Project
3040 Erwin Road
Durham, NC 27705
(919) 383-6687

OHIO

Breast Cancer Detection Center
Logan Hall Basement
Cincinnati General Hospital
234 Goodman Street
Cincinnati, OH 45267
(513) 872-5335

OKLAHOMA

Breast Cancer Center
711 East Stanton Young Boulevard
Oklahoma City, OK 73104

Oklahoma Hospital's Breast Cancer Control
  Network
Oklahoma Medical Research Foundation
825 Northeast 13th Street
Oklahoma City, OK 73104
(405) 235-8331, Ext 460

OREGON

Breast Cancer Screening Center
2222 Northwest Lovejoy Street
Suite 171
Portland, OR 97210
(503) 229-7292

PENNSYLVANIA

Breast Cancer Demonstration Project
Albert Einstein Medical Center
Old York and Tabor Roads
Philadelphia, PA 19141
(215) 455-8400, Ext. 11

Breast Cancer Detection Center
Department of Radiology
Temple University Hospital
3401 North Broad Street
Philadelphia, PA 19140
(215) 221-4206

Breast Cancer Detection Center
Hill Building
Second Floor, Room 430
3515 Fifth Avenue
Pittsburgh, PA 15213
(412) 624-2671

839

Fox Chase Cancer Center
The American Oncologic Hospital
Central and Shelmire Avenues
Philadelphia, PA 19111
(215) 722-1900, Ext. 302

RHODE ISLAND

Breast Cancer Detection Project
Multiphasic Screening Center
593 Eddy Street
Providence, RI 02902
(401) 277-8201

TENNESSEE

Vanderbilt Breast Cancer Detection Center
110 Baker Building
110-21st Avenue South
Nashville, TN 37203
(615) 322-3495

TEXAS

Breast Cancer Detection Center of
   St. Joseph's Hospital
2000 Crawford
Houston, TX 77002
(713) 659-8626

VERMONT

University of Vermont
College of Medicine
Burlington, VT 05401
(802) 656-2563

WASHINGTON

Breast Cancer Detection Center
1323 Spring Street
Seattle, WA 98104
(206) 322-0500

WISCONSIN

Breast Cancer Detection Center
8700 West Wisconsin Avenue
Milwaukee, WI 53226
(414) 257-5200

National Surgical Adjuvant Project for Breast and Bowel Cancers (NSABP)†

NSABP Headquarters Office
3550 Terrace Street
Room 914, Scaife Hall
Pittsburgh, PA 15261
(412/624-2671)

Bernard Fisher, M.D., Project Chairman
Lisa Begg Marino, R.N., M.S., Executive Director

1. ALBANY REGIONAL CANCER CENTER

   P. O. Box 8538
   Albany, NY 12208
   (518/489-2607)
   *Dr. Thomas J. Cunningham (Med. Oncol.)
   Dr. Richard R. Caradonna (Med. Oncol.)
   Dr. Robert R. Sponzo (Med. Oncol.)
   Ms. Barbara Demyan

2. ALBERT EINSTEIN COLLEGE OF MEDICINE

   Van Etten Hospital, Room 5C21
   1300 Morris Park Avenue
   Bronx, NY 10461
   (212/430-3063)
   *Dr. Herbert Volk (Surgeon)
   Dr. George Escher (Medical Oncologist)
   Dr. Barry Kaplan (Medical Oncologist)
   Dr. Frank Stratford (Surgeon)
   Ms. Giovanna Cavasotto
   Ms. Margot Wulf
   Ms. Dolores McCaffrey, RN

   Jacobi Hospital
   Pelham Parkway & Eastchester Road
   Bronx, NY 10461
   (212/430-5716)
   Dr. Nino Carnevale (Surgeon)
   Dr. John Molnar (Pathologist)

   Hospital of the Albert Einstein College
     of Medicine
   1825 Eastchester Road, 1—92
   Bronx, NY 10461
   (212/430-2922)
   Dr. Jay Bosworth (Radiation
     Oncologist)

3. ALBERT EINSTEIN MEDICAL CENTER

   1335 W. Tabor Road
   Philadelphia, PA 19141
   (215/329-0700)
   *Dr. Stanley Levick (Hematol./Oncol.)
   Dr. Kenneth M. Algazy (Hematol./
     Oncol.)
   Dr. Agit M. Desai (Hematol./Oncol.)
   Dr. Leonard J. Levick (Hematol./
     Oncol.)
   Ms. Carol Massa

†See "Treatment" in breast cancer section.   *Principal Investigator

4. ALLENTOWN HOSPITAL/
    ALLENTOWN SACRED HEART
    HOSPITAL CENTER

    1730 Chew Street
    Allentown, PA 18104
    (215/433-6691)
    *Dr. David Prager (Medical Oncologist)
    Dr. Joseph Prorok (Surgeon)
    Dr. Robert Post (Medical Oncologist)
    Dr. Nathan Silon (Radiation
        Oncologist)
    Dr. Lloyd E. Barron, II (Medical
        Oncologist)
    Dr. Alexander Nedwich (Pathologist)
    Ms. Lois Ronca

    2200 Hamilton Street
    Allentown, PA 18104
    Dr. Milton Friedberg (Surgeon)

    1210 S. Cedar Crest Boulevard
    Allentown, PA 18105
    (215/821-2050)
    Dr. John Shane (Pathologist)
    Dr. Michael Scarlotto (Pathologist)
    Dr. Raymond Rachman (Pathologist)

5. BAPTIST MEMORIAL HOSPITAL

    1000 Moreno Street
    Pensacola, FL 32501
    (904/434-4785)
    *Dr. Edward Knight (Medical
        Oncologist)
    Dr. Joseph Weaver (Medical
        Oncologist)
    Dr. Paul Meadows (Radiation
        Oncologist)
    Dr. Albert Drlicka (Pathologist)
    Ms. Neena Tennant, P.A.

    5149 North 9th Avenue
    Pensacola, FL 32504
    (904/434-4785)
    Dr. Russell Lowery (Surgeon)
    Dr. Manuel Lopez (Clin. Immun.)

6. BAY MEMORIAL MEDICAL
    CENTER/GULF COAST
    COMMUNITY HOSPITAL

    717 East 7th Street
    Panama City, FL 32401
    (904/769-9408)
    *Dr. Wm. Gregory Bruce (Surgeon)

    527 N. Palo Alto Street
    Panama City, FL 32401
    (904/769-0088)
    Dr. Craig A. Usas (Radiation Oncol.)

    449 Magnolia Avenue
    Panama City, FL 32401
    (904/763-0260)
    Dr. Robert L. Hellman (Pathologist)
    Dr. William A. Sybers (Pathologist)

7. BERKSHIRE MEDICAL CENTER

    725 North Street
    Pittsfield, MA 01201
    (413/499-4161)
    *Dr. Jesse Spector (Hematol./
        Oncology)
    *Dr. Harvey Zimbler (Hematol./
        Oncology)
    Dr. Jeffrey Ross (Pathology)
    Ms. Judith Tremblay, R.N.

    276 South Street
    Pittsfield, MA 01201
    Dr. Michael Ciborski (Surgeon)
    Dr. Roy T. Walchenbach (Surgeon)

    197 South Street
    Pittsfield, MA 01201
    Dr. Robert Tracy (Surgeon)
    Dr. Gerald Haidak (Surgeon)
    Dr. Clement C. Curd (Surgeon)

    East Street Medical Building
    Pittsfield, MA 01201
    Dr. Wynn Sayman (Surgeon)
    Dr. Ralph Zupanec (Surgeon)

    Doctors' Building
    Hospital Avenue
    North Adams, MA 01247
    Dr. Frank Eddy (Surgeon)

    123 Union Street
    Bennington, VT 05201
    Dr. Oakley Frost (Surgeon)

8. BOSTON UNIVERSITY

    75 East Newton Street
    Boston, MA 02118
    (617/247-5224)

*Dr. Peter J. Deckers (Surgeon)
*Dr. Merrill I. Feldman (Radiation
  Oncol.)
Dr. Neil S. Yeston (Surgeon)
Dr. Peter Mozden (Surgeon)
Dr. Philip Gordon (Pathologist)

720 Harrison Avenue
Boston, MA 02118
(617/247-5610)
Dr. Jack Evjy (Medical Oncologist)
Dr. Donna Barnard (Surgeon)
Dr. Harvey Finkel (Hematology/
  Oncology)
Ms. Mary Beth Prendergast, R.N., M.S.
Ms. Janet Scanlon, R.N., B.S.

199 Chelmsford Street
Chelmsford, MA 01824
(617/256-6511)
Dr. Maurice Huckins (Surgeon)

Lowell General Hospital
Lowell, MA 01854
(617/458-6604)
Dr. Negi Mohammed (Radiation
  Oncol.)

9. CALGARY CANCER CENTER

2104 2nd Street, S.W.
Calgary, Alberta T5S 1S5
CANADA
(403/263-0770)
*Dr. L. Martin Jerry (Clinical
  Immunologist)
Dr. Peter Geggie (Medical Oncologist)
Dr. Ian Scott Brown (Radiation
  Oncologist)
Dr. Keith Arthur (Radiation
  Oncologist)
Ms. Marilyn Morimoto, R.N.

Foothills Hospital
1403 29th Street, N.W.
Calgary, Alberta
CANADA
Dr. Peter Cruse (Surgeon)
Dr. Donald Wallace (Medical
  Oncologist)
Dr. Fred Alexander (Pathologist)

10. CROSS CANCER INSTITUTE

11560 University Avenue
Edmonton, Alberta T6G 122
CANADA
(403/432-8771)

*Dr. Sandy Paterson (Medical
  Oncologist)
Dr. Alan Lees (Radiation Oncologist)
Dr. Harry Hyde (Surgeon)
Miss Debbie Schinnour, R.N.

11. DANIEL FREEMAN HOSPITAL

323 N. Prairie Avenue, Suite 222
Inglewood, CA 90301
(213/674-0050)
*Dr. Elliott Hinkes (Medical
  Oncologist)
Dr. Richard Small (Radiation
  Oncologist)
Dr. Raouf Yuja (Pathologist)

333 N. Prairie Avenue
Inglewood, CA 90301
(213/674-7050)
Ms. Patricia Lee, R.N.
Ms. Cecelia C. Flick, R.N.

12. DEKALB GENERAL HOSPITAL

2701 N. Decatur Road
Decatur, GA 30022
(404/282-4444)
Dr. Frank Matthews (Pathologist)
Mr. Ken Arnold
Ms. Linda Sheivlhud

755 Columbia Drive
Decatur, GA 30033
(404/373-3196)
*Dr. S. Angier Wills (Surgeon)

13. DENVER GENERAL HOSPITAL

8th Avenue & Cherokee Street
Denver, CO 80204
(303/893-6000)
Dr. Joseph Preston (Pathologist)
Dr. Don Clarke (Pathologist)
Ms. Donna Meiselbaugh, R.N.

843

4200 East Ninth Avenue
Denver, CO 80220
(303/893-7024)
*Dr. George E. Moore (Surgeon)
Dr. Ralph Gerner (Surgeon)

West Ninth Street
Denver, CO 80204
(303/893-7024)
Dr. Franklin B. Johnson (Radiation
  Oncol.)

14. DOWNSTATE MEDICAL CENTER

445 Lenox Road
Box 23
Brooklyn, NY 11203
(212/270-2401)

450 Clarkson Avenue
Brooklyn, NY 11203
(212/270-2401)
*Dr. Bernard Gardner (Surgeon)
Dr. Antonio Alfonso (Surgeon)
Dr. Julian Rosenthal (Medical
  Oncologist)
Dr. Joseph Bohorquez (Radiation
  Oncol.)
Dr. Anthony Nicastri (Pathologist)
Dr. Yale Rosen (Pathologist)
Dr. Sameer Rafla (Radiation Oncol.)
Ms. Rosemary Scocozzo

451 Clarkson Avenue
Brooklyn, NY 11203
(212/638-7100)

Dr. Joseph Newman (Clinical
  Immunologist)

15. EAST LANSING, MICHIGAN STATE
UNIVERSITY

Department of Medicine
B-220 Life Sciences
East Lansing, MI 48824
(517/353-6625)
*Dr. Leif Suhrland (Medical
  Oncologist)
Ms. Ruth Duncanson, R.N.

B-437 Clinical Sciences
East Lansing, MI 48824
(517/353-5490)
Dr. Raphael de los Santos (Surgeon)

E.W. Sparrow Hospital
1215 East Michigan Avenue
Lansing, MI 48912
(517/487-6111)
Dr. Clyde Spencer (Radiation
  Oncologist)
Dr. Ralph Edminister (Pathologist)

16. ELLIS FISCHEL STATE CANCER
HOSPITAL

Business Loop 70 & Garth Avenue
Columbia, MO 65201
(314/443-3103)
Ms. Donna Meyer

Business Loop 30
Garth Avenue
Columbia, MO 65201
(314/443-3103)
*Dr. William Johnston (Surgeon)
Dr. Nestor Canoy (Radiation
  Oncologist)
Dr. Carl Kardinal (Medical Oncologist)
Dr. Carlos Perez-Mesa (Pathologist)

17. GEISINGER MEDICAL CENTER

Danville, PA 17821
(717/275-6201)
*Dr. C.W. Konvolinka (Surgeon)
Dr. Bert Bernath (Medical Oncologist)
Dr. David Beiler (Radiation Oncologist)
Dr. C. James Favino (Pathologist)
Dr. M. Fleetwood (Clinical
  Immunologist)
Mrs. Audrey Brocious
Ms. Phyllis Holdren
Ms. Patricia Porter, R.N.

18. GROUP HEALTH MEDICAL
CENTER

201 16th Avenue, East
Seattle, WA 98112
(206/326-6262)
200 15th Avenue, East
Seattle, WA 98112
(206/326-6262)
*Dr. Robert Bourdeau (Surgeon)
Dr. S. W. Douglas (Medical Oncologist)
Dr. I. I. Schuldberg (Pathologist)
Dr. E. R. Clarke (Medical Oncologist)

Dr. Thomas W. Johnson (Radiation
Oncol.)
Ms. Sherri Ann Strite

19. HARBOR GENERAL HOSPITAL

1000 West Carson Street
Torrance, CA 90509
(213/328-2380)
*Dr. David State (Surgeon)
*Dr. M. Michael Shabot (Surgeon)
Dr. Jerome Block (Medical Oncologist)
Dr. Frank Hirose (Pathologist)
Ms. Susan Rizzo

20. HENNEPIN COUNTY MEDICAL
CENTER

701 Park
Minneapolis, MN 55415
(612/347-2121)
*Dr. Claude R. Hitchcock (Surgeon)
Dr. John I. Coe (Pathologist)
Ms. Phyllis Anderson

900 South 8th Street
Minneapolis, MN 55404
(612/347-4187)
Dr. Manucher Azad (Radiation
Oncologist)

21. HÔPITAL FRANCO-MUSULMAN

93000 Bobigny
FRANCE
(843-40-04)
*Professor Lucien Israel (Medical
Oncol.)
Dr. Richard Edelstein (Medical Oncol.)
Dr. Alain DePierre (Medical
Oncologist)
Dr. Jacques Aguilera (Medical
Oncologist)

10, Avenue de l'Opéra
Paris, 1
FRANCE
Dr. Jacques Reynier (Surgeon)

National Cancer Institute
Bethesda, MD 10014
(301/496-1567)
Dr. Coston Berard (Pathologist)

22. HÔPITAL L'HÔTEL-DIEU DE
QUÉBEC

11, Côte du Palais
Québec, G1R 2J6 CANADA
(418/694-5352)
*Dr. Louis Dionne (Surgeon)
Dr. Antoine Kibrite (Surgeon)
Dr. Jacques Laverdiere (Radiation
Oncol.)
Dr. Real Lagace (Pathologist)
Ms. Marjolaine Berube

23. JEFFERSON HOSPITAL

11th Walnut Street
Philadelphia, PA 19107
(215/829-6000)
Dr. Arthur Patchefsky (Pathologist)

111 South 11th Street
Philadelphia, PA 19107
(215/928-6952)
*Dr. Arthur Weiss (Medical
Oncologist)
Ms. Linda Doroba

24. JEWISH GENERAL HOSPITAL

3755 Côte St. Catherine Road
Montreal, Québec H3T 1A4
CANADA
(514/342-3504)
*Dr. Richard Margolese (Surgeon)
Dr. Claude LaChance (Pathologist)
Dr. Mark Wainberg (Clinical
Immunologist)
Mrs. Karen Koenig
Ms. Fran Marzinotto

1650 Cedar Avenue
Montreal, Québec H3G 1A4
CANADA
(514/937-6011)
Dr. Julio Guerra (Radiation
Oncologist)

25. KAISER PERMANENTE, HARBOR
CITY

1050 West Pacific Coast Highway
Harbor City, CA 90710
(213/325-5111)
*Dr. Eugene Pollack (Surgeon)

Dr. John Rowe (Pathologist)
Dr. James Grossman (Medical
    Oncologist)
Ms. Ethhel Richardson

26. KAISER PERMANENTE,
     PORTLAND

5055 North Greeley Avenue
Portland, OR 97232
(503/282-8421)
Dr. Robert McFarlane (Surgeon)
Dr. Edward Ariniello (Surgeon)
Dr. T. Tseun Chan (Pathologist) III

2606 Northeast Broadway
Portland, OR 97232
(503/282-8421)
*Dr. Andrew Glass (Medical
    Oncologist)
Ms. Marge Erwin, R.N.
Ms. Nancy Hayes, R.N.
Ms. Alice Gemmet

700 N.E. 47th Avenue
Portland, OR 97232
(503/297-4411)
Dr. John Molendyk (Radiation
    Oncologist)

9205 S.W. Barnes Road
Portland, OR 97229
(503/297-4411)
Dr. Richard Lowy (Radiation
    Oncologist)

2801 Gatenbein
Portland, OR 97232
(503/280-4161)
Dr. Norman Willis (Radiation
    Oncologist)

27. KAISER PERMANENTE, SAN
     DIEGO

4647 Zion Avenue
San Diego, CA 92120
(714/563-3186)
*Dr. Thomas Campbell (Medical
    Oncologist)
Dr. Marvin Nicola (Pathologist)
Ms. Barbara House, P.A.

5110 N. Edgemont
Los Angeles, CA 90027
(714/563-7186)
Dr. A. Robert Kagan (Radiation
    Oncologist)

28. LAHEY CLINIC FOUNDATION

605 Commonwealth Avenue
Boston, MA 02215
(617/262-4900)
*Dr. Richard Oberfield (Medical
    Oncologist)
Dr. Blake Cady (Surgeon)
Dr. Joyce McCaffrey (Medical
    Oncologist)
Dr. John Wolff (Medical Oncologist)
Dr. Ferdinand Salzman (Radiation
    Oncologist)
Dr. Theodore Lo (Radiation
    Oncologist)
Dr. Elton Watkins (Clinical
    Immunologist)
Ms. Terry Hamilton
Ms. Elaine Costello, R.N.

29. LETTERMAN ARMY MEDICAL
     CENTER

Presidio of San Francisco
San Francisco, CA 94129
(415/561-2232)
*Dr. David Gandara (Hem./Onc.)
Dr. John Hutton (Surgeon)
Dr. William R. Starke (Pathologist)
Dr. James Congdon (Oncology Fellow-
    NRMC)
Ms. Cynthia Clark

30. LOUISIANA STATE UNIVERSITY

1542 Tulane Avenue
New Orleans, LA 70112
(504/568-4750)
*Dr. Isidore Cohn (Surgeon)
*Dr. Robert Beazley (Surgeon)
Dr. Edgar Hull (Medical Oncologist)
Dr. Joseph Schlosser (Radiation
    Oncologist)
Dr. Ronald Welsh (Surgeon)
Ms. Sydney Gardberg
Ms. Janet Bradford, R.N.

31. LOUISIANA STATE UNIVERSITY
(SHREVEPORT)

School of Medicine
P. O. Box 33932
Shreveport, LA 71130
(318/226-3306)
*Dr. Leonard I. Goldman (Surgeon)
Dr. Ronald Golinger (Surgeon)
Dr. Darryl Williams (Hematologist/
Oncol.)
Dr. Allan Miller (Medical Oncologist)
Dr. James Thomson (Radiation
Oncologist)

32. LYNN HOSPITAL

212 Boston Street
Lynn, MA 01904
(617/598-5100)
*Dr. Lester Tobin (Medical Oncologist)
Dr. Edward Braun (Medical
Oncologist)
Dr. Calvin Dorsey (Surgeon)
Dr. Robert Sloane (Surgeon)
Dr. Donald Perlman (Surgeon)
Dr. Emei Shen (Pathologist)
Dr. Sabin Levenson (Surgeon)
Ms. Catherine Vigeant, R.N.

33. MAIMONIDES MEDICAL CENTER

4802 Tenth Avenue
Brooklyn, NY 11219
(212/853-1200)
*Dr. George Degenshein (Surgeon)
Dr. Jerome Applebaum (Medical
Oncologist)
Dr. Stanley Minkowitz (Pathologist)
Ms. Noreen Katz

450 Clarkson Avenue
Brooklyn, NY 11203
(212/270-1593)
Dr. Joseph Bohorquez (Radiation
Oncologist)

34. MANITOBA CANCER
FOUNDATION

700 Bannatyne Avenue
Winnipeg, Manitoba R3E 0V9
CANADA

(204/786-4731)
*Dr. David Bowman (Medical
Oncologist)
Dr. Martin Levitt (Medical Oncologist)
Dr. Donald Penner (Pathologist)
Dr. David Owen (Pathologist)
Dr. David Beatty (Surgeon)
Dr. James Gillies (Radiation
Oncologist)
Ms. Janice Lutz, R.N.
Ms. Else Johnson
Ms. Kerry McConnell, R.N.

35. MARTIN LUTHER HOSPITAL

1761 West Romneya Drive
Suite G & H
Anaheim, CA 92801
(714/533-2280)
*Dr. Jack Brook (Medical Oncologist)
Dr. Lakshminarayanan Subramanyam
(Med. Onc.)

241 Avenida Santa Dorotea
La Habra, CA 90630
(714/870-6772)
Dr. Leonida Zaharia (Medical
Oncologist)

Placentia-Linda Community Hospital
1301 Rose Drive
Placentia, CA 92670
(714/993-2000)
Dr. Spencer B. Gilbert (Pathologist)

36. McGILL UNIVERSITY

1650 Cedar Avenue
Montreal, Québec H3G 1A4
CANADA
(514/937-6011)
*Dr. Phil Gold (Clinical Immunologist)

37. MEDICAL COLLEGE OF
PENNSYLVANIA

3300 Henry Avenue
Philadelphia, PA 19129
(215/842-6000)
*Dr. James Bassett (Surgeon)
Dr. John Clark (Surgeon)
Dr. Subhash C. Bansal (Surgeon)
Dr. Joanne Overleese (Surgeon)

847

Dr. Janet Parker (Radiation Oncologist)
Dr. Gerald Justh (Pathologist)
Ms. Cindy Tepper

38. MEDICAL COLLEGE OF VIRGINIA

1200 East Broad Street
Richmond, VA 23298
(804/770-5221)
*Dr. Walter Lawrence (Surgeon)
Dr. Wade Smith (Medical Oncologist)
Dr. E. Richard King (Radiation
   Oncologist)
Dr. Saul Kay (Pathologist)
Ms. Barbara Satterwhite, R.N.
Ms. Linda Keener, R.N.

39. MEDICAL COLLEGE OF WISCONSIN

8700 West Wisconsin Avenue
Milwaukee, WI 53226
(414/257-5936)
*Dr. William Donegan (Surgeon)
Dr. James Cox (Radiation Oncologist)
Dr. Lawrence Clowery (Pathologist)
Dr. Frank Jones (Surgeon)
Dr. Richard M. Hansen (Med.
   Oncologist)
Ms. Colleen Beaman, R.N.
Ms. Maureen Koehler

2025 East Newport Avenue
Milwaukee, WI 53211
(414/272-3816)
Dr. Wayne Boulanger (Surgeon)

3321 North Maryland Avenue
Milwaukee, WI 53211
(414/964-5100)
Dr. Lyle R. Heim (Clinical
   Immunologist)

40. MEMORIAL CANCER RESEARCH FOUNDATION

3828 Hughes Avenue
Culver City, CA 90230
(213/836-7000)
Dr. Irwin Grossman (Radiation
   Oncologist)
Dr. Victor Rosen (Pathologist)
Dr. Jacob Turner (Pathologist)

9808 Venice Boulevard
Culver City, CA 90230
(213/559-3550)
*Dr. David Plotkin (Medical
   Oncologist)
Ms. Deborah Medoff

9808 Venice Boulevard
Culver City, CA 90230
(213/836-3104)
Dr. Gerald Glantz (Surgeon)

8733 Beverly Boulevard
Los Angeles, CA 90048
(213/652-8990)
Dr. Morris Freidin (Surgeon)

9400 Brighton Way
Beverly Hills, CA 90210
(213/276-6157)
Dr. Alexander Korn (Surgeon)

11860 Wilshire Boulevard
West Los Angeles, CA 90025
(213/478-1177)
Dr. Rafael Rodriguez (Surgeon)

540 North Central Avenue
Glendale, CA 91203
(213/247-5440)
Dr. Donald Bogdon (Medical
   Oncologist)
Dr. John Gunnell (Medical Oncologist)
Dr. Gilbert Hum (Medical Oncologist)
Dr. Cary Gota (Medical Oncologist)

3440 Lomita
Torrance, CA 90505
(213/530-3813)
Dr. Stephen Lemkin (Medical
   Oncologist)
Dr. Malin R. Dollinger (Medical
   Oncologist)
Dr. Lowell Greenberg (Medical
   Oncologist)
Dr. Stuart Wong (Medical Oncologist)

2001 4th Avenue
San Diego, CA 92101
(714/234-6261)
Dr. Thomas Lehar (Medical
   Oncologist)
Dr. Donald Newman (Medical
   Oncologist)

Dr. Donald Balfour (Medical Oncologist)

41. MICHAEL REESE HOSPITAL

29th & South Ellis Avenue
Chicago, IL 60616
(312/791-2000)
*Dr. Richard Desser (Medical Oncologist)
Dr. Richard Evans (Surgeon)
Dr. Arthur Mitchel (Surgeon)
Dr. Ram K. Goyal (Radiation Oncologist)
Dr. Wendy Recant (Pathologist)
Ms. Rhonda Shackelford
Ms. Dellie Chan, R.N.

42. MONTEFIORE HOSPITAL & MEDICAL CENTER

111 East 210th Street
Bronx, NY 10467
(212/920-5411)
*Dr. Richard Rosen (Surgeon)
Dr. Edward Greenwald (Medical Oncologist)
Dr. Mark Markham (Medical Oncologist)
Dr. Flora Mincer (Radiation Oncologist)
Dr. Norwin Becker (Pathologist)
Ms. Beatrice Markham

43. MONTREAL GENERAL HOSPITAL

1650 Cedar Avenue
Montreal, Québec H3G 1A4
CANADA
(514/937-6011)
*Dr. John MacFarlane (Surgeon)
Dr. J. D. Palmer (Surgeon)
Dr. Michael Thirlwell (Medical Oncologist)
Dr. Julio Guerra (Radiation Oncologist)
Dr. T. N. Roman (Radiation Oncologist)
Dr. Lawrence Hampson (Surgeon)
Dr. W. P. Duguid (Pathologist)
Dr. D. M. P. Thomson (Clinical Immunologist)
Ms. Lucy Cristofanilli
Ms. Monica MacDonald, R.N.

44. MOUNT SINAI HOSPITAL OF CLEVELAND

University Circle
Cleveland, OH 44106
(216/795-6000)
*Dr. Sidney Sachs (Surgeon)
Dr. Louis H. Levine (Pathologist)
Dr. Richard Bornstein (Medical Oncologist)
Dr. Norman Berman (Radiation Oncologist)
Ms. Sherri Reynolds, R.N.
Ms. Phyllis Hall

45. NAVAL REGIONAL MEDICAL CENTER

8750 Mountain Boulevard
Oakland, CA 94627
(415/639-2017)
*Dr. Richard M. Deaner (Surgeon)
Dr. John J. Stoltenberg (Surgeon)
Dr. Michael L. Smith (Surgeon)
Dr. Robert L. Donnell (Medical Oncologist)
Dr. Gary W. Zelles (Surgeon)
Dr. David Karp (Radiation Oncologist)
Dr. Philip Vogt (Pathologist)
Ms. Joan Jackson

46. ONTARIO CANCER FOUNDATION

Civic Hospital Division
Ottawa Civic Hospital
Ottawa, K1Y 4E9 CANADA
(613/728-2745)
*Dr. James Devitt (Surgeon)
*Dr. David J. Klaassen (Medical Oncologist)
Dr. G.E. Catton (Radiation Oncologist)
Dr. E. Liepa (Pathologist)
Ms. Terry Clayton

47. PENNSYLVANIA HOSPITAL

320 South 9th Street
Philadelphia, PA 19107
(215/829-3583)
*Dr. Harvey Lerner (Surgeon)

8th & Spruce Streets
Philadelphia, PA 19107
(215/829-5000)

849

Dr. Dominic DeLaurentis (Surgeon)
Dr. John Glassburn (Radiation
  Oncologist)
Dr. S. Prasasvinichai (Radiation Oncol.)
Dr. Else Olen (Pathologist)
Ms. Ellen Marcovitz
Ms. Kate Godwin, R.N.

48. PONDVILLE HOSPITAL

P. O. Box 111
Walpole, MA 02801
(617/762-6837)
*Dr. Leo Stolbach (Medical Oncologist)
Dr. Carol Amick (Pathologist)
Dr. C. William Kaiser (Surgeon)
Ms. Donna Cardellecchio, R.N.

Lemeul Shattuck Hospital
170 Morton Street
Jamaica Plain, MA 02130
(617/522-8400)
Dr. Joseph Cohen (Medical Oncologist)
Dr. Charles Rosenbaum (Medical
  Oncologist)

New England Medical Center
171 Harrison Avenue
Boston, MA 02111
(617/956-5144)
Dr. Larry Nathanson (Medical
  Oncologist)

49. ROYAL VICTORIA HOSPITAL

687 Pine Avenue West
Montreal, Québec H3A 1A1
CANADA
(514/842-1251)
*Dr. Henry Shibata (Surgeon)
Dr. Giles Tremblay (Pathologist)
Dr. Juergen Knaack (Pathologist)
Dr. Harry Himal (Surgeon)
Dr. Guerin Dorval (Clinical
  Immunologist)
Dr. Samuel Solomon (Endocrinologist)
Ms. Chris Soucie, R.N.

1650 Cedar Avenue
Montreal, Québec H3G 1A4
CANADA
(514/842-1251)
Dr. Julio Guerra (Radiation Oncologist)

50. RUSH PRESBYTERIAN-ST. LUKE'S
MEDICAL CENTER

1753 West Congress Parkway
Chicago, IL 60612
(312/942-5000)
*Dr. Steven Economou (Surgeon)
*Dr. Janet Wolter (Medical Oncologist)
Dr. Arthur Rossof (Clinical
  Immunologist)

1725 West Harrison
Chicago, IL 60612
(312/942-5755)
Dr. Frank Hendrickson (Radiation
  Oncologist)
Dr. Anupam Routh (Radiation
  Oncologist)
Dr. Edmund Pellettiere (Pathologist)
Ms. Susan Kotrba

51. SAGINAW COOPERATIVE
HOSPITALS, INC.

1000 Houghton Avenue
Saginaw, MI 48602
(517/771-6893)
Dr. William Rice (Surgeon)
Dr. Paul Colligan (Pathologist)
Dr. Robert Powers (Surgeon)
Dr. Charles Koucky (Surgeon)
Ms. Marie Johnson, R.N.

Michigan State University
Life Sciences Building—220
East Lansing, MI 48824
*Dr. Nikolay Dimitrov (Medical
  Oncologist)

52. ST. LUC HOSPITAL

1058 St. Denis Street
Montreal, Québec
CANADA
(514/285-1525)
*Dr. Roger Poisson (Surgeon)
Dr. Pierre Franche Bois (Surgeon)
Dr. Jean Cote (Pathologist)
Dr. Claude Thout (Hematologist)
Dr. Louis Perron (Hematologist)
Ms. Odette Rivard, R.N.

Maisonneuve Hospital
Montreal, CANADA
(514/285-1525)
Dr. Jean Philip Mercier
(Radiotherapist)

53. ST. LUKE'S HOSPITAL

44th & Wornall Road
Kansas City, MO 64111
(816/932-2000)
Dr. Ralph R. Hall (Medical Oncologist)
Dr. John Rippey (Pathologist)
Ms. Peggy Brinkman, R.N.

4320 Wornall Road
Kansas City, MO 64111
(816/753-7400)
*Dr. Paul Koontz (Surgeon)
Dr. Karl H. Hanson (Medical
Oncologist)
Dr. Joe L. Rector (Radiation
Oncologist)

54. ST. MICHAEL'S HOSPITAL

30 Bond Street
Toronto, M5B 1WB
CANADA
(416/360-4245)
Dr. Ken R. Butler (Medical Oncologist)
Dr. M. B. Garvey (Medical Oncologist)
Dr. Ara Chalvardjian (Pathologist)
Dr. Dennis William Jirsch (Surgeon)
Dr. Arthur Leznoff (Clinical
Immunologist)

55 Queen Street East
Toronto, M5C 1R5
CANADA
(416/367-9670)
*Dr. Leo Mahoney (Surgeon)
Ms. Ruth Rowden
Ms. Ann Harrington, R.N.
Ms. Kathleen Arthurs

Princess Margaret Hospital
500 Sherbourne Street
Toronto, M4X 1K9 CANADA
(416/924-0671)
Dr. Roy Clark (Radiation Oncologist)

55. ST. VINCENT'S HOSPITAL,
INDIANAPOLIS

2001 West 86th Street
Indianapolis, IN 46260
(317/871-2345)
Dr. James Sullivan (Pathologist)
Dr. Marvin Melton (Pathologist)

8402 Harcourt Road
Indianapolis, IN 46260
(317/259-7138)
*Dr. John Cavins (Medical Oncologist)
Dr. Joseph C. Finneran (Surgeon)
Ms. Jodi Friedmeyer
Ms. Maggie McMann, R.N.

56. ST. VINCENT'S HOSPITAL, NEW
YORK

153 West 11th Street
New York, NY 10011
(212/620-1234)
*Dr. Thomas Nealon (Surgeon)
Dr. Carlo E. Grossi (Surgeon)
Dr. William R. Grace (Medical
Oncologist)
Dr. George Schwarz (Radiation
Oncologist)
Dr. Ilona Toth (Pathologist)
Dr. Patrick McKenna (Clinical
Immunologist)
Ms. Rita Murphy

57. SOUTH NASSAU COMMUNITIES
HOSPITAL

2445 Oceanside Road
Oceanside, NY 11572
(516/764-2600)
*Dr. Nicholas LiCalzi (Surgeon)
Dr. Bong Kim (Radiation Oncologist)
Dr. Ahmed Khapra (Pathologist)
Dr. Maurice Goldenhar (Clinical
Immunol.)
Ms. Margaret Bowra
Ms. Marie Peters, R.N.

1703 Merrick Avenue
Freeport, NY 11566
(516/378-3311)
Dr. Ronald Primis (Medical
Oncologist)

498 North Brookside Avenue
Freeport, NY 11520
(516/379-0790)
Dr. Sanford Pariser (Medical
  Oncologist)

446 Foxhurst Road
Oceanside, NY 11572
(516/764-2120)
Dr. Stanley Hyman (Clinical
  Immunologist)

58. TULANE UNIVERSITY

1430 Tulane Avenue
New Orleans, LA 70112
(504/588-5110)
*Dr. Edward Krementz (Surgeon)
*Dr. Carl Sutherland (Surgeon)
Dr. H. Nina Dhurandhar (Pathologist)
Dr. Joseph Schlosser (Radiation
  Oncologist)
Ms. Debbie Tuminello, R.N.

59. UNIVERSITY OF CALIFORNIA,
     SAN DIEGO

225 West Dickinson Street
San Diego, CA 92103
(714/294-6222)
*Dr. Yosef Pilch (Surgeon)
Dr. Robert Barone (Surgeon)
Dr. John Mendelsohn (Medical
  Oncologist)
Dr. Joella F. Utley (Radiation
  Oncologist)
Dr. Sidney Saltzstein (Pathologist)
Ms. Mary C. Sooy
Ms. Becky Trangenstein, R.N.

60. U.S. NAVAL HOSPITAL, SAN DIEGO

San Diego, CA 92134
(714/233-2022)
*Dr. George Looney (Surgeon)
Dr. Frederic Sanford (Radiation
  Oncologist)
Dr. Harry Long (Medical Oncologist)
Ms. Jo Gann
Ms. Jane Brownfield

61. UNIVERSITY OF FLORIDA (JHEP)

320 Prudential Drive
Suite 511
Jacksonville, FL 32207
(904/399-0818)
*Dr. Neil Abramson (Medical
  Oncologist)

Barrs Street & St. Johns Avenue
Jacksonville, FL 32204
904/398-7751)
Dr. Matthew Patterson (Pathologist)

1842 King Street
Jacksonville, FL 32204
(904/388-5452)
Dr. Harry Reinstine (Surgeon)

800 Prudential Drive
Jacksonville, FL 32207
(904/398-3511)
Dr. Bhojraj Paryani (Radiation
  Oncologist)
Ms. Jacque DeLuca

University Hospital of Jacksonville
655 West Eighth Street
Jacksonville, FL 32209
(904/358-3272)
Dr. Luis Urdaneta (Surgeon)
Dr. Sam E. Stephenson, Jr. (Surgeon)
Dr. Victoria Medina (Radiation
  Oncologist)
Dr. Rosilie Saffos (Pathologist)
Ms. Judy Kosinski
Ms. Pamela Martin, R.N.
Ms. Judith Kidd, R.N., B.S.

62. UNIVERSITY OF IOWA

University Hospitals
Iowa City, IA 52240
(319/356-3584)
*Dr. Peter Jochimsen (Surgeon)
Dr. Michael Corder (Medical
  Oncologist)
Dr. Barry Sherman (Medical
  Oncologist)
Dr. Hamed Tewfik (Radiation
  Oncologist)
Dr. Howard Latourette (Radiation
  Oncologist)
Dr. Frederic Stamler (Pathologist)

Dr. Joseph Skibba (Surgeon)
Ms. Vicki Drennan
Ms. Judith Gust, R.N.
Ms. Donna Olson
Ms. Susan Gorrell

McFarland Clinic
12th and Douglas
Ames, IA 50010
(515/232-4530)
Dr. S. Donald Zaentz (Internist)

717 A Avenue NE
Cedar Rapids, IA 52402
(319/364-0225)
Dr. Campbell F. Watts (Surgeon)

210 North Linden Street
Lamoni, IA 50140
(515/784-3371)
Dr. Norman Nelson (General Practice)

610 North 4th Street
Burmington, IA 52601
(319/753-5444)
Dr. John E. McGee (Oby./Gyn.)

204 North Jefferson
Mt. Pleasant, IA 52641
(319/385-4631)
Dr. Ernest Lerner (Internal Medicine)

204 Arch Street
Burlington, IA 52601
Dr. Theodore T. Mazur (Surgeon)

3319 Spring Street
Davenport, IA 52807
Dr. Charles R. Fesenmeyer (Surgeon)

63. UNIVERSITY OF MARYLAND

22 South Greene Street
Baltimore, MD 21201
(301/528-5835)
*Dr. E. George Elias (Surgeon)
Dr. Mukund S. Didolkar (Surgeon)
Dr. Don M. Morris (Surgeon)
Dr. Ill Soo Kim (Radiation Oncologist)
Dr. Meyer Reuben Heyman (Medical
   Oncologist)
Ms. Teri Zentai
Ms. Sally Bonczhowski, R.N.

64. UNIVERSITY OF PITTSBURGH

3550 Terrace Street
Pittsburgh, PA 15261
(412/624-2671)
*Dr. Bernard Fisher (Surgeon)

Adjuvant Therapy Center
3515 Fifth Avenue
Pittsburgh, PA 15213
(412/624-6221)
Ms. Mary Ketner, R.N.
Ms. Susan Encke, R.N.
Ms. Debra Pollak, R.N.
Ms. Lisa Begg Marino, R.N., M.S.
Ms. Debbie Kolcun
Ms. Wendy Kramer

Shadyside Hospital
5230 Centre Avenue
Pittsburgh, PA 15232
(412/622-2121)
Dr. Edwin R. Fisher (Pathologist)
Dr. Alka Sharad Palekar (Pathologist)
Dr. Morgan McCoy, II (Pathology
   Fellow)
Ms. Marion Siebert

Presbyterian-University Hospital
230 Lothrop Street
Pittsburgh, PA 15213
(412/647-2345)
Dr. Robert B. Atwell (Surgeon)
Dr. Leon Barnes (Pathologist)
Dr. George Benz (Surgeon)
Dr. Melvin Deutsch (Radiation
   Oncologist)
Dr. Edward W. Jew (Surgeon)
Dr. Jon Lloyd (Surgeon)
Dr. Scott Williams (Surgeon)
Dr. John W. Smith (Surgeon)
Dr. Edward Longabaugh (Surgeon)
Dr. Charles Watson (Surgeon)
Dr. William Watson (Surgeon)
Dr. Marshall Webster (Surgeon)

Western Pennsylvania Hospital
4800 Friendship Avenue
Pittsburgh, PA 15224
(412/682-4200)
Dr. William Cooper (Internal
   Medicine)
Dr. William L. Chapman (Internal
   Medicine)

Dr. E. Ralph Erickson (Pathologist)
Dr. John Hill (Internal Medicine)
Dr. Charles Strodes (Internal Medicine)
Dr. Herbert Jacob (Internal Medicine)
Dr. Harold Semins (Surgeon)

Allegheny General Hospital
320 E. North Avenue
Pittsburgh, PA 15212
(412/237-3630
Dr. Robert Hartsock (Pathologist)
Dr. M. B. Javan (Surgeon)
Dr. Wayne Pfrimmer (Hematol./
  Oncology)
Dr. Reginald Pugh (Hematol./
  Oncology)
Dr. Lewis Schiffer (Hematol./
  Oncology)
Dr. Bernard Zidar (Hematol./
  Oncology)
Ms. Colleen Murphy

Montefiore Hospital
3459 Fifth Avenue
Pittsburgh, PA 15213
(142/683-1100)
Dr. Stuart Chetlin (Surgeon)
Dr. Stanley Hirsch (Surgeon)
Dr. Samuel Jacobs (Medical
  Oncologist)
Dr. Gerald Kaufer (Surgeon)
Dr. Charles Lebovitz (Surgeon)
Dr. Harvey Mendelow (Pathologist)

Radiology Associates of Erie
104 East Second Street
Fifth Floor
Erie, PA 16507
(814/459-5000)
Dr. Jay Jenkins (Medical Oncologist)
Dr. Peter M. Scibetta (Radiation
  Oncologist)
Ms. Linda Callahan, R.N.
Ms. Pauline Asmer

Hamot Medical Center
201 State Street
Erie, PA 16512
(814/455-6711 x220)
Dr. John Fust (Pathologist)

St. Vincent's Health Center
232 West 25th Street
Erie, PA 16512
(814/459-4000)
Dr. Robert Renz (Pathologist)

Sewickley Valley Hospital
700 Borad Street
Sewickley, PA 15143
(412/741-2700)
Dr. Daniel Brooks (Surgeon)
Dr. Alfred Doyle (Medical Oncologist)
Dr. Clarence Miller (Pathologist)

Magee Womens Hospital
Forbes and Halket Streets
Pittsburgh, PA 15213
(412/647-2345)
Dr. John Parsons (Radiation
  Oncologist)
Dr. Arthur Murphy (Surgeon)
Dr. Bernard Klionsky (Pathologist)
Dr. Alan Kunschner (Surgeon)
Dr. Thomas Allen (Surgeon)
Dr. Rupert Friday (Gynecologist)

South Side Hospital
South 20th & Jane Streets
Pittsburgh, PA 15203
(412/481-3300)
Dr. Robert E. Gregory (Surgeon)
Dr. Leonard Myers (Pathologist)

Westmoreland Hospital
532 West Pittsburgh Street
Greensburg, PA 15601
(412/837-0100)
Dr. Joseph Gall (Hematol./Oncology)
Dr. James Dull (Surgeon)
Dr. Doris Maxwell (Surgeon)
Dr. T. K. Morrow (Pathologist)

McKeesport Hospital
1500 Fifth Avenue
McKeesport, PA 15132
(412/664-2000)
Dr. Frank Bondi (Surgeon)
Dr. Perry C. Martineau (Pathologist)

Mercy Hospital
Stevenson and Locust Streets
Pittsburgh, PA 15219
(412/232-8111)
Dr. Jeanne Cooper (Pathologist)
Dr. Charles E. Copeland

Citizen's General Hospital
651 Fourth Avenue
New Kensington, PA 15068
(412/337-3541)
Dr. Charles Graff (Surgeon)

Dr. Herman Klieger (Pathologist)
Dr. Jonathan Schwartz (Surgeon)
Dr. Douglas F. Brady (Surgeon)

Columbia Hospital
Penn Avenue and West Street
Pittsburgh, PA 15221
(412/247-2424)
Dr. Edward Waisbrot (Surgeon)
Dr. Donald H. Quint (Pathologist)

Monongahela Valley Hospital
West Chess Street
Monongahela, PA 15068
(412/258-4800)
Dr. John Brandon (Pathologist)
Dr. Edgar C. Cordero (Surgeon)

North Hills Passavant Hospital
9100 Babcock Boulevard
Pittsburgh, PA 15237
(412/931-3840)
Dr. William A. Altenhoff (Surgeon)
Dr. Herbert Anderson (Pathologist)
Dr. Harry M. Null (Surgeon)

Central Medical Pavillion
1400 Centre Avenue
Pittsburgh, PA 15219
(412/562-3000)
Dr. Joseph Finegold (Surgeon)
Dr. Cyril Wecht (Pathologist)

Suburban General Hospital
S. Jackson Avenue
Pittsburgh, PA 15202
(412/734-1800)
Dr. Donald D. Davis (Surgeon)
Dr. Sanford Edberg (Pathologist)

Bashline Memorial Hospital
516 Oakland Avenue
Grove City, PA 16127
(412/458-9400)
Dr. Don L. Bashline (Surgeon)
Dr. Helga Nallathambe (Pathologist)

Butler Hospital
East Brady Street Extension
Butler, PA 16001
(412/283-6666)
Dr. Paul Maust (Surgeon)
Dr. A. M. Tirrello (Pathologist)

Sharon Hospital
740 E. State Street
Sharon, PA 16146
(412/981-1700)
Dr. Ravi Sachdeva (Surgeon)
Dr. Donald Cohen (Pathologist)

Medical Center of Beaver Falls, Inc.
Beaver Falls Unit
Beaver Falls, PA 15010
(412/843-6000)
Dr. Prisco T. Evangelista (Surgeon)
Dr. Jack Right (Pathologist)

Andrew Kaul Memorial Hospital
St. Mary's, PA 15857
(814/467-6611)
Dr. Paul Myers (Surgeon)
Dr. Dennis A. Sharky (Pathologist)

65. UNIVERSITY OF ROCHESTER

Box 704
601 Elmwood Avenue
Rochester, NY 14642
(716/275-3924)
Dr. John Bennett (Medical Oncologist)
Dr. Thomas Bonfiglio (Pathologist)
Ms. Joanne Greenwood

335 Mt. Vernon Avenue
Rochester, NY 14620
(716/271-3300)
*Dr. Edwin Savlov (Surgeon)
Dr. Eileen Paterson (Radiation
   Oncologist)

South Avenue at Bellvue Drive
Rochester, NY 14620
(716/473-2300)
Dr. Sidney Sobel (Radiation Oncologist)

66. UNIVERSITY OF TEXAS HEALTH
     CENTER AT SAN ANTONIO

7703 Floyd Curl Drive
San Antonio, TX 78284
(512/696-6151)
*Dr. A. B. Cruz (Surgeon)
*Dr. J. Bradley Aust (Surgeon)
Dr. George Bannayan (Pathologist)
Dr. Daniel Thor (Clinical
   Immunologist)

Dr. Joaquin Mira (Radiation
Oncologist)
Ms. Mary Lou Guerrero
Ms. Jody Sapp, R.N.

Division of Oncology
Department of Medicine
7703 Floyd Curl Drive
San Antonio, TX 78284
(512/696-9660)
Dr. Robert Livingston (Medical
Oncologist)
Dr. Richard Reed (Medical Oncologist)

67. UNIVERSITY OF VERMONT

Given Building
Burlington, VT 05401
(802/656-2563)
*Dr. Roger Foster (Surgeon)
Dr. Carleton Haines (Surgeon)
Dr. Richard Albertini (Clinical
Immunologist)
Ms. Cheryl Richard
Ms. Patti Sheridan, R.N.
Ms. Mabel Hills, R.N.

Burgess Residence
Burlington, VT 05401
(802/656-3724)
Dr. Jerome Yates (Medical Oncologist)

Medical Alumni Building
Burlington, VT 05401
(802/656-3506)
Dr. Roy Korson (Pathologist)

Mary Fletcher Unit
Burlington, VT 05401
(802/656-3501)
Dr. James Gagnon (Radiation
Oncologist)
Dr. Adrian R. Bourque (Radiation
Oncologist)

68. VALLEY HOSPITAL

Linwood & N. Van Dien Avenues
Ridgewood, NJ 07541
(201/445-4900)
Dr. Paul Hartman (Radiation
Oncologist)
Dr. William Green (Pathologist)
Ms. Wanda Borgen

130 Prospect Street
Ridgewood, NJ 07540
(201/444-6640)
*Dr. Hugh Auchincloss (Surgeon)

530 N. Maple Avenue
Ridgewood, NJ 07540
(201/445-2725)
Dr. Allen Chinitz (Medical Oncologist)

385 Maple Street
Ridgewood, NJ 07450
(201/652-2800)
*Dr. Harold Bruck (Surgeon)

69. WASHINGTON UNIVERSITY

660 South Euclid
St. Louis, MO 63110
(314/494-8775)
*Dr. Marc Wallack (Surgeon)
Dr. Harvey Butcher (Surgeon)
Dr. Gordon Philpott (Surgeon)
Dr. Geoffrey Herzig (Medical
Oncologist)

510 South Kings Highway
St. Louis, MO 63110
(314/454-2134)
Dr. Carlos Perez (Radiation Oncologist)
Dr. John Bedwinek (Radiation
Oncologist)

4960 Audubon Avenue
St. Louis, MO 63310
(314/454-3420)
Dr. Walter Bauer (Pathologist)
Ms. Peggy Nelson, R.N.
Ms. Debbie Dieterichs, R.N.
Ms. Gail Farley, R.N.
Ms. Diane Bohner, R.N.

4989 Barnes Hospital
St. Louis, MO 63110
(314/454-3420)
Ms. Betty Williamson

70. WEST HILLS HOSPITAL

7301 Medical Center Drive
Suite 501
Canoga Park, CA 91307
(713/703-7421)
*Dr. Ronald Citronbaum (Medical
Oncologist)

71. WEST SUBURBAN HOSPITAL

    518 North Austin Boulevard
    Oak Park, IL 60302
    (312/383-6200)
    *Dr. Everett Nicholas (Surgeon)
    Dr. Stanley V. Hoover (Radiation
      Oncologist)
    Dr. Frederick I. Volini (Pathologist)
    Ms. Ann Gallagher

72. WILMINGTON MEDICAL CENTER

    Carpenter Memorial Clinic
    Chestnut and Broom Streets
    Wilmington, DE 19899
    (302/428-1212)
    *Dr. Robert Frelick (Medical
      Oncologist)

Dr. Leslie Whitney (Surgeon)
Dr. Siamak Samii (Medical Oncologist)
Dr. Irving Berkowitz (Medical
  Oncologist)
Dr. Timothy Wozniak (Medical
  Oncologist)
Dr. Donald Tilton (Radiation
  Oncologist)
Dr. Patrick Ashley (Pathologist)
Dr. Yogi Patel (Medical Oncologist)
Dr. Carlo Cuccia (Radiation
  Oncologist)
Dr. Anita Hodson (Clinical
  Immunologist)
Dr. Emerson Gledhill (Surgeon)
Ms. Alice Kyle, R.N.
Ms. Sara Ortalani, R.N.
Ms. Doris Hatfield, R.N.
Ms. Joanne Tully Cossman, R.N.

Cancer Information Service Hot-Lines*

CALIFORNIA:	southern part—area codes 213, 714, 805: 1-800-252-9066 rest of state: 213-226-2374
COLORADO:	1-800-332-1850
CONNECTICUT:	1-800-922-0824
DELAWARE:	1-800-523-3586
FLORIDA:	1-800-432-5953 in Dade County: 305-547-6920 for Spanish-speaking callers: 1-800-432-5955 for Spanish-speaking callers in Dade County: 305-547-6960
HAWAII:	Oahu—536-0111 (neighboring islands—ask operator for Enterprise 6702)
ILLINOIS:	800-972-0586
MAINE:	800-225-7034
MARYLAND:	800-492-1444
MASSACHUSETTS:	1-800-952-7420
MINNESOTA:	1-800-582-5262
MONTANA:	1-800-525-0231
NEW HAMPSHIRE:	1-800-225-7034

*See p. 693.

NEW JERSEY:	800-523-3586
NEW MEXICO:	1-800-525-0231
NEW YORK STATE	1-800-462-7255
NEW YORK CITY:	212-794-7982
NORTH CAROLINA:	800-672-0943
PENNSYLVANIA:	1-800-822-3963
TEXAS	1-800-392-2040
VERMONT:	1-800-225-7034
WASHINGTON, D.C. metropolitan area:	202-232-2833
WASHINGTON STATE:	1-800-552-7212
WISCONSIN:	800-362-8038
WYOMING:	1-800-525-0231
ALL OTHER AREAS (except Alaska):	800-638-6994

Comprehensive Cancer-Care Centers Sponsored by the National Cancer Institute*

ALABAMA:

Comprehensive Cancer Center
University of Alabama in Birmingham
University Station
Birmingham, AL 35294
205-934-5077

Cancer Communication Office
205-934-2651

CALIFORNIA:

Los Angeles County — University of
    Southern California Comprehensive
    Cancer Center
2025 Zonal Avenue
Los Angeles, CA 90033
213-226-2008

Director, Office of Cancer Communications
213-226-2371

UCLA — Jonsson Comprehensive Cancer
    Center
UCLA School of Medicine
924 Westwood Boulevard, Suite 650
Los Angeles, CA 90024
213-825-5268
213-825-5412

*See p. 679.

COLORADO:

Colorado Regional Cancer Center, Inc.
165 Cook Street
Denver, CO 80206
303-320-5921

Director, Education and Information
303-320-5921

CONNECTICUT:

Yale University Comprehensive Cancer
    Center
333 Cedar Street
New Haven, CT 06510
203-432-4122

Program Manager
203-436-3779

DISTRICT OF COLUMBIA:

Georgetown University/Howard University
    Comprehensive Cancer Center
Vincent T. Lombardi Cancer Research
    Center

861

Georgetown University
3800 Reservoir Road, N.W.
Washington, DC 20007
202-625-7066
and
Howard University Cancer Research Center
Department of Oncology
2041 Georgia Avenue, N.W.
Washington, DC 20060
202-745-1406

Cancer Coordinating
Council for Metropolitan Washington
202-797-8876

FLORIDA:

Comprehensive Cancer Center for the State
  of Florida
University of Miami School of Medicine/
  Jackson Memorial Medical Center
Centre House, Roof Garden
1400 N.W. 10th Ave.
Miami, FL 33136
305-547-6758

Cancer Information Service
305-547-6678

ILLINOIS:

Illinois Cancer Council (includes
  Northwestern University Cancer Center,
  University of Chicago Cancer Research
  Center, Rush-Presbyterian-St. Luke's
  Medical Center, University of Illinois and
  several other health organizations)
37 S. Wabash Avenue
Chicago, IL 60603
312-346-9813

Cancer Information Service
302-346-9813

MARYLAND:

Johns Hopkins Comprehensive Cancer
  Center
600 N. Wolfe Street
Baltimore, MD 21205
301-955-3300

Communications Director
301-955-3636

MASSACHUSETTS:

Sidney Farber Cancer Institute
44 Binney Street
Boston, MA 02115
617-732-3555

Communications Officer
617-732-3150

MICHIGAN:

Comprehensive Cancer Center of
  Metropolitan Detroit (includes the
  Michigan Cancer Foundation and Wayne
  State University)
110 East Warren Street
Detroit, MI 48201
313-833-0710

MINNESOTA:

Charles G. Moertel, M.D., Director
Mayo Comprehensive Cancer Center
200 First Street, S.W.
Rochester, MN 55901
507-282-3261

Communications Specialist
507-284-8285

NEW YORK:

Memorial Sloan-Kettering Cancer Center
1275 York Avenue
New York, NY 10021
212-794-7646

Director, Office of Cancer Communications
212-794-7982

Rosewell Park Memorial Institute
666 Elm Street
Buffalo, NY 14263
716-845-5770

Cancer Control Communications Officer
716-845-4402

NORTH CAROLINA:

Duke University Comprehensive Cancer
  Center
P.O. Box 3814
Durham, NC 27710
919-684-2282

Director, Cancer Control Program
919-286-2214

OHIO:

The Ohio State University Comprehensive
  Cancer Center
357 McCampbell Hall
1580 Cannon Drive
Columbus, OH 43210
614-422-5022

Cancer Center Communications Office
614-422-5022

PENNSYLVANIA:

Fox Chase/University of Pennsylvania
  Comprehensive Cancer Center
7701 Burholme Avenue
Philadelphia, PA 19111
215-728-2717

Communications Coordinator
215-728-2700

TEXAS:

The University of Texas System Cancer
  Center
M.D. Anderson Hospital and Tumor
  Institute
6723 Bertner Avenue
Houston, TX 77030
713-792-3000

Cancer Information Service
Program Administrator
713-792-3363

WASHINGTON:

Fred Hutchinson Cancer Research Center
1124 Columbia Street
Seattle, WA 98104
206-292-2930

Communications Officer
206-292-6301

WISCONSIN:

The University of Wisconsin Clinical Cancer
  Center
Clinical Science Center
600 Highland Avenue
Madison, WI 53705
608-263-5404

Public Affairs Coordinator
608-262-0046

863

Clinical and Nonclinical Cancer Centers Sponsored by NCI***

CALIFORNIA:

Dr. Steven K. Carter*
Director, Northern California
Cancer Program
770 Welch Road, Suite 190
Palo Alto, CA 94304
415-497-5353

Dr. Henry S. Kaplan**
Maureen Lyles D'Ambrogio Professor of
   Radiology
Director, Cancer Biology Research
   Laboratory
Stanford University Medical Center
Stanford, CA 94305
415-497-7313
415-497-5055

Dr. C. Arthur Knight**
Chairman, Department of Molecular
   Biology
Director, Virus Laboratory
University of California
Berkeley, CA 94720
415-642-7057

*Clinical Cancer Center
**Nonclinical Cancer Center

Dr. Gordon H. Sato**
University of California
P.O. Box 109
La Jolla, CA 92037
714-452-3095

Dr. F.M. Huennekens**
Chairman, Department of Biochemistry
Director, Specialized Cancer Center
Scripps Clinic and Research Foundation
10666 N. Torrey Pines Road
La Jolla, CA 92037
714-455-9100, ext. 338

Dr. Willian R. Clark**
Associate Professor in Biology
Department of Biology
University of California
Los Angeles, CA 90024
213-825-7684

Dr. Walter Eckhart**
Associate Research Professor
Armand Hammer Center for Cancer Biology
The Salk Institute
P.O. Box 1809
San Diego, CA 92112
714-453-4100, ext. 386

***See p. 679.

865

GEORGIA:

Dr. Charles H. Huguley, Jr., Director*
Emory University Cancer Center
Rm. 606F, Emory University Hospital
Atlanta, GA 30322
404-329-7016

HAWAII:

Dr. Lawrence H. Piette, Director*
Cancer Center of Hawaii
University of Hawaii at Manoa
1997 East-West Road
Honolulu, HI 96822
808-948-7173
808-948-7246

IDAHO:

Dr. Charles E. Smith*
Medical Director
Mountain States Tumor Institute
151 East Bannock
Boise, ID 83702
208-345-1780

KANSAS:

Dr. James T. Lowman, Director*
Mid-America Cancer Center Program
The University of Kansas Medical Center
College of Health Sciences & Hospital
Rainbow Boulevard at 39th
Kansas City, KS 66103
913-588-5700

MASSACHUSETTS:

Dr. Sidney R. Cooperband, Director*
Boston University Cancer Research Center
80 East Concord Street
Boston, MA 02118
617-247-6075

Dr. Mahlon B. Hoagland**
President and Scientific Director
Worcester Foundation for Experimental
  Biology, Inc.
222 Maple Avenue
Shrewsbury, MA 01545
617-842-8921

MISSOURI:

Missouri Cancer Programs, Inc.*
115 Business Loop 70 West
Columbia, MO 65201
314-449-3945

Dr. Samuel B. Guze**
Director of Cancer Centers
Washington University School of Medicine
660 South Euclid Avenue
St. Louis, MO 63110
314-454-3013

NEW JERSEY:

Dr. Jacques R. Fresco, Director**
Basic Science Cancer Center
Princeton University
Frick Chemical Laboratory
Princeton, NJ 08540
609-452-3927

NEW MEXICO:

Dr. Morton M. Kligerman, Director*
Cancer Research and Treatment Center
University of New Mexico
Albuquerque, NM 87131
505-277-2151

NEW YORK:

Dr. Leonard Weiss, Director*
Department of Experimental Pathology
Roswell Park Memorial Institute
Cancer Cell Center
666 Elm Street
Buffalo, NY 14263
716-845-3311

Dr. Harry Eagle, Director*
Cancer Research Center
Albert Einstein College of Medicine
1300 Morris Park Avenue
Bronx, NY 10461
212-430-2302
212-792-2233

Dr. Vincent P. Hollander, Director*
Research Institute for Skeletomuscular
  Diseases
Hospital for Joint Diseases and Medical
  Center
1919 Madison Avenue
New York, NY 10035
212-876-7222

Dr. Paul A. Marks, Director*
Columbia University Cancer Research
  Center
College of Physicians & Surgeons
701 West 168th Street
New York, NY 10032
212-694-3807
212-694-4138

Dr. H. Sherwood Lawrence*
Professor & Head, Infectious Disease &
  Immunology Division
Department of Medicine
New York University Medical Center
550 First Avenue
New York, NY 10016
212-679-3200

Dr. Robert A. Cooper, Jr., Director*
University of Rochester Cancer Center
601 Elmwood Avenue
Rochester, NY 14642
716-275-4865

Dr. Norton Nelson**
Professor and Chairman
Department of Environmental Medicine
New York University Medical Center
550 First Avenue
New York, NY 10016
212-679-3200, ext. 2881

Dr. Ernst L. Wynder**
President and Medical Director
American Health Foundation
1370 Avenue of the Americas
New York, NY 10019
212-489-8700

NORTH CAROLINA:

Dr. Joseph S. Pagano, Director*
Cancer Research Center
University of North Carolina
Box 3, Swing Building 217H
Chapel Hill, NC 27514
919-966-1183
919-966-3036

Dr. Charles L. Spurr*
Director, Oncology Research Center
Bowman Gray School of Medicine
300 South Hawthorne Road
Winston-Salem, NC 27103
919-727-4464

OHIO:

Dr. Arthur Flynn, Director*
The Cancer Center, Inc.
11000 Cedar Avenue
Cleveland, OH 44106
216-421-7300

Dr. Earle C. Gregg**
Professor of Radiology (Physics)
University Hospitals
2065 Adelbert Road
Cleveland, OH 44106
216-444-3522

OKLAHOMA:

Dr. G. Bennett Humphrey, Director*
Oklahoma Cancer Center
University of Oklahoma Health Sciences
  Center
P.O. Box 26901
Oklahoma City, OK 73190
405-271-4485

PENNSYLVANIA:

Dr. Fred Rapp, Professor and Chairman**
Department of Microbiology
The Pennsylvania State University College
  of Medicine
Hershey, PA 17033
717-534-8253

867

Dr. Hilary Koprowsi, Director**
The Wistar Institute of Anatomy and
  Biology
36th Street at Spruce
Philadelphia, PA 19104
215-387-6700, ext. 201

Dr. Peter N. Magee, Director**
Fels Research Institute
Temple University Medical School
3420 N. Broad Street
Philadelphia, PA 19140
215-221-4312

PUERTO RICO:

Dr. Enrique Perez-Santiago*
Director, Puerto Rico Cancer Center
University of Puerto Rico
Medical Sciences Campus
G.P.O. Box 5067
San Juan, PR 00936
809-763-2443
809-765-2363

RHODE ISLAND:

Dr. Paul Calabresi*
Physician-in-Chief
Roger Williams General Hospital
825 Chalkstone Avenue
Providence, RI 02908
401-456-2070

TENNESSEE:

Dr. James J. Nickson, Director*
Memphis Regional Cancer Center
800 Madison Avenue
Memphis, TN 38163
901-528-5739

Dr. Alvin M. Mauer, Medical Center*
St. Jude Children's Research Hospital
332 North Lauderdale
Memphis, TN 38101
901-525-8381, ext. 271

TEXAS:

Dr. Eugene P. Frenkel*
Director, Cancer Center
University of Texas Health Science Center
5323 Harry Hines Boulevard
Dallas, TX 75235
214-688-2182

Dr. William C. Levin, President*
The University of Texas Medical Branch
Administrative Building, Suite 646
Galveston, TX 77550
713-765-1902

VIRGINIA:

Dr. Walter Lawrence, Jr.*
MCV/VCU Cancer Center
Box 37 MCV Station
Medical College of Virginia
Virginia Commonwealth University
Richmond, VA 23298
804-770-7682
804-770-7476

WISCONSIN:

Dr. Donald Pinkel*
Professor & Chairman
Department of Pediatrics
Medical College of Wisconsin
1700 West Wisconsin Avenue
Milwaukee, WI 53233
414-344-7100, ext. 374

Cancer Programs Approved by the American College of Surgeons as of Sept. 1, 1980*

ALABAMA

Birmingham
University of Alabama Hospitals
Veterans Administration Hospital

Mobile
University of South Alabama Medical
  Center

Tuskegee
Veterans Administration Hospital

ALASKA

Anchorage
Alaska Hospital and Medical Center
Providence Hospital
USPHS Alaska Native Medical Center

Fairbanks
Fairbanks Memorial Hospital

ARIZONA

Flagstaff
Flagstaff Hospital and Medical Center of
  Northern Arizona

Mesa
Desert Samaritan Hospital & Health Center
Mesa Lutheran Hospital

Phoenix
Good Samaritan Hospital
Maricopa County General Hospital
Memorial Hospital
Veterans Administration Medical Center

Scottsdale
Scottsdale Memorial Hospital

Tucson
Tucson Medical Center
University Hospital
Veterans Administration Medical Center

ARKANSAS

Fayetteville
Washington Regional Medical Center

Little Rock
University Hospital
Veterans Administration Hospital

Texarkana
St. Michael Hospital

*See p. 720.

869

CALIFORNIA

Alhambra
Alhambra Community Hospital

Anaheim
Anaheim Memorial Hospital
Martin Luther Hospital Medical Center

Arcadia
Methodist Hospital of Southern California

Bakersfield
Kern Medical Center
San Joaquin Community Hospital

Bellflower
Bellwood General Hospital
Kaiser Foundation Hospital

Berkeley
Alta Bates Hospital
Herrick Memorial Hospital

Burbank
St. Joseph Medical Center

Canoga Park
West Hills Medical Center

Concord
Mount Diablo Hospital Medical Center

Covina
Inter-Community Hospital

Culver City
Dr. David Brotman Memorial Hospital

Duarte
City of Hope National Medical Center

Fontana
Kaiser Foundation Hospital

Fountain Valley
Fountain Valley Community Hospital

Fresno
Fresno Community Hospital and Medical
    Center
Valley Children's Hospital
Veterans Administration Medical Center

Glendale
Glendale Adventist Medical Center
Glendale Community Hospital

Granada Hills
Granada Hills Community Hospital

Harbor City
Kaiser Foundation Hospital

Imola
Napa State Hospital

Inglewood
Centinela Medical Center
Daniel Freeman Memorial Hospital

La Jolla
Green Hospital of Scripps Clinic
Scripps Memorial Hospital

La Mesa
Grossmont District Hospital

Laguna Hills
Southern Orange County Cancer Program
Saddleback Community Hospital

Livermore
Veterans Administration Medical Center

Loma Linda
Loma Linda University Medical Center

Long Beach
Long Beach Community Hospital
Los Altos Hospital
Memorial Hospital Medical Center of Long
    Beach
Naval Regional Medical Center
St. Mary Medical Center—Bauer Hospital

Los Angeles
California Hospital Medical Center
Children's Hospital of Los Angeles
Hollywood Presbyterian Medical Center
Hospital of the Good Samaritan
Kaiser Foundation Hospital—Cadillac
Kaiser Foundation Hospital—Sunset
Los Angeles County—USC Medical Center
Martin Luther King, Jr. General Hospital
Orthopaedic Hospital
Queen of Angels Hospital
St. Vincent's Medical Center
UCLA Hospital
White Memorial Medical Center

Lynwood
St. Francis Medical Center

Martinez
Veterans Administration Medical Center

Mission Viejo
Mission Community Hospital

Modesto
Memorial Hospitals Association

Montebello
Beverly Hospital

Monterey Park
Garfield Medical Center

Newport Beach
Hoag Memorial Hospital—Presbyterian

Northridge
Northridge Hospital Foundation

Oakland
Naval Medical Center
Samuel Merritt Hospital

Oceanside
Tri-City Hospital

Orange
St. Joseph Hospital
University of California Irvine Medical
    Center

Oxnard
St. John's Hospital

Palm Springs
Desert Hospital

Panorama City
Kaiser Foundation Hospital

Pasadena
Huntington Memorial Hospital
St. Luke's Hospital of Pasadena

Pomona
Pomona Valley Community Hospital

Redlands
Redlands Community Hospital

Redondo Beach
South Bay Hospital

Redwood City
Sequoia Hospital

Riverside
Parkview Community Hospital
Riverside Community Hospital
Riverside General Hospital—University
    Medical Center

Sacramento
Mercy Hospital
Sutter Community Hospitals of Sacramento
University of California—Davis Medical
    Center

San Bernardino
St. Bernadine Hospital
San Bernardino County Medical Center

San Clemente
San Clemente General Hospital

San Diego
Children's Hospital & Health Center
Donald Sharp Memorial Community
    Hospital
Kaiser Foundation Hospital
Mercy Hospital and Medical Center
Naval Regional Medical Center
University Hospital

San Dimas
Tri-Hospital Cancer Program
    Foothill Presbyterian Hospital,
    Glendora
    Glendora Community Hospital,
    Glendora
    San Dimas Community Hospital,
    San Dimas
    West Covina Hospital, *West Covina*

San Francisco
French Hospital/Medical Center
Letterman Army Medical Center
Mount Zion Hospital and Medical Center
Ralph K. Davies Medical Center/Franklin
    Hospital
St. Francis Memorial Hospital
St. Mary's Hospital and Medical Center
San Francisco General Hospital Medical
    Center
USPHS Hospital
University of California Hospitals and
    Clinics
Veterans Administration Medical Center

San Gabriel
Community Hospital of San Gabriel

San Jose
O'Connor Hospital
San Jose Hospital
Santa Clara Valley Medical Center

San Pablo
Brookside Hospital

San Pedro
San Pedro and Peninsula Hospital

Santa Ana
Santa Ana—Tustin Community Hospital

Santa Barbara
Santa Barbara Cottage Hospital

Santa Monica
St. John's Hospital and Health Center
The Santa Monica Hospital Medical Center

Stockton
Dameron Hospital

Thousand Oaks
Los Robles Regional Medical Center

Torrance
Los Angeles County Harbor—UCLA
   Medical Center
Torrance Memorial Hospital Medical Center

Travis AFB
David Grant USAF Medical Center

Upland
San Antonio Community Hospital

Van Nuys
Valley Presbyterian Hospital

Visalia
Kaweah Delta District Hospital

Walnut Creek
John Muir Memorial Hospital

Whittier
Presbyterian Intercommunity Hospital

COLORADO

Colorado Springs
Penrose Hospital

Denver
American Cancer Research Center and
   Hospital, *Lakewood*
Fitzsimons Army Medical Center
Porter/Swedish Cancer Program
   Porter Memorial Hospital
   Swedish Medical Center, *Englewood*
Presbyterian Medical Center
Rose Medical Center
St. Anthony Hospital Systems
St. Joseph Hospital
St. Luke's Hospital
University of Colorado Medical Center—
   Colorado General Hospital
Veterans Administration Medical Center

Fort Carson
US Army Hospital

Fort Collins
Poudre Valley Memorial Hospital

Greeley
Weld County General Hospital

Longmont
Longmont United Hospital

Montrose
Montrose Memorial Hospital

Pueblo
St. Mary—Corwin Hospital

USAF Academy
USAF Academy Hospital

Wheat Ridge
Lutheran Medical Center

CONNECTICUT

Bridgeport
Bridgeport Hospital
Park City Hospital
St. Vincent's Medical Center

Danbury
Danbury Hospital

Derby
Griffin Hospital

Farmington
University of Connecticut Health Center—
   John Dempsey Hospital

Greenwich
Greenwich Hospital Association

Groton
Naval Submarine Medical Center

Hartford
Hartford Hospital
Mount Sinai Hospital
St. Francis Hospital and Medical Center

Meriden
Meriden-Wallingford Hospital

New Haven
Hospital of St. Raphael
Yale-New Haven Hospital

Norwalk
Norwalk Hospital

'Norwich
The William W. Backus Hospital

Stamford
St. Joseph Hospital
Stamford Hospital

Torrington
Charlotte Hungerford Hospital

Waterbury
St. Mary's Hospital
Waterbury Hospital

DELAWARE

Lewes
Beebe Hospital of Sussex County

Wilmington
Veterans Administration Center
Wilmington Medical Center

DISTRICT OF COLUMBIA

Washington
Children's Hospital National Medical Center
Georgetown University Hospital
Greater Southeast Community Hospital
Howard University Hospital
Walter Reed Army Medical Center

FLORIDA

Daytona Beach
Halifax Hospital Medical Center

Dunedin
Mease Hospital and Clinic

Gainesville
Shands Teaching Hospital and Clinic

Jacksonville
Memorial Hospital of Jacksonville
Naval Regional Medical Center
St. Vincent's Medical Center
University Hospital of Jacksonville

Miami
James M. Jackson Memorial Hospital

Pensacola
Naval Aerospace and Regional Medical
  Center
West Florida Hospital

Tallahassee
Tallahassee Memorial Hospital

Tampa
St. Joseph's Hospital
Tampa General Hospital

GEORGIA

Albany
Phoebe Putney Memorial Hospital

Americus
Americus and Sumter County Hospital

Austell
Cobb General Hospital

Atlanta
Crawford W. Long Memorial Hospital of
  Emory University
Emory University Hospital
Georgia Baptist Medical Center
Grady Memorial Hospital
Piedmont Hospital
St. Joseph's Hospital
West Paces Ferry Hospital

Augusta
Eugene Talmadge Memorial Hospital
University Hospital

Columbus
Medical Center

873

Dalton
Hamilton Memorial Hospital

Decatur
De Kalb General Hospital
Veterans Administration Hospital, Atlanta

East Point
South Fulton Hospital

Fort Benning
Martin Army Hospital

Fort Gordon
Dwight D. Eisenhower Army Medical
 Center

Gainesville
Northeast Georgia Medical Center

La Grange
West Georgia Medical Center/Enoch
 Callaway Cancer Clinic

Macon
Medical Center of Central Georgia

Savannah
Memorial Medical Center

Tifton
Tift General Hospital

HAWAII

Honolulu
Kaiser Foundation Hospital
Kapiolani Hospital
Kuakini Medical Center
Queen's Medical Center
St. Francis Hospital
Tripler Army Medical Center

IDAHO

Boise
St. Luke's Hospital & Mountain States
 Tumor Institute

Lewiston
St. Joseph's Hospital

Nampa
Mercy Medical Center

Twin Falls
Magic Valley Memorial Hospital

ILLINOIS

Arlington Heights
Northwest Community Hospital

Aurora
Copley Memorial Hospital

Berwyn
Mac Neal Memorial Hospital

Carbondale
Memorial Hospital of Carbondale

Chicago
Bethesda Hospital
Central Community Hospital
Children's Memorial Hospital
Columbus Hospital
Cook County Hospital
Edgewater Hospital
Franklin Boulevard Community Hospital
Holy Cross Hospital
Illinois Masonic Medical Center
Louis A. Weiss Memorial Hospital
Mercy Hospital and Medical Center
Mount Sinai Hospital Medical Center
Northwestern Memorial Hospital
Ravenswood Hospital Medical Center
Rush-Presbyterian-St. Luke's Medical
 Center
St. Elizabeth's Hospital
St. Joseph Hospital
St. Mary of Nazareth Hospital Center
Swedish Covenant Hospital
University of Chicago Hospitals and Clinics
University of Illinois Hospital
Veterans Administration West Side Hospital

Chicago Heights
St. James Hospital

Danville
Lakeview Medical Center
Saint Elizabeth Hospital

Decatur
Decatur Memorial Hospital

Effingham
St. Anthony's Memorial Hospital

Elgin
St. Joseph Hospital
Sherman Hospital

Elk Grove Village
Alexian Brothers Medical Center

Elmhurst
Memorial Hospital of DuPage County

Evanston
Evanston Hospital
St. Francis Hospital of Evanston

Evergreen Park
Little Company of Mary Hospital

Great Lakes
Naval Regional Medical Center

Harvey
Ingalls Memorial Hospital

Hines
Veterans Administration Medical Center

Hinsdale
Hinsdale Sanitarium and Hospital

Kankakee
St. Mary's Hospital of Kankakee

Lake Forest
Lake Forest Hospital

Libertyville
Condell Memorial Hospital

Maywood
Foster G. McGaw Hospital

McHenry
McHenry Hospital

Moline
Lutheran Hospital

Oak Lawn
Christ Hospital

Oak Park
West Suburban Hospital

Park Ridge
Lutheran General Hospital

Peoria
Methodist Medical Center of Illinois
St. Francis Hospital Medical Center

Quincy
Blessing Hospital
St. Mary Hospital

Rockford
Rockford Memorial Hospital
St. Anthony Hospital Medical Center
Swedish-American Hospital

Skokie
Skokie Valley Community Hospital

Sterling
Community General Hospital

Streator
St. Mary's Hospital

Urbana
Carle Foundation Hospital

INDIANA

Bluffton
Caylor-Nickel Hospital

Evansville
Deaconess Hospital
Welborn Memorial Baptist Hospital

Gary
Methodist Hospital of Gary

Hammond
St. Margaret Hospital

Indianapolis
Community Hospital of Indianapolis
Methodist Hospital of Indiana
St. Vincent Hospital and Health Care Center

Lafayette
St. Elizabeth Hospital Medical Center

Terre Haute
Terre Haute Regional Hospital
Union Hospital

Vincennes
Good Samaritan Hospital

IOWA

Des Moines
Iowa Methodist Medical Center
Mercy Hospital
Veterans Administration Hospital

875

Dubuque
Finley Hospital
Mercy Health Center—St. Joseph's Unit
Xavier Hospital

Iowa City
University of Iowa Hospitals and Clinics

KANSAS

Fort Riley
Irwin Army Hospital

Hays
Hadley Regional Medical Center
St. Anthony Hospital

Kansas City
Bethany Medical Center
University of Kansas Medical Center

Manhattan
Memorial/St. Mary Hospitals Cancer
  Program
  Memorial Hospital
  The Saint Mary Hospital

Wichita
St. Francis Hospital
St. Joseph Medical Center
Veterans Administration Medical and
  Regional Office Center
Wesley Medical Center

KENTUCKY

Fort Campbell
United States Army Hospital

Lexington
Good Samaritan Hospital
University Hospital

Louisville
Highlands Baptist Hospital
Louisville General Hospital
Norton Children's Hospitals
  Children's Hospital Unit
  Norton Memorial Infirmary Unit
Veterans Administration Medical Center

Madisonville
Hopkins County Hospital

LOUISIANA

Alexandria
Alexandria Tumor Registry Program
  Rapides General Hospital
  St. Frances Cabrini Hospital

Eunice
Moosa Memorial Hospital

Lake Charles
St. Patrick Hospital of Lake Charles

New Orleans
Charity Hospital of Louisiana at New
  Orleans
Touro Infirmary
USPHS Hospital
Veterans Administration Hospital

Shreveport
Louisiana State University Hospital
Veterans Administration Medical Center

MAINE

Augusta
Augusta General Hospital

Bangor
Eastern Maine Medical Center

Lewiston
Central Maine General Hospital
St. Mary's General Hospital

Norway
Stephens Memorial Hospital

Portland
Maine Medical Center

Presque Isle
Arthur Gould Memorial Hospital

Rockland
Penobscot Bay Medical Center

Togus
Veterans Administration Medical Center

Waterville
Mid-Maine Medical Center

MARYLAND

Andrews A.F. Base
Malcolm Grow USAF Medical Center

Baltimore
Franklin Square Hospital
Greater Baltimore Medical Center
Johns Hopkins Hospital
St. Joseph Hospital
Sinai Hospital of Baltimore
South Baltimore General Hospital
USPHS Hospital
University of Maryland Hospital

Bethesda
National Naval Medical Center

Leonardtown
St. Mary's Hospital

Salisbury
Peninsula General Hospital

Towson
St. Joseph Hospital

MASSACHUSETTS

Boston
Beth Israel Hospital
Boston City Hospital
Children's Hospital Medical Center
Faulkner Hospital, *Jamaica Plain*
Lahey Clinic Foundation
New England Deaconess Hospital
Peter Bent Brigham Hospital
St. Elizabeth's Hospital of Boston, *Brighton*
USPHS Hospital, *Brighton*
University Hospital
Veterans Administration Medical Center,
   Jamaica Plain

Brockton
Brockton Hospital
Cardinal Cushing General Hospital

Cambridge
Mount Auburn Hospital

Chelsea
Lawrence F. Quigley Memorial Hospital,
   Soldier's Home in Massachusetts

Concord
Emerson Hospital

Danvers
Hunt Memorial Hospital

Framingham
Framingham Union Hospital

Holyoke
Holyoke Hospital
Providence Hospital

Hyannis
Cape Cod Hospital

Lynn
Lynn Hospital

Medford
Lawrence Memorial Hospital

Newton Lower Falls
Newton-Wellesley Hospital

North Adams
North Adams Regional Hospital

Northampton
The Cooley Dickenson Hospital

Norwood
Norwood Hospital

Pittsfield
Berkshire Medical Center

Salem
Salem Hospital

Springfield
Baystate Medical Center
Mercy Hospital

Stoughton
Goddard Memorial Hospital

Walpole
Pondville Hospital

Waltham
Waltham Hospital

Winchester
Winchester Hospital

Worcester
St. Vincent Hospital
The Memorial Hospital
Worcester City Hospital

MICHIGAN

Allen Park
Veterans Administration Hospital

Ann Arbor
St. Joseph Mercy Hospital
University Hospital

Battle Creek
Calhoun Country Medical Society Cancer
  Program
  Battle Creek Sanitarium Hospital
  Community Hospital Association
  Leila Y. Post Montgomery Hospital

Dearborn
Oakwood Hospital

Detroit
Detroit General Hospital
Harper-Grace Hospitals
Henry Ford Hospital

Flint
Hurley Medical Center
St. Joseph Hospital

Grand Rapids
Blodgett Memorial Medical Center
Butterworth Hospital
Ferguson-Droste-Ferguson Hospital
St. Mary's Hospital

Lansing
Edward W. Sparrow Hospital

Menominee
Marinette, Wi-Menominee Cancer Program
Menominee County-Lloyd Hospital

Muskegon
Hackley Hospital and Medical Center

Rochester
Crittenton Hospital

Royal Oak
William Beaumont Hospital

Southfield
Providence Hospital

MINNESOTA

Crookston
Riverview Hospital Association

Fergus Falls
Lake Region Hospital

Grand Rapids
Itasca Memorial Hospital

Hibbing
Hibbing General Hospital

Minneapolis
Abbott-Northwestern Hospital
Children's Health Center & Hospital
Metropolitan Medical Center
St. Mary's Hospital
University of Minnesota Hospitals and
  Clinics
Veterans Administration Hospital

Moorhead
St. Ansgar Hospital

Rochester
Mayo Clinic

St. Louis Park
Methodist Hospital

MISSISSIPPI

Biloxi
Howard Memorial Hospital
Veterans Administration Hospital

Hattiesburg
Forrest County General Hospital

Jackson
University Hospital
Veterans Administration Medical Center

Keesler
USAF Medical Center

Vicksburg
Mercy Regional Medical Center

MISSOURI

Cape Girardeau
St. Francis Medical Center
Southeast Missouri Hospital

878

Columbia
Ellis Fischel State Cancer Hospital

Fort Leonard Wood
U.S. General Leonard Wood Army Hospital

Kansas City
Baptist Memorial Hospital
Menorah Medical Center
St. Luke's Hospital
Trinity Lutheran Hospital
Truman Medical Center

Poplar Bluff
Doctors Regional Medical Center

St. Louis
Deaconess Hospital
Incarnate Word Hospital
Jewish Hospital of St. Louis
St. Anthony's Medical Center
St. Louis Children's Hospital
St. Mary's Health Center

Sikeston
Missouri Delta Community Hospital

MONTANA

Butte
St. James Community Hospital
    Mary Swift Memorial Tumor Clinic

NEBRASKA

Lincoln
Lincoln General Hospital
Veterans Administration Medical Center

Omaha
Archbishop Bergan Mercy Hospital
Bishop Clarkson Memorial Hospital
Immanuel Medical Center
Nebraska Methodist Hospital
St. Joseph Hospital
University of Nebraska, Hospital & Clinics

NEW HAMPSHIRE

Exeter
Exeter Hospital

Hanover
Mary Hitchcock Memorial Hospital

Keene
Cheshire Hospital

Manchester
Catholic Medical Center
Elliot Hospital

Portsmouth
Portsmouth Hospital

Rochester
Frisbie Memorial Hospital

NEW JERSEY

Atlantic City
Atlantic City Medical Center

Belleville
Clara Maass Memorial Hospital

Camden
West Jersey Hospital System

Denville
St. Clare's Hospital

East Orange
Veterans Administration Medical Center

Elizabeth
Elizabeth General Hospital and
    Dispensary, Wuester Clinic

Englewood
Englewood Hospital

Green Brook
Raritan Valley Hospital

Hackensack
Hackensack Hospital

Hackettstown
Hackettstown Community Hospital

Livingston
St. Barnabas Medical Center

Montclair
The Mountainside Hospital

Morristown
Morristown Memorial Hospital

Mount Holly
Burlington County Memorial Hospital

Neptune
Jersey Shore Medical Center Fitkin Hospital

Newark
Newark Beth Israel Medical Center

Newton
Newton Memorial Hospital

Orange
The Hospital Center at Orange

Passaic
Beth Israel Hospital

Paterson
St. Joseph's Hospital and Medical Center

Phillipsburg
Warren Hospital

Plainfield
Muhlenberg Hospital

Princeton
The Medical Center at Princeton

Somerville
Somerset Hospital Medical Center

Trenton
St. Francis Medical Center

Woodbury
Underwood-Memorial Hospital

NEW MEXICO

Albuquerque
Bernalillo Medical Center
Lovelace Medical Center
St. Joseph Hospital
Veterans Administration Medical Center

NEW YORK

Albany
Veterans Administration Hospital

Amityville
Brunswick Hospital Center

Binghamton
Our Lady of Lourdes Memorial Hospital

Buffalo
Children's Hospital of Buffalo
Deaconess Hospital of Buffalo
Erie County Medical Center
Roswell Park Memorial Institute
Veterans Administration Medical Center

Castle Point
Veterans Administration Medical Center

Cobleskill
Community Hospital of Schoharie County

Cooperstown
Mary Imogene Basset Hospital

East Meadow
Nassau County Medical Center

Elmira
Arnot-Ogden Memorial Hospital

Glen Cove
Community Hospital at Glen Cove

Johnson City
Charles S. Wilson Memorial Hospital

Kenmore
Kenmore Mercy Hospital

Manhasset
North Shore University Hospital

Mineola
Nassau Hospital

Mount Kisco
Northern Westchester Hospital Center

Mount Vernon
Mount Vernon Hospital

New Hyde Park
Long Island Jewish Medical Center

New Rochelle
New Rochelle Hospital Medical Center

New York City
Bronx *(Mailing address: Bronx)*
  Bronx-Lebanon Hospital Center
  Misericordia Hospital Medical Center
  Montefiore Hospital and Medical
    Center
  Veterans Administration Medical Center

880

Brooklyn *(Mailing address: Brooklyn)*
Brooklyn-Cumberland Medical Center
Jewish Hospital & Medical Center of
Brooklyn
Long Island College Hospital
Lutheran Medical Center
St. John's Episcopal Hospital
State University of New York, Downstate
Medical Center and
Kings County Hospital Center
Wyckoff Heights Hospital
The Methodist Hospital
Manhattan *(Mailing address: New York)*
Beekman-Downtown Hospital
Bellevue Hospital Center
Beth Israel Medical Center
Cabrini Health Care Center
Harlem Hospital Center
Manhattancal Center
Cabrini Health Care Center
Harlem Hospital Center
Manhattan Eye, Ear and
Throat Hospital
Memorial Sloan-Kettering Cancer Center
New York Infirmary
New York University Medical Center
University Hospital
St. Clare's Hospital and Health Center
St. Luke's Hospital Center
St. Vincent's Hospital and Medical
Center of New York
The New York Hospital
Veterans Administration Medical Center
Queens *(Mailing addresses: Astoria,
Edgemere, Elmhurst, Far Rockaway,
Flushing, Forest Hills, Glen Oaks, Hollis,
Jackson Heights, Jamaica, Kew Gardens,
Little Neck, Long Island City, Queens
Village, St. Albans, and Whitestone)*
Booth Memorial Medical Center, *Flushing*
Flushing Hospital and Medical Center
Flushing
LaGuardia Hospital, *Forest Hills*
Jamaica Hospital, *Jamaica*
Mary Immaculate Hospital, Division of
the Catholic Medical Center of Brook-
lyn and Queens, *Jamaica*
Queens Hospital Center, *Jamaica*
St. John's Queens Hospital,
Division of the Catholic Medical

Center of Brooklyn and Queens,
Elmhurst
Richmond *(Mailing address: Staten Island)*
Doctors' Hospital of Staten Island
St. Vincent's Medical Center of
Richmond
Staten Island Hospital
USPHS Hospital

Nyack
Nyack Hospital

Oceanside
South Nassau Communities Hospital

Patchogue
Brookhaven Memorial Hospital Medical
Center

Plainview
Central General Hospital

Port Jefferson
John T. Mather Memorial Hospital and St.
Charles Hospital

Port Jervis
St. Francis Hospital of Port Jervis

Poughkeepsie
Vassar Brothers Hospital

Rochester
The Genesee Hospital
Highland Hospital of Rochester
Park Ridge Hospital
Rochester St. Mary's Hospital of the Sisters
of Charity

Rockville Centre
Mercy Hospital

Saratoga Springs
Saratoga Hospital

Schenectady
Ellis Hospital

Syracuse
St. Joseph's Hospital Health Center
University Hospital of Upstate Medical
Center

Walton
Delaware Valley Hospital

881

NORTH CAROLINA

Asheville
Veterans Administration Hospital

Camp LeJeune
Naval Regional Medical Center

Chapel Hill
North Carolina Memorial Hospital

Durham
Duke University Medical Center
Veterans Administration Medical Center

Shelby
Cleveland Memorial Hospital

Valdese
Valdese General Hospital

Winston-Salem
North Carolina Baptist Hospital

NORTH DAKOTA

Fargo
St. John's Hospital
St. Luke's Hospital-Fargo Clinic

Grand Forks
The United Hospital

Minot
St. Joseph's Hospital

Rugby
Good Samaritan Hospital Association

Williston
Mercy Hospital

OHIO

Akron
Akron City Hospital
Akron General Medical Center

Cincinnati
Children's Hospital Medical Center
Good Samaritan Hospital
Jewish Hospital of Cincinnati
University of Cincinnati Medical Center,
   Cincinnati General Hospital

Cleveland
Cleveland Clinic Hospital
Deaconess Hospital of Cleveland
Huron Road Hospital
Lutheran Medical Center
St. Alexis Hospital

Columbus
Children's Hospital
Ohio State University Hospitals
The Hawkes Hospital of Mount Carmel
   Mount Carmel Medical Center
   Mount Carmel East Hospital

Dayton
Good Samaritan Hospital and
   Health Center
Miami Valley Hospital
St. Elizabeth Medical Center
Veterans Administration Center

Dover
Union Hospital Association

Kettering
Kettering Medical Center

Mayfield Heights
Hillcrest Hospital

Sandusky
Good Samaritan Hospital

Springfield
Springfield-Urbana Cancer Program
   Community Hospital/Springfield and
      Clark County
   Mercy Medical Center
   Mercy Memorial Hospital, *Urbana*

Sylvania
Flower Hospital

Toledo
Medical College of Ohio Hospital
Toledo Hospital

Wright-Patterson AFB
USAF Medical Center

Youngstown
Youngstown Hospital Association

882

OKLAHOMA

Ada
Valley View Hospital

Ardmore
Memorial Hospital of Southern Oklahoma

Bartlesville
Jane Phillips Episcopal Memorial Medical
  Center

Chickasha
Grady Memorial Hospital

Oklahoma City
Baptist Medical Center of Oklahoma
Mercy Health Center
Oklahoma Children's Memorial Hospital
Presbyterian Hospital
St. Anthony Hospital
University Hospital & Clinics

Okmulgee
Okmulgee Memorial Hospital Authority

Shattuck
Newman Memorial Hospital

Shawnee
Shawnee Medical Center Hospital

Tulsa
Hillcrest Medical Center
Saint Francis Hospital
St. John's Medical Center

OREGON

Albany
Albany General Hospital

Bend
St. Charles Medical Center

Coos Bay
Bay Area Hospital

Corvallis
Good Samaritan Hospital

Eugene
Sacred Heart General Hospital

Grants Pass
Josephine General Hospital

Medford
Medford Tumor Clinic Cancer Program
  Providence Hospital
  Rogue Valley Memorial Hospital

Oregon City
Willamette Falls Community Hospital

Pendleton
St. Anthony Hospital

Portland
Emanuel Hospital
Good Samaritan Hospital and Medical
  Center
Kaiser Foundation Hospitals, Oregon Region
Physicians and Surgeons Hospital
Portland Adventist Medical Center
Providence Medical Center
St. Vincent Hospital and Medical Center
University of Oregon Health Sciences
  Center Hospital and Clinics
Veterans Administration Hospital

Salem
Salem Hospital

Tualatin
Meridian Park Hospital

PENNSYLVANIA

Allentown
Allentown Hospital Association
Allentown and Sacred Heart Hospital Center
Sacred Heart Hospital

Altoona
Altoona Hospital
Mercy Hospital

Bethlehem
St. Luke's Hospital

Bryn Mawr
Bryn Mawr Hospital

Dansville
Geisinger Medical Center

Easton
Easton Hospital

Erie ·
Hamot Medical Center

Greensburg
Westmoreland Hospital Association

Johnstown
Conemaugh Valley Memorial Hospital

Lancaster
Lancaster General Hospital
St. Joseph Hospital

Latrobe
Latrobe Area Hospital

Lewistown
Lewistown Hospital

McKeesport
McKeesport Hospital

Natrona Heights
Allegheny Valley Hospital

Norristown
Montgomery Hospital
Sacred Heart Hospital

Paoli
Paoli Memorial Hospital

Philadelphia
Albert Einstein Medical Center—Northern
   Division
American Oncologic Hospital
Children's Hospital of Philadelphia
Episcopal Hospital
Fox Chase Medical Center
Graduate Hospital of the University of
   Pennsylvania
Hahnemann Medical College and Hospital
Hospital of the University of Pennsylvania
Jeanes Hospital
Lankenau Hospital
Medical College of Pennsylvania and
   Hospital
Mercy Catholic Medical Center
Naval Regional Medical Center
Presbyterian-University of Pennsylvania
   Medical Center
Temple University Hospital
Thomas Jefferson University Hospital

Pittsburgh
Allegheny General Hospital
Children's Hospital of Pittsburgh
Magee-Women's Hospital
Mercy Hospital of Pittsburgh
St. Francis General Hospital
St. Margaret Memorial Hospital

Pottsville
Pottsville Hospital and Warne Clinic

Reading
The Reading Hospital and Medical Center

Sayre
Robert Packer Hospital

Scranton
Mercy Hospital

Sellersville
Grandview Hospital

State College
Centre Community Hospital

West Chester
Chester County Hospital

Wilkes-Barre
Veterans Administration Hospital
Wilkes-Barre General Hospital

York
York Hospital

RHODE ISLAND

Newport
Naval Regional Medical Center

SOUTH CAROLINA

Anderson
Anderson Memorial Hospital

Beaufort
Naval Hospital

Charleston
Medical University of South Carolina
   Hospital

Columbia
Richland Memorial Hospital
South Carolina Baptist Hospital
Veterans Administration Medical Center

Florence
McLeod Memorial Hospital

Fort Jackson
Moncrief Army Hospital

Greenwood
Self Memorial Hospital

Spartanburg
Spartanburg General Hospital

SOUTH DAKOTA

Aberdeen
St. Luke's Hospital

Watertown
Memorial Medical Center

Yankton
Sacred Heart Hospital

TENNESSEE

Bristol
Bristol Memorial Hospital

Johnson City
Memorial Hospital
Veterans Administration Center

Memphis
Baptist Memorial Hospital
Methodist Hospital
St. Jude Children's Research Hospital
University of Tennessee/City of Memphis
  Hospitals

Millington
Naval Regional Medical Center of Memphis

Nashville
George W. Hubbard Hospital of Meharry
  Medical College
Nashville Metropolitan General Hospital
Vanderbilt University Hospital

TEXAS

Amarillo
Panhandle Regional Tumor Clinic and
  Registry
  High Plains Baptist Hospital
  Northwest Texas Hospital
  St. Anthony's Hospital
  Deaf Smith General Hospital, *Hereford*

Big Spring
Malone-Hogan Hospital
Veterans Administration Hospital

Corpus Christi
Memorial Medical Center
Naval Regional Medical Center
Spohn Hospital

Dallas
Baylor University Medical Center
Methodist Hospitals of Dallas
Parkland Memorial Hospital
St. Paul Hospital
Veterans Administration Medical Center

El Paso
R. E. Thomason General Hospital
William Beaumont Army Medical Center

Fort Sam Houston
Brooke Army Medical Center

Fort Worth
John Peter Smith Hospital
St. Joseph's Hospital

Galveston
University of Texas Medical Branch
  Hospitals

Houston
Ben Taub General Hospital
Park Plaza Hospital
Rosewood General Hospital
St. Elizabeth Hospital
St. Joseph Hospital
Texas Children's Hospital
The University of Texas, M. D. Anderson
  Hospital and Tumor Institute

Kerrville
Veterans Administration Hospital

885

Lubbock
Highland Hospital
Methodist Hospital

Plainview
Central Plains General Hospital

San Antonio
Bexar County Hospital District
Santa Rosa Medical Center

Stephenville
Stephenville Hospital

Temple
King's Daughters Hospital
Scott and White Memorial Hospital
Veterans Administration Center

Texarkana
St. Michael Hospital

Waco
Hillcrest Baptist Hospital
Providence Hospital

Wharton
Gulf Coast Medical Center

UTAH

Salt Lake City
Latter-Day Saints Hospital
University of Utah Medical Center
Veterans Administration Hospital

VERMONT

Burlington
Medical Center Hospital of Vermont

Randolph
Gifford Memorial Hospital

VIRGINIA

Big Stone Gap
Lonesome Pine Hospital

Charlottesville
University of Virginia Hospitals

Clifton Forge
Emmett Memorial Hospital

Danville
The Memorial Hospital

Falls Church
Fairfax Hospital

Hampton
Veterans Administration Medical Center

Harrisonburg
Rockingham Memorial Hospital

Leesburg
Loudoun Memorial Hospital

Lynchburg
Lynchburg General-Marshall Lodge
   Hospitals
Virginia Baptist Hospital

Norfolk
DePaul Hospital
Norfolk General Hospital

Portsmouth
Naval Regional Medical Center

Richmond
Medical College of Virginia Hospitals
St. Luke's Hospital
St. Mary's Hospital

Roanoke
Community Hospital of Roanoke Valley
Roanoke Memorial Hospital

Salem
Lewis-Gale Hospital
Veterans Administration Hospital

Winchester
Winchester Memorial Hospital

WASHINGTON

Aberdeen
Aberdeen Cancer Program
   Grays Harbor Community Hospital
   St. Joseph Hospital

Bellevue
Overlake Memorial Hospital

Bellingham
St. Joseph Hospital
St. Luke's General Hospital

Bremerton
Naval Regional Medical Center

Everett
General Hospital of Everett and Providence
 Hospital

Kirkland
Evergreen General Hospital

Mount Vernon
Skagit Valley Hospital

Olympia
St. Peter Hospital

Seattle
Children's Orthopedic Hospital & Medical
 Center
Doctor Hospital
Group Health Hospital of Puget Sound
Northwest Hospital
Providence Medical Center
Swedish Hospital Medical Center
University Hospital
Virginia Mason Hospital

Sedro Woolley
United General Hospital

Spokane
Deaconess Hospital
Sacred Heart Medical Center

Tacoma
Madigan Army Medical Center
Tacoma General Hospital

Walla Walla
St. Mary Community Hospital

Wenatchee
Wenatchee Valley Clinic

WEST VIRGINIA

Beckley
Appalachian Regional Hospital

Charleston
Charleston Area Medical Center

Clarksburg
Veterans Administration Hospital

Elkins
Davis Memorial Hospital
Memorial General Hospital Association

Huntington
St. Mary's Hospital
Veterans Administration Medical Center

Kingwood
Preston Memorial Hospital

Man
Man Appalachian Regional Hospital

Montgomery
Montgomery General Hospital

Morgantown
West Virginia University Hospital

Philippi
Broaddus Hospital

Wheeling
Ohio Valley Medical Center

WISCONSIN

Appleton
St. Elizabeth Hospital

Cudahy
Trinity Memorial Hospital

Eau Claire
Luther Hospital
Sacred Heart Hospital

Fond du Lac
St. Agnes Hospital

Green Bay
St. Vincent Hospital

Janesville
Mercy Hospital of Janesville

La Crosse
La Crosse Lutheran Hospital
St. Francis Hospital

Madison
Madison General Hospital
Methodist Hospital
St. Mary's Hospital Medical Center
University of Wisconsin Hospitals

Manitowoc
Holy Family Hospital

Marinette
Marinette-Menominee, MI Cancer Program
Marinette General Hospital

Marshfield
Marshfield Clinic

Milwaukee
Columbia Hospital
Deaconess Hospital
Milwaukee County General Hospital
Mount Sinai Medical Center
St. Francis Hospital
St. Joseph's Hospital
St. Luke's Hospital
St. Mary's Hospital

Monroe
St. Clare Hospital of Monroe

Oshkosh
Mercy Medical Center

Watertown
Watertown Memorial Hospital

Wausau
Wausau Hospital Center

Wood
Veterans Administration Center

WYOMING

Cheyenne
De Paul Hospital
Memorial Hospital of Laramie County

PUERTO RICO

Ponce
Clinica Oncologica Andres Grilasca
Hospital De Damas

San German
Hospital De La Concepcion

San Juan
I. Gonzales Martinez Oncologic Hospital
University District Hospital
Veterans Administration Center & Hospital

Index of Symptoms

Most medical books, including both those written for lay readers and those written for professionals, aren't very helpful if you want to know what diseases could be causing a particular symptom. In order to find the cause of a symptom, you must either already have a fairly good idea of what diseases could cause the symptom in the first place or else devote hours to a difficult and frustrating search through the text. To remedy this situation, we have included the following index of symptoms.

This index is by no means complete, for gynecological diseases may produce a wide variety of symptoms. It would be impossible to catalog all of them. Also, some of the symptoms produced by gynecological diseases are nonspecific. For example, a number of the conditions described in this book can cause a fever, but so can a wide variety of other diseases that have no relation to a woman's reproductive organs. For practical reasons, we have limited our index to the following categories of symptoms:

□ Symptoms Related to the Vulva
  Itching and Burning of the External Genitals
  Sores, Lumps, Rashes or Growths on the Vulva
  White Patches on, or a Whitish Appearance of, the Vulvar Skin
□ Symptoms Related to the Vagina
  Growths, Lumps or Protrusions on the Vaginal Wall or at the Vaginal Opening
  Sores or Red Areas on the Vaginal Walls
  Painful Intercourse
  Vaginal Discharges
□ Symptoms Related to the Cervix
  Changes in the Shape of the Cervical Os

This index is not meant to take the place of the doctor. Don't fool yourself into thinking that you can diagnose or treat yourself, for accurate diagnosis is not usually based on the presence of a single symptom. The exact nature of the symptom, the presence or absence of other symptoms, the medical history and the findings of physical exams and laboratory tests may be necessary. If, for example, you have a nipple discharge, the doctor will want to examine the discharge microscopically. If s/he finds the discharge is composed of breast milk, s/he will want to proceed differently from the way s/he would if the discharge were composed of pus. If you have a milky nipple discharge, the doctor will want to pay close attention to your medical history, especially to your childbirth experiences. If your milky discharge is accompanied by an absence of menstrual periods, the presence of this symptom will also aid the doctor in diagnosis. Many factors, then, come into play, and a simple index like this one cannot hope to cover the complexities in diagnosis. It can, however, help you to identify a group of possible causes for your symptom and to become well-informed about the possibilities and the necessity for certain diagnostic procedures.

Symptoms Related to the Vulva

Itching and Burning of the External Genitals

Itching and burning of the external genitals can be a symptom of virtually every vulvar disease. Most itching or burning is due to some form of vulvitis or to the discharge from a vaginal infection. Sexually transmitted diseases are also a common cause of itching and burning of the outer genitals. Less frequently, other problems may cause these symptoms. Any of the following diseases may give rise to vulvar itching or burning:

Vulvitis (*see* p. 237)
Postmenopausal vulvitis (*see* p. 244)

Sores, Lumps, Rashes or Growths on the Vulva

The skin of the vulva, like the skin anywhere else on the body, is subject to a number of sores, lumps and bumps. Any of the diseases that cause itching and burning (see above) can lead to scratching, which in turn can lead to rashes and the formation of vesicles, or pimplelike blisters. In addition there are a number of sexually transmitted diseases, vulvar diseases and other conditions that can cause sores, lumps, rashes or growths on the vulva, such as:

Lymphopathia venereum (*see* p. 566)
Other sexually transmitted diseases (*see* pp. 567-69)

White Patches on or a Whitish Appearance of the Vulvar Skin

White patches on or a whitish hue to the vulvar skin can be caused by any of the diseases that can cause itching and burning of the vulvar skin (see above). The itching and burning lead to scratching, which can cause a white appearance. In addition, the following diseases can cause this symptom:

Postmenopausal vulvitis (*see* p. 244)
Depigmentation (*see* p. 252)
Vulvar dystrophy (*see* pp. 257-58)

Symptoms Related to the Vagina

Growths, Lumps or Protrusions on the Vaginal Wall or at the Vaginal Opening

A number of different conditions can cause these symptoms, including:

Bartholinitis (*see* p. 247)
Skeneitis (*see* pp. 248-49)
Imperforate hymen (*see* pp. 250-51)
Vulvar cysts at the vaginal opening (*see* pp. 253-54)
Benign solid tumors of the vulva located at the vaginal opening (*see* pp. 254-56)
Cystocele and urethrocele (*see* pp. 296-97)
Rectocele and entrocele (*see* p. 300)
Benign tumors of the vagina (*see* pp. 307-308)
Vaginal adenosis (*see* pp. 309-10)
Clear cell adenocarcinoma (*see* p. 313)
Cancer of the vagina (*see* pp. 316-17)
Endometriosis (*see* pp. 375-77)
Prolapse of the uterus, vagina and cervix (*see* p. 400)

Sores or Red Areas on the Vaginal Walls

Women who practice vaginal self-exam may notice sores or red areas on the vaginal walls. These are usually related to such infectious diseases as vaginitis (*see* pp. 272-79) or sexually transmitted diseases (*see* pp. 536-69). Other conditions can also cause these symptoms. Any of the following conditions may be responsible:

Trich (*see* pp. 280-81)
Yeast infections (*see* pp. 287-88)
Hemophilus (*see* pp. 290-91)
Nonspecific vaginitis (*see* p. 292)
Postmenopausal vaginitis (*see* p. 244)
Lacerations of the vagina (*see* p. 295)

Fistulas (*see* p. 303)
Vaginal adenosis (*see* pp. 309-10)
Clear cell adenocarcinoma (*see* p. 313)
Cancer of the vagina (*see* pp. 316-17)
Gonorrhea (*see* p. 544)
Herpes (*see* p. 550)
Syphilis (*see* pp. 556-57)
Granuloma inguinale (*see* p. 564)
Chancroid (*see* p. 565)
Lymphopathia venereum (*see* p. 566)
Other sexually transmitted diseases (*see* pp. 567-69)

Painful Intercourse

The medical term for painful intercourse is "dyspareunia." Painful intercourse may be associated with attempts to place the penis in the vagina or with deep thrusting during intercourse.

The vulvar, vaginal or cervical tissues may become inflamed, and friction from the penis may further irritate these tissues. Any of the following conditions may cause inflammation of the vulvar, vaginal or cervical tissues and make intercourse painful:

Vulvitis (*see* pp. 239-40)
Postmenopausal vulvitis (*see* p. 244)
Bartholinitis (*see* p. 247)
Skeneitis (*see* pp. 248-49)
Vulvar dystrophy (*see* p. 258)
  Trich (*see* p. 281), Yeast infections (*see* p. 287), Hemophilus (*see* p. 291), Nonspecific vaginitis (*see* p. 292), Postmenopausal vaginitis (*see* p. 244)

Cervicitis (*see* p. 327)

Other Sexually Transmitted Diseases (*see* pp. 567-69)
  Gonorrhea (*see* pp. 544-45), Herpes (*see* p. 551), Syphilis (*see* pp. 556-57), Genital warts (*see* p. 562), Granuloma inguinale (*see* p. 564), Chancroid (*see* p. 565), Lymphopathia venereum (*see* p. 556), Other sexually transmitted diseases (*see* pp. 567-69)

Painful intercourse may also be caused by anatomical abnormalities, such as:

Imperforate hymen (*see* pp. 250-51)
Vaginal stenosis (*see* p. 293)
Congenital absence of the lower part of the vagina (*see* p. 306)
Transverse vaginal septum (*see* p. 306)
Septate vagina (*see* p. 306)

Vaginismus (*see* pp. 301-302), a spasm of the vaginal muscles, can cause pain on intercourse. Infections of the urinary tract may also make intercourse painful. If a woman has not been sufficiently aroused and lubricated prior to intercourse, the penis may irritate the dry tissues.

Although most women with tipped uteri (*see* pp. 395-99) do not have problems, some women whose uteri are tipped do experience pain on deep thrusting. Such pain may also be due to pelvic inflammatory disease (*see* pp. 372-76). Endometriosis (*see* pp. 373-86) can likewise cause pain on deep thrusting, and if the endometriosis involves the vagina or vulva, any attempt at intercourse may be painful.

Other pelvic conditions can cause pain, and sometimes intercourse may aggravate this pain. For instance, physiologic cysts on the ovaries (*see* pp. 441-43) may rupture during intercourse, causing pain. Indeed, any tumor on a pelvic organ could result in pain during intercourse (see abdominal pain below).

Vaginal Discharge

It is normal to have some amount of vaginal discharge. Normal vaginal discharge tends to be clear to somewhat milky in color and may leave a slightly yellowish stain on the underclothes. The texture, consistency and amount of the vaginal discharge varies according to the stage of the menstrual cycle and the state of sexual excitement. Becoming familiar with your vaginal discharge will help you to recognize abnormal discharges.

The most common cause of vaginal discharge is vaginitis (*see* pp. 272-73). The nature of the discharge may give a clue as to what type of vaginitis you have. For instance, trich (*see* pp. 281-82) tends to produce a discharge with a yellow or green tinge, although it may also be gray or white. The trich discharge is apt to be thin and watery, although in mixed infections it may be thick and creamy. It is often frothy (that is, it has tiny bubbles in it) and tends to smell rather fishy. Yeast infections (*see* pp. 287-88) often cause a cottage-cheese-like discharge—a whitish discharge that is watery, with thick, curdlike clumps of cheesy material. It often smells like fermenting yeast. Hemophilus (*see* pp. 290-91) discharge tends to be rather abundant and smell bad. It may look like a thin, gray, flour paste. Any of these discharges may cause itching and burning of the external genitals.

Although the various types of vaginitis tend to have characteristic appearances, appearances can be deceiving. Another organism may be responsible, or the infection may be a mixed one. The symptoms of one form of vaginitis may mask those of another. Other forms of vaginitis, cervical infections, pelvic infections and sexually transmitted diseases can also cause abnormal vaginal discharges and include:

Nonspecific vaginitis (*see* p. 292)
Postmenopausal vaginitis (*see* p. 244)
Cervicitis (*see* p. 326)
Cervical erosions (*see* p. 330)
Pelvic inflammatory disease (*see* p. 370)
Gonorrhea (*see* p. 544)
Herpes (*see* p. 550)
Syphilis (*see* p. 556)
Genital warts (*see* p. 562)
Granuloma inguinale (*see* p. 564)

Chancroid (*see* p. 565)
Lymphopathia venereum (*see* p. 566)
Other sexually transmitted diseases (*see* pp. 567-69)

In addition to infections, there are other conditions that can cause an abnormal vaginal discharge, including any of the following:

Vaginal adenosis (*see* pp. 309-10)
Clear cell adenocarcinoma (*see* p. 313)
Cancer of the vagina (*see* p. 316)
Cervical polyps (*see* pp. 332-33)
Dysplasia (*see* p. 282)
Carcinoma in situ (*see* p. 264)
Cervical cancer (*see* p. 352)
Uterine fibroids (*see* pp. 406-407)
Endometrial polyps (*see* p. 412)
Benign tumors of the Fallopian tube (*see* p. 413)
Uterine cancer (*see* p. 422)
Cancer of the Fallopian tubes (*see* p. 433)

An object left in the vagina too long (tampon, diaphragm, cervical cap, pessary) can cause a foul-smelling discharge. The strings of an IUD may irritate the cervical glands, causing an increase in the amount of vaginal discharge. The hormones in the Pill can stimulate the cervical glands and may also result in an increase in vaginal discharge. Some women have a brownish discharge at the end of their menstrual cycle. This discharge is old blood still being shed.

If the vaginal discharge has a pink or brown tinge, this may indicate that there is blood in the discharge. Bloody discharges are discussed under the symptom index heading Abnormal Uterine Bleeding.

Symptoms Related to the Cervix

Changes in the Shape of the Cervical Os

The cervical os may change in appearance, but this is not necessarily a sign that something is wrong, for the os changes over the course of the menstrual cycle and over the course of a woman's lifetime. At the time of ovulation and the time of the menstrual flow, the os is apt to be more dilated. Before childbirth the os usually appears as a small round indentation in the center of the cervix. After childbirth it is apt to look more like a short vertical slit. Other variations in the shape of the os on an otherwise normal cervix may be due to growths or clumps protruding through the os (see below) or to cervical lacerations (*see* pp. 335-37). The os may be entirely closed up due to cervical stenosis (*see* pp. 338-40) or cervicitis (*see* pp. 325-29).

Growths or Clumps of Tissue Protruding Through the Cervical Opening.

Women who practice speculum self-exam may see clumps of tissue or growths protruding through the cervix. Conditions that can cause this include:

895

Sores, Cysts, Lumps, Red or White Areas on the Cervix

Women who practice self-exam may notice sores, lumps, cysts or red or white areas on the cervix. Most often these are the result of infections of the vagina and cervix, sexually transmitted diseases or cervical erosions and eversions. Any of the following conditions may result in these symptoms:

Symptoms Related to the Breast

Breast Lumps and Other Abnormalities in the Shape or Appearance of the Breast.

A lump or thickening in the breast is an important symptom. In addition, the following signs or symptoms in the breast deserve attention:

□ A depressed or bulging area in the skin or any change in the shape or symmetry of the breast

- A thickening on the skin of the breast that may feel warm to the touch
- Dilated veins in the breast. Some women normally have visible bluish-colored veins in their breasts; however, the appearance of such veins in a woman who has not had them previously or a change in the appearance of such veins in a woman who has previously had them calls for medical attention
- A change in the texture or color of the skin of the breast. The appearance of areas of skin with the texture of an orange peel, a condition known as peau d'orange, is particularly important
- Any change in the condition of the nipple or the areola. Changes in the size or shape, skin texture or direction in which the nipple points, retraction of the nipple, cracks in the nipple or scaling of the skin around the nipple are important
- Discharge from the nipple (see Nipple Discharge below)
- A lump in the axilla (armpit)
- A sore on the breast or nipple that does not heal
- Hot, swollen or sore breast
- Unusual ache or pain that persists

These signs and symptoms may be caused by either a benign or malignant condition, such as:

Cystic disease of the breast (*see* pp. 477-78)
Mastitis (*see* p. 480)
Fat necrosis (*see* p. 481)
Fibroadenomas (*see* pp. 482-83)
Cystosarcoma phyllodes (*see* p. 484)
Lipomas and other benign, soft tumors of the breast (*see* p. 485)
Mammary duct ectasia (*see* p. 486)
Breast cancer (*see* p. 497)

Nipple Discharge

Nipple discharge is sometimes, but not always, a sign that something is wrong. On occasion, newborn babies secrete milk from the breast. The same kind of secretions may occur at puberty, and some women produce a milky secretion at certain points in their menstrual cycles. These types of secretions may be due to temporary hormone fluctuations and may therefore not be anything serious. Some women, especially those that have had more than one child, secrete breast milk during pregnancy. Women who are breast-feeding may have a spontaneous trickle or even a flow of breast milk at times when the infant is not actually sucking on the nipple. While this may be distressing, it is generally not serious. Some women produce breast milk even when they are not pregnant or breast-feeding, and this condition, known as galactorrhea (*see* pp. 487-91), may be due serious underlying problem. The causes of galactorrhea are discussed in detail under that heading.

In addition to milk, there are a number of other types of discharge that may be expressed or may flow spontaneously from the nipple. The color, texture and consistency of these discharges vary. Red, brown or black discharges may

897

indicate that either fresh or old blood is present in the discharge. The discharge may also be white, green, yellow or gray. A number of breast diseases may be responsible for nipple discharges, including:

Cystic disease (*see* p. 476)
Mastitis (*see* p. 480)
Intraductal papillomas (*see* p. 485)
Mammary duct ectasia (*see* p. 486)
Breast cancer (*see* p. 497)

Symptoms Related to the Menstrual Cycle

Abnormal Menstrual Periods, Bleeding Between Periods or Any Abnormal Uterine Bleeding

Irregularities in menstrual bleeding may occur at the time of puberty. The periods may be spaced irregularly or may be unusually heavy or light. These irregularities are normal during this period of life, when the menstrual cycle is just gearing up. Unless the bleeding is especially profuse (soaking more than 6-8 pads or tampons a day) there is no need for concern, since it takes a few years before most girls' periods become regular.

Irregularities in menstrual bleeding also occur at the end of the reproductive cycle, when a woman's menstrual cycle is gearing down. Some women menstruate normally until they come to an abrupt stop; others experience a gradual decrease in the volume of flow and longer times in between periods; still others have irregularly spaced periods interspersed with times when they have normal periods. All these patterns are considered normal. If however, there is a heavy, gushing flow, periods that last longer than usual, periods that occur more frequently than every 21 days or bleeding that starts again a year or more after the last period, this may be a sign that something is wrong.

Irregular menstrual periods may also occur in women during their menstruating years. The length of the cycle and the duration and amount of the flow may vary from month to month, even in a normal, healthy woman. But persistent or severe abnormalities may be a sign that something is wrong.

Bleeding between the periods and other types of abnormal bleeding may occur in any age group and may or may not be serious.

There are a wide variety of conditions that can cause these symptoms. These causes are discussed under the heading Abnormal Uterine Bleeding (*see* pp. 602-607), and a chart of causes is included there (*see* p. 604).

Absence of Menstrual Periods

The absence of menstrual periods is called amenorrhea. If a girl hasn't had her first period by the expected age, she is said to have primary amenorrhea. If a woman who has previously menstruated stops having her periods, she is said to have secondary amenorrhea.

Although amenorrhea is a symptom of disease and not a disease itself, it is frequently the absence of menstruation that brings the woman to the doctor. Since amenorrhea may be the symptom of any of a number of underlying diseases, some of which are not strictly gynecologic in nature, diagnosis is largely a process of elimination. For these reasons we have included a discussion of amenorrhea (*see* pp. 581-601) in the reference section on diseases. A chart on the possible causes of this symptom is given there (*see* p. 583).

Hot Flashes and Symptoms that Occur at the Time of Menopause

Hot flashes, or flushes, are intense sensations of heat that are not uncommon among women who are experiencing a natural or a premature menopause (*see* pp. 612-14). Some women experience them temporarily following hysterectomy, even if the ovaries have not been removed. The exact cause is unknown. Possible causes for hot flashes, osteoporosis, the drying of urinary and vaginal tissues, depression, changes in sex drive and other symptoms that may occur at the time of menopause are discussed under the heading Menopausal Problems (*see* pp. 608-12).

Menstrual Cramps

Menstrual cramps are not uncommon; almost every woman experiences them at some time in her life. Sometimes the cramps are the result of a specific underlying disease. Sometimes no cause can be found. Although menstrual cramps are actually a symptom and not a disease, we have included a section on menstrual cramps (*see* pp. 575-81) in the reference section on disease. Possible causes for this symptom are detailed there.

Premenstrual Pain, Weight Gain, Breast Tenderness, Mood Changes and Other Symptoms That Occur in Relation to the Menstrual Cycle

Women experience a wide variety of symptoms in relation to their menstrual cycles. Most of these occur in the days preceding the menstrual cycle, so these symptoms are termed "premenstrual syndrome," or PMS for short. There are many theories to explain PMS. A description of the type of symptoms associated with PMS and possible causes is given under the heading Premenstrual Syndrome (*see* pp. 573-75).

Infertility and Sterility

These conditions are often thought of as diseases in and of themselves, for the inabilility to get pregnant is what causes a woman to seek medical help. Actually, these conditions are the symptom or aftermath of some underlying disease or abnormality. Although these conditions are in a sense symptoms, we have devoted a section in the reference section on diseases to these conditions.

Detailed information about the possible causes is given there under the heading Infertility and Sterility (*see* pp. 622-34).

Abdominal Pain

Abdominal pain may be a symptom of literally hundreds of conditions that have nothing to do with gynecological problems, including kidney stones and gallstones, urinary tract problems, appendicitis, ulcers and other gastric disturbances, benign or malignant tumors, colitis and other infections in the abdominal cavity, to name just a few. The following gynecological conditions described in this book can cause abdominal pain:

Index

and ovarian pregnancies, 653
and pelvic inflammatory disease, 372
and perforation of uterus, 125, 126
postcoital, 216-217
and pregnancy, 127-129
problems and disadvantages, 121-122
removal of, 121
safety, 81, 122
and subsequent fertility, 129-130
test prior to insertion of, 118
types of, 114-115, 116, 117
See also IUD strings
IUD strings, 119, 121, 124
and cervical erosion and eversion, 330
and pregnancy, 128-129
Ives. *See* Syphilis

J

Jaundice, and Pill, 108
Joint Commission on Accreditation of Hospitals (JCAH), 699-700

K

Karyotype test
and testicular feminization, 598
and Turner's syndrome, 595
Kidney infections. *See* Bladder and kidney infections
Klinefelter's syndrome, and sperm production, 627
Kraurosis vulvae. *See* Vulvar dystrophy
Kwell, and crabs, 560

L

Labia, agglutination of, 252
Labia majora, 24

Labia minora, 25
Lacerations
cervical, *see* Cervical lacerations
of vagina, vulva, and perineum, 294-295
Lactation. *See* Milk secretion
Laetrile, 690-692
Laminaria rods, 202, 209
Lamp, for gynecological self-exam, 19
Laparoscopic tubal ligation, 186-188
Laparoscopy, 740-741
and menstrual cramps, 578-579
and ovarian cancer, 471
and pelvic inflammatory disease, 378, 383
and recovery of IUD, 126
Laparotomy, and pelvic scar tissue, 623-624
Laser therapy, and vaginal cancer, 322
Leiofibroma. *See* Fibromas
Leiomyofibromas. *See* Fibromas
Leiomyomas. *See* Lipomas of breast; Uterine fibroids
Leiomyomata uteri. *See* Uterine fibroids
Lesbians, health care for, 225
Leukemia, and chemotherapy, 688
Leukoderma, 251-252
Leukoplakia of cervix, 341
Leukoplakia of vulva. *See* Vulvar dystrophy
LGV. *See* Lymphogranuloma venereum
LH, 58
LH test, 599-600
LHRF, 58
Lichen sclerosus, 257, 258, 260
Ligament resection, and menstrual cramps, 580-581
Lipids, and Pill, 110-111
Lipoma fibrosom. *See* Fibromas
Lipomas of breast, 484-485. *See also* Fibromas
Lippes Loop, 115
Liver function, and amenorrhea, 591
Liver tumors, and Pill, 107
Lobes of breast, 43

National Surgical Adjuvant Project for
    Breast and Bowel Cancers
    (NSABP), 518-520, 841-857
Natural family planning, 160-176
    advantages, 175
    disadvantages and problems, 175-
        176
    sources for information on, 174-175
    use of, 173-174
    See also Basal body temperature;
        Rhythm method; Cervical
        mucus method
Nausea and vomiting, and Pill, 105
Needle-aspiration, and diagnosis of
    cystic disease of breast, 479
Needle biopsy, 505-506
    of breast, 475
Neisseria gonorrhea. *See* Gonococcus
Nephritis, and amenorrhea, 591
Nephrostomy, 304
Neurectomy, and endometriosis,384
Neurodermatitis of vulva, 242-243
Neurofibromas of vulva, 255
Nevi. *See* Nevus
Nevus of vulva, 256
NFP. *See* Natural family planning
Nipples, 43
    changes in, 474, 897
    discharge from, 48, 891-898, *see also*
        Galactorrhea
    and intraductal papillomas, 485
    inverted, 43
    See also Breast self-exam
Nitrimidazone, and trich, 285
Nits, 559-560
Noncancerous tumors of tubes. *See*
    Benign tumors of Fallopian tubes
Noninvasive carcinoma. *See* Carcinoma
    in situ
Nonspecific vaginitis, 292. *See also*
    Hemophilus
Nurse-practitioners, 225-226
    and fertility work-ups, 631
Nurses, as source of information on
    doctors, 222-223

Nutrition
    and premenstrual syndrome, 574
    and repeated miscarriages, 644
    See also Diet

O

Obesity, and uterine cancer, 419
OC's. *See* Pill
Oligomenorrhea. *See* Abnormal uterine
    bleeding
Oophorectomy, 721-723
    and advanced breast cancer, 530-531
    and premature menopause, 613
Oophoritis. *See* Pelvic inflammatory
    disease
Oral contraceptives. *See* Pill
Oral-genital sex
    and chancroid, 564
    and diaphragms, 137-138
    and flavored spermicide, 131
    and genital warts, 562
    and gonorrhea, 544, 547
    and herpes, 549
    and infections, 76
    and syphilis, 555, 558
Organic birth control. *See* Natural
    family planning
Organic brain disease, and
    hypothalamic amenorrhea, 586-
    587
Orgasms
    and clitoris, 26
    and hysterectomy, 715
    vaginal ballooning during, 131, 132
    and vulvectomy, 711-712
Osteoporosis, 59
    and estrogen replacement therapy,
        765-766
    and exercise, 610
    and menopause, 610-611, 613
    and premature menopause, 613
Ovarian cancer, 459-472
    diagnosis of, 462-465

P